Physiological Aspects
of
Clinical
Neuro-Ophthalmology

Physiological Aspects of Clinical Neuro-Ophthalmology

Edited by
C. Kennard
and
F. Clifford Rose

London
CHAPMAN AND HALL

First published in 1988 by
Chapman and Hall Ltd
11 New Fetter Lane, London EC4P 4EE

Printed in Great Britain at
The University Press, Cambridge

ISBN 0 412 29110 X

British Library Cataloguing in Publication Data

Physiological aspects of clinical neuro-
ophthalmology.
1. Neuro-ophthalmology
I. Kennard, Christopher II. Rose, F. Clifford
616.7'62 RE725

ISBN 0-412-29110-X

Contents

Contributors

Jurgen Bolz PhD
Laboratory of Neurobiology
The Rockefeller University
1230 York Avenue
New York
New York 10021 USA

Thomas M. Bosley MD
Neuro-ophthalmology Service
Wills Eye Hospital and
Department of Neurology
Hospital of the University of
Pennsylvania
Philadelphia
PA, USA

Thomas Brandt MD
Ludwig-Maximilians-Universität
München
Klinikum Grosshadern
Neurologische Klinik
8000 München 70
Marchioninistrasse 15
W. Germany

Ulrich Büttner MD
Ludwig-Maximilians-Universität
München
Klinikum Grosshadern
8000 München 70
Marchioninistrasse 15
W. Germany

J.A. Büttner-Ennever PhD
Institut für Neuropathologie der
Universität Munchen
8000 München 2
Thalkirchner Strasse 36
W. Germany

A.J. Chitty
MRC Cognitive Neuroscience
Research Group
University of St Andrews
St Andrews
Fife KY16 9JU

H. Collewijn PhD
Department of Physiology I
Erasmus Universiteit Rotterdam
Postbus 1738
3000 DR Rotterdam
The Netherlands

E. de Haan
MRC Neuropsychology Unit
Radcliffe Infirmary
Woodstock Road
Oxford

Ennio De Renzi MD
Clinica Neurologica della
Universitá di Modena
Policlinico
Via del Pozzo 71
41100 Modena
Italy

Marianne Dieterich MD
Neurological Clinic
Klinikum Grosshadern
University of Munich
8000 München 70
W. Germany

C.J.K. Ellis MD, MRCP
Consultant Neurologist
Poole General Hospital
Longfleet Road
Poole
Dorset BH15 2JB

L. Ferman PhD
Department of Physiology I
Erasmus Universiteit Rotterdam
Postbus 1738
3000 DR Rotterdam
The Netherlands

Lars Frisén MD, PhD
Department of Ophthalmology
University of Göteborg
Sahlgren's Hospital
S-413 45 Göteborg
Sweden

J.M. Gibson MD, MRCP
Senior Registrar in Neurology
Royal Victoria Hospital
Grosvenor Road
Belfast BT12 6BA

Charles D. Gilbert MD, PhD
The Rockefeller University
1230 York Avenue
New York
New York 10021
USA

R.W. Guillery FRS
Dr Lee's Professor of Anatomy
Department of Human Anatomy
University of Oxford
South Parks Road
Oxford OX1 3QX

M.H. Harries PhD
MRC Cognitive Neuroscience
Research Group
University of St Andrews
St Andrews
Fife KY16 9JU

Sohan Singh Hayreh MD, PhD, DSc, FRCS
Professor of Ophthalmology
The University of Iowa Hospitals
and Clinics
Department of Ophthalmology
Iowa City
Iowa 52242
USA

Alfred Huber MD
Professor of Ophthalmology
University of Zurich
Zurich
Switzerland

G.W. Humphreys PhD
Department of Psychology
Birkbeck College
University of London
Malet Street
London WC1E 7HX

Edward L. Keller PhD
Smith Kettlewell Eye Research Foundation
and
University of California
Berkeley
2232 Webster Street
San Francisco
California 94115
USA

Christopher Kennard PhD, MRCP
Consultant Neurologist
The London Hospital
Whitechapel
London E1 1BB

G. Kommerell MD
Klinikum der Albert-Ludwigs-Universität
Universitäts Augenklinik
Abteilung Neuroophthalmologie und Schielbehandlung
7800 Freiburg
Killianstrasse 5
W. Germany

R. John Leigh MD
Associate Professor of Neurology
Case Western Reserve University
Department of Neurology
University Hospitals
Cleveland
Ohio 44106
USA

W.I. McDonald PhD, FRCP
University Department of Clinical Neurology
Institute of Neurology
The National Hospital
Queen Square
London WC1N 3BG

A.J. Mistlin
MRC Cognitive Neuroscience Research Group
University of St Andrews
St Andrews
Fife KY16 9JU

F. Newcombe PhD
MRC Neuropsychology Unit
Radcliffe Infirmary
Woodstock Road
Oxford

D.I. Perrett PhD
MRC Cognitive Neuroscience Research Group, Psychology Lab.
University of St Andrews
St Andrews
Fife KY16 9JU

Charles Pierrot-Deseilligny MD
Hôpital de la Salpêtrière
47 Blvd de l'Hôpital
75651 Paris
Cedex 13
France

M.J. Riddoch PhD
Department of Paramedical Sciences
North East London Polytechnic
Romford Road
London E15 4LZ

F. Clifford Rose FRCP
Director, Academic Unit of Neuroscience
Charing Cross and Westminster Medical School
University of London
London W6 8RF

R. Ross Russell MD, FRCP
Consultant Physician
Department of Neurology
St Thomas' Hospital
Lambeth Palace Road
London SE1 7EH

K.H. Ruddock PhD
Imperial College of Science and Technology
The Blackett Laboratory
Prince Consort Road
London SW7 2BZ

M.D. Sanders FRCP, FRCS
Consultant Neuro-ophthalmologist
The National Hospital for Nervous Diseases
Queen Square
London WC1N 3BG

Shirley A. Smith PhD
Department of Clinical Pharmacology
St Thomas' Hospital
University of London
Lambeth Palace Road
London SE1 7EH

Stephen E. Smith DM
Department of Clinical Pharmacology
St Thomas' Hospital
University of London
Lambeth Palace Road
London SE1 7EH

H. Stanley Thompson MD
Professor of Ophthalmology
University of Iowa
Iowa City
Iowa
USA

Ronald J. Tusa MD, PhD
Department of Neurology
Meyer 2-147
The Johns Hopkins Hospital
Baltimore
Maryland 21205
USA

Joel M. Weinstein MD
Assistant Professor of Ophthalmology, Neurology and Neurosurgery
Medical School
University of Wisconsin–Madison
Department of Ophthalmology
F4/338 Clinical Science Center
600 Highland Avenue
Madison
Wisconsin 53792
USA

Torsten N. Wiesel PhD
Laboratory of Neurobiology
The Rockefeller University
1230 York Avenue
New York
New York 10021
USA

Semir Zeki PhD

Professor of Neurobiology
University College London
Department of Anatomy and
Embryology
Gower Street
London WC1E 6BT

Thomas J. Zweifel OD

Clinical Assistant Professor of
Neurology
Medical College of Wisconsin
Milwaukee
Wisconsin
USA

Preface

About half of all the afferent fibres projecting to the brain are from the eye, a fact which indicates the primacy of vision amongst the special senses. It is not surprising, therefore, that study of the visual system, including eye movements, has received considerable attention from basic neuroscientists. This relatively recent escalation of interest has been matched by an ever-increasing volume of research into aspects of altered visual function encountered in pathological states in man. For this reason, there is an increasing need for clinical neurologists and basic neuroscientists to discuss areas of common interest and such an international group was invited to attend a meeting in July 1986 to discuss 'Physiological Aspects of Clinical Neuro-Ophthalmology' at the Medical Society of London, funded by the Mansell Bequest. Participants were asked to prepare a chapter in their area of expertise emphasizing neuro-anatomical and neurophysiological aspects and, where possible, relate this to pathophysiological mechanisms involved in clinical disease.

The resulting compilation, which covers a wide area dealing both with visual processing and the control of eye movements, will be of interest to ophthalmologists and neurologists in training, practising neuro-ophthalmologists who wish to update their knowledge of the basic mechanisms underlying many of the common conditions which they routinely examine, and basic neurobiologists in the visual sciences.

C. Kennard

F. Clifford Rose

London 1987

Part I

The Visual Pathways

CHAPTER 1

Visual acuity and visual field tests: psychophysical versus pathophysical objectives

LARS FRISÉN

1.1 Introduction

Clinical use of acuity and visual field tests dates back more than one century. The principles laid down by the early pioneers, Frans Cornelis Donders (1818–89), Albrecht von Graefe (1828–1870), Herman Snellen (1834–1908), Edmond Landolt (1846–1926) and Jannik Bjerrum (1851–1920), have been manipulated, permutated and refined in innumerable ways, but the original ideas have stood the test of time remarkably well: these early investigators would easily feel at home with today's clinical routines. Even the recent entry of computers onto the clinical scene has not really changed the nature of acuity or visual field tests.

What has changed, of course, is clinical experience, and the clinical database is still growing briskly. Understanding has also been broadened by the immense advances in experimental physiology, at least in a general sense. Unfortunately, the techniques used by experimental physiologists have little in common with clinical techniques. Experimental studies on disturbances comparable to those encountered in man are, as yet, very few, and further, species differences hamper direct transfer of knowledge from experimental animals to man.

A much closer bond exists in the field of experimental psychophysics, i.e. the quantitative study of links between various physical stimuli and perception but, again, there are many important differences in favoured techniques, and the major role in psychophysics of advanced (and sometimes contested) mathematical modelling handicaps fruitful exchange. Psychophysical tools like Fourier transforms in space and time domains, mathematical filtering procedures, and abstract channel concepts, are presently worlds apart from the clinician's morphologically centred background. However, the psychophysicist's reliance on statistical logic for unambiguous definition of results could and should find its place also in clinical routines.

The clinician usually performs his examinations with other questions in mind than an improved understanding of what governs normal perception: his principal interest is detecting and monitoring any injuries or lesions. Consequently, his measurements should directly reflect the actual degree of damage sustained by the visual system. Hence, the goal of clinical examinations is not really a psychophysical one, even if the tests themselves can be labelled psychophysical. It may be useful to introduce a specific term to emphasize the quite specialized clinical objectives, namely 'pathophysics', to designate the quantitative assessment of injury by psychophysical measurements of function.

1.2 A pathophysics preamble

The difference between psychophysical and pathophysical viewpoints can be illustrated as follows.

Both acuity and visual field tests furnish quantitative information on the visual performance of the tested subject, as reflected by his responses to sets of test targets. The measurements are obtained under carefully defined conditions, at least nominally. Hence, acuity and field tests meet minimum criteria for psychophysical tests. But, what bearings have the results on the state of the visual system? For instance, what is the meaning of an acuity measurement of, say, 0.5 (20/40)? This is easily identified as an abnormal result, but how severely affected is the visual system? Is 0.25 (20/80) twice as bad? Or, in the case of visual field measurements, what is the meaning of, say, a 10 degree localized bulge in a perimetric isopter, or a 5 dB increase in a static threshold? Again, these are easily recognized as abnormal results but what do they tell about the severity of the underlying lesion? Is a 20 degree bulge or a 10 dB threshold elevation the consequence of twice the amount of damage? Providing answers to these types of questions is the task of pathophysics.

A potentially controversial aspect of the pathophysical concept is the definition of severity of lesions. Is it actually possible to quantify all different pathogenetic mechanisms, and to compare, quantitatively, their different effects? The answer to this specific question is, at least for the time being, negative. A provisional solution is to express the degree of damage, irrespective of the actual mechanism, as the *functionally equivalent damage* to a quantifiable reference mechanism. For the visual system, I suggest *disconnection of retinal output channels* (ganglion cells) as the reference lesion. It will be shown below that the proportion of *functional* output channels can be predicted from certain vision measurements. It is proposed that any other cause of visual loss, or any combination of causes, can be matched by a numerically and spatially appropriate disconnection of output channels. Accordingly, the severity of these other lesions, or combinations of lesions, can be expressed as that extent of disconnection which produces the same test result. Taking an arbitrary retinopathy as an example, with acuity reduced to, say, 0.5, how severe is the damage? According to the above proposal, it is equivalent to that degree of foveal output channel disconnection which produces the same acuity level. It will be shown below that the matching degree of disconnection can be estimated to 85%.

The above proposals naturally require validation, and presumably also revision. It is not unlikely, for instance, that there exist forms of visual impairment which cannot be mimicked by disconnecting retinal output channels. These first proposals are primarily meant to serve as seeds for a potentially fruitful evolution of pathophysical ideas and tools.

This chapter attempts to illuminate psychophysical and pathophysical aspects of clinical acuity and visual field tests, and also examines the question of what we as clinicians really want from our tests. Because of their different operating modes and applications, the two types of tests are best treated separately. Only the briefest of backgrounds will be sketched, the reader being referred to broader reviews for detail. A highly recommended introduction to experimental physiology and psychophysics is Barlow and Mollon's *The Senses* (1982). For more psychophysical detail, see Kelly and Burbeck (1984). Westheimer's (1965) and Lit's (1968) reviews of normal acuity are already classical. Clinically oriented acuity reviews above textbook level seem to be lacking, but for visual fields, Greve's (1973) and Frisén's (1979a) reviews complement each other. The proceedings of the International Perimetric Society (published in *Documenta Ophthalmologica Proceedings Series*, volumes 14, 19, 26, 35 and 42) are excellent sources for additional information.

1.3 Visual acuity

1.3.1 DEFINITIONS

Visual acuity is a measure of the visual capacity to resolve small detail at high contrast. There are two major test approaches: one involves alignment, e.g. of the vernier variety, and the other involves identification of a target characteristic, e.g. the position of the opening in a broken ring. Tests belonging to the latter category, or ordinary acuity tests, normally supply results that can be loosely compared with the dimensions of the foveal receptor matrix. Alignment acuity is much better, and is often termed 'hyperacuity' (see Westheimer, 1979b, for a review), but clinical experience with these tests is minimal (Enoch, Essock and Williams, 1984).

Clinical tradition strongly favours a very limited number of ordinary acuity test objects, or optotypes. Letter optotypes in rows are by far the most common. Although letter stroke width is held to be the critical detail, same-size letters with same-width strokes may have quite different legibility (Sloan, Rowland and Altman, 1952; Hedin and Olsson, 1984), presumably due to complex interactions between letter components, where angles of branching, length and radii of arcs, and proximity factors all play important roles. Hence, it is not really surprising that even modern charts produced according to established rules may give divergent results (Frisén, 1986).

An obvious solution to this problem is to use a single optotype, and present it in different orientations. Tumbling Es and Cs are classical examples, but it is difficult both to read rows composed of such optotypes, and to check the responses. The simple expedient of presenting Es or Cs singly has the important drawback of changing the nature of the test task, and impairing diagnostic yield.

Many other types of test targets have been suggested but found little favour with clinicians. Letter optotypes have always prevailed, and will presumably continue to do so, because of the easily understood test task, the easy checking of responses, and the link to activities of daily life. The rapidity of the test, and the small cost of equipment, are additional major advantages. Letter tests could be improved by manipulating typefaces so as to obtain the same legibility for all letters. Preferably, legibility should be identical to that of the uniquely well-defined and well-known Landolt's C, as proposed by the NRC/NAS (1980) Working Group 39. Ironically, this group accepts the so-called Sloan series of letters as an exact equivalent, notwithstanding the demonstration of quite unequal legibility by the original investigators (Sloan, Rowland and Altman,

1952). The argument that average *line* legibility is constant is incompatible with acuity's threshold nature (see below).

Typeface adjustment for equal legibility should also allow precise comparisons of results obtained with letters from different alphabets. The powerful graphics capabilities of modern personal computers should make such an adaptation a relatively straightforward task. Incidentally, there are many good reasons to stay with a computer display, and to let the computer do the actual testing (see below).

Infants and small children require other types of tests and, although currently a very active research field (Simons, 1983) they fall outside the scope of this chapter.

1.3.2 DESIGNATIONS OF VISUAL ACUITY

There are two common modes of designating results, namely in decimal and Snellen notations. The former, introduced by Ferdinand Monoyer (1836–1912), utilizes the inverse of the visual angle (in minutes of arc) subtended by the stroke width. Hence, an optotype with a stroke subtending an angle of 1′ is designated 1.0, while a stroke of 2′ corresponds to 0.5, and 4′ to 0.25. The Snellen notation, which actually was proposed by Donders, gives a more vivid picture, by introducing an element of distance. The reference distance is usually 20 ft (originally Paris ft). A letter with a stroke width subtending 1′ at 20 ft is designated 20/20. A letter twice as large subtends the same visual angle at 40 ft and is designated 20/40. Doubling the size again requires doubling of the distance to preserve the reference visual angle: this target is designated 20/80.

The rationale for these designations has been challenged innumerable times, but without enduring success (Ogle, 1953; Westheimer, 1979a), which is unfortunate, because the classical notations tend to conserve erroneous views of what is normal and abnormal, and are poorly compatible with statistical logic. A neutral designation like minimum angle of resolution, MAR, is vastly superior. A useful alternative is to adopt a decibel (dB) notation, which is currently acquiring a firm footing among computerized perimeters. Here, it could relate any visual angle A to a selected reference angle R in the following way:

$$A = 10 \times \log_{10}(A/R)\,\text{dB}$$

Assuming a reference angle R of 1′, a 2′ angle would be designated $10 \times \log_{10}(2/1) = 10 \times 0.3010 = 3\,\text{dB}$, and 4′ $10 \times 0.6020 = 6\,\text{dB}$. A particular advantage of this system is that round decibel steps (0, 1, 2, 3 . . ., corresponding to a scale factor of $10^{0.1} = 1.259$) are nearly optimal for most clinical purposes (Ogle, 1953; NRC/NAS, 1980).

Another problem in describing visual acuity is that acuity cannot be well characterized by a single number. Everyday clinical experience powerfully illustrates acuity's threshold nature: most tested subjects are capable of reading at least a few lines without errors, but as the difficulty of the task increases, the number of errors also increases (Fig. 1.1). Performance defines a frequency-of-seeing curve. It is usually suggested that acuity is designated as the smallest optotypes which can be read 100% or 90% correct. While superficially reasonable, these are actually very harsh criteria, which give undue weight to single, random errors, and underestimate acuity. From statistical points of view, there are many advantages in estimating a 50% correct criterion. A fractional criterion is the only way of assessing acuity precisely: like most measurable characteristics of man, acuity does not naturally come in round numbers. Acceptance of this fact should put an end to the eternal discussions of the best labelling of lines on acuity charts.

Whatever the threshold level actually selected, performance also needs to be described with a measure relating to the variation about the frequency-of-seeing curve, e.g. a confidence interval, to be fully defined.

True threshold measurements are very simple to obtain, even with printed acuity charts. All that is needed is a chart with a suitable scale factor and rows of fine enough letters. The number of correct responses

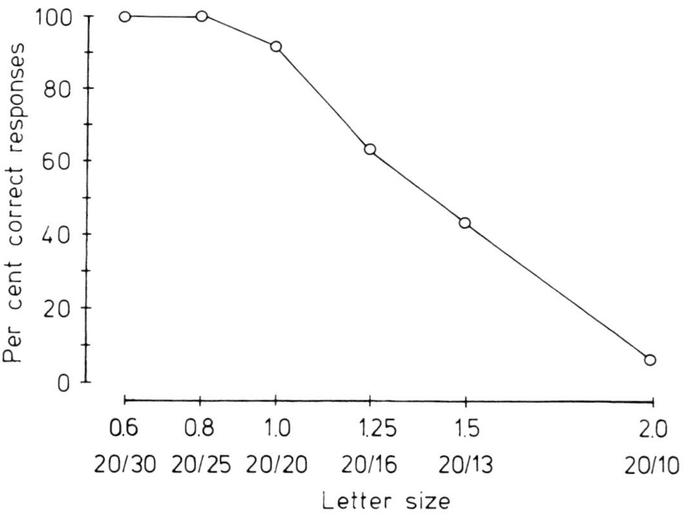

Fig. 1.1 A typical result of an ordinary acuity test, using rows of letters: the proportion of correct responses decreases with increasing difficulty of the task. Letter size is given in both decimal and Snellen notation.

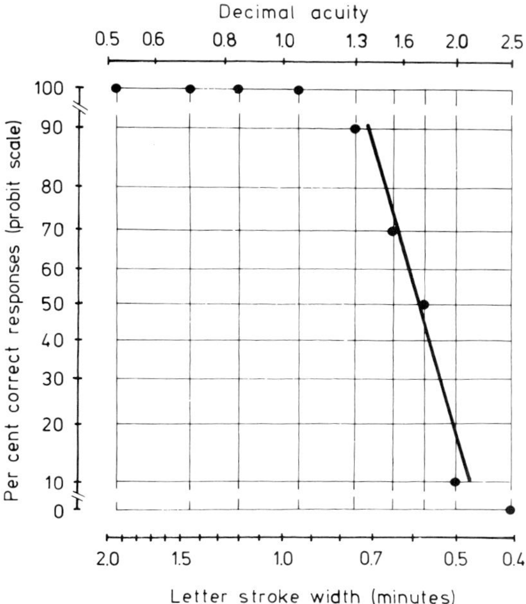

Fig. 1.2 A typical result of an ordinary acuity test, using rows of letters: the proportion of correct responses has been plotted on a probit scale, and the visual angle of letter strokes on a logarithmic scale. 0 and 100% are not defined in the probit scale. The transformations result in a linear frequency-of-seeing curve, which allows direct estimation of any desired threshold level. In this example, the 50% level is 0.58 minutes of arc (1.72, 20/12). (Redrawn from Frisén and Frisén, 1976.)

are counted for each line. The results can then be entered in a properly scaled diagram, and analysed graphically to obtain any desired threshold level (Fig. 1.2). Or, still better, ever new combinations of well-calibrated optotypes, appropriately stepped in size, might be displayed on the screen of a personal computer. The computer could also do a formal statistical analysis at lightning speed, and provide a printed record of all details (Timberlake, Mainster and Schepens, 1980).

1.3.3 NORMAL LIMITS FOR LETTERS IN ROWS

As already indicated, the results of a visual acuity test are critically dependent on the actual test task, and the criteria used. A faultless study of letter-row acuity in a large group of normals remains to be done. Normal letter-row acuity is unknown to this day but a reasonably close approximation is summarized in Fig. 1.3. It is immediately obvious that

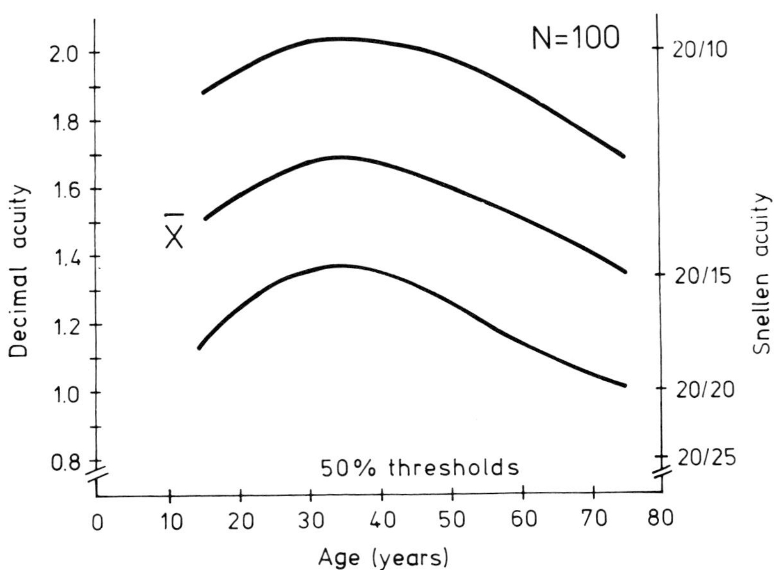

Fig. 1.3 Normal visual acuity for letters in rows (50% threshold level) as a function of age. The curves represent average acuity and 95% confidence intervals. (Redrawn from Frisén and Frisén, 1976.)

acuity varies considerably between normal individuals, even if corrected for age, and that it is rare for normal individuals to have an acuity level of only 1.0 (20/20). Hence, it is perfectly legitimate to complain of impaired acuity, and still with ease read letters at the conventional limit of normal performance. Use of test charts without smaller targets guarantees inability to recognize the first stages in acuity loss. Similarly, erroneous views of what is normal may create false impressions of the diagnostic utility of other types of central vision tests. It is wise to examine the basis for comparison whenever a test is held capable of revealing 'subclinical' or 'hidden' visual loss. Deplorably, the basis is not infrequently only a simple statement like 'normal' or 'near normal' acuity.

1.3.4 PATHOGENESIS OF ACUITY IMPAIRMENT

Whilst it would not be possible to discuss all the clinical conditions capable of affecting visual acuity, not least because the precise mechanism of visual loss is rarely well understood, mechanisms fall under one or more of the following broad headings:

1. Optical faults
2. Destruction, dysfunction or dislocation of foveal cones
3. Transmission disturbances within the retina and the visual pathways
4. Cortical lesions
5. Faulty eye movements

Not surprisingly, optical faults have been the subject of many careful quantitative studies (e.g. Prince and Fry, 1957): after all, acuity tests are first and foremost used as aids in the assessment and correction of refractive errors. Much less is known about the effects of other types of optical faults, e.g. corneal opacities and cataracts, a deficiency of knowledge partly attributable to the lack of techniques for gauging the optical fault itself. Predictions of acuity from clinical examinations of the state of the optical media are notoriously unreliable.

The effects on visual acuity of destruction, dysfunction or dislocation of foveal cones are poorly known. Understanding how normal cones govern normal acuity is a first step towards insight. Intuitively, there should exist a relationship between cone spatial density, and the *minimum separabile*. Herman von Helmholtz (1821–1894) had already argued that resolution is limited by the need of differential stimulation within a cone triplet. Hence, within a row of three cones, the flanking cones should be excited to a higher level than the intervening one. Unfortunately, this simple reasoning cannot account for acuity's threshold nature: the mere existence of a threshold indicates the operation of additional factors. These include: quantum statistics, internal noise, variations in pupil size and accommodation, and eye movements. More intangible factors are also involved, e.g. how certain the tested subject needs to be to acknowledge a weak stimulus. Therefore, investigations of any relationship between resolution and retinal morphology must involve statistical logic. Equally important, the relationship must be shown to apply also for altered cone separations. The retinal disorder, macular oedema, offers a unique natural model for such an analysis.

Retinal oedema is nearly always associated with dysmetropsia, i.e. an apparent change in size of the perceived image, of which micropsia is the most common. In unilateral macular oedema, an object appears smaller than when viewed by the normal eye. Micropsia can be explained by dislocation of cones (Fig. 1.4). Since unilateral micropsia also can be measured, it is possible to estimate the change in cone separation relative to the fellow eye. Parallel measurements of visual resolution have revealed a simple proportionality (a linear regression through the origin) between receptor separation, and the *minimum separabile*, over a range of receptor dislocations (Frisén and Frisén, 1979). Because of the operation

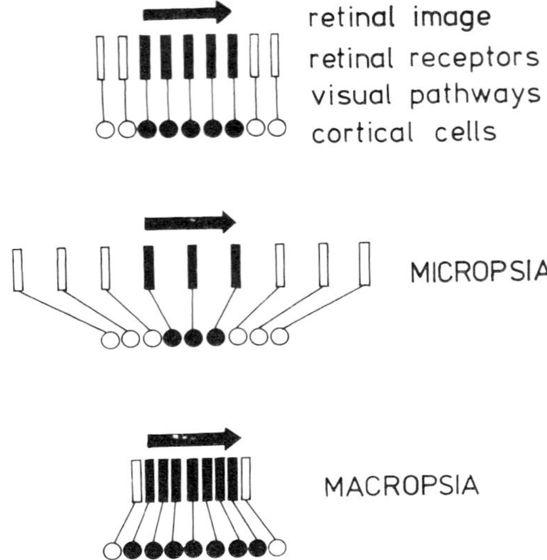

Fig. 1.4 Schematic explanation of how a changed separation of foveal cones may cause dysmetropsia. One and the same retinal image excites five foveo-cortical visual channels in the normal eye (top), but three channels in an eye with macular oedema (middle), and seven in an eye with abnormally tightly crowded cones (bottom). Being unaware of the altered positions of the foveal cones, the brain is bound to misinterpret the size of the retinal image, with resulting micropsia and macropsia, respectively.

of additional factors influencing acuity, as exemplified above, the magnitude of the direction coefficient is inaccessible to an anatomical interpretation.

Interestingly, a proportional relationship appears to apply also to tactile resolution and the spatial density of cutaneous receptors (for review, see Johansson and Vallbo, 1983).

The relationship just described indicates that there are one-to-one links between the foveal cones and the more proximal elements in the foveo-cortical neural channels. Whilst there is anatomical support for this single-chain model (Polyak, 1941, p. 425; Missotten, 1974), there is also evidence that one and the same foveal cone may be in contact with other elements in the complex retinal circuitry (Polyak, 1941, p. 431). Apparently, any such side connections serve purposes other than recognition of fine detail at high contrast, e.g. they might be called into play by moving retinal images or at low luminance levels.

The proportionality model can be shown to apply also to the extrafoveal retina, at least up to 80 degrees of eccentricity (Frisén and Frisén, 1976). Extrafoveally, the model does not involve cone density, but ganglion cell density, which is not unexpected, as the input units, the cones, outnumber by far the output units, the ganglion cells. Changing the emphasis to ganglion cells does not imply a fundamental difference between foveal and extrafoveal acuity-limiting factors: it is the spatial density of *output units* that limits acuity in both cases. The fovea is a special case chiefly because of its one-to-one input–output connections.

Returning to retinal disease, the linear model may also be applied to disorders other than macular oedema. Two requirements need to be fulfilled: one is that the separation between normally functioning foveal cones is different from normal, e.g. by destruction of part of the cone population. The other is that functional cones are uniformly distributed: clearly, localized destruction might leave islands within the fovea with normal receptor density. Such islands might be capable of upholding normal acuity.

It is currently impossible to predict quantitatively how acuity may change with diseases which do not alter the spatial density of working cones, but instead change their orientation, their quantum-conversion efficiency, or their signal propagation.

Turning to the visual pathways, analysis becomes much simpler. Failure of foveal transmission channels can be viewed as a disconnection of the corresponding cones. Acuity will then be determined by the spatial density of the remaining, non-disconnected cones.

This reasoning is directly applicable to optic nerve lesions (Frisén and Quigley, 1984), but how is acuity affected in chiasmal lesions? The answer is most easily obtained by dealing first with the effect of a more remote injury, namely occipital lobectomy, which results in complete blindless if bilateral, but does not change acuity at all if unilateral (Dubois-Poulsen *et al.*, 1952; Frisén, 1980). Hence, each fovea must project to both occipital lobes, and in such a fashion that loss of one projection does not affect the spatial density of still-connected foveal cones. This, then, means that the fovea, contrary to classical belief, must have two non-overlapping outflows: one destined for the ipsilateral cortex, and one destined to the contralateral cortex. Either one suffices to uphold normal acuity.

As with unilateral occipital lobectomy, all other single retrochiasmal lesions of the visual pathways spare acuity. Retrochiasmal lesions must be bilateral in order to affect both foveal projections. Acuity will then be determined by the degree of damage suffered by the less-injured side, and it will be the same in both eyes.

Turning back to the chiasm, it is now clear that acuity should remain normal as long as one foveal outflow from each eye remains intact, i.e. as long as only crossing fibres are affected. Once non-crossing fibres are also involved, acuity will fail. Actually, acuity is rarely spared at the time of clinical presentation, if measured carefully enough (Frisén, 1980). The acuity loss is usually asymmetrical, reflecting lateral asymmetry of the underlying lesion.

Finally, disorders of eye motility are well known to be capable of impairing acuity, and this is true both for reduced, and for excessive, eye movements. Quantitative studies seem to be lacking as yet.

1.3.5 ACUITY PATHOPHYSICS

At the present state of knowledge, acuity measurements can quantitatively predict only two types of abnormality. One is the degree of ametropia, the other is the proportion of functional visual channels in diseases which destroy or disconnect foveal cones. When combined with micropsia measurements, it is also possible to predict the anatomical severity of unilateral macular oedema.

Predicting channel loss requires that the cone disconnection is uniformly distributed over the fovea. If this requirement is fulfilled, the relationship assumes the general form

$$\text{functional channel fraction} = k \times (\text{VA})^2$$

where k is a constant, and VA is acuity in decimal designation. k appears to average about 0.6. Figure 1.5 gives the same relationship graphically. Note that this is a general expression only, with unknown confidence intervals. If confidence intervals could be calculated, they would presumably be quite wide because of the wide variability of acuity even in normals (Fig. 1.3). This leads to variation also in the magnitude of k. As an average, however, it can be seen that so-called normal visual acuity (1.0, or 20/20) can be upheld with a 41% loss of neural channels, and that 'one-half normal acuity' (0.5, 20/40) requires no more than 15%. Acuity 0.25 (20/80) is more than twice as bad as 0.5 in terms of lesion extent: it requires no more than 3.7% of the original complement of channels. If nothing else, these calculations give some life to the otherwise quite meaningless numbers used for describing acuity and acuity loss.

The monotonous nature of the relationship between acuity and channel density indicates that acuity has no redundancy. Every channel contributes, and loss of even one single channel impairs acuity, albeit in a minuscule way. This indicates that acuity measurements, properly performed and evaluated, are powerful tools for diagnosing certain types of visual system lesions. In particular, acuity tests are very useful for detecting and quantifying lesions that may change the spatial density of foveo-cortical neural channels in more than one half of the fovea, i.e. lesions situated between the fovea anteriorly, and the optic chiasm posteriorly. On the other hand, foveal acuity tests are useless for diagnosing unilateral retrochiasmal lesions.

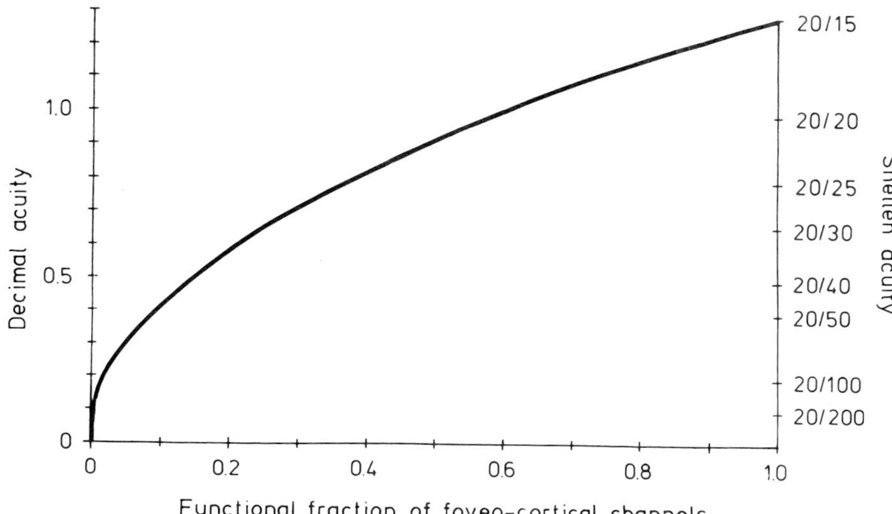

Fig. 1.5 The general form of the relationship between number of working foveo-cortical neural channels (expressed as a fraction of normal), and visual acuity (assuming a normal acuity of 1.3). (Redrawn form Frisén and Quigley, 1984.)

1.3.6 ACUITY AS A REFERENCE PATHOPHYSICAL MEASUREMENT

A tool for defining the pathophysical lesion equivalent must meet several demands. Most important is the measurement of a non-redundant function. High validity, reliability, sensitivity and specificity, are additional requirements. Acuity tests score high in all these regards, if carefully controlled and carefully executed.

A reference test tool naturally should use precisely defined test conditions. Again, Landolt's C, or exactly equivalent letter optotypes, presented at standardized background and surround luminances, appear close to ideal from the practical point of view. So-called sinusoidal gratings are strongly favoured by psychophysicists and an increasing number of clinical investigators; they have several advantages, particularly when investigating the role of contrast in resolution. Unfortunately, the pathophysics of resolution at low contrast are poorly understood, so that, for the present, it seems best to stay with high contrast.

High-contrast gratings can be used as acuity targets but the resolution criterion must then be very carefully defined, because perception of the grating elements changes in a peculiar way with increasing spatial frequency (number of cycles per degree of angle). Grating elements can usually be seen to fill the full test field as long as the spatial frequency is clearly supraliminal, which is not the case when the threshold is being approached: the higher the frequency is made, the smaller becomes the part of the test field where grating elements can be seen. The patch of visible elements is centred on the point of fixation, and the patch moves with changes in gaze direction. The diameter of the patch decreases with increasing spatial frequency, until it finally disappears. This phenomenon, of course, is a reflection of the monotonous increase of resolution thresholds with increasing distance from the fovea, and is an unwanted complication in the assessment of acuity.

The only serious limitation of ordinary acuity tests is their insensitivity to single retrochiasmal visual pathway lesions but, as shown by Aubert and Foerster as long ago as 1857, it is also possible to measure acuity in peripheral vision. Such measurements should allow the assessment of severity of any lesion, irrespective of its position in the visual pathways. Unfortunately, practically useful methods for assessing acuity in peripheral vision are lacking. Some approaches currently being explored are reviewed below.

1.4 Visual fields

1.4.1 DEFINITIONS

The visual field is that part of exterior space from which the eye can perceive light. In practice, this is measured monocularly by means of a perimeter, an instrument that uses typically a hemispherical background, or cupola, with a fixating mark at the pole, and means for displaying a spot of light in selected locations on the uniformly illuminated background. The test spot usually subtends less than one degree of angle at the eye, which is centred in the cupola opening. Spot luminance can be varied within wide limits under operator control, to assess 'differential light sensitivity'. Actually, the test task probes pattern and contrast sensitivity simultaneously (Regan and Beverley, 1983), and has no simple relationship to acuity tasks (Aulhorn, 1964; Johnson, Keltner and Balestrery, 1978; Lie, 1980).

There are two major test procedures. One – static perimetry – employs static stimuli, and varies spot luminance in each location to find the threshold level. The other – kinetic perimetry – depends on the normally monotonous increase in thresholds with increasing eccentricity in the field. Here, the light spot is moved more or less centripetally from an area where it cannot be seen, until perception is signalled. If this is repeated from several different directions, the ensemble of loci of perception defines a curve of equal visibility, or an isopter. Other light spots define other isopters, smaller or larger, depending on the contrast level. As performed manually, neither technique provides well-defined threshold values: in practice, reproducible thresholding requires computer control. Static and kinetic perimetry are not mutually exclusive. On the contrary, there is much to speak for a combination of the two with kinetic perimetry for broad outlines, and static perimetry for filling in of detail.

Because of the huge extent of the normal visual field, and the limited endurance of the subject under test, it is impossible to chart the full visual field in minute detail in one sitting. Instead, the field is sampled in a limited number of locations, typically perhaps 50 or 100. Optimum distribution of tested locations requires much practical training and a good deal of insight into the complexities of various types of field defects. Actually, manual perimetry is probably the most intellectually demanding test in the ophthalmologist's arsenal (Frisén, 1979a). Ironically, it is at the same time an utterly boring test for the patient. Because of the difficulties of finding gifted perimetrists (cf. Trobe *et al.*, 1980), and the expense of their labour, there has been an intensive development of automated perimeters (Heijl and Krakau, 1975; Fankhauser, 1979; and others), the overwhelming majority of which are static perimeters. Some approach the test problem by brute computer force, working with a patience and endurance that exceeds by far that of the average patient. Others may to some degree mimic a human operator, by virtue of partially adaptive software (Haeberlin and Fankhauser, 1980), but the beautiful diagrams produced at the end of the examination may be difficult to reproduce in repeat examinations (Wilensky and Joondeph, 1984; Keltner, Johnson and Lewis, 1985). Judging the qualities of computerized perimeters is very difficult (Greve, 1982; Flanagan *et al.*, 1984; Drance and Anderson, 1985; Keltner and Johnson, 1986), and much development remains to be done.

Modern perimetry is nearly exclusively achromatic. Colour perimetry poses demands that are difficult to meet with current equipment (Hedin and Verriest, 1981). A recent report indicates a close correlation between chromatic and achromatic visual loss (Hart and Burde, 1985).

In addition to these and similar quantitative techniques, clinicians often use informal qualitative 'confrontation' tests when screening for visual field defects, particularly those that may occur with neurological disease (e.g. Trobe *et al.*, 1981). In the right hands, these tests may be quite useful, but in the wrong hands the results may be disastrous. This is the strength and the weakness of confrontation tests, which fall outside the scope of this chapter.

1.4.2 DESIGNATING RESULTS

Most modern perimeters use test targets conforming with the series devised originally by Goldmann (1945). Surface area is varied with a step factor of 4: the smallest target, designated 0, is $1/16\,mm^2$. Target size III ($4\,mm^2$) seems to be the most common in computerized routines, and subtends a visual angle of about 0.5 degree. Size is usually kept constant as long as possible. Instead, luminance is varied, usually with a step factor of $10^{0.1}$, or 1 dB. Unfortunately, manufacturers often define the starting point of the decibel scale in different ways. Background luminances are also often different, so that comparison of results between instruments may be difficult.

1.4.3 NORMAL LIMITS

Detection of minor visual field abnormalities requires precise knowledge of what is normal, which is actually hard to define, particularly in manual, kinetic perimetry, the most common examination technique. While tables of average isopters have been published, normal variability, both between and within tested subjects and examiners, is so large that only major deviations from normal can be detected in this way. Instead, examiners depend on the recognition of abnormalities of isopter shape. The magnitude of the minimum abnormality that can be detected this way is not known. Objective techniques of known power have been described (Frisén and Frisén, 1975; Hart, 1981) but they have been unable to make inroads into clinical routines.

Better references are available for static perimetry, which is less plagued by examiner variability than is kinetic perimetry, but variability within and between individuals remains high (Jacobs and Patterson, 1985; Wild *et al.*, 1986), and tabulated references apply only to limited numbers of target sizes, test locations and age categories. It is difficult to know how to use normal references: strict adherence to, say, averages identifies exactly one half the population of normal subjects as abnormal. Hence, recognition of minor defects is still difficult, and has unknown power. Actually, power may be better in kinetic perimetry because the shape of normal isopters goes back to general symmetry conditions within the eye: such references are largely lost in static perimetry. Small deviations from normal may also be concealed in the heavily interpolated and coarsely stepped grey-scale charts produced by some automatic perimeters. The situation is better for some of the advanced automated instruments, which apply statistical logic for recognizing abnormality (Flammer *et al.*, 1985). The qualities of such analyses ultimately depends on the quality of the normal references.

1.4.4 PATHOGENESIS OF FIELD DEFECTS

The common feature of all perimetric defects (but not necessarily of all visual field defects) is elevation of thresholds. Different types of defects can be discerned on the basis of spatial distribution and magnitude of threshold elevations. The principle of retinotopy adequately explains how spatial distribution of defects comes about, and requires no comment here. It is much more difficult to understand how threshold elevations come about. Actually, it is difficult to understand the background even for normal perimetric thresholds, in spite of decades of ardent collection of data on the effect of various permutations of test variables. While the normal decline in sensitivity with increasing eccentricity roughly mimics the decline in cone spatial density, at least for certain targets and certain backgrounds, this really affords little insight because cones vastly outnumber output (ganglion) cells. This forcefully indicates that several cones must converge on one and the same ganglion cell, to form so-called receptive fields. The convergence factor and the spatial extent of receptive fields is known to vary with the distance from the fovea.

While many factors influencing sensitivity of receptive fields are known from experimental studies, what ultimately determines receptive field sensitivity in the perimetric situation is poorly understood. It is still more difficult to understand what determines thresholds within overlapping receptive fields – it is believed that 30 or more receptive fields may overlap in any given extrafoveal retinal locus (e.g. Fischer, 1973; Peichl and Wässle, 1979), and that neighbouring ganglion cells interact with each other (Mastronarde, 1983). An intriguing possibility is that there is a good deal of specialization in trigger features among receptive fields, so that each, when properly triggered, sends its own 'caricature' of the visual world upstream, along parallel channels, but this is a controversial subject (Barlow, 1972; Lennie, 1980; Kelly and Burbeck, 1984). Much work remains to be done to understand how the visual system normally sets its perimetric thresholds; how pathophysiological mechanisms may raise perimetric thresholds is still more elusive. Acuity thresholds are less enigmatic because they depend on central comparisons of activation in more than one retinal locus: ignorance of what is compared is not equally devastating here.

Meanwhile, an immense database has been built up on various clinical conditions which may be associated with threshold elevations. Broadly speaking, they seem to fall under the same main headings that were used in the analysis of acuity loss above.

1.4.5 PATHOPHYSICS OF PERIMETRY

Results of field tests can be manipulated quantitatively in several ways, e.g. by determining the area enclosed by isopters (e.g. Weleber and Tobler, 1986), or by calculating various indices (Brechner and Whalen, 1984; Flammer *et al.*, 1985; van den Berg *et al.*, 1985; and others). Because of lack of understanding of threshold-setting mechanisms, there is no way of relating these or other representations of perimetric results to the state of the visual system, except in general, qualitative terms. *Hence, the severity of any lesions cannot reliably be estimated from perimetric measurements.* Even qualitative evaluations, e.g. in the form of ranking, can be misleading. Ranking seems to be reasonably safe only within repeat examinations done in the same individual. Comparisons between individuals may be unsafe, unless the number of ranking levels is very small, or the comparison involves diseases with precisely predictable modes of progression (Frisén, 1980).

The lack of understanding also means that the important question of redundancy cannot be answered with any degree of precision. However, parallel evaluations of visual fields and the state of the retinal ganglion cell axons (by ophthalmoscopy or histopathology) indicate that redundancy does exist in perimetry (Frisén, 1979b,c; Quigley, 1985). The visual system apparently has what in neurological parlance is termed a 'safety factor', i.e. the system can sustain damage without affecting perimetric results (Fig. 1.6). A more sceptical interpretation is that perimetry leaves something to be desired.

One way of improving this situation might be to use other types of perimetric targets. Targets measuring acuity are potentially the most useful, because of the reasonably well-understood relationship between resolution thresholds and channel spatial density, and the lack of redundancy. Unfortunately, measuring resolution in peripheral vision is a very demanding and time-consuming task. Nevertheless, the approach is workable, and the first results indicate that resolution is affected at an earlier stage of disease than is simple contrast sensitivity, at least in the only disease – glaucoma – so far studied relatively extensively (Phelps, 1985; cf. also Heron, Milner and Regan, 1975). However, clinical acceptance of acuity-related perimetry demands simpler equipment, simplified test tasks and a radically shortened test duration, which might be realized by using so-called vanishing optotypes in a computer-graphics display (Fig. 1.7). Vanishing optotypes have the peculiar property of closely approximated detection and resolution thresholds, i.e. they are either resolvable, or invisible (Howland, Ginsburg and Campbell, 1978; Frisén, 1986), which allows rapid and confident bracketing of thresholds.

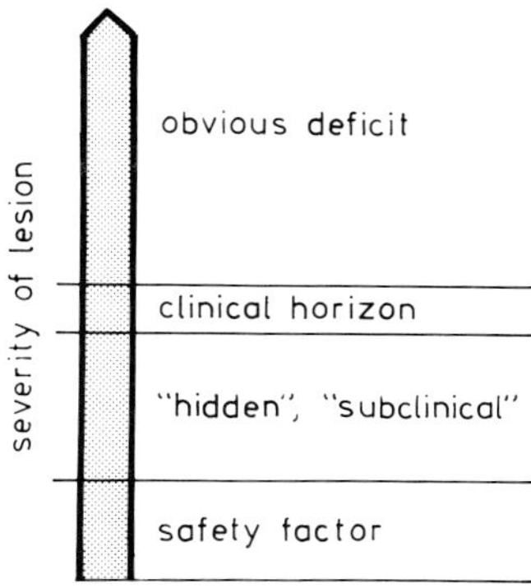

Fig. 1.6 Schematic representation of different obstacles to psychophysical detection of a visual system lesion. Proportions are arbitrary. A safety factor is said to exist if the system can sustain damage without showing a functional corollary. 'Hidden' or 'subclinical' visual loss is often said to exist if an ordinary acuity or visual field test does not reveal damage, in contrast to some other type of test. Like other obstacles, the clinical horizon depends on the qualities of testing techniques and how well normal limits are known.

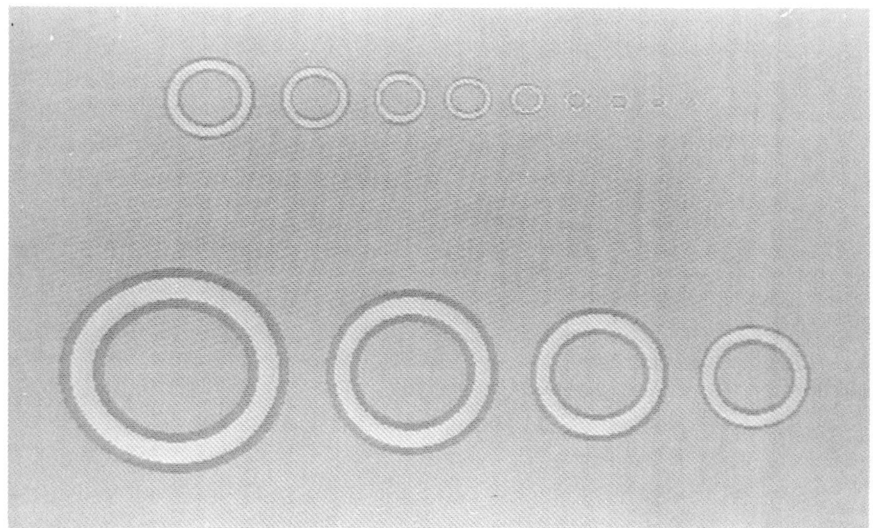

Fig. 1.7. A series of 'vanishing' test targets produced by computer graphics for a visual field screener (L. Frisén, presented at 6th International Neuro-Ophthalmology Society meeting, Hakone, June 9 – 14, 1986). Note how changes in viewing distance alter the number of visible targets: the so-called high-pass spatial frequency filtering (Howland, Ginsburg and Campbell, 1978) causes a close appositioning of detection and resolution thresholds.

Another approach to visual field testing with a pathophysical potential is 'layer-by-layer perimetry' (Enoch, 1978), which is currently a laboratory procedure.

1.5 Concluding remarks

As mentioned in the introduction, clinical acuity and visual field tests have stood the test of time well, i.e. they have not changed very much since first described more than a century ago. Unfortunately, at least in this context, standing the test of time implies little more than resistance to change: it certainly does not guarantee that the original procedures meet modern demands. What, then, are modern demands? What do we clinicians really want from acuity and field tests? Or more neutrally, if we could start anew, how would we like to test central and peripheral vision? This very legitimate question is actually difficult to answer, because there are so many different demands involved, and many compromises have to be made. The following is an attempt towards a list of desirable general properties:

1. Measurements should be interpretable in quantitative pathophysical terms.
2. Statistical indices of quality of results should be provided for every examination.
3. Sensitivity and specificity must be optimally balanced for *early* stages of disease (advanced stages rarely present problems even with poor techniques).
4. Test duration should be carefully balanced for optimum quality of results, and preferably geared to the individual subject's capacity.
5. Tests should ensure subject's attention, e.g. by feedback devices, and by intelligible result presentations.
6. Demands on examiner proficiency and training must be realistic.
7. Test terminology should be neutral, without historical ties.
8. Measurements should have a bearing on activities of daily life so that any practical handicap can be predicted.

From what has been stated above, it is apparent that both acuity and visual field tests as routinely performed in the clinic fail to meet many of these demands. The situation is worst for manual visual field tests because of the shortage of skilled perimetrists. Some of the computer-based field tests fare better, but they are far from ideal and, at the present level of understanding, prospects for useful standardization of perimetry seem to be bleak.

Immediate prospects for improvement are better with central vision acuity tests, which seem to require only small changes (standardization of optotype legibility and of background and surround luminances, statistical evaluation, neutral terminology) to meet basic demands.

A further desirable development would be to test both central and peripheral vision in identical or at least comparable ways, perhaps even with the same equipment. Computer graphics may prove to be the best approach to such a unitary ideal.

References

Aubert, H. and Foerster, R. (1857) Beiträge zur Kenntniss des indirecten Sehens. I. Untersuchungen über den Raumsinn der Retina. *Arch. Ophthalmol.*, **3**, 1–37.

Aulhorn, E. (1964) Über die Beziehung zwischen Lichtsinn und Sehschärfe. *Albrecht von Graefe's Arch. Ophthalmol.*, **167**, 4–74.

Barlow, H.B. (1972) Single units and sensation: a neuron doctrine for perceptual psychology? *Perception*, **1**, 371–94.

Barlow, H.B. and Mollon, J.D. (eds) (1982) *The Senses*. Cambridge University Press, Cambridge.

Brechner, R.J. and Whalen, R.W. (1984) Creation of the transformed Q statistic probability distribution to aid in the detection of abnormal computerized visual fields. *Ophthalmol. Surg.*, **15**, 833–6.

Drance, S.M. and Anderson, D. (eds) (1985) *Automatic Perimetry in Glaucoma. A Practical Guide*. Grune and Stratton, Orlando.

Dubois-Poulsen, A., Magis, C., de Ajuriaguerra, J. and Hecaen, H. (1952) Les conséquences visuelles de la lobectomie occipitale chez l'homme. *Ann. Oculist*, **185**, 305–47.

Enoch, J.M. (1978) Quantitative layer-by-layer perimetry. *Invest. Ophthalmol. Vis. Sci.*, **17**, 208–57.

Enoch, J.M., Essock, E.A. and Williams, R.A. (1984) Relating vernier acuity and Snellen acuity in specific clinical applications. *Doc. Ophthalmol.*, **58**, 71–7.

Fankhauser, F. (1979) Problems related to the design of automatic perimeters. *Doc. Ophthalmol.*, **47**, 89–138.

Fischer, B. (1973) Overlap of receptive field centers and representation of the visual field in the cat's optic tract. *Vision Res.*, **13**, 2113–20.

Flammer, J., Drance, S.M., Augustiny, L. and Funkhouser, A. (1985) Quantification of glaucomatous visual field defects with automated perimetry. *Invest. Ophthalmol. Vis. Sci.*, **26**, 176–81.

Flanagan, J.G., Wild, J.M., Barnes, D.A., Gilmartin, B.A., Good, P.A. and Crews, S.J. (1984) The qualitative comparative analysis of the visual field using computer assisted, semi-automated and manual instrumentation: I Scoring system. *Doc. Ophthalmol.*, **58**, 319–24.

Frisén, L. (1979a) Cornerstones of perimetric strategy, in *Topics in Neuro-ophthalmology* (eds H.S. Thompson, R. Daroff, L. Frisén, J.S. Glaser and M.D. Sanders). Williams and Wilkins, Baltimore, pp. 3–19.

Frisén, L. (1979b) Ophthalmoscopic evaluation of the retinal nerve fiber layer in neuro-ophthalmologic conditions, in *Neuro-Ophthalmology: Focus 1980* (ed. J.L. Smith). Masson, New York, pp. 53–67.
Frisén, L. (1979c) Funduscopic correlates of visual field defects due to lesions of the anterior visual pathway. *Doc. Ophthalmol. Proc. Ser.*, **19**, 5–16.
Frisén, L. (1980) The neurology of visual acuity. *Brain*, **103**, 639–70.
Frisén, L. (1986) Vanishing optotypes. A new type of acuity test letters. *Arch. Ophthalmol.*, **104**, 1194–8.
Frisén, L. and Frisén, M. (1975) Objective recognition of abnormal isopters. *Acta Ophthalmol.*, **53**, 378–92.
Frisén, L. and Frisén, M. (1976) A simple relationship between the probability distribution of visual acuity and the density of retinal output channels. *Acta Ophthalmol.*, **54**, 437–44.
Frisén, L. and Frisén, M. (1979) Micropsia and visual acuity in macular edema. A study of the neuroretinal basis of visual acuity. *Albrecht von Graefe's Arch. Klin. Exp. Ophthalmol.*, **210**, 69–77.
Frisén, L. and Frisén, M. (1981) How good is normal visual acuity? A study of letter acuity thresholds as a function of age. *Albrecht von Graefe's Arch. Klin. Exp. Ophthalmol.*, **215**, 149–57.
Frisén, L. and Quigley, H.A. (1984) Visual acuity in optic atrophy. A quantitative clinicopathological study. *Graefe's Arch. Clin. Exp. Ophthalmol.*, **222**, 71–4.
Goldmann, H. (1945) Ein selbstregistrierandes Projektionsperimeter. *Ophthalmologica*, **109**, 71–9.
Greve, E.L. (1973) Single and multiple stimulus static perimetry in glaucoma: the two phases of perimetry. *Doc. Ophthalmol.*, **36**, 1–355.
Greve, E.L. (1982) Performance of computer assisted perimeters. *Doc. Ophthalmol. Proc. Ser.*, **53**, 343–80.
Haeberlin, H. and Fankhauser, F. (1980) Adaptive programs for analysis of the visual field by automatic perimetry – basic problems and solutions. Efforts oriented towards the realization of the generalized spatially adaptive Octopus program SAPRO. *Doc. Ophthalmol. Proc. Ser.*, **50**, 123–41.
Hart. W.M. (1981) Computer processing of visual data. II. Automated pattern analysis of glaucomatous visual fields. *Arch. Ophthalmol.*, **99**, 133–6.
Hart, W.H. and Burde, R.M. (1985) Color contrast perimetry. The spatial distribution of color defects in optic nerve and retinal diseases. *Ophthalmology*, **92**, 768–76.
Hedin, A. and Olsson, K. (1984) Letter legibility and the construction of a new visual acuity chart. *Ophthalmologica*, **189**, 147–56.
Hedin, A. and Verriest, G. (1981) Is clinical colour perimetry useful? *Doc. Ophthalmol. Proc. Ser.*, **26**, 161–84.
Heijl, A. and Krakau, C.E.T. (1975) An automatic static perimeter, design and pilot study. *Acta Ophthalmol.*, **53**, 293–310.
Heron, J.R., Milner, B.A. and Regan, D. (1975) Measurement of acuity variations within the central visual field by neurological lesions. *J. Neurol. Neurosurg. Psychiat.*, **38**, 356–62.
Howland, B., Ginsburg, A. and Campbell, F. (1978) High-pass spatial frequency letters as clinical optotypes. *Vision Res.*, **18**, 1063–6.

Jacobs, N.A. and Patterson, I.H. (1985) Variability of the hill of vision and its significance in automated perimetry. *Br. J. Ophthalmol.*, **69**, 824–6.

Johansson, R.S. and Vallbo, B. (1983) Tactile sensory coding in the glabrous skin of the human hand. *Trends Neurosci.*, **6**, 27–32.

Johnson, C.A., Keltner, J.L. and Balestrery, F. (1978) Effects of target size and eccentricity on visual detection and resolution. *Vision Res.*, **18**, 1217–22.

Kelly, D.H. and Burbeck, C.A. (1984) Critical problems in spatial vision. *CRC Crit. Rev. Biomed. Eng.*, **10**, 125–77.

Keltner, J.L., Johnson, C.A. and Lewis, R.A. (1985) Quantitative office perimetry. *Ophthalmology*, **92**, 862–72.

Keltner, J.L. and Johnson, C.A. (1986) Current status of automated perimetry. Is the ideal automated perimeter available? *Arch. Ophthalmol.*, **104**, 347–9.

Lennie, P. (1980) Parallel visual pathways: a review. *Vision Res.*, **20**, 561–94.

Lie, I. (1980) Visual detection and resolution as a function of retinal locus. *Vision Res.*, **20**, 967–74.

Lit, A. (1968) Visual acuity. *Ann. Rev. Psychol.*, **19**, 115–54.

Mastronarde, D.N. (1983) Interactions between ganglion cells in cat retina. *J. Neurophysiol.*, **49**, 350–65.

Missotten, L. (1974) Estimation of the ratio of cones to neurons in the fovea of the human retina. *Invest. Ophthalmol.*, **13**, 1045–9.

NRC/NAS Working Group 39 (1980) Recommended standard procedures for the clinical measurement and specification of visual acuity. *Adv. Ophthalmol.*, **41**, 103–48.

Ogle, K.N. (1953) On the problem of an international nomenclature for designating visual acuity. *Am. J. Ophthalmol.*, **36**, 909–21.

Peichl, L. and Wässle, H. (1979) Size, scatter and coverage of ganglion cell receptive field centres in the cat retina. *J. Physiol.*, **291**, 117–41.

Phelps, C.D. (1985) Acuity perimetry and glaucoma. *Trans. Am. Ophthalmol. Soc.*, **84**, 1–63.

Polyak, S.L. (1941) *The Retina*. University of Chicago Press, Chicago.

Prince, J.H. and Fry, G.A. (1957) The effects of spherical ametropia and astigmatism on visual acuity. *Br. J. Physiol. Optics*, **14**, 190–203.

Quigley, H.A. (1985) Better methods in glaucoma diagnosis. *Arch. Ophthalmol.*, **103**, 186–9.

Regan, D. and Beverley, K.I. (1983) Visual fields described by contrast sensitivity, by acuity, and by relative sensitivity to different orientations. *Invest. Ophthalmol. Vis. Sci.*, **24**, 754–9.

Simons, K. (1983) Visual acuity norms in young children. *Surv. Ophthalmol.*, **28**, 84–92.

Sloan, L.L., Rowland, W.M. and Altman, A. (1952) Comparison of three types of test target for the measurement of visual acuity. *Quart. Rev. Ophthalmol.*, **8**, 4–16.

Timberlake, G.T., Mainster, M.A. and Schepens, C.L. (1980) Automated clinical visual testing. *Am. J. Ophthalmol.*, **90**, 369–73.

Trobe, J.D., Acosta, P.C., Shuster, J.J. and Krischer, J.P. (1980) An evaluation of the accuracy of office perimetry. *Am. J. Ophthalmol.*, **90**, 654–60.

Trobe, J.D., Acosta, P.C., Krischer, J.P. and Trick, G.L. (1981) Confrontation visual field techniques in the detection of anterior visual pathway lesions. *Ann. Neurol.*, **10**, 28–34.

van den Berg, T.J.T.P., van Spronsen, R., van Veenendaal, W.G. and Bakker, D. (1985) Psychophysics of intensity discrimination in relation to defect volume examination on the scoperimeter. *Doc. Ophthalmol. Proc. Ser.*, **42**, 147–51.

Weleber, R.G. and Tobler, W.R. (1986) Computerized quantitative analysis of kinetic visual fields. *Am. J. Ophthalmol.*, **101**, 461–8.

Westheimer, G. (1965) Visual acuity. *Ann. Rev. Psychol.*, **16**, 359–80.

Westheimer, G. (1979a) Scaling of visual acuity measurements. *Arch. Ophthalmol.*, **97**, 327–30.

Westheimer, G. (1979b) The spatial sense of the eye. *Invest. Ophthalmol. Vis. Sci.*, **18**, 893–912.

Wild, J.M., Wood, J.M., Flanagan, J.G., Good, P.A. and Crews, S.J. (1986) The interpretation of the differential threshold in the central visual field. *Doc. Ophthalmol.*, **62**, 191–202.

Wilensky, J.T. and Joondeph, B.C. (1984) Variation in visual field measurement with an automated perimeter. *Am. J. Ophthalmol.*, **97**, 328–31.

CHAPTER 2

Psychophysical testing of normal and abnormal visual function

K.H. RUDDOCK

2.1 Introduction

Abnormal visual function in man is usually assessed by some form of psychophysical test, often applied in combination with other non-invasive techniques, such as recording of electrical activity (ERG and VEP), and with CT scanning to examine the location and extent of any lesion. In this chapter, I review a number of psychophysical methods, some newly developed (Ruddock, 1982; 1983), and I describe the results of their application in the study of abnormal responses. The interpretation of these results requires consideration of structural and functional organization of the primate visual pathways derived from experiments on non-human species, and pertinent features of this organization are reviewed briefly in the next section.

2.2 Representations of the visual field and single cell responses in primate visual pathways

Ablation studies on the macaque reveal that at least three retinal projections are implicated in the perception of light stimuli, namely the geniculo-striate and collicular pathways and the accessory optic tract. The last appears to mediate discrimination between light and darkness when all other visual discriminations are absent (Pasik and Pasik, 1971), but it is the other two which subserve the responses under consideration in this chapter. It has been proposed that these two pathways perform complementary roles, the collicular projection being responsible for the control of eye-movements made in response to visual stimuli and the geniculostriate projection for the fine discrimination between stimulus parameters such as colour and spatial pattern (Sprague, 1966; Schneider, 1969). Such division of function is not, however, maintained post-operatively in the macaque where recovery of function occurs if either the striate cortex or superior colliculus remains intact (Weiskrantz, 1972), with permanent losses observed when corresponding regions of *both* neural centres are ablated (Mohler and Wurtz, 1977). Both these projection pathways carry topographical representations of the visual field, that on the striate cortex being the first of a series of contiguous field mappings, extending through the prestriate cortex, immediately anterior to the striate cortex (see Chapter 6). The visual field defects in man caused by lesions occurring at different points along the striate pathway have been described in detail, e.g. by Teuber, Battersby and Bender (1960). The determination of visual field defects and the nature of residual vision within these regions is considered in the case studies of Section 2.4.

Electrophysiological responses of single neurones in these pathways have been extensively investigated, and certain general features can be identified. Three principal classes of retinal ganglion cell, designated X-, Y- and W-, have been distinguished (Enroth-Cugell and Robson, 1966; Stone and Hoffmann, 1972). In primates, X-cells project exclusively to the lateral geniculate nucleus (LGN); they have small receptive fields, are organized concentrically in centre-surround antagonistic regions and yield narrow-band spectral responses which tend to be sustained during stimulation. Y-type cells project to both the LGN and the superior colliculus; they also have centre-surround antagonistic receptive fields, which are larger than those of X-type cells, and they yield broad-band spectral responses with prominent transients elicited by changes in stimulus illumination. W-cells have the slowest conduction velocities of the three groups, but are otherwise somewhat inhomogeneous in response characteristics. Some have receptive fields which yield both 'on' and 'off' responses, and are suppressed by contrast change of either polarity. These and other W-response types are reviewed by Stone (1983).

Single cells located in the superficial layer of the superior colliculus respond selectively to flashed and rapidly moving stimuli, have large receptive fields and are insensitive to stimulus orientation (Schiller and Koerner, 1971; Goldberg and Wurtz, 1972). Neurones of the LGN yield response patterns similar to those of retinal X- and Y-type ganglion cells, but new response features are observed in recordings made from neurones of the striate and prestriate cortex. In the striate, one group of cells which maintain centre-surround antagonism in their receptive fields, are markedly wavelength selective in response and are monocularly driven (Gouras, 1974). Many other cells, however, respond selectively to elongated stimuli, such as bars and edges, orientated to within some ±20° of a preferred direction, which varies from cell to cell (Hubel and Wiesel, 1962, 1968). They are in the main binocularly driven, and two principal classes are generally recognized; simple cells, with receptive fields composed of separate, mutually antagonistic regions, and complex cells the receptive fields of which receive co-extensive antagonistic inputs. The latter are selectively stimulated by moving stimuli, in some cases requiring movement in a particular direction.

The outstanding feature of prestriate functional organization is that cells selectively sensitive to one particular stimulus parameter tend to be grouped into a single representation of the visual field. Thus in V2 and V3, immediately adjacent to the striate area V1, some 80–90% of neurones are selectively sensitive to stimulus orientation, while very few are selective in their response to stimulus colour or direction of movement. Similarly in V4, some 60% of cells respond selectively depending on stimulus colour, and in V5, about 90% are sensitive to direction of stimulus movement (Zeki, 1978). This division of function according to anatomical location has great significance for the interpretation of certain visual abnormalities in man. Cells with an even higher degree of stimulus specificity have been recorded in the superior temporal sulcus of the macaque cortex. These are responsive selectively to anatomical features such as hands and faces (Perrett *et al.*, 1984–5).

2.3 Psychophysical methods

There are several psychophysical functions which are widely used in the description of abnormal visual performance. They rest on the measurement of visual sensitivity in detection of a target or in discrimination between stimuli, and can be conveniently listed according to the stimulus parameter used in their determination. In each case, I also describe briefly the specification of the stimulus parameter itself.

2.3.1 AVERAGE ILLUMINATION

Average illumination is specified in units of radiometric flux (e.g. μwatts m^{-2}), photometric flux (e.g. lumens m^{-2}) or, as in this chapter, in the units of retinal illumination, the Troland, defined as the product (luminance in candelas m^{-2} × pupil area in mm^2). The mean illumination level of the stimulus sets the sensitivity of the eye in detection of a simple target, as is illustrated in Fig. 2.1. Thus it is usual to determine sensitivity functions with reference to a constant illumination level.

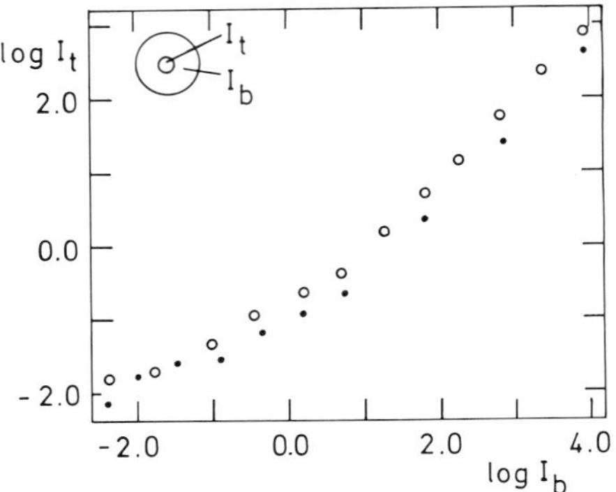

Fig. 2.1 Experimental values of the illumination, I_t, required for detection of a circular target (diameter 1°), presented in a 0.5 s on, 0.5 s off cycle against a circular background (diameter 7°) of illumination I_B. Illumination levels are expressed in log trolands; data for two subjects.

2.3.2 SPATIAL DISTRIBUTION

Spatial distribution of the light stimulus is expressed as the angular size (in degrees) subtended at the eye. Periodic patterns, such as gratings consisting of alternate dark and light bars, are described by their periodicity (in cycles per degree, Fig. 2.2). Sinusoidal distributions of light are specified by a single frequency, whereas square-waveform gratings are composed of an infinite series of sinusoids, with a corresponding infinite range of spatial frequencies. The degree to which the stimulus illumination varies about the mean is specified by the contrast level, defined as $(I_{max} - I_{min})(I_{max} + I_{min})^{-1}$ (see Fig. 2.2). It is also usual to specify the direction of orientation for elongated one-dimensional stimuli such as bars and gratings (e.g. 45° to the vertical meridian).

Spatial resolution, as measured by acuity tests, defines visual performance in the discrimination of spatial patterns. A more general description of spatial response is provided by the measurement of the contrast threshold at which a sinusoidal grating can just be detected (Fig. 2.3).

2.3.3 TEMPORAL CHARACTERISTICS

The temporal characteristics of the stimulus are defined by the duration of a single flash, by the temporal frequency (in hertz) of a sinusoidally modulated stimulus, or by the periodicity of any other periodic wave-

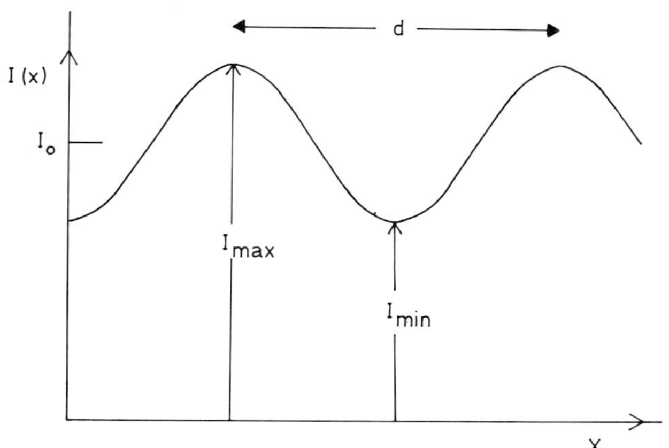

Fig. 2.2 Illumination, I(x), of a one-dimensional sinusoidal grating plotted against distance, x, along the grating. I_o is the mean, I_{max} the maximum and I_{min} the minimum illumination level. d denotes the wavelength and the periodicity is defined in terms of the spatial frequency given e.g. as d^{-1} cycles deg^{-1}.

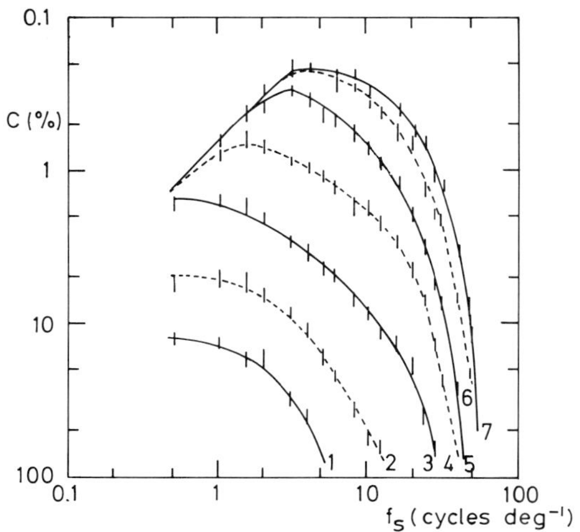

Fig. 2.3 The contrast level, defined as $(I_{max}-I_{min})(I_{max}+I_{min})^{-1}\times 100\%$, required for detection of a sinusoidal grating of spatial frequency f_s. Each curve refers to a different mean illumination, I_o, increasing in steps of ×10 from 0.0009 trolands (1) to 900 trolands (7). (After van Nes and Bouman, 1967).

form. The modulation depth of a temporally modulated stimulus is defined in a manner similar to that of spatial contrast, as $(I_{max} - I_{min})(I_{max} + I_{min})^{-1}$. A common measure of temporal response is the critical fusion frequency (CFF), defined as the frequency at which flicker can just no longer be detected in a fully (100%) modulated stimulus (Fig. 2.4). A more comprehensive description of temporal response is provided by the modulation transfer function of the visual system (Fig. 2.5).

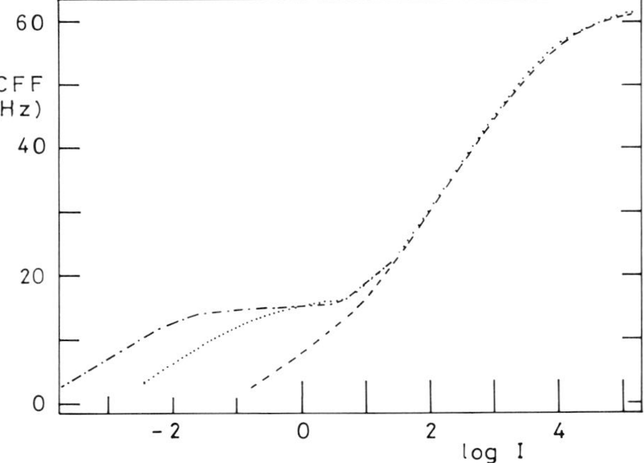

Fig. 2.4 Critical fusion frequency (CFF) plotted as a function of retinal illumination I (log trolands) for a circular field (diameter 19°). At lower illuminations, different stimulus wavelengths yield different values, according to their effectiveness in stimulation of the rod system (450 nm .–.–.–.; 575 nm ..... and 670 nm – – – –). (After Hecht and Schlaer, 1936.)

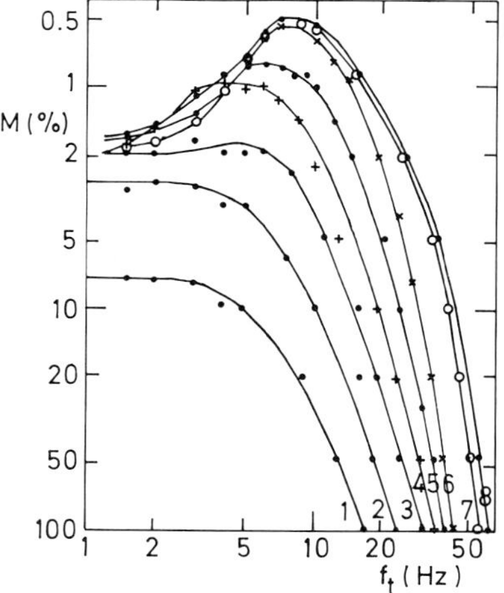

Fig. 2.5 Modulation depth (%) required for detection of sinusoidal flicker of frequency f_t in a small circular field (diameter 2°) on a large surround (diameter 60°). Each curve refers to a different mean illumination, I_o, increasing from 0.375 (1), 1(2), 3.75(3), 10(4), 37.5(5), 100(6), 1000(7) to 10 000 trolands (8) (After de Lange, 1958.)

A different form of temporal response is obtained by measurement of thresholds for detection of targets moving at constant velocity, measured in deg s^{-1} (see Fig. 2.6). Movement can be simulated by sequential presentation of flashed stationary targets separated in space, the resulting sensation usually being called ϕ-motion (Fig. 2.7), although several different kinds of apparent motion are distinguished (Wertheimer, 1912).

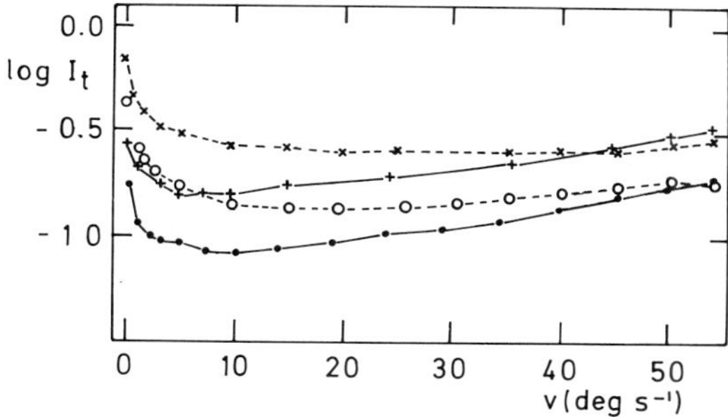

Fig. 2.6 Illumination, I_t (log trolands), required for detection of a circular target (diameter 3.5°), moving along the horizontal meridian at constant velocity v (deg s^{-1}). The target was displaced through 8° at the centre of a circular background (diameter 17°; illumination 0.5 log trolands). Data for foveal viewing (● and +), and for presentation 30° off axis (o and x); different symbols refer to two subjects. (After Barbur and Ruddock, 1980.)

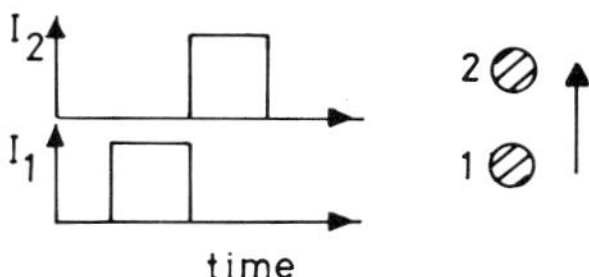

Fig. 2.7 Successive presentation of two targets, displaced with respect to each other, produces apparent movement from that presented first to the second, as indicated by the arrow (I_1 and I_2 denote the illuminations of the two targets, as a function of time, t).

2.3.4 SPECTRAL CHARACTERISTICS

The spectral characteristics of a light stimulus are defined completely by the spectral distribution of the flux emitted from a source or reflected by a surface. In the simplest case, a quasi-monochromatic stimulus is defined by its wavelength (in nanometres) plus the half width of the associated waveband (typically several nm). More complex spectral distributions can be defined in terms of normal trivariant colour vision, as defined by standardized data (Commission Internationale d'éclairage (CIE), 1931).

In this system, colour quality is given by two co-ordinates x and y (Fig. 2.8) and quantity by a third co-ordinate, Y (see Wright, 1960, for a detailed exposition).

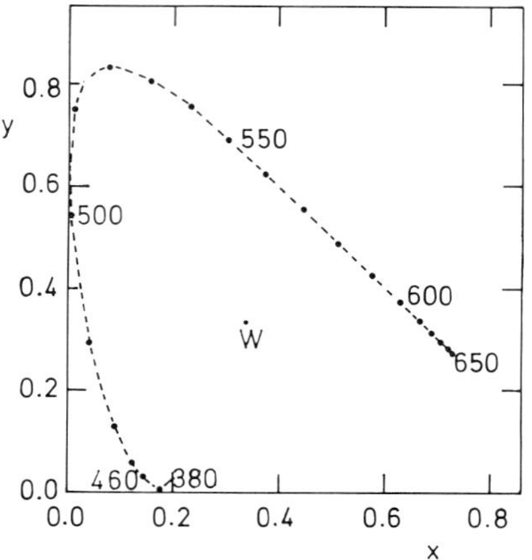

Fig. 2.8 The CIE chromaticity diagram showing the x-y co-ordinates of spectral stimuli (denoted by wavelength in nm) and white light stimuli (denoted W).

The functions described in Sections 2.3.1–2.3.4 above are all measures of overall visual performance and although useful in the description of functional losses which occur in defective vision, they have restricted value in identifying the underlying mechanisms. Other, more-specialized methods have been developed for the investigation of specific response mechanisms and I summarize below those employed in the case studies of Section 2.4.

2.3.5 BACKGROUND MODULATION METHOD

This was developed for the study of spatial and temporal responses of visual mechanisms involved in the detection of moving targets. The principle of the method rests on the change in sensitivity for detection of moving targets caused by the introduction of spatial and/or temporal modulation in the background field (see Fig. 2.9). As the target parameters are unchanged in any set of measurements, the effect of modulating the background is attributed to its influence on the visual mechanism responsible for detection of that particular target. In practice, two types of visual mechanism are revealed in these experiments, one with high spatial frequency and low-pass (sustained) temporal response, and the other with low spatial frequency and band-pass (transient)

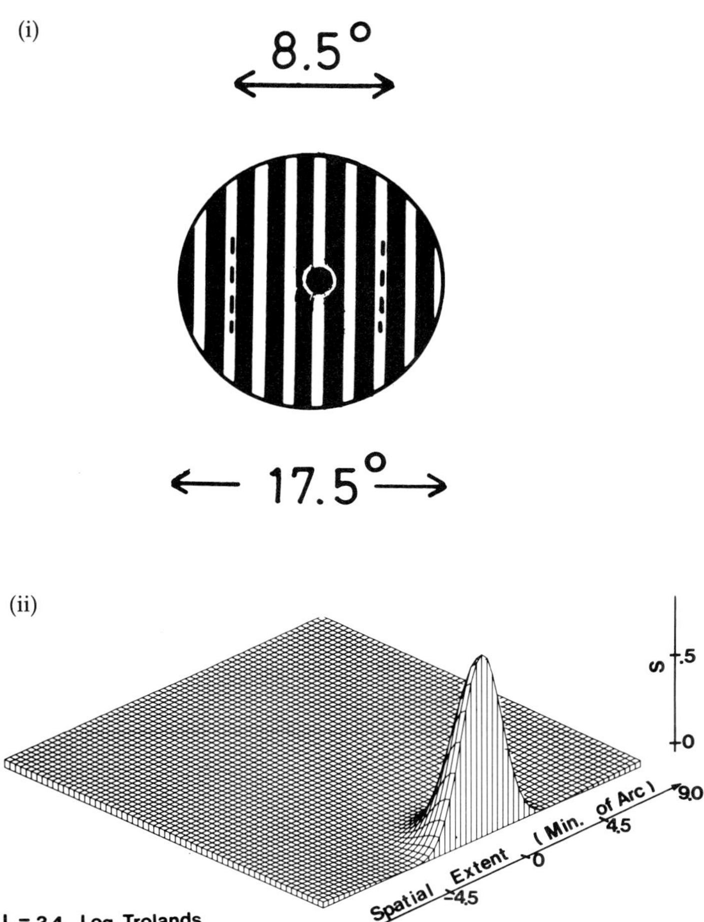

Fig. 2.9 (i) The background modulation method for determination of spatial and temporal response characteristics. The circular target moves across the modulated background, and threshold is measured as a function of background modulation frequency (in this case, spatial). (ii) The spatial sensitivity of the ST1 filter, shown in cross-section, recorded for a mean background illumination of 3.4 log trolands. Note the circular symmetry and centre-surround antagonistic organization. (After Barbur and Ruddock, 1980.)

temporal response. They are known respectively as spatio-temporal (ST) mechanisms 1 and 2. These mechanisms have circularly symmetric spatial organization (Fig. 2.9) and their properties are essentially independent of the target parameters, such as size and velocity. They appear to act as general filters of the retinal image and Holliday and Ruddock (1983) argued that they correspond to X- (ST1) and Y- (ST2) mechanisms located in the prestriate pathways. Their responses can be represented by a network, as illustrated in Fig. 2.10, and they show selective changes in cases of amblyopia (Section 2.4.1) and optic neuritis.

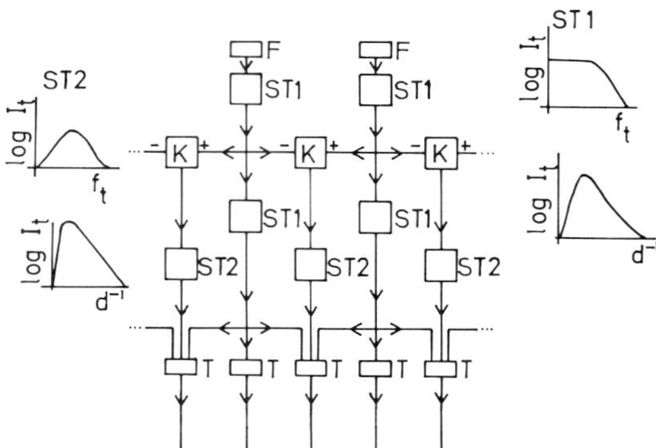

Fig. 2.10 Network representation of the early stages of filtering by the visual system, showing interaction between the two filters ST1 and ST2, via the units K. F represents the Fechner filter, which determines simple threshold of the kind shown in Fig. 2.1, and T the threshold device for the two filters. The characteristics of the two filters, illustrated to the left and right of the network, are expressed in terms of illumination, I_t, required for detection of the moving target, plotted against the spatial, d^{-1}, or temporal frequency, f_t, of the background.

2.3.6 ORIENTATION SENSITIVE RESPONSES

The activity of orientation sensitive mechanisms in human vision are readily demonstrated by adaptation methods. The apparent width of bars in a grating changes immediately following adaptation to a grating of different bar-width, and this phenomenon, first demonstrated by Blakemore and Sutton (1969), provides evidence of width and orientation selective visual mechanisms. Subsequently, it was established that the dark and light bars in the gratings adapt independently of each other (Burton, Naghshineh and Ruddock, 1977; de Valois, 1977). Thus there are two independent mechanisms, one sensitive to positive contrast components of the retinal image (the light bars) and the other to the negative contrast components of the retinal image (the dark bars).

The band-width and orientation selectivity of such adaptation mechanisms have been extensively studied by measurement of contrast threshold for detection of a grating. The contrast required for detection of a test grating is raised transiently following several minutes of (nonlocalized) adaptation to a high contrast grating of similar width and orientation (Fig. 2.11) (Gilinsky, 1968; Pantle and Sekuler, 1968; Blakemore and Campbell, 1969). The characteristics of this response are obtained by measuring the change in contrast for a fixed test grating and for various adaptation parameters.

Results indicate the activity of visual mechanisms tuned to within ±20°

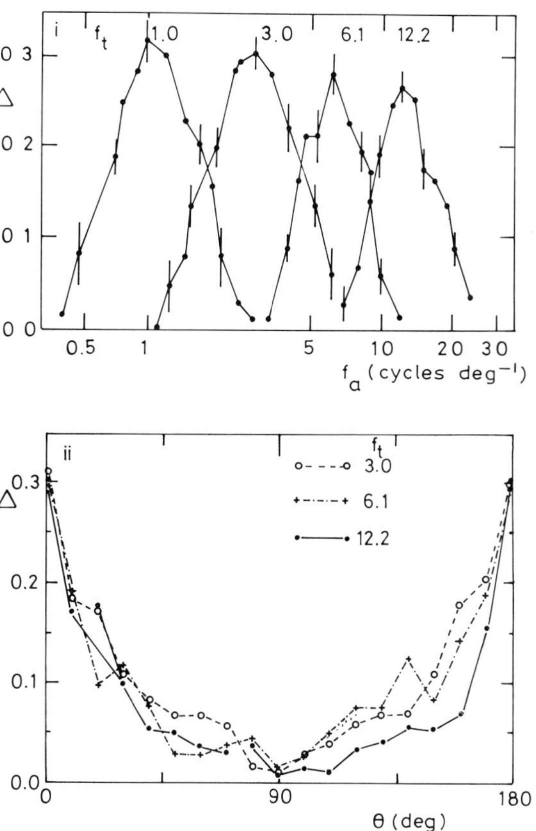

Fig. 2.11 (i) Increase in illumination (or contrast), △, required for detection of a sinusoidal test grating, following adaptation to a high contrast grating of spatial frequency, f_a, orientated parallel to the test. Responses are given for four test gratings, of different spatial frequencies as denoted on the figure (in cycles deg^{-1}). Note that in each case, △ is maximum when the test and adaptation gratings are matched in spatial frequency. (ii) The increase in threshold, △, for detection of a test grating following adaptation to a high contrast grating, orientated at angle θ relative to the test. Data are given for three spatial frequencies of the test and adaptation gratings, which were matched in each case. (After Maudarbocus and Ruddock, 1973.)

and with spatial frequency band-width of about 2 octaves. There are multiple mechanisms, as is revealed by the fact that frequency response curves always peak at the frequency of the test grating. The mechanisms are located centrally, as the adaptation effects are transferred from one eye to the other.

2.3.7 DISCRIMINATION OF SIMPLE GEOMETRIC PATTERNS

This has been studied directly using visual fields of the kind illustrated in Fig. 2.12. The subject is asked to detect a single target element, which differs from the large number of identical background elements by a single parameter, such as orientation. Detection of the target is signalled by pressing a button, and the time elapsed between presentation and detection of the target is logged. Both the locations of the background elements and that of the target are randomized from presentation to presentation as also is the value of the target parameter under study (e.g. its angle of orientation). Different classes of target element give strongly characteristic orientation discrimination data (Fig. 2.13) and the discrimination can also be measured by the time, $T_{\frac{1}{2}}$, required for 50% probability of detecting a given target (Fig. 2.14). This direct method of discrimination measurement can be applied to a variety of parameters associated

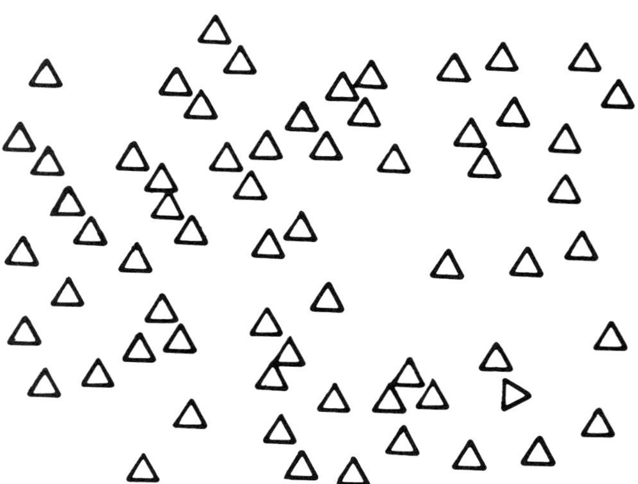

Fig. 2.12 Visual field consisting of a number of identical, randomly distributed and non-interesting background elements, △, and a single target element differentiated from the others, in this case by its orientation.

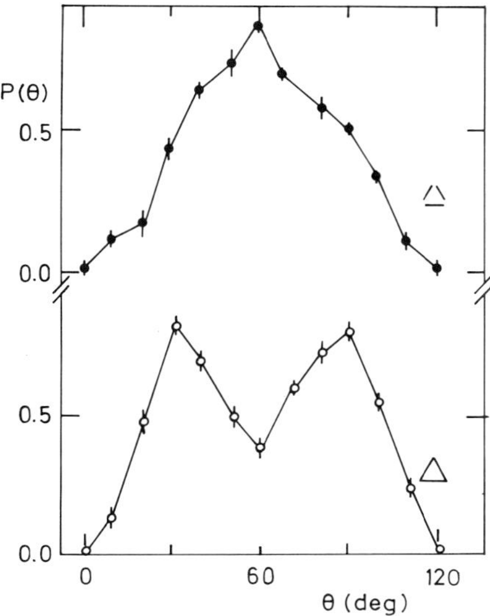

Fig. 2.13 Probability P(θ) for detection, within 1.0 s of presentation, of a target orientated at angle θ relative to the background elements △ or △ (as marked).

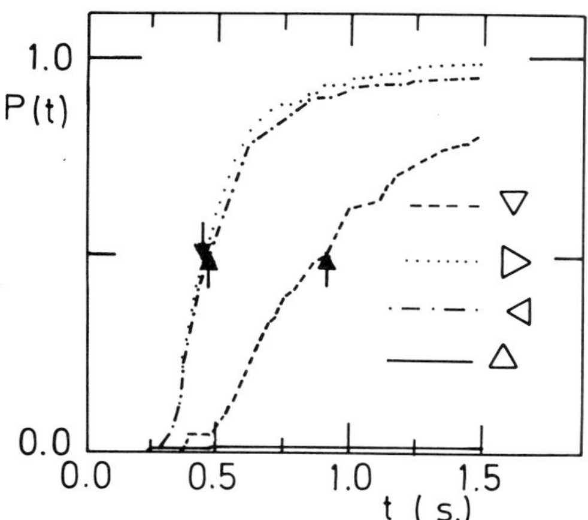

Fig. 2.14 Probability, P(t) for detection of a target within time, t, following presentation of the stimulus (Fig. 2.12). Results are given for four target orientations 30°(◁), 60°(▽), 90°(▷) and the 'null' target, which matches the background, 0°(△). The time, $T_{\frac{1}{2}}$, required for 50% probability is denoted by the arrows.

with spatial structure, including orientation, magnification and texture. It has proved particularly useful in the investigation of subjects suffering abnormal pattern discrimination and form agnosia (Section 2.4.5).

2.4 Case studies

In this section I present the results of psychophysical studies performed on a number of subjects, the group as a whole including examples of several visual abnormalities. The results are collected according to the defects which they describe.

2.4.1 AMBLYOPIA

Amblyopia is the term given to loss of visual resolution due to changes in the neural pathways and is usually caused by strabismus or large refractive error in one eye, suffered during the period of critical development. The critical period in man is generally reckoned to be less than 7 years of age and treatment traditionally consists of occlusion (i.e. patching) of the normal eye. The nature of the underlying neural mechanism is still the subject of debate. The modified pattern of binocular input to the striate cortex which is induced by suture of one eye (Wiesel and Hubel, 1963; Hubel, Wiesel and Levay, 1977) has encouraged wide speculation that amblyopia is of cortical origin. Ikeda and her co-workers have, however, demonstrated that in cats with surgically induced strabismus, the X-, but not Y-type retinal ganglion and geniculate nerve cells lose spatial resolution (Ikeda, 1980; Ikeda and Tremain, 1978).

Application of the background modulation method reveals marked changes in the spatial response of the ST1, but not the ST2 mechanism, and the temporal responses also remain unchanged (Fig. 2.15). The change in the ST1 spatial frequency response corresponds to an increase in the spatial dimensions of the mechanism, that is, a decrease in its spatial resolution (Fig. 2.16). One unexpected result was that in subjects who had received patching treatment, but not in the others, the ST1 spatial response is abnormal in the 'normal' as well as in the amblyopic eye. To the extent that the ST mechanisms can be associated with prestriate neuronal activity, these results support the findings of Ikeda and her co-workers in showing selective changes in the ST1 mechanisms, with its X-type response characteristics, rather than in the Y-type ST2 mechanism. The changes in ST1 do not, however, account completely for the losses in visual acuity, with which they correlate only weakly in measurements for a group of subjects (Grounds, Holliday and Ruddock, 1983).

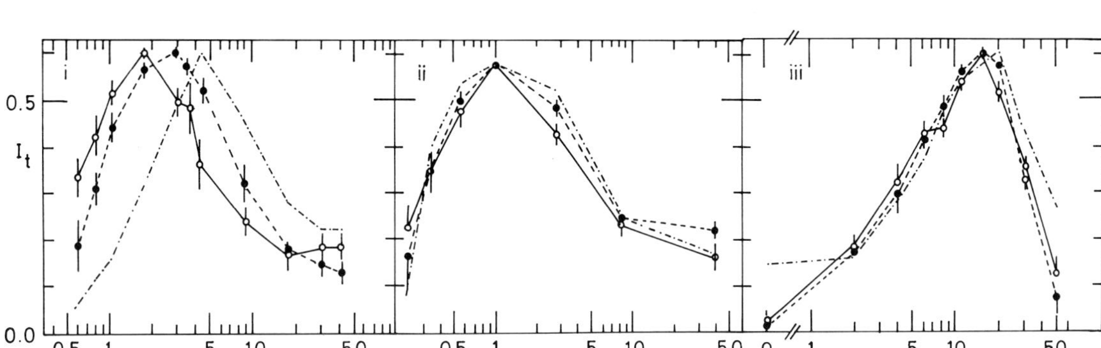

Fig. 2.15 Data for spatio-temporal filtering in subjects suffering amblyopia. (i) ST1 spatial responses. Average data for seven normal subjects (–.–.–.) and the 'normal' eyes (●–––●–) and abnormal eyes (○–○–) of 12 strabismic amblyopes. (ii) ST2 spatial responses. Average data for six normal subjects (–.–.–.) and the 'normal' eyes (●–––●–) and abnormal eyes (○–○–) of nine amblyopes. (iii) ST2 temporal responses. Average values for five normal subjects (.–.–.–.) and for the 'normal' eyes (●–––●–) and abnormal eyes (○–○–) of nine amblyopes. In each case, threshold illumination, I_t, for detection of a moving target is plotted against spatial (f_s) or temporal (f_t) frequency. Note that only (i) shows any differences between normal and amblyopic data. (After Grounds, Holliday and Ruddock, 1983.)

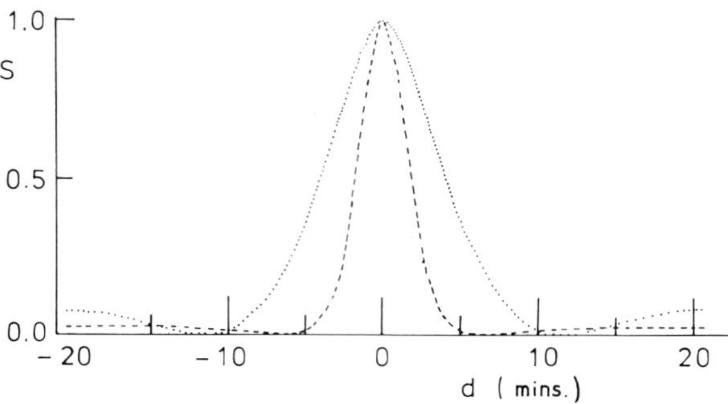

Fig. 2.16 The spatial distribution of the ST1 response mechanism (in cross-section); average data of the seven normal subjects (– – –) and of the 'abnormal' eyes of the 12 strabismic amblyopes, (. . . . .) taken from Fig. 2.15.

2.4.2 HEMIANOPIA AND QUADRANTANOPIA

Lesions of the post-chiasmal pathways frequently give rise to loss of visual sensitivity, extending over large areas of the visual field, and are homonymous for the two eyes. The losses sometimes affect one quadrant or one-half of the visual field and the cases considered here fall into one or other of those categories. Of 25 such subjects examined, five were able to detect transient, localized changes of illumination within the visual field defect. Detection threshold for moving targets decreases as target velocity increases, although it always remains abnormally high (Fig. 2.17). CFF values for the corresponding regions are, however, depressed, thus demonstrating that they do not provide a reliable monitor of transient vision, but rather reflect the high threshold detection levels (see also Section 2.4.3). A particularly important feature of residual vision within these field defects is that it permits accurate location of the targets, but not pattern recognition. For example, spatial discrimination for displacement of two targets which generate apparent motion (Fig. 2.7) is essentially normal (Fig. 2.18). The subjects are, however, unable to distinguish between a single target and a pair of targets presented simultaneously at a separation of 7°, well above that required for discrimination of their displacement. Thus residual vision in these subjects is mediated by a mechanism which signals target location, but not spatial pattern. In terms of the functional division of the visual pathways, this corresponds to activity in the 'where' system, and it is speculated that residual vision in these subjects reflects activity in the collicular projection.

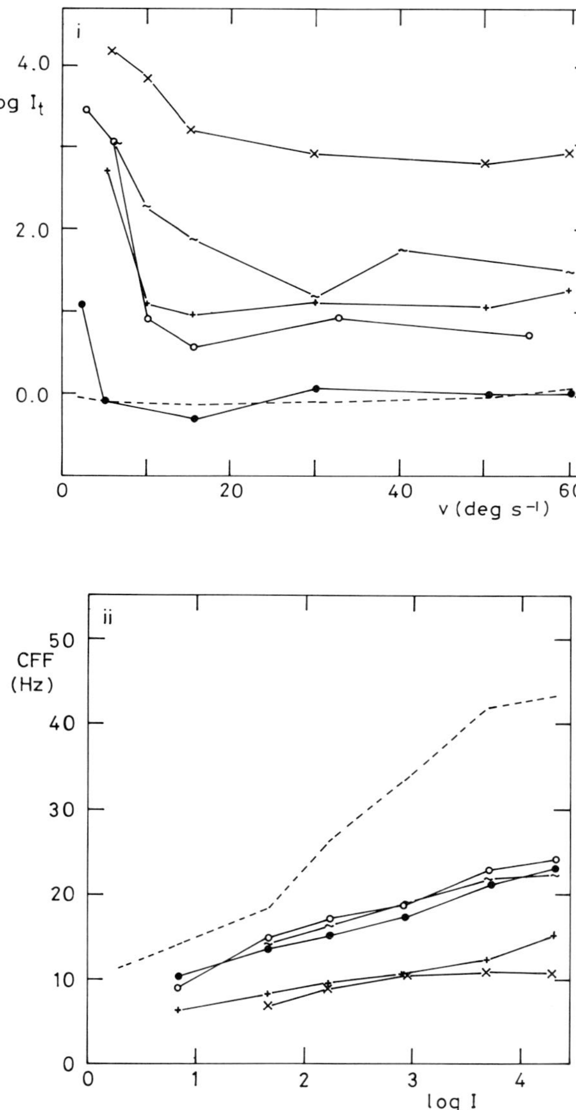

Fig. 2.17 (i) Threshold illumination, I_t, for detection of a circular target (diameter 3.5°) moving along the horizontal meridian at v deg s^{-1}. Data are for five subjects suffering damage to the striate cortex, leading to 'blindness' in the contralateral field. The broken line denotes the mean data for the normal fields of the same subjects. (ii) CFF values for the 'blind' fields of the same five subjects, measured for a circular field (diameter 5.5°) of illumination I (in log trolands) superimposed on a uniform background of illumination 0.75 log troland. The broken line denotes the mean value for their normal fields.

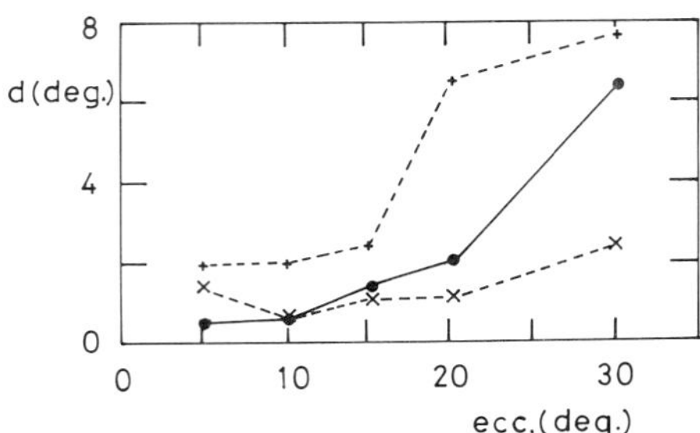

Fig. 2.18 The separation, d, of two circular targets (diameter 1°) required for 90% probability of correct discrimination of the displacement direction (left to right, or vice versa), when the two targets are presented sequentially for 800 ms each (see Fig. 2.7). (After Blythe *et al.*, 1986a.)

2.4.3 PERSEVERATION

Critchley (1951) used the term perseveration to describe the abnormal spread of sensation beyond the physical limits, either spatial or temporal, of the stimulus. Two forms of temporal disturbance can be distinguished, one characterized by systematic persistence of visual sensation after stimulation and the other by the occurrence of sensation in the absence of immediate stimulation. The latter occurs unpredictably and is therefore difficult to study, whereas the former is a consistent phenomenon and can be examined psychophysically. I describe results for a single subject FB, who experiences vivid after-images persisting for periods of up to several minutes after viewing even moderately bright lights. The most significant finding is that the increment threshold for detection of a target superimposed on a background field is raised for some 15 s after the background is removed (Fig. 2.19), whereas for normal subjects it falls rapidly within 100 ms. This period of decreased threshold sensitivity is not as extended as the after-images themselves, but provides an objective demonstration of abnormal visual function. It increases as either the illumination level or the duration of the background increases (Fig. 2.20). The after-images maintain the spatial structure of the stimuli which give rise to them, except that spatial frequencies of $\geqslant 10$ cycles deg^{-1} are absent. Thus after-images produced by gratings match in appearance the structure of the stimulus grating for as long as they remain visible. The after-images have the same colour appearance ($x = 0.411$, $y = 0.476$; $Y < 42.5$) regardless of the stimulus colour which produces them, and they exhibit no temporal modulation, even if elicited by flashed or moving stimuli. It might appear at first sight that such after-images may be caused either by abnormal adaptation of a kind similar to that which

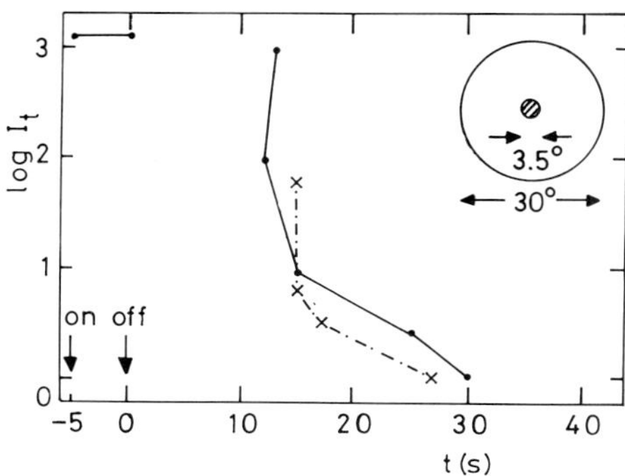

Fig. 2.19 Threshold illumination, I_t (log trolands), for detection of a circular target (diameter 3.5°) following 5 s viewing of a circular stimulus (diameter, 30°, illumination 2.9 log trolands). Full circles: both stimuli presented to the same eye; Crosses: the two stimuli presented one to each eye. Subject FB. For normal subjects, threshold recovery occurs within 100 ms.

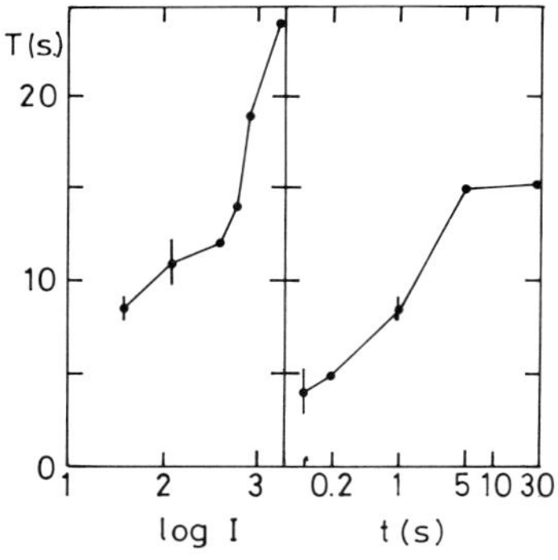

Fig. 2.20 T, the time at which log I_t (Fig. 2.19) falls to half its level during presentation of the 30° field. T is plotted against the illumination, I (log trolands), and against the duration of presentation, t, of the 30° field. Subject FB. (After Blythe *et al.*, 1986b.)

produces normal light adaptation effects or by abnormal temporal responses. In normal vision, however, increases in increment thresholds produced by light adaptation are strictly monocular, whereas the raised thresholds observed for FB can be transferred from one eye to the other (Fig. 2.19 crosses). Further her temporal sensitivity, measured either for detection of moving targets or in terms of critical fusion frequency, is essentially normal. Thus, psychophysical methods demonstrate objectively the effects of prolonged visual sensation, and also provide evidence regarding the underlying mechanism. The results indicate that FB's after-images are caused by prolonged activity following stimulation in central neural mechanisms sensitive to spatial pattern. After-images in some other cases of perseveration exhibit colour effects and temporal variation, and appear to involve abnormal activity in response mechanisms not implicated in FB's case (See Blythe *et al.*, 1986b, for a review).

2.4.4 VISUAL EXTINCTION

The rapid fading, or 'extinction', of visual sensation during maintained stimulation is the converse of perseveration, and is frequently observed in subjects with lesions of the posterior parietal lobe, at the border with the occipital lobe (Bender, 1946). Its study by psychophysical methods is illustrated for the case of a single subject GJ, with a tumour in the parieto-occipital cortex, demonstrated both by CT scan and in post-mortem autopsy (Fig. 2.21). She reported that during voluntary fixation, there was rapid fading of images located in the right visual hemifield, contralateral to the tumour. Under transient presentation, colour vision, stereoscopy and spatial resolution in the right hemifield were normal, but under fixation sustained images faded rapidly, giving a grey, uniform

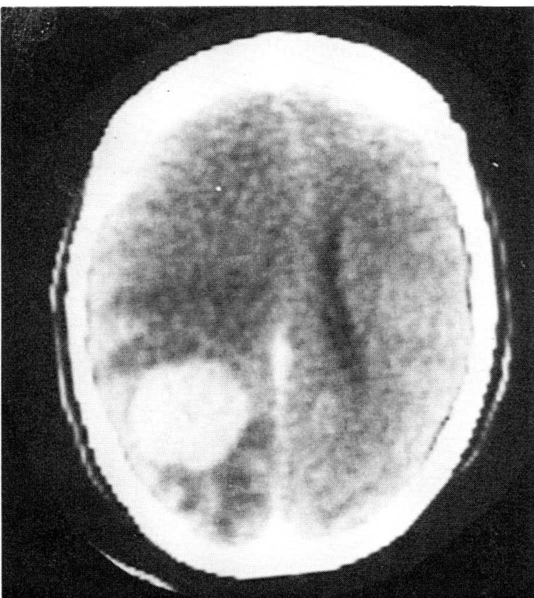

Fig. 2.21 CT X-ray scan showing a large enhancing lesion in the left parieto-occipital region with surrounding oedema. Subject GJ.

sensation lacking all the normal response attributes, and the phenomenon as described by the subject herself is similar to the fading of stabilized retinal images (Ditchburn and Ginsburg, 1952). Fading of the image was demonstrated by measurement of threshold illumination for detection of a moving grating as a function of grating velocity (Fig. 2.22). At low velocity, GJ's threshold is raised significantly above normal, but as velocity increases to 8 deg s^{-1}, it approaches the normal value. The rapid fading of retinal images caused by parietal lobe lesions is significant in demonstrating that maintenance of visual sensation under voluntary fixation is dependent on normal cortical function.

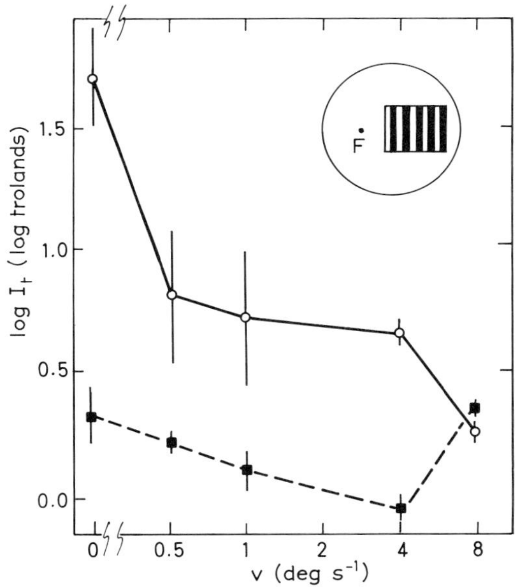

Fig. 2.22 Threshold illumination, I_t (log troland) for detection of a vertically orientated grating (1 cycle deg^{-1}) the bars of which moved with constant velocity v deg s^{-1}. The target was located with its near edge 3° off-axis in the right hemifield, and was superimposed on a uniform background (diameter 15°) of illumination 2.5 log trolands (see inset). Data for GJ (open circles) and normal subject PS (full squares). (After Holliday, Kennard and Ruddock, 1985.)

2.4.5 ABNORMAL PATTERN RECOGNITION

A number of studies have been carried out on subjects who are incapable of pattern discrimination and recognition, yet have normal spatial resolution. Although such conditions are usually classed as form agnosia, there is considerable diversity both in the response characteristics of different subjects and in the interpretations of such deficits offered by the various investigations (Geschwind, 1965; Warrington, 1985; Humphreys and Riddoch, 1987). One critical issue concerns the persistence of low level visual discriminations in form agnosia, and in this section I examine discrimination of simple geometrical shapes by two subjects who exhibit abnormal pattern discrimination. One subject, AP has a mild defect, possibly dyslexic in origin, whilst the other, HJA, suffers a particularly severe loss of pattern recognition and discrimination (Humphreys and Riddoch, 1984).

AP, a graduate mathematician, often confuses mathematical symbols, e.g. $\cup$ with $\cap$, makes frequent errors of spelling and was unable to read or write until her teens. Her discrimination of magnification, measured by the methods described in Section 2.3.7, is normal, but for some shapes, her discrimination of orientation is abnormal. This is illustrated in Fig. 2.23, which shows that her responses for elements △ are normal, whereas those for elements △ are markedly anomalous, approximating to the normal data for elements △. The experiments therefore provide objective evidence of abnormal image processing by AP's visual system, and imply that those mechanisms responsible for associating lines into two-dimensional images behave abnormally (see Ike and Ruddock, 1987, for a fuller discussion).

The second subject, HJA, experienced general loss of pattern

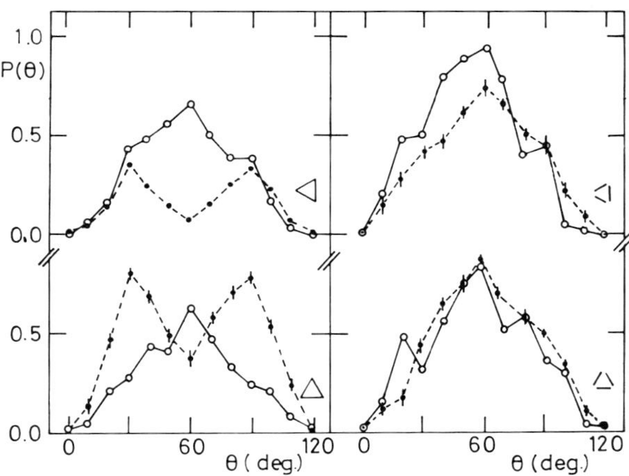

Fig. 2.23 Probability P(θ), for detection within 1.0 s, of a target orientated at angle θ relative to the various background elements, as denoted in the figure. Each background consisted of 60 randomly distributed elements. Data for AP (open circles) and a group of normal subjects. (After Ike and Ruddock, 1987.)

recognition following a stroke, suffered post-operatively some five years ago. Despite having normal spatial resolution, he recognizes visually neither common objects nor highly specific, but familiar, images such as the faces of close relatives. His responses to the multi-element discrimination patterns (Fig. 2.24) exhibit a particularly sharp distinction between two levels of visual processing. For single lines, |, or even quasi-single lines, ⋮, his response times $T_{\frac{1}{2}}$ for detection of the target are essentially normal, whereas for two-dimensional elements, they become very much slower than those of even naïve normal subjects, with quasi-linear patterns such as |||| giving intermediate results. The data of Fig. 2.24 all refer to detection of orientation change, and show that he is particularly poor at extracting targets which form the mirror image of the triangular elements (e.g. △→▽). In other experiments, he was asked to detect triangular elements of the same orientation, but different in structure from the background triangles, which were always △. The results demonstrated that even with marked differences between target and background, he was unable to perform the task normally, and it is possible to order different types of target according to difficulty of detection, i.e. according to the value of $T_{\frac{1}{2}}$. Some examples are given in Fig. 2.25, and define different targets in order of increasing discriminability. As well as providing a well defined basis for comparison between different agnosic subjects, such experiments also yield results which are important in the analysis of pattern recognition in normal subjects.

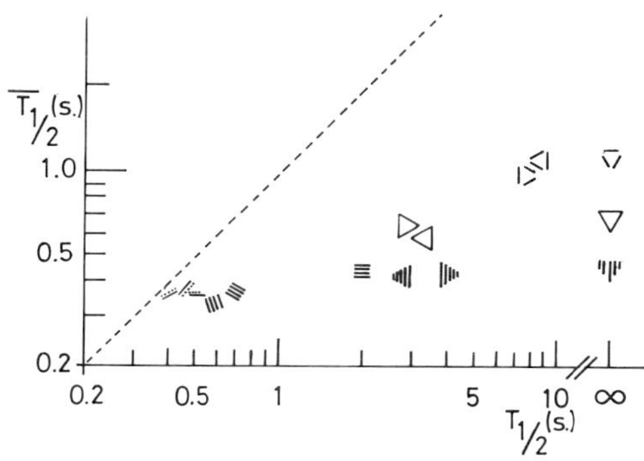

Fig. 2.24 Discrimination of different target elements, as illustrated in the figure, presented in a background of 20 similar elements, orientated in an upright position (i.e. |, ⋮, △, △, ≜ and ⦀). Values of the time, $T_{\frac{1}{2}}$, required for 50% probability of detection (see Fig. 2.14) for subject HJA, are plotted against $\overline{T}_{\frac{1}{2}}$, the average value for the three normal subjects. (After Bromley *et al*, 1986.)

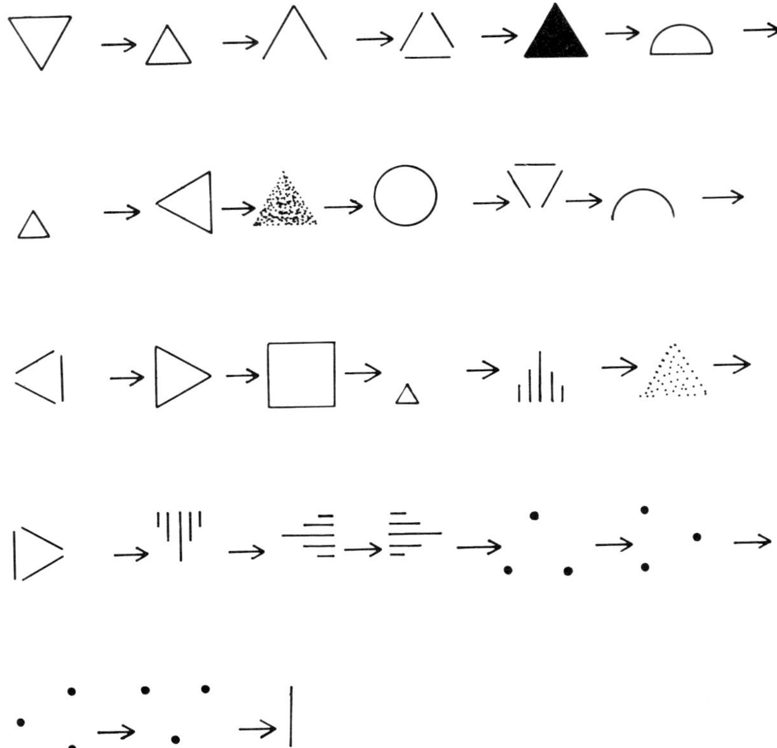

Fig. 2.25 The relative order of difficulty with which HJA discriminates the targets shown from a background of 20 elements △, the size of which was that of the top left target.

2.5 Colour vision deficiencies

Congenital colour vision deficiencies have been extensively investigated psychophysically (e.g. Wright, 1946) and the underlying changes in the cone photopigments are documented even at molecular level (Nathans *et al.*, 1986). The small group of unilateral congenital defects (e.g. Judd, 1948; Bender *et al.*, 1972) set a puzzle for geneticists, and merit further study with reference to modern views on prestriate organization. Lesions of the central pathways can give rise to achromatopsia which, as in the case of HJA described above, is frequently associated with defective pattern recognition (Meadows, 1974).

I describe here a different phenomenon, exhibited by a single subject MW, to date the only known case of this kind. Under achromatic conditions, his vision is entirely normal, but in monochromatic and particularly red lights, he suffers considerable loss of spatial resolution. This low acuity results from the spread of sensation beyond the area of stimulation, which results in a 'steely-grey' sensation. Within this area, his detection and perception of visual stimuli, even those which otherwise elicit normal responses, are suppressed (Fig. 2.26). The extent of the inhibitory area increases as either the saturation or the luminance of the coloured stimulus increase, and it occurs mainly, but not exclusively, with red and purple stimuli. The inhibitory influence of coloured stimuli is apparent even in detection of incremental flashes, which is, however, normal for white light (Fig. 2.27). His VEPs are normal for red stimuli

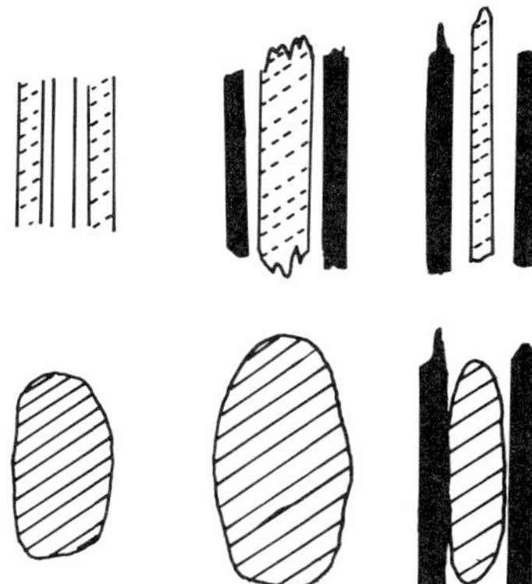

Fig. 2.26 Stimuli consisting of black and red bars shown in the top row as full black and hatched areas respectively, as represented by MW (bottom row). The hatched areas in the bottom row appeared as 'silver-grey with a metallic sheen'. (After Hendricks, Holliday and Ruddock, 1981.)

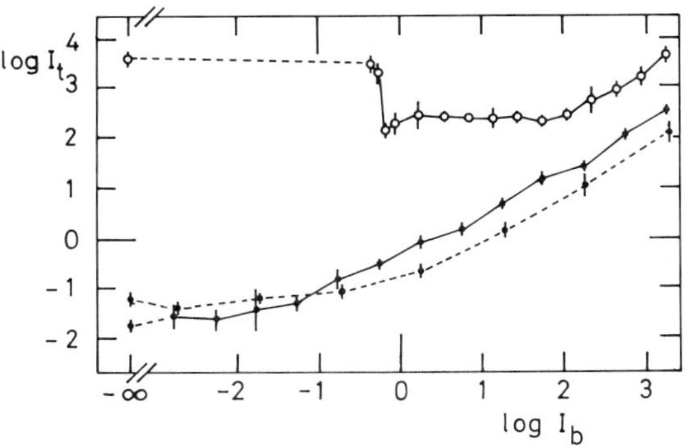

Fig. 2.27 Threshold illumination, I_t, for detection of a circular spot (diameter 1°), presented in a 0.5 s on, 0.5 s off cycle against a background of uniform illumination I_b (expressed in log trolands). Data for MW (o) and two normal subjects. (After Bender and Ruddock, 1974.)

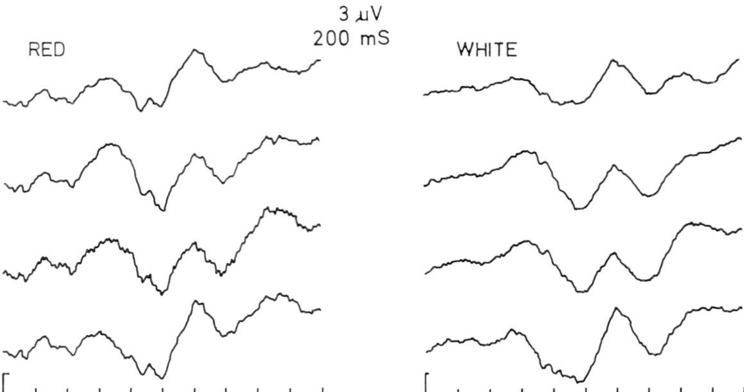

Fig. 2.28 Visually evoked potentials recorded from the occipital cortex in response to alternating red and white or black and white chequer-board patterns. Subject MW was unable to detect the former, but the evoked potentials are similar to those obtained for the latter.

which he cannot perceive (Fig. 2.28) and a further indication of central involvement is that he can recognize stereoscopic images constructed from two-colour random-dot patterns (Julesz, 1971), even though the red component image is not resolved.

MW's defect is highly colour specific, as in contrast to many cases of achromotopsia he has no loss of other visual function. It therefore offers striking evidence that in the central visual pathways, colour is processed independently of other stimulus parameters.

Acknowledgements

I acknowledge with thanks the time and effort made by the various subjects whose responses are described, and for the many contributions of my co-workers. The research described was supported in part by research grants awarded jointly to Dr C. Kennard (London Hospital) and myself by the Jules Thorne Charitable Trust and the Wellcome Trust.

References

Barbur, J.L. and Ruddock, K.H. (1980) Spatial characteristics of movement detection mechanisms in human vision. I. Achromatic mechanisms. *Biol. Cyber.*, **37**, 77–92.

Bender, B.G. and Ruddock, K.H. (1974) The characteristics of a visual defect associated with abnormal responses to both colour and luminance. *Vision Res.*, **14**, 383–93.

Bender, B.G., Ruddock, K.H., de Vries-de Mol, E.C. and Went, L.N. (1972) The colour vision characteristics of an observer with unilateral defective colour vision: results and analysis. *Vision Res.*, **12**, 2035–57.

Bender, M.B. (1946) Changes in sensory adaptation time and after-sensation with lesions of the parietal lobe. *Arch. Neurol. Psychiat.*, **55**, 299–319.

Blakemore, C. and Campbell, F.W. (1969) On the existence of neurones in the human visual system selectively sensitive to the orientation and size of retinal images. *J. Physiol. (Lond.)*, **203**, 237–60.

Blakemore, C. and Sutton, P. (1969) Size adaptation: a new after effect. *Science, NY*, **166**, 245–7.

Blythe, I.M., Bromley, J.M., Kennard, C. and Ruddock, K.H. (1986a) Visual discrimination of target displacement remains after damage to the striate cortex in humans. *Nature (Lond.)*, **320**, 619–21.

Blythe, I.M., Bromley, J.M., Ruddock, K.H., Kennard, C. and Traub, M. (1986b) A study of systematic visual perseveration involving central mechanisms. *Brain*, **109**, 661–75.

Bromley, J.M., Humphreys, G.J., Javadnia, A., Riddoch, M.J. and Ruddock, K.H. (1986) Pattern discrimination in a human subject suffering visual agnosia. *J. Physiol. (Lond.)*, **377**, 67.

Burton, G.J., Naghshineh, S. and Ruddock, K.H. (1977) Processing by the human visual system of the light and dark contrast components of the retinal image. *Biol. Cyber.*, **27**, 189–97.

Critchley, M. (1951) Types of visual perseveration: 'paliopsia' and 'illusory visual spread'. *Brain*, **74**, 267–99.

Ditchburn, R.W. and Ginsburg, B.L. (1952) Vision with stabilised retinal images. *Nature (Lond.)*, **170**, 36–7.

Enroth-Cugell, C. and Robson, G.J. (1966) The contrast sensitivity of retinal ganglion cells of the cat. *J. Physiol. (Lond.)*, **187**, 517–52.

Geschwind, N. (1965) Disconnection syndromes in animals and man. *Brain*, **88**, 237–94 and 585–644.

Gilinsky, A.S. (1968) Orientation-specific effects of patterns of adaptating light on visual acuity. *J. Opt. Soc. Am.*, **58**, 13–18.

Goldberg, M.E. and Wurtz, R.H. (1972) Activity of the superior colliculus in behaving monkeys. I. Visual receptive fields of single neurons. *J. Neurophysiol.*, **35**, 542–59.

Gouras, P. (1974) Opponent-colour cells in different layers of foveal striate cortex. *J. Physiol. (Lond.)*, **238**, 583–602.

Grounds, A.R., Holliday, I.E. and Ruddock, K.H. (1983) Two spatio-temporal filters in human vision. 2. Selective modification in amblyopia, albinism and hemianopia. *Biol. Cyber.*, **47**, 191–201.

Hecht, S. and Schlaer S. (1936) Intermittent stimulation by light **V**. The relation between intensity and critical frequency for different parts of the spectrum. *J. Gen. Physiol.*, **19**, 965–77.

Hendricks, I.M., Holliday, I.E. and Ruddock, K.H. (1981) A new class of visual defect: spreading inhibition elicited by chromatic light stimuli. *Brain*, **104**, 813–40.

Holliday, I.E. and Ruddock, K.H. (1983) Two spatio-temporal filters in human vision. I. Temporal and spatial frequency response characteristics. *Biol. Cyber.*, **47**, 173–90.

Holliday, I.E., Kennard, C. and Ruddock, K.H. (1985) Rapid fading of visual sensations in a subject with a parietal-occipital tumour. *Ophthal. Physiol. Opt.*, **5**, 149–56.

Hubel, D.H. and Wiesel, T.N. (1962) Receptive fields, binocular interaction and functional architecture in the cat's visual cortex. *J. Physiol. (Lond.)*, **160**, 106–54.

Hubel, D.H. and Wiesel, T.N. (1968) Receptive fields and functional architecture of monkey striate cortex. *J. Physiol. (Lond.)*, **195**, 215–43.

Hubel, D.H., Wiesel, T.N. and Levay, S. (1977) Plasticity of ocular dominance columns in monkey striate cortex. *Phil. Trans. R. Soc. Lond. B.*, **278**, 377–409.

Humphreys, G.J. and Riddoch, M.J. (1987) The fractionation of visual agnosia, in *Visual Object Processing: A Cognitive Neurophysiological Approach* (eds G.J. Humphreys and M.J. Riddoch). Erlbaum, New York, pp. 281–306.

Ike, E.E. and Ruddock, K.H. (1987) Visual discrimination for simple geometrical patterns. 2. Atypical responses in a subject suffering difficulties with pattern recognition. *Spatial Vision* **2**, 31–7.

Ike, E.E., Ruddock, K.H. and Skinner, P. (1987) Visual discrimination for simple geometrical patterns. I. Measurements for multiple element stimuli. *Spatial Vision* **2**, 13–29.

Ike, E.E., Ruddock, K.H. and Skinner, P. (1986) Visual discrimination for simple geometrical patterns. I. Measurements for multiple element stimuli. *Spatial Vision* (in press).

Ikeda, H. (1980) Visual acuity – its development and amblyopia. Edridge-Green Lecture 1979. *J. R. Soc. Med.*, **73**, 546–55.

Ikeda, H. and Tremain, K.E. (1978) Development of spatial resolving power of lateral geniculate neurones in kittens. *Exp. Brain Res.*, **31**, 193–206.

Judd, D.B. (1948) Colour perceptions of deuteranopic and protanopic observers. *J. Res. Nat. Bur. Stand.*, **41**, 247–71.

Julesz, B. (1971) *Foundations of Cyclopean Vision*. University Press, Chicago.

Lange, H. de (1958) Research into the dynamic nature of fovea cortex system with intermittent and modulated light. I Attenuation characteristics with white and colored light. *J. Opt. Soc. Am.*, **48**, 777–84.

Maudarbocus, A.Y. and Ruddock, K.H. (1973) Non-linearity of visual signals in relation to shape-sensitive adaptation responses. *Vision Res.*, **13**, 1713–37.

Meadows, J.C. (1974) Disturbed perception of colours associated with localized cerebral lesions. *Brain*, **97**, 615–32.

Mohler, C.W. and Wurtz, R.H. (1977) Role of striate cortex and superior colliculus in visual guidance of saccadic eye movements in monkeys. *J. Neurophysiol.*, **40**, 74–94.

Nathans, J., Piantanida, T.P., Eddy, R.L., Shows, T.B. and Hogness, D. (1986) Molecular genetics of inherited variation in human color vision. *Science, NY*, **232**, 203–10.

van Nes, F.L. and Bouman, M.A. (1967) Spatial modulation transfer in the human eye. *J. Opt. Soc. Am.*, **57**, 401–6.

Pantle, A. and Sekuler, R.W. (1968) Size-detecting mechanisms in human vision. *Science, NY*, **162**, 1146–8.

Pasik, T. and Pasik, P. (1971) The visual world of monkeys deprived of striate cortex: effective stimulus parameters and the importance of the accessory optic system. *Vision Res. Suppl.*, **3**, 419–33.

Perrett, D.I., Smith, P.A.J., Potter, D.D., Mistlin, A.J., Head, A.S., Milner, A.D. and Jeeves, M.A. (1984–5) Visual cells in the temporal cortex sensitive to face view and gaze direction. *Proc. R. Soc. Lond. B.*, **223**, 293–317.

Ruddock, K.H. (1982) Psychophysical studies on subjects with visual defects. Edridge-Green Lecture 1981. *J. R. Soc. Med.*, **75**, 315–22.

Ruddock, K.H. (1983) Visual mechanisms for the analysis of spatial pattern. *Ophthal. Physiol. Opt.*, **3**, 93–119.

Schiller, P. and Koerner, F. (1971) Discharge characteristics of single units in superior colliculus of the alert rhesus monkey. *J. Neurophysiol.*, **34**, 920–36.

Schneider, G. (1969) Two visual systems. *Science, NY*, **163**, 895–902.

Sprague, J.M. (1966) Interaction of cortex and superior colliculus in mediation of visual guided behaviour in the cat. *Science, NY*, **153**, 1544–7.

Stone, J. (1983) *Parallel Processing in the Visual System*. Plenum, New York, pp. 39–41.

Stone, J. and Hoffmann, K.P. (1972) Very slow conducting ganglion cells in the cat's retina: a major, new functional type? *Brain Res.*, **43**, 610–16.

Teuber, H.L., Battersby, W.S. and Bender, M.B. (1960) *Visual Field Defects after Penetrating Wounds of the Brain*. Harvard University Press, Cambridge, MA.

de Valois, K.K. (1977) Independence of black and white: phase specific adaptation. *Vision Res.*, **17**, 209–15.

Warrington, E.K. (1985) Agnosia: the impairment of object recognition in *Handbook of Clinical Neurology*, **1**, *Clinical Neuropsychology* (ed. J.A.M. Frederiks), Elsevier, Amsterdam, pp. 333–49.

Weiskrantz, L. (1972) Behavioural analysis of the monkey's visual nervous system. *Proc. R. Soc. Lond. B.*, **182**, 427–55.

Wertheimer, M. (1912) Experimentelle Studien über das Sehen von Bewegung. *Z. Psychol.*, **61**, 161–265.

Wiesel, T.N. and Hubel, D.H. (1963) Single cell responses in striate cortex of kittens deprived of vision in one eye. *J. Neurophysiol.*, **26**, 1003–17.

Wright, W.D. (1946) *Researches on Normal and Defective Colour Vision*. Kimpton, London.

Wright, W.D. (1960) *Measurement of Colour*. Hilger, London.

Zeki, S. (1978) Uniformity and diversity of structure and function in rhesus monkey prestriate visual cortex. *J. Physiol. (Lond.)*, **277**, 273–90.

CHAPTER 3

Retinal representations in prethalamic visual pathways

R.W. GUILLERY

The classical view of retinal representations in the optic nerve and tract was summarized by Polyak, 1957 (see Fig. 3.1), and this is still generally regarded as an accurate account of the condition that obtains in mammals with a significant binocular field of view. In Fig. 3.1 each optic nerve is shown as carrying an orderly representation of the visual field seen by one eye, and each tract as carrying a single binocular representation of the contralateral hemifield. One surprising feature of this scheme is that the two hemifields, one from each eye, are brought together to form a single fused representation in the tract only to be separated again in the lateral geniculate nucleus, where the components from each eye terminate in separate layers (not shown in the figure). A problem from the contemporary point of view is that the process of matching the maps cannot be regarded as a simple developmental process. Axons from homonymous points on the retinae must run together in the tract even though these two points are not matched in terms of the symmetry of the developing organism and cannot be matched in terms of visual field co-ordinates since, at the relevant developmental stage, there is no visual field: the eyes are closed and the receptors have not yet developed. That is, if the accuracy of the classical scheme is accepted, then a developmental mechanism must be postulated for bringing the maps into register, but such a mechanism would serve no defined useful end for the survival of the organism. As far as is known, there are no significant binocular interactions between impulses travelling in the axons of the tract, so that

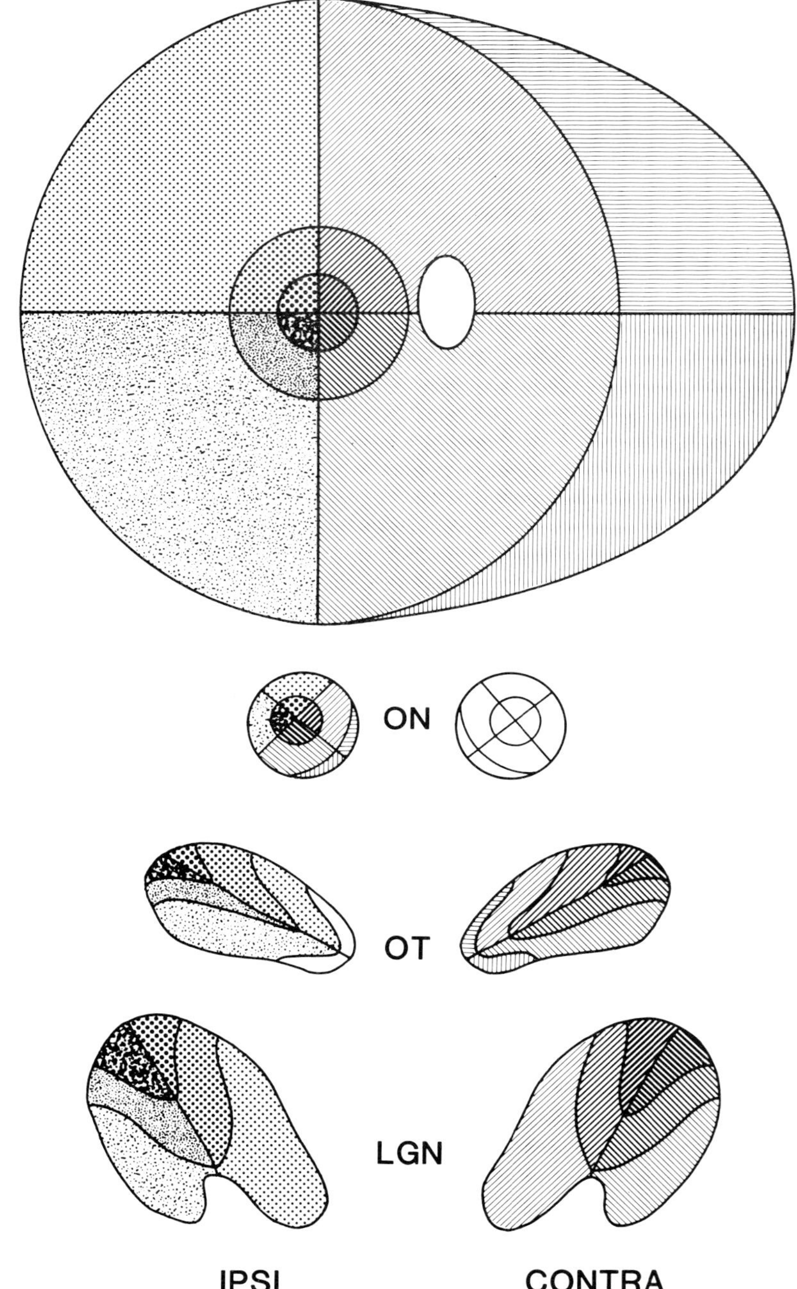

ON
OT
LGN
IPSI
CONTRA

neighbour relationships in the tract are not likely to be of functional significance.

My interest in the optic tract was first stimulated by a consideration of the albino abnormality. In albino mammals a significant component of the retinofugal pathway from the temporal retina does not stay on its own side as is normal, but instead crosses in the optic chiasm. The details of this abnormality have been worked out most clearly for cats (Guillery and Kaas, 1971; Kaas and Guillery, 1973; Shatz, 1974; Stone, Campion and Leicester, 1978; Cooper and Pettigrew, 1978; Creel, Hendrickson and Leventhal, 1982) but there is good evidence for believing that a comparable abnormality of the chiasmatic pathway occurs in all albino mammals in which the retinal melanin is significantly reduced, including primates (Lund, 1965; Creel, 1971; Guillery, 1974; Guillery *et al.*, 1984). Some years ago Mason studied the mapping of the retina in the optic tracts of such abnormal animals. She used Siamese cats, which have a hypopigmented retina due to the action of an allele of the albino series (the *c* locus), and in which the abnormal central maps in the lateral geniculate nucleus and visual cortex had been clearly defined by earlier studies. Her results were surprisingly difficult to interpret, so much so that they have never been published in full. Two points puzzled us. One was that the mapping definable in the optic tracts of normal and of Siamese cats was far from accurate. By making limited retinal lesions and then plotting the distribution of degenerating axons in the optic tract, she showed that even quite small retinal lesions produced degeneration that was widely scattered throughout the tract, with just a tendency to concentrate in one part of the tract. The second puzzle was that although the abnormal fibres from the temporal retina were in the wrong tract, they seemed to be mapped in roughly the appropriate part of the tract. We had not expected this. The abnormal fibres must approach the optic tract from the wrong side since they enter the tract medially from the chiasm, instead of laterally from the temporal part of the optic nerve; yet, on Mason's evidence, they pass to roughly the right part of the tract, not to the medial part of the tract where one could reasonably have expected to find them. It was difficult to propose a developmental mechanism that could produce such a result.

Fig. 3.1 Schema of the retinal maps in the human optic nerve (ON), optic tract (OT) and lateral geniculate nucleus (LGN). The retina is represented at the top of the figure with the fovea indicated by the crossing of the vertical and horizontal meridians and the optic disc shown in white. Nasal retina is to the right, temporal retina to the left, and the portion of the retina that looks at the monocular crescent of the visual field is represented as the part of the retina furthest to the right. Note that the separation of the ipsilateral and contralateral components in the laminae of the dorsal lateral geniculate nucleus is not shown in this schema. (Modified from Polyak (1957).)

At about the time that these studies of the Siamese cat's optic tract were being done, Horton, Greenwood and Hubel (1979) published a short paper that seemed to indicate quite clearly that there was no retinotopic map in the normal cat's optic nerve or tract. They injected a small amount of horseradish peroxidase into the lateral geniculate nucleus and labelled eight retinal ganglion cells with this enzyme, which is transported retrogradely down the axons so that the cells and their axons are labelled. They showed that these eight axons did not maintain neighbour relationships in their central course, but took rather widely divergent paths. From this result and from Mason's observations, it can be concluded that there is not an accurate mapping in the central pathways. Mason's observations suggested that there is a rough mapping, which was apparent when relatively large numbers of fibres were involved but which might be lost when relatively few fibres were being traced.

Further clues as to the nature of this rough mapping were already available in the 1970s in published studies of the optic nerve and tract of cats, although they had never been interpreted in terms of the classical notion of accurate maps being represented in the central pathways. It was known that fibres of different diameters were mingled in the optic nerve (van Crevel and Verhaart, 1963; Donovan, 1967) but were segregated in the optic tract (Bishop, Jeremy and Lance, 1953; Bishop and Clare, 1955; Chang, 1956). In the optic tract the finer fibres were described as occupying the deep parts of the tract whereas the coarser fibres lay more superficially, nearer the pia. Clearly, such a segregation of fibre diameter classes in the tract, but not in the nerve, must reflect some major rearrangement of the maps, if indeed there are maps; but neither the possibility of such a rearrangement, nor its nature had been considered in any detail by earlier investigators.

One further piece of evidence contributed to our reinterpretation of fibre order in the cat's optic tract. Polley, who had been studying the cat's retinofugal pathways for many years in Chicago, showed me that there is a dorsal part of the optic tract in cats that is essentially free of uncrossed axons. This 'pure crossed' crescent was intriguing because it did not occupy the part of the tract in which one might expect the representation of the monocular crescent of the visual field to lie. We were able to show that the monocular crescent of the visual field is represented ventrally in the tract (Torrealba *et al.*, 1982); that is, lesions of peripheral nasal retina produce degeneration in the ventral, but not the dorsal, parts of the cat's optic tract. So we had to ask what this dorsal pure crossed component might be mapping, or how it might relate to the classical map, which still provided our only conceptual framework.

We briefly considered the possibility that the pure crossed component might represent a fibre group that is seen in normal non-primate mammals but that seems to have been entirely lost in primates. This is a crossed component from the temporal retina, which goes mainly to the superior colliculus (e.g. Harting and Guillery, 1976; Wässle and Illing, 1980), but our experimental evidence did not support this logically rather appealing interpretation. The fibres from the contralateral temporal retina mapped through the whole cross-section of the optic tract in a normal cat.

At this point Torrealba, and later Eysel, undertook a detailed study of the fibre arrangement in the tract in terms of retinal maps, and we also started to look more closely at the distribution of fibre diameter classes in the tract (Guillery *et al.*, 1982; Torrealba *et al.*, 1982). The combination of the two approaches led us to a quite different view of fibre arrangements in the optic tract of cats, namely that fibres are arranged in the tract in an order that represents the time of their arrival in the tract during development. The deepest fibres in the tract are the oldest, the most superficial, nearest to the pia, are the youngest.

Stimulated by this interpretation, Walsh undertook studies of early development of the cat's retina and showed that different classes of ganglion cell are produced as distinct waves, each in a rough central peripheral order (Walsh *et al.*, 1983; Walsh and Polley, 1985). Consequently, if the fibres in the tract are arranged according to the time of arrival, there should be several partially overlapping visual field maps, each representing a distinct class of retinal ganglion cell (Fig. 3.2 and see below for details).

This interpretation, that fibre order in the tract represents developmental order was new for mammals but had long been recognized for amphibians (Herrick, 1942; Gaze and Grant, 1978), where the retina develops in a strictly concentric sequence so that the newest fibres represent the most peripheral retina. Hence the chronological order is also a retinotopic order. In a developing frog the retina has to be used for vision as it grows, starting from the early stages of a mobile tadpole. Rings of new retina are added to the outside of a functioning retina, and corresponding layers of new axons are added to the pial surface of the optic tract. In a mammal the retina is non-functional as it develops, since the eyes do not open until after all the ganglion cells have formed. The developmental order is not a strictly central-peripheral order (see below) and the chronological order of ganglion cell development is consequently not a strict retinotopic order.

Before considering the evidence on which we based our view that fibre order in the optic tract represents a chronological order, it is worth pointing out that this interpretation accommodates the two problems mentioned earlier. One was that there is a rough retinal map in the tract but that it is surprisingly inaccurate compared to fish or frog. This can be

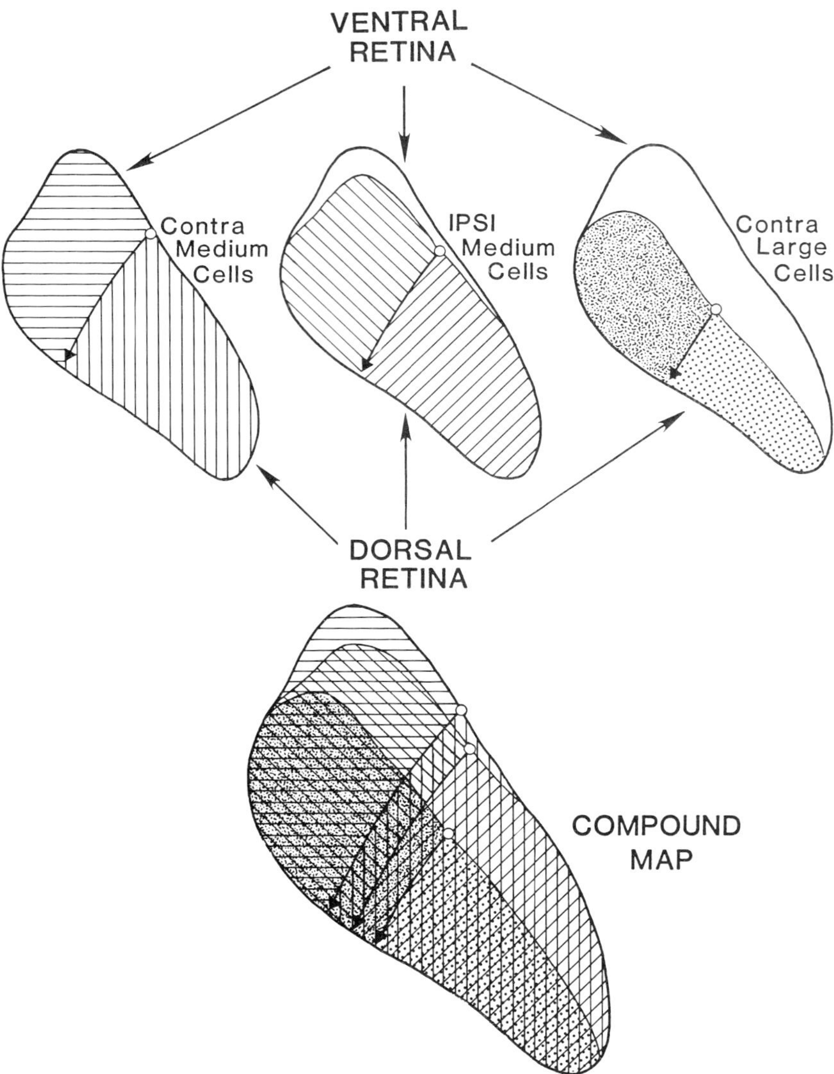

Fig. 3.2 Schematic representation of a section cut transverse to the fibres of the optic tract of a cat. The medium-sized axons of the medium-sized (X) cells from the contralateral eye are distributed throughout the tract as shown in the upper left figure, in which the ventral retinal fibres are represented by horizontal shading, the dorsal retinal fibres by vertical shading, the area centralis is shown as a small circle and the horizontal meridian as an arrow. The distribution of the medium-sized (X-) axons from the ipsilateral eye is shown in the top centre and the distribution of large (Y-) axons from the contralateral eye is shown in the top right figure. The distribution of the uncrossed large axons is not shown, nor is that of the smallest (W-) axons. The formation of several partially overlapping maps in the tract is shown at the bottom of the figure. (Modified from Torrealba *et al.* (1982).)

seen as reflecting the extent to which in mammals retinal development is not under severe functional restraints to follow a strict central peripheral order since the mammal does not need a functioning retina until well after all the retinofugal axons have entered the tract. The second problem concerned the apparently normal position of the abnormally crossed retinofugal axons of Siamese cats, which can also be seen as an expected outcome if the abnormal fibres develop at the normal time. Although they are in the wrong tract they will still pass to their chronologically appropriate position.

Our studies of the cat's optic tract showed that there are three axon diameter classes distinguishable on the basis of their distribution in the optic tract rather than the two described by earlier investigations. The deepest parts of the tract are occupied primarily by medium-sized axons (2–4 μm in diameter). The thickest fibres (4 μm plus in diameter) lie in the superficial half of the tract, and the thinnest fibres (less than 1.5 μm in diameter) are scattered throughout most parts of the tract, but are densest immediately beneath the pia (Guillery *et al.*, 1982). These three axon diameter classes can be related to three functionally and morphologically distinct types of retinal ganglion cell which had been previously described and characterized by others as X-cells, Y-cells and W-cells, having axonal conduction velocities in the medium, fast and slow ranges respectively (see Rodieck, 1979; Sherman and Spear, 1982; Stone, 1983, for details of the X, Y, W classification). Since conduction velocity and axon diameter are directly related, the categorization of cell types in terms of axon diameters in the tract was relatively straightforward, although the details, especially regarding possible sub-classes of W-cell are beyond the scope of this brief review.

When small quantities of horseradish peroxidase were deposited in the optic tract, the retinal ganglion cells having axons in that part of the tract could be labelled by the retrograde transport of the enzyme. It became clear that each class of retinal ganglion cell has an independent, imprecise, yet roughly topographic map in the tract. These several maps are not in register in the tract. Not only is the Y-cell map displaced relative to the X-cell map, but in addition the ipsilateral map is displaced relative to the contralateral map (see Fig. 3.2).

The arrangement of fibres seen in the tract behind the optic chiasm is maintained throughout the further central course of the fibres. The crossed fibres end more deeply in the lateral geniculate nucleus than do the uncrossed fibres, and the axons of W-cells end more superficially in the lateral geniculate nucleus and superior colliculus than do the X- and Y-cells. In so far as the X- and Y-pathways are separated in their central termination, the Y-axons are nearer the pia than the X-axons, in accordance with their position in the tract. It appears as though during development the layering of fibres in the tract might determine the layering of the terminals centrally.

The studies of early retinal development undertaken by Walsh *et al.*, 1983 (and see Walsh and Polley, 1985) used tritiated thymidine to mark the stage at which nerve cells are generated ('neuronal birthdating') and showed that the medium-sized X-cells are born earliest, the large Y-cells are born later and the smallest W-cells are born throughout the relevant developmental stages but are produced primarily as a late wave. That is, position in the tract relates closely to age: as we have seen, X-cell axons lie deepest, Y-cell axons lie more superficially and W-cell axons are scattered throughout the tract but form a particularly dense population superficially. In terms of their birthdates the cell classes form partially overlapping populations and in terms of position in the tract the cell classes form partially overlapping maps (Fig. 3.2). The relationship between the crossed and the uncrossed components can also be related to birthdates. Ganglion cells in the nasal retina are born somewhat earlier than those in the temporal retina and the discrepancy is greatest for the ventral parts of the retina (Walsh and Polley, 1985). The pure crossed crescent that Polley had observed in the optic tract is made up predominantly of fibres from the ventral retina (Torrealba *et al.*, 1982; and see Fig. 3.2). The displacement of the ipsilateral map relative to the contralateral map thus matches evidence obtained from birthdating to a significant extent.

It could be argued that the close relationship between birthdates and fibre order in the optic tract represents a neat correlation but that it tells us little about the actual development of the optic tract. There is no good reason for believing that axons of first-born ganglion cells must also reach the optic tract first. Different ganglion cell classes could have different axonal growth rates.

More direct evidence about the development of the optic tract was obtained by Walsh in ferrets, carnivores that have a retinofugal pathway generally similar to the cat's (Walsh and Guillery, 1985). Retinofugal axons were labelled by intraocular injections of axonally labelled tracers early in intrauterine development, before all the ganglion cells had formed. It was shown that after short survival periods of about 24 hours all the axons in the tract were labelled whereas after longer survival periods only the deepest fibres were labelled, the superficial zone of unlabelled fibres increasing with the length of the survival. The interpretation of this differential labelling was that the unlabelled axons were formed after the label had ceased to be available for making the ganglion cells and that these unlabelled axons nearest the pia were therefore the youngest. Walsh (1986) also showed that the change in fibre order, from one that is roughly retinotopic close to the eye, to the age-related order seen in the tract, occurs distal to chiasm, roughly where in a fetal ferret the optic nerve passes through the optic foramen.

All the evidence presented above relates to the cat and ferret. The question arises whether the change from a retinotopic to a temporal order applies to other mammals, including, of course, ourselves. Hoyt and Luis (1963) described a rearrangement of fibres according to size in the optic chiasm of the monkey, and noted that larger fibres tend to move to inferior, or superficial parts of the optic tract. Since we have seen a change from a retinotopic to a temporal order in frogs and cats it may be reasonable to suppose that this is a general feature of vertebrate development, but it should be added that the temporal order in the frog is also a retinotopic order because the retina grows as an orderly series of concentric rings. We do not know how the primate retina grows in terms of the precise central: peripheral sequence, nor do we know whether different retinal cell types that are found in primates (see, for example, Leventhal, Rodieck and Dreher, 1981; Perry, Oehler and Cowey, 1984) develop at different times, as they do in the cat. We do know that the magnocellular geniculate layers, which lie nearest the pia are innervated by thicker, more rapidly conducting axons (Sherman *et al.*, 1976; Schiller and Malpeli, 1978) and there is evidence that these axons come from a distinctive class of retinal ganglion cell. Reese (Reese and Guillery, 1987) has been studying the optic tract and optic nerve of adult monkeys and from his preliminary evidence it is clear that there is a non-homogeneous distribution of fibre diameter types in the nerve and tract. It also appears that there is a change in fibre order comparable to that seen in cats. In the tract, the coarser fibres destined for the magnocellular layers are segregated, lying nearer the surface.

From a comparative point of view one would like to postulate that in primates as in other vertebrates the order in the tract represents the order of axonal arrival in the tract, and that this is related to the birthdates of the relevant ganglion cells. The evidence supporting such a point of view is not yet complete. Critical experiments of the type done in cats and ferrets will prove difficult and expensive to do in primates. The demonstration of different birthdates for different classes of ganglion cell would be feasible and would provide significant further evidence for the view of the organization of the optic tract summarized here.

From a clinician's point of view a different approach may be more practical and more interesting. If there is a separation of functionally distinct fibre classes in the optic tract but not in the optic nerve, then it should be possible to demonstrate a differential effect of lesions for the tract that cannot be seen in the nerve. On the view I am proposing, one would expect to find that partial lesions of the optic nerve produce a visual field defect that includes all aspects of visual function, whereas a partial lesion of the tract *could* produce a differential involvement of the parvocellular pathway (colour, high acuity) relative to the magnocellular pathway, or could produce non-homonymous, that is, incongruous visual field defects. Clearly, one must exclude lesions that by their nature affect different fibre classes differentially.

There are some indications in the literature that lesions of the optic tract may occasionally produce results that fit such a proposal. Most strikingly, it has been reported that visual field defects produced by partial tract lesions are incongruous (Bender and Bodis-Wollner, 1978; Savino *et al.*, 1978; Newman and Miller, 1983). The incongruity can be quite marked, to a degree that suggests the crossed and uncrossed pathways may be distinctly out of register in the tract. In terms of the developmental interpretation proposed here this would imply that nasal and temporal retina develop at significantly different stages.

Bender and Bodis-Wollner (1978) also note that tract lesions can produce a dissociation of visual functions, an amblyopia for colour or form appearing earlier than do defects of vision for moving targets. This is interpreted as indicating that pathways concerned with distinct functions are segregated in the tract. A further step is to suggest that these pathways develop at different fetal stages and to propose this as the reason for the segregation.

One can, given appropriate methods and an awareness of the problems, expect to take the analysis further. Visual functions such as pupillary or eye movement control may have afferent components consisting largely of one ganglion cell class, developing roughly at one stage and, therefore, probably localized to one part of the tract. These, too, may then be affected by partial tract lesions. Almost any dissociation of function produced by a partial lesion will tend to favour the developmental hypothesis proposed here and to argue against the classical view of two precisely in-register maps of visual hemifields.

Acknowledgements

I thank B. Reese for helpful comments on a first draft; G. Davies and R. Taylor for the typing.

References

Bender, M.B. and Bodis-Wollner, I. (1978) Visual dysfunctions in optic tract lesions. *Ann. Neurol.*, **3**, 187–93.

Bishop, G.H. and Clare, M.H. (1955) Organization and distribution of fibers in the optic tract of the cat. *J. Comp. Neurol.*, **103**, 209–304.

Bishop, P.O., Jeremy, D. and Lance, J.W. (1953) The optic nerve. Properties of a central tract. *J. Physiol. (Lond.)*, **121**, 415–32.

Chang, H.T. (1956) Fibre groups in primary optic pathway of cat. *J. Neurophysiol.*, **19**, 224–31.

Cooper, M.L. and Pettigrew, J.D. (1978) The retinothalamic pathways in Siamese cats. *J. Comp. Neurol.*, **187**, 313–48.

Creel, D.J. (1971) Visual anomaly associated with albinism in the cat. *Nature (Lond.)*, **231**, 465–6.

Creel, D.J., Hendrickson, A.E. and Leventhal, A.G. (1982) Retinal projections in tyrosinase-negative albino cats. *J. Neurosci.*, **2**, 907–17.

Crevel, H. van and Verhaart, W.J.C. (1963) The rate of secondary degeneration in the central nervous system II. The optic nerve of the cat. *J. Anat. (Lond.)*, **97**, 451–64.

Donovan, A. (1967) The nerve fibre composition of the cat optic nerve. *J. Anat.*, **101**, 1–11.

Gaze, R.M. and Grant, P. (1978) The diencephalic course of regenerating retinotectal fibres in *Xenopus* tadpoles. *J. Embryol. Exp. Morphol.*, **44**, 201–16.

Guillery, R.W. (1974) Visual pathways in albinos. *Sci. Am.*, **230**, 44–54.

Guillery, R.W. and Kaas, J.H. (1971) A study of normal and congenitally abnormal retino-geniculate projections in cats. *J. Comp. Neurol.*, **143**, 73–100.

Guillery, R.W., Hickey, T.L., Kaas, J.H., Felleman, D.J., DeBruyns, E.J. and Sparks, D.L. (1984) Abnormal central visual pathways in the brain of an albino green monkey (*Cercopithecus aethiops*). *J. Comp. Neurol.*, **226**, 165–83.

Guillery, R.W., Polley, E.H. and Torrealba, F. (1982) The arrangement of axons according to fiber diameter in the optic tract of the cat. *J. Neurosci.*, **2**, 714–21.

Harting, J.K. and Guillery, R.W. (1976) Organization of retinocollicular pathways in the cat. *J. Comp. Neurol.*, **166**, 133–44.

Herrick, C.J. (1942) Optic and postoptic systems in the brain of *Amblystoma tigrinum*. *J. Comp. Neurol.*, **77**, 191–353.

Horton, J.C., Greenwood, M.M. and Hubel, D.H. (1979) Non-retinotopic arrangement of fibers in cat optic nerve. *Nature*, **282**, 720–2.

Hoyt, W.F. and Luis, O. (1963) The primate chiasm. *Arch. Ophthalmol.*, **70**, 113–29.

Kaas, J.H. and Guillery, R.W. (1973) The transfer of abnormal visual field representations from the dorsal lateral geniculate nucleus to the visual cortex in Siamese cats. *Brain Res.*, **59**, 61–95.

Leventhal, A., Rodieck, R.W. and Dreher, B. (1981) Retinal ganglion cell classes in the old world monkey: morphology and central projections. *Science*, **213**, 1139–42.

Lund, R.D. (1965) Uncrossed visual pathways in hooded and albino rats. *Science*, **149**, 1506–7.

Newman, S.A. and Miller, N.R. (1983) Optic tract syndrome. Neuro-ophthalmologic considerations. *Arch. Ophthalmol.*, **101**, 1241–50.

Perry, V.H., Oehler, R. and Cowey, A. (1984) Retinal ganglion cells that project to the dorsal lateral geniculate nucleus in the macaque monkey. *Neuroscience*, **12**, 1101–23.

Polyak, S. (1957) *The Vertebrate Visual System*. University of Chicago Press, Chicago.

Reese, B.E. and Guillery, R.W. (1987) Distribution of axons according to diameter in the monkey's optic tract. *J. Comp. Neurol.*, **260**, 453–60.

Rodieck, R.W. (1979) Visual pathways. *Ann. Rev. Neurosci.*, **2**, 193–225.

Savino, P.J., Paris, M., Schatz, N.J., Orr, L.S. and Corbett, J.J. (1978) Optic tract syndrome. A review of 21 patients. *Arch. Ophthalmol.*, **96**, 656–63.

Schiller, P.H. and Malpeli, J.G. (1978) Functional specificity of lateral geniculate nucleus laminae of the rhesus monkey. *J. Neurophysiol.*, **41**, 788–97.

Shatz, C.J. (1974) A comparison of visual pathways in Boston and Midwestern Siamese cats. *J. Comp. Neurol.*, **171**, 205–28.

Sherman, S.M. and Spear, P.D. (1982) Organization of the visual pathways in normal and visually deprived cats. *Physiol. Rev.*, **62**, 738–855.

Sherman, S.M., Wilson, J.R., Kaas, J.H. and Webb, S.V. (1976) X- and Y-cells in the dorsal lateral geniculate nucleus of the owl monkey (*Aotus trivisgatus*). *Science*, **192**, 475–7.

Stone, J. (1983) *Parallel Processing in the Visual System*. Plenum, New York.

Stone, J., Campion, J.E. and Leicester, J. (1978) The naso-temporal division of the retina in the Siamese cat. *J. Comp. Neurol.*, **180**, 783–98.

Torrealba, F., Guillery, R.W., Eysel, U., Polley, E.H. and Mason, C.A. (1982) Studies of retinal representations within the cat's optic tract. *J. Comp. Neurol.*, **211**, 377–96.

Walsh, C. (1986) Age-related fiber order in the ferret's optic nerve and optic chiasm. *J. Neurosci.*, **6**, 1635–42.

Walsh, C. and Guillery, R.W. (1985) Age-related fiber order in the optic tract of the ferret. *J. Neurosci.*, **5**, 3061–70.

Walsh, C. and Polley, E.H. (1985) The topography of ganglion cell production in the cat's retina. *J. Neurosci.*, **5**, 741–50.

Walsh, C., Polley, E.H., Hickey, T.L. and Guillery, R.W. (1983) Generation of cat retinal ganglion cells in relation to central pathways. *Nature*, **302**, 611–14.

Wässle, H. and Illing, R.-B. (1980) The retinal projection to the superior colliculus in the cat: a quantitative study with HRP. *J. Comp. Neurol.*, **190**, 333–46.

CHAPTER 4

Physiology and pathology of the optic chiasm

THOMAS M. BOSLEY

4.1 Introduction

Lesions of the anterior afferent visual system are diagnosed clinically by the presence of a relative afferent pupillary defect and specific types of visual field loss. Lesions of the optic chiasm, for example, classically cause temporal hemianopias while lesions of the optic tract cause non-congruous homonymous visual field loss. The clinical characteristics of chiasmal syndromes are already well described, and the discussion in this chapter will centre on new physiological information, new diagnostic tools and new clinical or experimental data confirming or expanding accepted observations.

The distinction between anatomy and physiology is a constant problem in a discussion of chiasmal syndromes. The anatomy of chiasmal dysfunction is usually more obvious than the physiology because chiasmal syndromes are caused by mass lesions at the base of the brain in the majority of cases. Neuro-ophthalmology is a clinical field, and discussions such as this cannot avoid an examination of new imaging tools that have radically changed our approach to the anatomic evaluation of this area of the brain. Nevertheless, neurophysiological changes must be more important than axonal destruction in most chiasmal syndromes because partial or full recovery of vision is quite common after surgical decompression or other therapy.

There are other reasons to consider physiological aspects of chiasmal syndromes. Regulation of chiasmal blood flow and the diseases that affect it are poorly understood. Why, for example, are acromegalics more at risk for chiasmal radiation vasculitis than are individuals with other types of peri-chiasmal compressive lesions? Even the types of visual field loss occurring in clinical chiasmal syndromes are more variable than previously realized. Ultimately, the perception of the visual world is a physiological phenomenon of the cerebral cortex, and loss of visual acuity or visual field must have physiological implications for those portions of the cortex predominantly involved in vision. Just what is deafferented visual cortex doing?

4.2 The normal optic chiasm

4.2.1 GROSS ANATOMY, HISTOLOGY AND PHYSIOLOGY

Nerve fibres making up the anterior afferent visual system arise from ganglion cells and traverse the nerve fibre layer lining the inner surface of the retina. These fibres divide into bundles prior to passing through the lamina cribrosa, and the entire optic nerve has a septate appearance because these small nerve fibre bundles remain intact as far back as the optic chiasm (Hoyt, 1962). Fibres from nasal and temporal retina begin to separate at the anterior angle of the chiasm and then divide into a crossed (nasal) segment that slightly outnumbers the uncrossed (temporal) segment (Kupfer, Chumbley and Downer, 1967). Fibres from the papillomacular bundle divide in a fashion similar to more peripheral fibres. Just as fibres from the papillomacular bundle make up a large proportion of the optic nerve, crossing fibres representing central vision make up a large proportion of the chiasm with perhaps a slightly greater representation posteriorly than anteriorly. Wilbrand (1926) claimed, and Hoyt and Luis (1962) confirmed, that ventral crossing fibres loop anteriorly into the terminal portion of the contralateral optic nerve (Wilbrand's knee) before turning posteriorly and laterally into the optic tract. These fibres are involved in lesions affecting the anterior angle of the chiasm, resulting in a junctional pattern of visual field loss with ipsilateral central and contralateral superotemporal scotomas.

Each optic tract contains axons from the ipsilateral temporal retina and the contralateral nasal retina, but these fibres are not completely mixed to form a single retinotopic representation of the contralateral visual field. The organization of the cat optic tract is discussed in Chapter 3.

The human optic chiasm is a flattened oblong structure formed by the union of the intracranial optic nerves at the base of the brain. It measures approximately 12 mm in transverse diameter, 8 mm in anteroposterior diameter and 4 mm in thickness. The intracranial optic nerves rise upwards from the optic canal in a plane inclined approximately 45° from the horizontal, and the optic chiasm is also oriented in this upward-sloping plane. Each optic tract emerges from the posterolateral angle of the chiasm and travels in front of the interpeduncular cistern and between the tuber cinereum and the anterior perforated substance before sweeping around the ipsilateral cerebral peduncle towards the lateral geniculate nuclei (LGN).

The optic chiasm forms part of the anterior–inferior wall of the third ventricle, and thus it is bounded posteriorly and superiorly by ventricular cerebrospinal fluid (CSF). The chiasmatic cistern lies anterior, inferior and posterior to the optic chiasm. It communicates laterally with each sylvian cistern and posterolaterally with the supratentorial portion of each ambient cistern. Anteriorly the chiasmatic cistern joins with the subarachnoid space extending between the two frontal lobes into the interhemispheric fissure, and posteriorly it merges with the interpeduncular cistern. The chiasm, therefore, is virtually surrounded by CSF.

The optic chiasm is located in the middle of the arterial circle of Willis, and its blood supply is quite diffuse. The lateral portion of the chiasm receives blood from a superior group of vessels arising from the anterior cerebral and anterior communicating arteries. The remainder of the chiasm is supplied by an inferior group of small vessels arising from the basilar, posterior communicating, posterior cerebral and internal carotid arteries (Bergland and Ray, 1969).

The primary role of neurones in the anterior afferent visual system is to transmit visual information to the LGN and beyond. The action potential frequencies and firing patterns of neurones in the optic nerves, optic chiasm and optic tracts have been studied carefully in experimental animals. In the cat, excitatory postsynaptic potentials of LGN neurones have the same statistical frequency characteristics as the discharge of optic nerve fibres, and these excitatory postsynaptic potentials are driven by retinal ganglion cells of the same functional type (Dubin and Cleland, 1977). The LGN receives strong afferent input from the striate cortex as well as the optic tracts, and firing patterns of LGN neurones are determined by neural activity both within the optic tract in the cat (Fourment *et al.*, 1984) and the visual cortex in the rat (Molotchnikoff, Tremblay and Lepore, 1984).

Visual information carried to the LGN by the anterior afferent visual system is obviously an important determinant of neural activity in the striate cortex. Hubel and Wiesel (1967) proved that the cat corpus callosum carries visual information from the contralateral visual cortex. Nevertheless, it has been shown recently that cat striate cortex deafferented by a complete lesion of the ipsilateral optic tract has almost no response to visual stimulation in either visual hemifield (Podell, Yinon and Hammer, 1984). It seems likely that the ipsilateral afferent visual system plays a similar dominant role in the activity of the human striate cortex.

4.2.2 NEURO-IMAGING OF THE NORMAL OPTIC CHIASM

The optic chiasm is a small structure, but it can be imaged reliably by high-resolution computed tomography (CT) because of the difference in X-ray attenuation between neural tissue and CSF (Hoyt, 1964; Amundsen and Newton, 1978). The chiasmal cistern is known radiologically as the suprasellar cistern (Dutton *et al.*, 1982; Kline, Vitek and Acker, 1983), which on high-resolution CT usually resembles a 5-pointed star because of extensions into (in clockwise order beginning anteriorly) the interhemispheric fissure, left sylvian cistern, left and right ambient cisterns, and right sylvian cistern (Fig. 4.1). If the interpeduncular cistern is visualized, a 6-pointed star is formed. Excellent coronal images can also be obtained, and high-resolution scanners may make three or four contiguous images through the suprasellar cistern in both transverse and coronal planes.

Magnetic resonance (MR) imaging is now available in many medical centres and offers an alternative technique for imaging the anterior afferent visual system. MR also takes advantage of different intensity signals generated by normal brain and cerebrospinal fluid. Contrast between grey matter, white matter and CSF is greater with MR than CT, but the spatial resolution of MR images generated in transverse and coronal planes is somewhat poorer than that of a high-resolution CT scan. Certain transverse MR images are inferior to transverse images of high-resolution CT in the region of the chiasm because they are degraded by computer-generated artefacts probably caused by movement in the great vessels of the circle of Willis and CSF.

Movement artefacts are not usually a problem in the coronal plane where MR is frequently superior to CT in demonstrating the suprasellar cistern bounded inferiorly by the sella and superiorly by a U-shaped structure consisting of the optic chiasm and hypothalamus (Fig. 4.2a). MR does not image bone or dental fillings so there are fewer computer-generated artefacts degrading these images than similar CT images. MR sagittal images have much higher resolution and contrast than reformated images obtained by CT (Fig. 4.2b). Both transverse and coronal planes can be used to image the entire course of the optic nerves, including the intracanalicular portions of the optic nerves which are seen poorly by CT. MR is clearly useful in imaging the optic chiasm (Daniels *et*

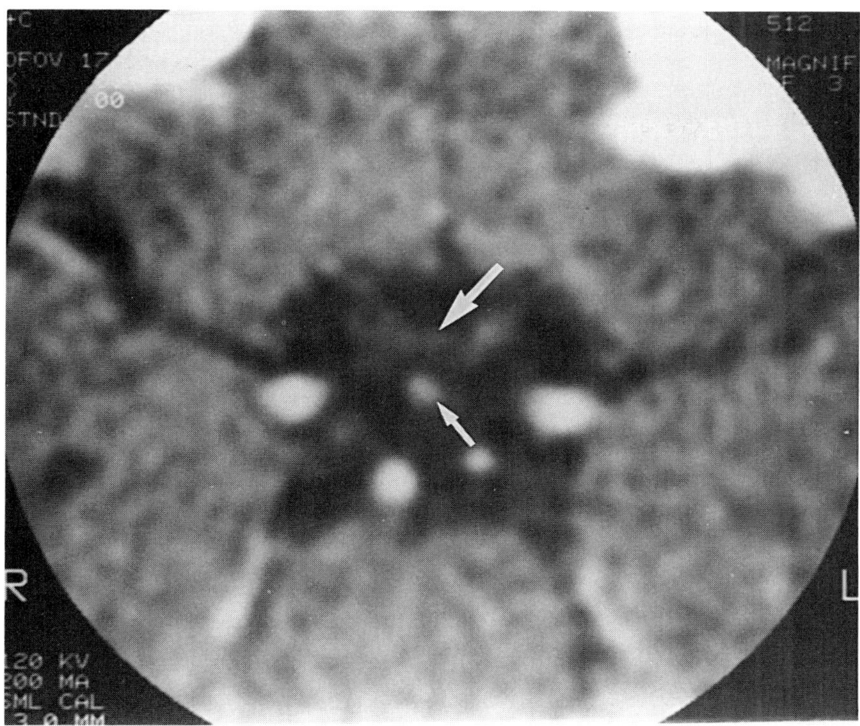

Fig. 4.1 High-resolution transverse CT with contrast of the suprasellar cistern as described. Optic chiasm is small transverse structure (long arrow) just anterior to enhancing pituitary infundibulum (short arrow). Larger enhancing structures are paired internal carotid arteries anteriorly and basilar artery posteriorly.

al., 1984; Hupp and Savino, 1986), but the quality of MR images varies widely from machine to machine, and the real clinical strengths of this technique in the peri-chiasmal region have yet to be completely delineated.

4.3 Pathology of the optic chiasm

4.3.1 CLINICAL SYNDROMES

Three-quarters of all compressive chiasmal syndromes cause a temporal hemianopic visual field defect in at least one eye (Elkington, 1968; Wilson and Falconer, 1968; Finn and Mount, 1974; Hollenhorst and Younge, 1976; Trobe, Tao and Schuster, 1984), but arcuate scotomas are also not infrequent in these patients (Trobe, Tao and Schuster, 1984). On very rare

(a)

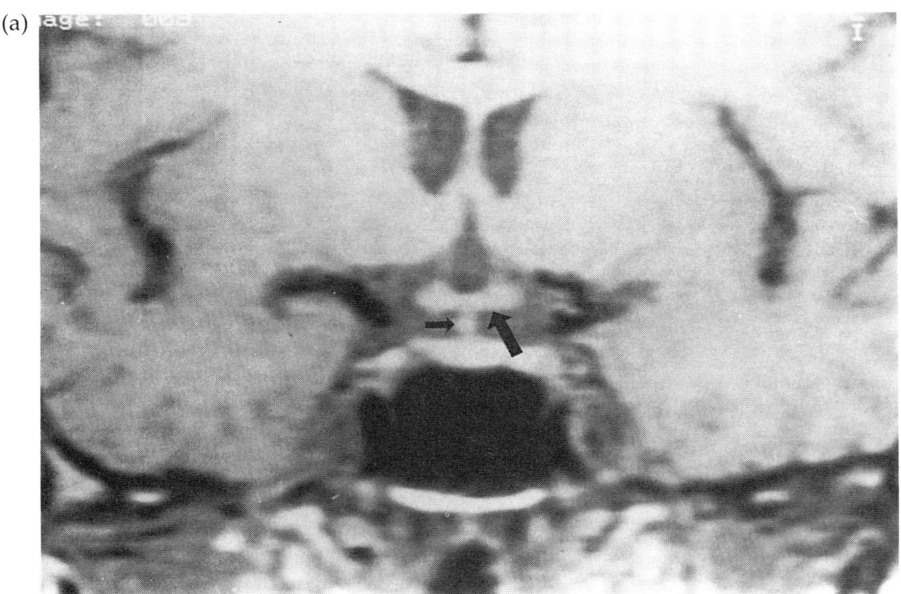

(b)

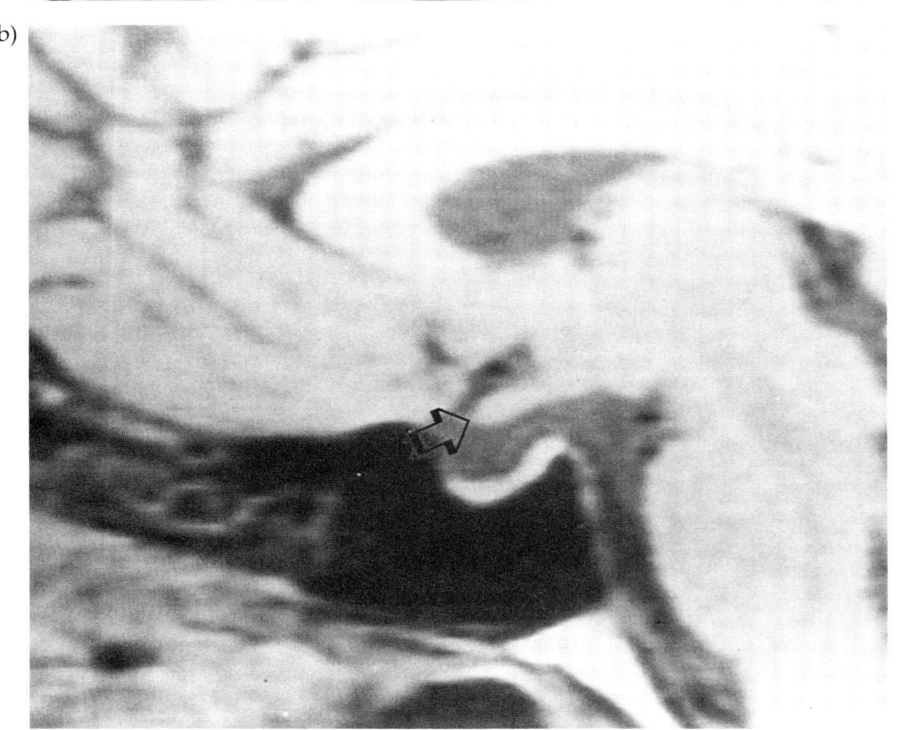

occasions arcuate scotomas may be the only evidence of intracranial optic nerve or chiasmal compression in patients who have not lost visual acuity and who have not developed temporal hemianopic visual field defects (Kline, 1981; Hupp *et al.*, 1986). This phenomenon probably occurs because of the continued division of the optic nerve throughout its course into nerve fibre bundles (Hoyt, 1962).

Asymmetric visual loss due to chiasmal compression is very common, and Trobe, Tao and Schuster (1984) found that the junctional pattern of visual field defects with ipsilateral central scotoma and contralateral temporal hemianopia was nearly as common (39%) as the classic bitemporal pattern (46%). All their patients had either a relative afferent pupillary defect or a hemianopia in at least one eye. There are, of course, other neurological symptoms that may accompany chiasmal syndromes (Table 4.1), and a careful history and neurological examination may well help to narrow the differential diagnosis prior to neuro-imaging.

Table 4.1 Neurological problems accompanying chiasmal syndromes

Hormonal abnormalities
Panhypopituitarism
Diabetes insipidus
Cranial nerve deficits
Anosmia (cranial nerve 1)
Diplopia (cranial nerves 3, 4, 6)
Facial numbness (cranial nerve 5)
Horner's Syndrome (oculo-sympathetics)
Local mass effect
Hydrocephalus (obstruction of Foramen of Monroe)
Cerebrospinal fluid rhinorrhoea (erosion through cranial floor)
Temporal lobe epilepsy (compression of temporal lobe)

4.3.2 DIFFERENTIAL DIAGNOSIS

The differential diagnosis of clinical chiasmal lesions can be divided into compressive lesions, non-compressive lesions and those abnormalities that mimic the chiasmal syndrome (Table 4.2). Mass lesions are by far the most common cause of chiasmal syndromes because the chiasm may be compressed by benign tumours of the surrounding tissues including the

Fig. 4.2 (a) Coronal MR through the sella and suprasellar cistern as described. Optic chiasm is well seen as transverse structure (long arrow) located immediately above pituitary gland (short arrow) and below the third ventricle (in the midline). Arteries of the circle of Willis are well seen because moving blood does not generate MR signals. (b) Sagittal MR through the midline showing optic chiasm (arrow) located above sella filled with CSF and below chiasmatic cistern.

Table 4.2 Differential diagnosis of chiasmal syndromes

- Compressive
  - Benign tumours
    - Pituitary adenoma
    - Meningioma
    - Craniopharyngioma
    - Optic nerve or chiasmal glioma
    - Epidermoid
    - Dermoid
  - Malignant tumours
    - Metastases to pituitary gland
    - Metastases to brain
    - Sinus tumours
  - Other
    - Chiasmal vascular malformation
    - Giant suprasellar aneurysm
    - Arachnoid cyst
    - Enlarged third ventricle
    - Colloid cyst of third ventricle
    - Mucopyocele
- Inflammatory
  - Idiopathic (possibly sarcoid) chiasmal inflammation
  - Demyelination
  - Radiation necrosis
  - Giant cell arteritis
  - Syphilis
  - Tuberculosis
  - Chronic meningitis
- Toxic
  - Ethclorvynol (Placidyl)
  - Pheniprazine (Catron)
- Traumatic chiasmal syndrome
- Lesions mimicking chiasmal syndromes
  - Tilted optic discs
  - Enlarged blind spots
  - Bilateral cecocentral scotomas
  - Glaucoma (rarely)
  - Chloroquine retinopathy
  - Sector retinitis pigmentosa

pituitary gland, the pituitary stalk and the meninges. Other masses, such as aneurysms of the major blood vessels, arachnoid cysts and tumours of the third ventricle, bone and chiasm itself, are less common. Metastases to the pituitary gland are not infrequent, but they rarely cause pituitary dysfunction or chiasmal compression (Max, Dick and Rottenberg, 1981; Duvall and Cullen, 1982). Chiasmal compression as the initial sign of malignant nasopharyngeal and sinus tumours or malignant primary tumours of the meninges is exceptional because these patients are much more likely to experience disturbances of extraocular motility prior to visual loss.

The optic chiasm may become involved in inflammatory processes, but clinically significant demyelinating disease occurs much less frequently in the optic chiasm than it does in the optic nerves (Spector, Glazer and Schatz, 1980). Ischaemic lesions of the optic chiasm and optic tracts are infrequent, and disorders that cause ischaemic damage in this region tend to be diffuse vasculitic processes (giant cell arteritis, radiation vasculitis) or diseases affecting multiple large vessels at the base of the brain (Moyamoya disease).

4.3.3 NEURO-IMAGING OF PERI-CHIASMAL LESIONS

Both CT and MR have proven extraordinarily useful in imaging mass lesions displacing or compressing the optic chiasm, not only because of their spatial resolution, but also because each adds a physiological component to anatomic imaging. Contrast enhancement alters the CT appearance of mass lesions with increased vascularity or transudation of certain blood components. MR, on the other hand, yields images determined by the micro-milieu of hydrogen atoms, which in turn may be altered by physiological characteristics of a mass and its blood supply.

Computed tomography appearance of masses in the suprasellar region has been well described (Greitz, 1975; Reich *et al.*, 1975; Naidich *et al.*, 1976; Gyldensted and Karle, 1977; Daniels *et al.*, 1980; Dutton *et al.*, 1982) and, if scans are performed on a high resolution machine in both transverse and coronal planes with an inter-image distance of no more than 1.5 mm, it is unlikely that a mass lesion large enough to compress the optic chiasm from above or below will be overlooked.

> Patient RO. This 33-year-old man complained of 7 months of declining vision OS. Visual acuity was 20/15 OU, but on the left there was a mild dyschromatopsia, afferent pupillary defect, and superior and inferior arcuate scotomas by Goldmann kinetic perimetry (Fig. 4.3a) CT showed a large, low-density mass lesion involving predominantly the left middle cranial fossa and extending into the suprasellar cistern and across the midline to the right anterior clinoid process (Fig. 4.3b). Vision returned to normal after surgical decompression of the epidermoid tumour.

Where some uncertainty remains, CT metrizamide cisternography may be able to distinguish normal suprasellar cistern from loculated CSF within an arachnoid cyst and other lesions isodense with CSF (Drayer *et al.*, 1979). The disadvantages of the technique are that a spinal tap is required and that intrathecal metrizamide may rarely cause confusion

(a)

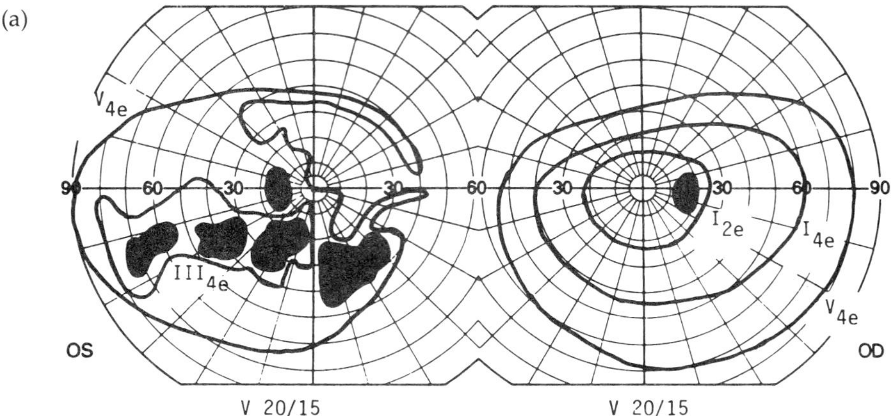

(b)

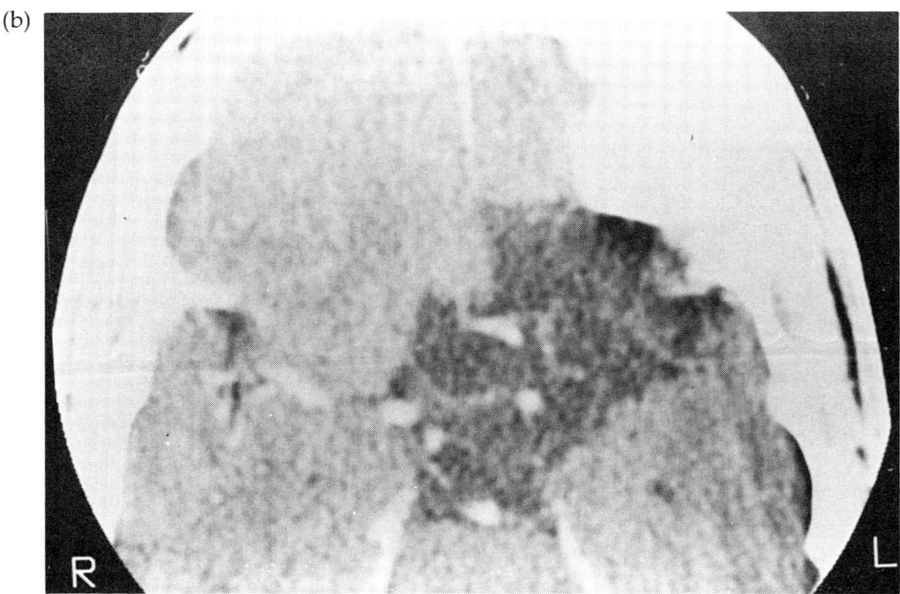

Fig. 4.3 (a) Goldmann kinetic perimetry of patient RO showing superior and inferior arcuate scotomas OS without loss of visual acuity. (b) Coronal CT with contrast through suprasellar cistern of same patient with epidermoid tumour seen as hypodense mass extending from left middle cranial fossa to left frontal fossa and suprasellar cistern. Optic chiasm is not seen. (Taken from Hupp and Savino, 1986.)

and seizures. CT may also be useful in the evaluation of certain non-compressive chiasmal syndromes, including demyelinating disease (Edwards, Gilmor and Franco, 1983), ischaemic disease of the chiasm (Lee, 1983; Ahmadi *et al.*, 1984) and chiasmal herniation into an empty sella (Bursztyn, Lavyne and Aisen, 1983).

Magnetic resonance imaging is a relatively new technique, but it is already apparent that MR will be superior to CT in diagnosing certain causes of chiasmal syndromes. Cystic collections of fluid may replace the suprasellar cistern and compress the chiasm without appearing particularly abnormal on CT. MR has the advantage of being able to detect subtle changes in protein concentration and other constituents of fluid and is usually able to distinguish normal CSF from abnormal fluid-filled structures. MR does not image bone, and certain abnormal structures within the perinasal sinuses contiguous with the planum sphenoidale may be better seen with MR. Flowing blood does not cause an MR signal, and the 'negative' image of the internal carotid arteries and its branches within and above the cavernous sinus is often superior to that of CT with contrast enhancement. MR can usually distinguish a suprasellar aneurysm from meningioma or pituitary adenoma without requiring an arteriogram.

Benign tumours at the base of the brain ordinarily have MR signal intensities similar to that of grey matter, making the full extent of a tumour difficult to determine. Sagittal images are sometimes useful in delineating the anatomic extent of such a mass. Fortunately, the relationship of tumour to chiasm is usually obvious because the signal intensity of white matter in the optic chiasm is different from that of most tumours. MR using a 1.5 Tesla superconducting magnet is very sensitive to small infarcts or haemorrhages within a mass such as a pituitary adenoma (Hackney *et al.*, 1986). These degenerative changes, when present, can help both in predicting the histology of a mass lesion and in understanding a sudden shift in the pace of clinical symptoms.

Patient MC. This 35-year-old woman had Nelson's syndrome after bilateral adrenalectomy 12 years previously for Cushing's syndrome. She had no visual symptoms, and neuro-ophthalmological examination was normal. CT showed a moderately large pituitary adenoma extending laterally into the left cavernous sinus and superiorly to the inferior border of the chiasm. One month after examination she developed a severe generalized headache with nausea and vomiting that resolved over 2 days with no focal neurological symptoms. Neuro-ophthalmological examination was again normal except for a subtle superior bitemporal hemianopia on Goldmann perimetry. Repeat CT (Fig. 4.4a) was unchanged, but MR (Fig. 4b and c) showed chiasm draped over the superior edge of the tumour and new

(a)

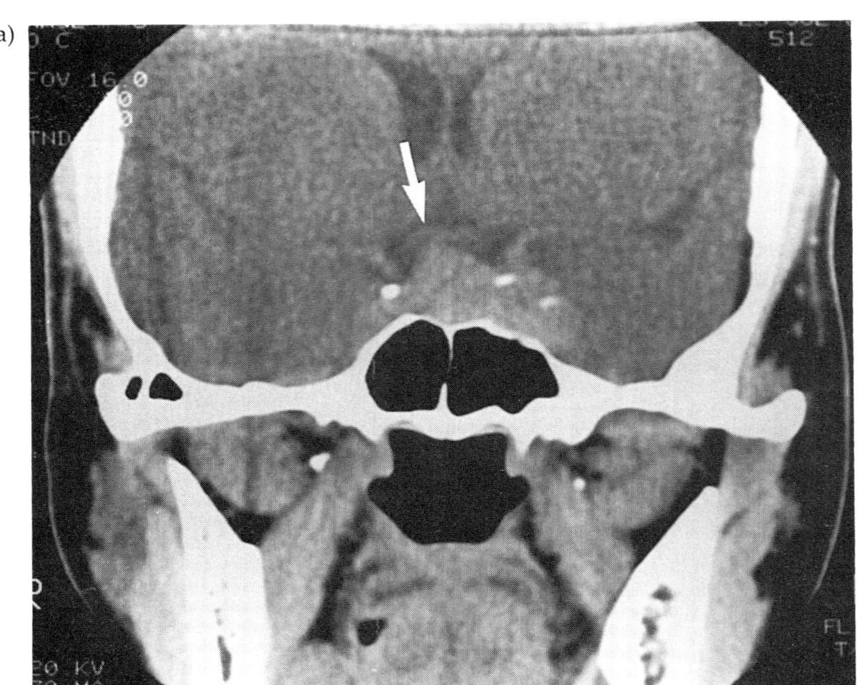

(b)

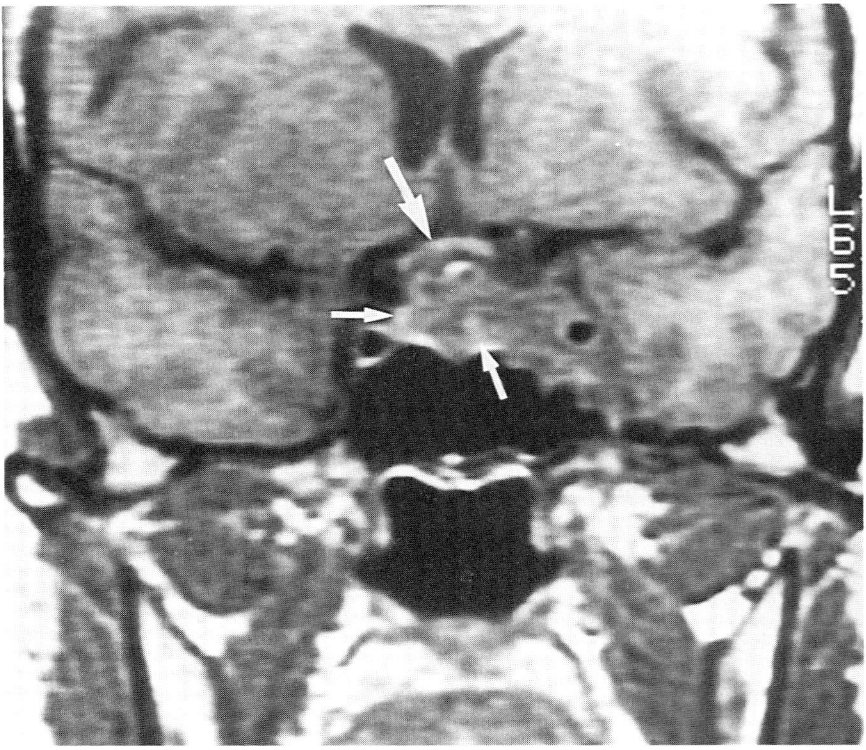

(c)

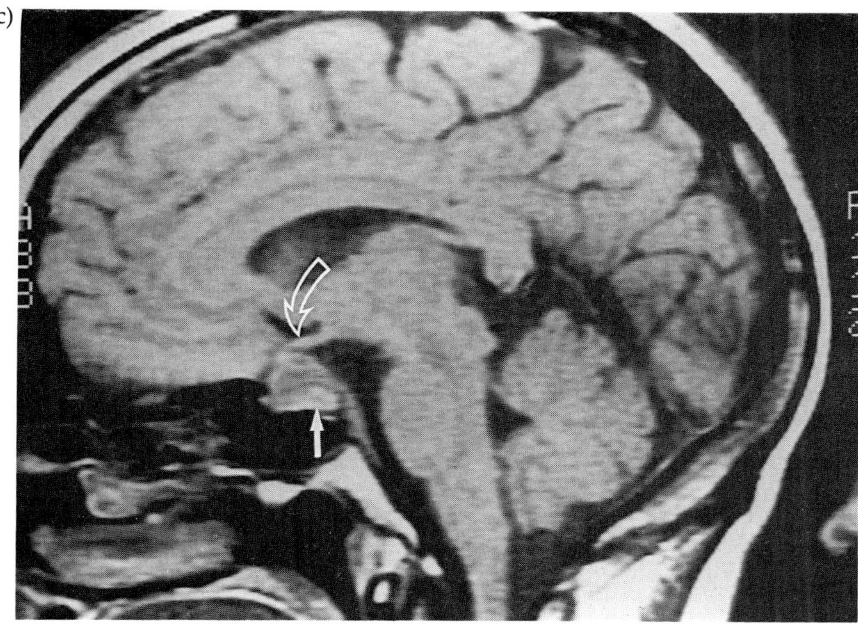

Fig. 4.4 (a) Coronal CT with contrast of patient MC through sella and suprasellar cistern demonstrating contrast enhancing pituitary adenoma extending up to inferior border of chiasm (arrow) and into left cavernous sinus. (b) Coronal MR of same patient through almost identical plane as (a) showing same tumour configuration. Optic chiasm (long arrow) is draped over superior aspect of tumour. Tumour is not homogeneous, but contains several small areas of high T2-intensity compatible with haemorrhages (short arrows). (c) Sagittal MR of same patient through midline plane similar to that of (b) showing pituitary adenoma elevating chiasm (long arrow). Note high-intensity signal at base of tumour indicating haemorrhage (short arrow).

haemorrhage within the tumour mass. The diagnosis of pituitary apoplexy was made, and the patient underwent uneventful trans-sphenoidal surgery with post-operative radiation therapy.

In clinical neuro-ophthalmology the distinction between a compressive and a non-compressive chiasmal syndrome can be made only by clinical imaging tools. In certain cases MR may be able to detect changes in signal intensity within the optic chiasm due to pathological processes that are considered non-compressive. MR is very sensitive to demyelination of cerebral white matter tracts, and chiasmal demyelination has also been reported occasionally (Grossman *et al.*, 1986). Small cerebral infarctions are also well seen with MR.

Some of the strengths of CT are the same as its weaknesses in relation to MR. CT images the base of the skull very well, and bony changes such as hyperostosis, remodelling and erosion may be important clues about a pathological process not available with MR. Likewise, calcium imaged by CT within a meningioma, aneurysm or craniopharyngioma may provide key information about the histology of a mass. CT contrast probes the vascular supply and vascular competence of a mass lesion, while similar information is not widely available with MR (Daniels *et al.*, 1984; Grossman *et al.*, 1986).

It is tempting to conclude that a normal CT scan is adequate to eliminate a compressive cause of a chiasmal syndrome (Foulds, Bronte-Stewart and McClure, 1983). The wary clinician should be cautious about making this assumption unless he is certain that the CT scan has been done on a high-resolution machine in the fashion described above. The CT scan should be reviewed personally to be sure that the suprasellar cistern was adequately imaged and that the scan was read correctly by the radiologist. An entirely normal high-quality CT means that the pursuit of a clinically obvious chiasmal syndrome must be taken at least one step further with a metrizamide CT scan or high-resolution MR. Neuro-imaging is not the only diagnostic tool available, and evaluation of the CSF and blood may well reveal evidence of an otherwise unsuspected inflammatory or infectious disease.

Non-compressive causes of clinical chiasmal syndromes are uncommon (Schatz and Schlezinger, 1976), but many are treatable. Toxic chiasmal syndromes usually respond to the removal of the toxin (Reynolds, Smith and McCrary, 1982). Syphilis, tuberculosis and other chronic meningitides may well improve with appropriate therapy. Giant cell arteritis (Crampton, 1959; Lee and Schatz, 1975) and other systemic vasculitides are treatable disorders that may on rare occasions cause chiasmal lesions. Finally, there are inflammatory chiasmal syndromes possibly related to sarcoid that do not follow the typical time course or recovery pattern of demyelinating disease and that frequently are steroid responsive (Ingestad and Stigmar, 1971; Kirkham, 1973).

Patient MH. This 33-year-old man complained of decreased vision in both eyes that had been progressive over the previous six months. Visual acuity was 20/40 OD and 20/25 OS with bilateral mild dyschromatopsias, right afferent pupillary defect and bitemporal visual field loss worse on the right. His evaluation included a normal CT scan, metrizamide CT, vasculitis studies, chest X-ray and cerebrospinal fluid evaluation, and the diagnosis of inflammatory chiasmal syndrome was made. He was treated with prednisone 80 mg daily on a tapering schedule over a period of months, and his vision returned to normal. Bitemporal visual loss recurred four months after discontinuing prednisone, and a repeat evaluation was again normal. Symptoms and signs again responded to steroid therapy.

4.3.4 RECOVERY OF VISION AFTER TREATMENT

Visual loss due to compressive chiasmal syndromes tends to improve after surgical decompression. Most patients with pituitary macroadenomas have improved vision after surgery while post-operative visual decline occurs in less than 10% (Wilson and Falconer, 1968; Tindall, McLanahan and Christy, 1977; Wilson and Dempsey, 1977). In operated suprasellar meningiomas, Finn and Mount (1974) and Gregorius, Hepler and Stern (1975) reported that more than 50% of patients had improved visual acuity and less than 15% showed worsening. Trobe, Tao and Schuster (1984) described a series of peri-chiasmal tumours including pituitary tumours, meningiomas, supraclinoid aneurysms and craniopharyngiomas, and documented an overall probability of improvement in visual function after operation of 43%. If the pre-operative visual acuity was 20/40 or better, the probability of full recovery of acuity was 89%, but the probability of full recovery fell to 17% if the pre-operative acuity was worse than 20/40. Visual recovery after surgery usually occurs almost immediately, but it may be delayed for as long as 10 weeks (Goldman *et al.*, 1985).

Patient RW. This 55-year-old man complained of gradually declining visual acuity in his left eye over the previous six months without other neurological or ophthalmological symptoms. Visual acuity was 20/25 OD and counting fingers at 3 feet OS with a striking left afferent pupillary defect, a small right superotemporal visual field defect, and dense cecocentral and temporal scotomas on the left. CT revealed a large, lobulated suprasellar mass (Fig. 4.5a and b) that was proven by arteriography to be a giant suprasellar aneurysm. After surgery, vision returned to 20/20 OU with full visual fields.

The physiological reasons for this rewarding recovery of visual acuity after treatment of compressive chiasmal lesions are unclear, but presumably compression stops electrical conduction in certain chiasmal neurones that are then able to resume functioning after surgery. Visual recovery is so rapid that it is unlikely that a regenerative process is involved.

Surgery is not necessary for the relief of chiasmal compression in at least one situation. Bromocriptine can decrease the size of prolactinomas (McGregor *et al.*, 1979; Wass *et al.*, 1982), and Moster *et al.* (1986) recently

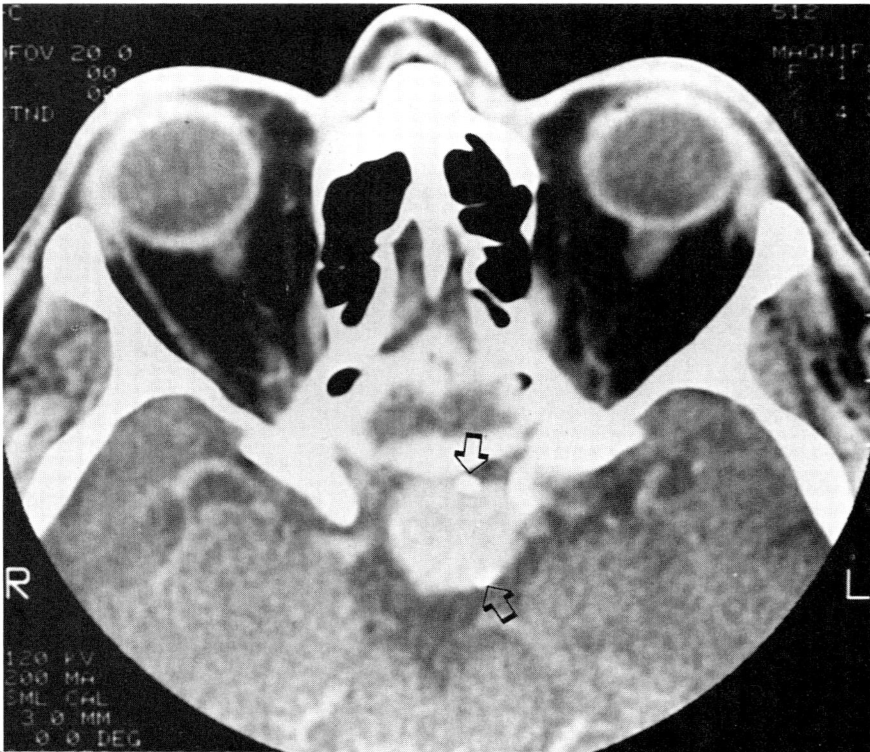

Fig. 4.5 (a) Transverse CT with contrast of patient RW reveals large, rounded, contrast enhancing mass within suprasellar cistern. Chiasm is not visible. Calcified areas at edge (arrows) of mass are typical within wall of an aneurysm.

reported that 9 of 10 patients with prolactin-producing macroadenomas treated with bromocriptine alone experienced improvement of visual field or visual acuity, sometimes within hours of beginning the medication. Two of these patients eventually underwent trans-sphenoidal surgery because of continued concern about their visual function, and neither improved post-operatively. These results imply that bromocriptine may well be the best means of correcting visual and hormonal function in patients with prolactin-producing tumours both acutely and chronically. The serum prolactin level is an important part of the pre-operative evaluation of a patient with a possible pituitary macroadenoma because most patients with non-prolactin-secreting tumours will require both trans-sphenoidal surgery and irradiation.

Surgery and irradiation may cause a delayed complication in certain

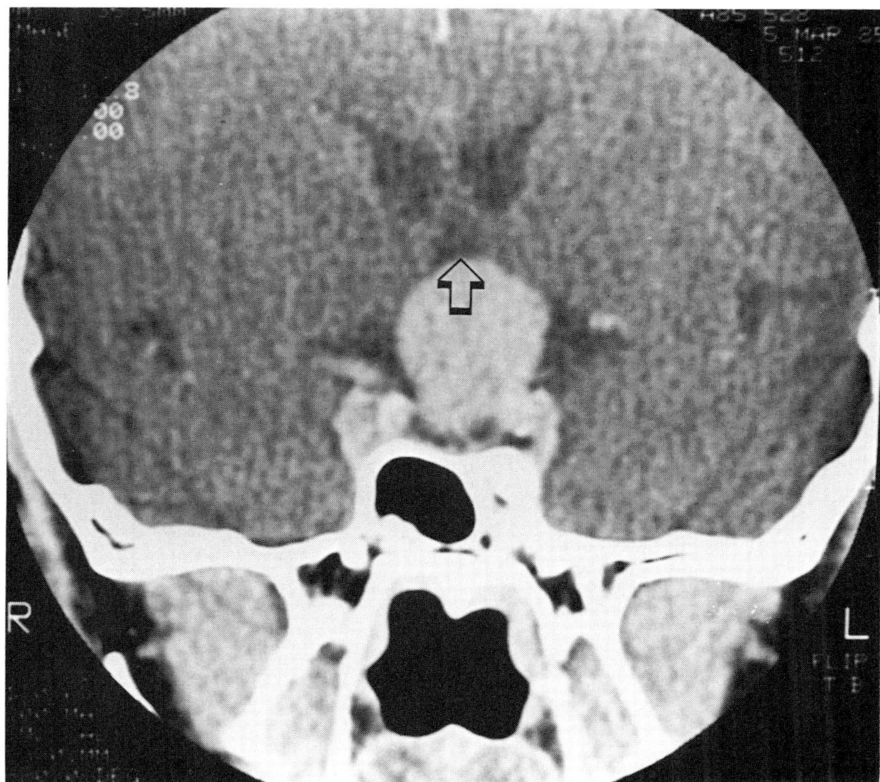

(b) Coronal CT with contrast of same patient shows that mass extends from sella through suprasellar cistern to indent the inferior border of the third ventricle (arrow).

patients with pituitary adenomas. Hammer (1983) reported that 4 of 87 patients with pituitary adenomas receiving post-operative radiation therapy suffered the tragic complication of chiasmal radiation vasculitis. Three of these four patients were acromegalics. Atkinson *et al.* (1979) reported that 4 of 23 irriadiated acromegalics experienced progressive visual loss unrelated to tumour growth. Radiation vasculitis of the optic chiasm is not limited to acromegalics (Harris and Levene, 1976; Aristizabal, Caldwell and Avila, 1977), but these reports agree with our experience at Wills Eye Hospital and imply that acromegalics have more chance of this devastating complication of radiation therapy than most other patients.

There is no apparent physiological reason why an elevated growth hormone level should place the optic chiasm and its vasculature in jeopardy after irradiation. The poor record of radiation necrosis must be compared to the results of trans-sphenoidal surgery alone, for Teasdale *et al.* (1982) reported no visual complications and no recurrent visual loss two years after trans-sphenoidal surgery in 28 acromegalics. Until more data are available, it may be wise to withhold radiation therapy in patients with chiasmal syndromes and elevated growth hormone levels.

4.3.5 POSITRON EMISSION TOMOGRAPHY

Positron emission tomography (PET) is a new technique yielding tomographic images of local cerebral glucose metabolism (corresponding to cortical energy consumption) or other physiological parameters such as brain oxygen metabolism or neurotransmitter receptor binding. We have used this technique to study glucose metabolism in the striate and visual association cortices of normal individuals receiving visual stimulation (Reivich *et al.*, 1985) and in individuals who have suffered ischaemic lesions affecting the optic radiations or visual cortex (Bosley *et al.*, 1985). We have recently performed several [^{18}F]-fluoro-2-deoxyglucose (FDG) positron emission tomographic studies looking at the effect of chiasmal damage on glucose uptake in primary and association visual cortex (Bosley *et al.*, 1987).

> Patient KJ. This 21-year-old man fell from a window during a college party three years previously sustaining a fracture through the roof of the left ethmoid sinus with a haematoma of the left frontal lobe and a traumatic chiasmal syndrome. His visual acuity was 20/20 OD and 20/60 OS with a left afferent pupillary defect and dense bitemporal hemianopia. The remainder of his neurological examination was significant only for a mild right hemiparesis. There was no clinical or radiological evidence of direct trauma to cortical visual areas.

Figure 4.6 is a PET image of brain glucose uptake in this patient with an asymmetric traumatic chiasmal syndrome. The right lateral geniculate body received neural input only from the temporal retina of the right eye because crossing fibres from the nasal field of the left eye were lost. The left lateral geniculate was more denervated than the right because some fibres from the ipsilateral temporal retina responsible for central vision were lost as well. Similarly, the right striate and visual association cortices were more completely innervated than cortical visual areas on the left.

The patient received monocular whole field visual stimulation to only the right eye with a pattern reversal chequerboard stimulus while the left eye was blindfolded. By patching the left eye, visual stimulation was delivered to the right lateral geniculate body and cortical visual areas while cortical visual areas on the left received no stimulation. Cortical

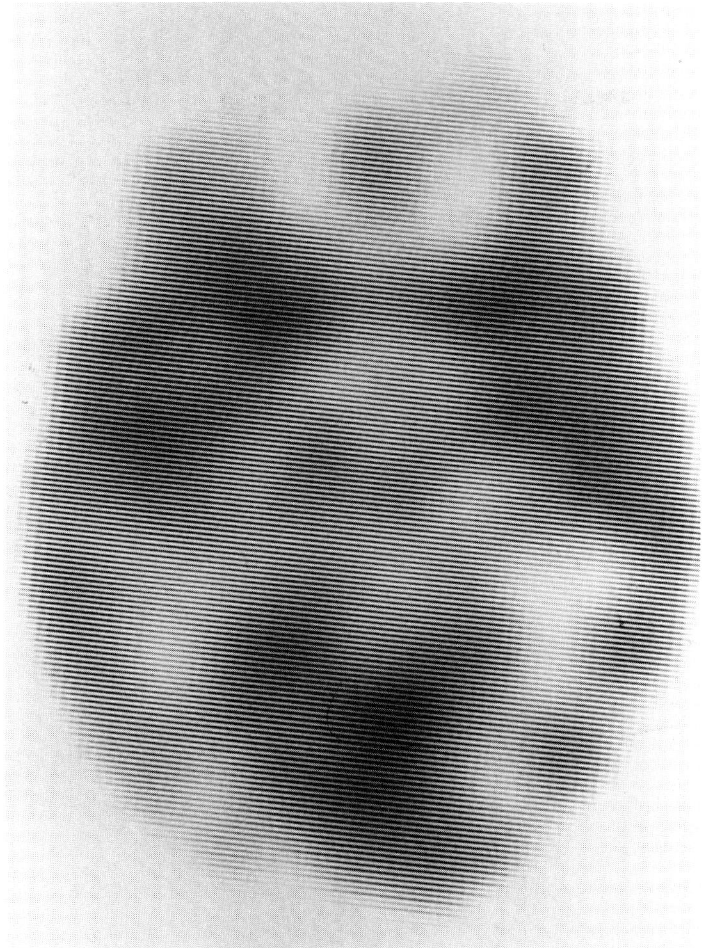

Fig. 4.6 FDG positron emission tomograph through level of striate and visual association cortex depicting local cerebral metabolic rates for glucose. Left side of brain on left side of image. Note more intense uptake of glucose into right striate and visual association cortex which received more innervation from anterior afferent visual system and more visual stimulation.

visual areas on the right metabolized glucose 10% (visual association cortex, anterior striate cortex) to 20% (posterior striate cortex) more rapidly than those on the left that were more denervated and that received no visual stimulation.

In patients studied so far it seems that visual stimulation with the chequerboard stimulus increases striate glucose uptake by approximately 10%. Of particular interest is the fact that intact innervation by the pregeniculate afferent visual system (independent of visual stimulation) may be responsible for as much as 40% of resting striate energy consumption. These results are compatible with previous reports in the cat (Bishop, Lovick and Williams, 1964), but this is the first demonstration in humans of the importance of background neural activity in the optic chiasm and anterior afferent visual system in modulating striate cortical activity.

4.4 The future

Clinicians today are fortunate to be able to obtain anatomical information about the peri-chiasmal region with an ease not dreamed of a generation ago. Most chiasmal syndromes are due to mass lesions, and most of these mass lesions can be imaged very well by CT and MR. With the power of neuro-imaging widely available, it is easy to become complacent, ignoring new rules that govern a new era: (1) high-resolution CT and MR scans have to be told to look at the chiasm very carefully in special ways; (2) not all compressive chiasmal lesions are easily imaged by CT alone; (3) low-resolution MR is no advance over CT in imaging the peri-chiasmal region; (4) the real advantages of high-resolution MR are not yet completely clear; and (5) there are a number of treatable non-compressive chiasmal syndromes that must be considered when CT and MR are normal.

Clinically relevant chiasmal anatomy is usually not a mystery today, and physiological questions have begun to take on more importance. Why do most compressive chiasmal syndromes improve after surgery? Why do some not improve? What is the full role of the anterior afferent visual system in transmitting visual information and modulating neural activity in the lateral geniculate and cortical visual areas? What is the cause of steroid-responsive chiasmal inflammation? Why do acromegalics seem more at risk for radiation-induced chiasmal vasculitis than other patients? Can MR, CT and PET be used in new ways to obtain physiological (as well as anatomical) information about the chiasm? Common anatomic lesions are now being dealt with in a relatively straightforward manner both diagnostically and therapeutically. We will almost certainly be able to treat both compressive and non-compressive chiasmal syndromes more effectively when we understand more about chiasmal neurophysiology and the regulation of chiasmal blood flow.

References

Ahmadi, J., Keane, J.R., McCormick, G.S., Fallis, R.J. and Miller, C.A. (1984) Ischemic chiasmal syndrome and hypopituitarism associated with progressive cerebro vascular occlussive disease. *Am. J. Neurorad.* **5**, 367–72.

Amundsen, P. and Newton, T.H. (1978) The subarachnoid cisterns, in *Radiology of the Skull and Brain* (eds T.H. Newton and D.G. Potts), Vol. 4. C.V. Mosby, St Louis, pp. 3588–711.

Aristizabal, S.A., Caldwell, W.L. and Avila, J. (1977) The relationship of time–dose fractionation factors to complications in the treatment of pituitary tumors by irradiation. *Int. J. Rad. Oncol. Biol. Phys.*, **2**, 667–73.

Atkinson, A.B., Allen, I.V., Gordon, D.S. *et al.* (1979) Progressive failure in acromegaly following external pituitary irradiation. *Clin. Endocrinol.*, **10**, 469–79.

Bergland, R. and Ray, B.S. (1969) The arterial supply of the human optic chiasm. *J. Neurosurg.*, **31**, 327–34.

Bishop, P.O., Lovick, W.R. and Williams, W.O. (1964) Statistical analysis of the dark discharge of lateral geniculate neurones. *J. Physiol.*, **170**, 598–612.

Bosley, T.M., Dann, R., Silver, F.L. *et al.* (1987) Lesions of the optic chiasm: positron emission tomography (in preparation).

Bosley, T.M., Rosenquist, A.C., Kushner, M., *et al.* (1985) Ischemic lesions of the occipital cortex and optic radiations: positron emission tomography. *Neurology*, **35**, 470–84.

Bursztyn, E.M., Lavyne, M.H. and Aisen, M. (1983) Empty sella syndrome with intrasellar herniation of the optic chiasm. *Am. J. Neurorad.*, **4**, 167–8.

Crampton, M.R. (1959) The visual changes in temporal (giant cell) arteritis. *Brain*, **82**, 377–90.

Daniels, D.L., Haughton, V.M., Williams, A.L. *et al.* (1980) Computed tomography of the optic chiasm. *Radiology*, **137**, 123–7.

Daniels, D.L., Herfkins, R., Gager, W.E. *et al.* (1984) Magnetic resonance imaging of the optic nerves and chiasm. *Radiology*, **152**, 79–83.

Drayer, B., Kaltah, J., Tosenbaum, A. *et al.* (1979) Diagnostic approaches to pituitary adenoma. *Neurology*, **29**, 161–9.

Dubin, M.W. and Cleland, B.G. (1977) The organization of visual inputs to interneurons of the lateral geniculate nucleus of the cat. *J. Neurophysiol.*, **9**, 410–27.

Dutton, J.J., Klingele, T.G., Burde, R.M. and Gado, M. (1982) Evaluation of the suprasellar cistern by computed tomography. *Ophthalmology*, **89**, 1220–5.

Duvall, J. and Cullen, J.F. (1982) Metastatic disease in the pituitary: Clinical features. *Trans. Ophthalmol. Soc. UK*, **102**, 481–6.

Edwards, M.K., Gilmor, R.L. and Franco, J.M. (1983) Computed tomography of chiasmal optic neuritis. *Am. J. Neurorad.*, **4**, 816–18.

Elkington, S.G. (1968) Pituitary adenoma: pre-operative symptomatology in a series of 260 patients. *Br. J. Ophthalmol.*, **52**, 322–8.

Finn, J.E. and Mount, L.A. (1974) Meningiomas of the tuberculum sellae and planum sphenoidale: a review of 83 cases. *Arch. Ophthalmol.*, **92**, 23–7.

Foulds, W.S., Bronte-Stewart, J. and McClure, E. (1983) Delayed diagnosis of optic nerve or chiasmal compression as a result of negative CT scanning. *Trans. Ophthalmol. Soc. UK*, **103**, 543–50.

Fourment, A., Hirsch, J.C., Marc, M.E. and Guidet, C. (1984) Modulation of postsynaptic activities of thalamic lateral geniculate neurons by spontaneous changes in number of retinal inputs in chronic cats. 1. Input–output relations. *Neuroscience*, **12**, 453–64.

Goldman, J.A., Hedges, T.R. III, Schucart, W. and Molitch, M.E. (1985) Delayed chiasmal decompression after transphenoidal operation for a pituitary adenoma. *Neurosurgery*, **17**, 962–4.

Gregorius, F.K., Hepler, R.S. and Stern, W.E. (1975) Loss and recovery of vision with suprasellar meningiomas. *J. Neurosurg.*, **42**, 69–75.

Greitz, T. (1975) Computer tomography for the diagnosis of intracranial tumors compared with other radiologic procedures. *Acta Radiol. Suppl.*, **346**, 14–20.

Grossman, R.I., Gonzalez-Scarano, F., Atlas, S.W., Galetta, S. and Silberberg, D.H. (1986) Multiple sclerosis: Gadolinium enhancement in MR imaging. *Radiology*, **161**, 721–5.

Gyldensted, C. and Karle, A. (1977) Computed tomography of intra and juxtasellar lesions. A radiographic study of 108 cases. *Neuroradiology*, **14**, 5–13.

Hackney, D.B., Savino, P.J., Grossman, R.I. *et al.* (1986) Degenerative changes in pituitary macroadenomas documented by magnetic resonance imaging. *Am. J. Neurorad.*, **7**, 544.

Hammer, H.M. (1983) Optic chiasmal radionecrosis. *Trans. Ophthalmol. Soc. UK*, **103**, 208–11.

Harris, J.R. and Levene, M.B. (1976) Visual complications following irradiation for pituitary adenomas and craniopharyngioma. *Radiology*, **120**, 167–71.

Hollenhorst, R.W. and Younge, B.R. (1976) Ocular manifestations of intrasellar and suprasellar tumors, in *Symposium on Neuro-ophthalmology* (eds R.M. Burde, J.S. Glazer, R.W. Hollenhorst, A. Jampolsky, N.J. Schatz, G.B. Udvarhelyi and H.J.L. Van Dike). C.V. Mosby, St Louis, pp. 191–207.

Hoyt, W.F. (1962) Anatomic considerations of arcuate scotomas associated with lesions of the optic chiasm. A Nauta exon degenerative study in the monkey. *Bull. Johns Hopkins Hosp.*, **111**, 57–71.

Hoyt, W.F. (1964) The human optic chiasm, in *Neuro-ophthalmology. Symposium of the University of Miami* (ed. J.L. Smith). Charles C. Thomas, Springfield, pp. 64–111.

Hoyt, W.F. and Luis, O. (1962) The primate chiasm: details of visual fiber organization studied by silver impregnation techniques. *Arch. Ophthalmol.*, **70**, 69–85.

Hubel, D.G. and Wiesel, T.N. (1967) Cortical and collosal connections concerned with the vertical meridian of visual fields in the cat. *J. Neurophysiol.*, **30**, 1561–73.

Hupp, S.L. and Savino, P.J. (1986) Imaging in neuro-ophthalmology, in *Ophthalmology Annual* (ed. R.D. Reinecke), Vol. II. Appleton-Century-Crofts, Norwalk, CT, pp. 51–82.

Hupp, S.L., Savino, P.J., Schatz, N.J., Sergott, R.C. and Bosley, T.M. (1986) Nerve fiber bundle visual field defects and intracranial mass lesions. *Can. J. Ophthalmol.* (in press).

Ingestad, R. and Stigmar, G. (1971) Sarcoidosis with ocular and hypothalamic pituitary manifestations. *Acta Ophthalmol.*, **49**, 1–10.

Kirkham, T.H. (1973) Neuro-ophthalmic presentations of sarcoidosis. *Proc. R. Soc. Med.*, **66**, 167–9.

Kline, L.B. (1981) Chiasmal compression without bitemporal hemianopia, in *Neuro-ophthalmology* (ed. J.L. Smith), Masson, New York, pp. 223–30.

Kline, L.B., Vitek, J.J. and Acker, J.D. (1983) Computed tomography in the evaluation of the optic chiasm. *Surv. Ophthalmol.*, **27**, 387–96.

Kupfer, C., Chumbley, L. and Downer, J. (1967) Quantitative histology of optic nerve, optic tract, and lateral geniculate nucleus in man. *J. Anat.*, **101**, 393–401.

Lee, F. (1983) Ischemic chiasma syndrome. *Am. J. Neurorad.*, **4**, 777–80.

Lee, K.F. and Schatz, N.J. (1975) Ischemic chiasmal syndrome. *Acta Radiol.* (*Suppl.*) (*Stockholm*), **347**, 131–47.

Mastronarde, D.N. (1984) Organization of the cat's optic tract as assessed by single axon recordings. *J. Comp. Neurol.*, **227**, 14–22.

Max, M.B., Dick, M.D.F. and Rottenberg, D.A. (1981) Pituitary metastasis. Incidence in cancer patients and clinical differentiation from pituitary adenoma. *Neurology*, **31**, 998–1002.

McGregor, A.M., Scanlon, M.F., Hall, K. Cook, D. and Hall, R. (1979) Reduction in size of a pituitary tumor by bromocriptine therapy. *N. Engl. J. Med.*, **300**, 291–3.

Molotchnikoff, S., Tremblay, F. and Lepore, F. (1984) The role of the visual cortex in response properties of lateral geniculate cells of rats. *Exp. Br. Res.*, **53**, 223–32.

Moster, M.L., Savino, P.J., Schatz, N.J., Snyder, P.J., Sergott, R.C. and Bosley, T.M. (1986) Visual function in patients with prolactinoma treated with bromocriptine. *Ophthalmology*, **92**, 1332–41.

Naidich, T.P., Pinto, R.S., Kushner, M.J. *et al.* (1976) Evaluation of sellar and parasellar masses by computed tomography. *Radiology*, **120**, 91–9.

Podell, M., Yinon, U. and Hammer, A. (1984) Properties of visual cortical cells of the intact and the deafferented hemisphere of unilateral optic tract sectioned acute and chronic adult cats. *Exp. Br. Res.*, **55**, 91–6.

Reich, N.E., Zelch, J.V., Alfidi, R.J. *et al.* (1975) Computer tomography and the detection of juxtasellar lesions. *Radiology*, **118**, 333–5.

Reivich, M., Kushner, M., Alavi, A. and Greenberg, J. (1985) Measurement of local cerebral glucose metabolism: Effect of pathology and functional stimulation, in *Cerebral Blood Flow and Metabolic Measurement* (eds S. Hoyer and A. Hartman). Springer-Verlag, Berlin, pp. 410–18.

Reynolds, W.D., Smith, J.L. and McCrary, J.A. (1982) Chiasmal optic neuritis. *J. Clin. Neuro-ophthalmol.*, **2**, 93–101.

Savino, P.J. (1986) The present role of magnetic resonance imaging in neuro-ophthalmology. *Can. J. Ophthalmol.*, **21**, 231–5.

Schatz, N.J. and Schlezinger, N.S. (1976) Non-compressive causes of chiasmal disease, in *Transactions of the New Orleans Academy of Ophthalmology* (*Symposium on Neuro-Ophthalmology*). C.V. Mosby, St Louis, pp. 90–7.

Spector, R.H., Glazer, J.S. and Schatz, N.J. (1980) Demyelinative chiasmal lesions. *Arch. Neurol.*, **37**, 757–62.

Teasdale, G.M., Hay, I.D., Beasttall, G.H. *et al.* (1982) Cryosurgery or microsurgery in the management of acromegaly. *J. Am. Med. Assoc.*, **247**, 1289–91.

Tindall, G., McLanahan, C. and Christy, J. (1977) Transphenoidal microsurgery for pituitary tumors, in *Neuro-ophthalmology Update* (ed. J.L. Smith). Masson, New York, pp. 227–39.

Trobe, J.D., Tao, A.H. and Schuster, J.J. (1984) Perichiasmal tumors: diagnostic and prognostic features. *Neurosurgery*, **15**, 391–9.

Wass, J.A.H., Williams, J., Charlesworth, M. *et al.* (1982) Bromocriptine in management of large pituitary tumors. *Br. Med. J.*, **284**, 1908–11.

Wilbrand, H.L. (1926) Schema des Verlaufs der Sehnervenfasern durch das Chiasma. *Z. Augenheilk.*, **59**, 135–44.

Wilson, C. and Dempsey, L. (1977) Neuro-ophthalmology and transphenoidal removal of pituitary adenomas, in *Neuro-ophthalmology Update* (ed. J.L. Smith). Masson, New York, pp. 221–6.

Wilson, P. and Falconer, M.A. (1968) Patterns of visual failure with pituitary tumors: clinical and radiologic correlations. *Br. J. Ophthalmol.*, **52**, 94–110.

CHAPTER 5

Mechanisms of processing in primary visual cortex

CHARLES D. GILBERT, JURGEN BOLZ AND TORSTEN N. WIESEL

As information from the retina is carried along the visual pathway, the visual image is analysed in terms of its various attributes and components. To do this, cortical cells have a number of specialized receptive field properties that are designed to perform specific functions, for example, the perception of form entails an analysis of contour – the border of an object is broken down into line segments of a particular orientation. Additional information about local curvature is obtained by a property known as end-inhibition. A cell showing this property is optimally activated by line segments of a given orientation and a restricted length. As the line is extended further, the cell's response diminishes. As a result, these cells respond better to curved lines than to long, straight lines. Other properties seen in the primary visual cortex include disparity sensitivity, which endow cells with the ability to determine the depth of an object in space, selectivity for direction of movement and colour.

Many of the properties described above are seen first in the primary visual cortex. The properties of the cortical input are much simpler. Cells in the lateral geniculate nucleus (LGN) have circularly symmetric receptive fields, and, by their antagonistic centre/surround receptive field structure, are sensitive to contrast in the visual environment. The receptive field properties that are unique to the cortex result from the spatial pattern of converging inputs and the balance between excitatory and inhibitory inputs. Even though the fundamental receptive field properties of cells in the primary visual cortex were described 25 years ago (Hubel and Wiesel, 1962), the mechanisms by which many of these properties are created remain a puzzle, but there is currently evidence accumulating that allows one to associate certain functional properties with particular cortical connections. In this chapter we will present one example of such an association.

The intrinsic cortical circuit consists of a stereotyped set of connections, including the presumed excitatory connections formed by spiny stellate and pyramidal cells, and inhibitory connections formed by smooth stellate cells. The excitatory connections form a sequence running from one cortical layer to the next. The principal ones in the cat include the input from the LGN to layer 4 of the cortex and a sequence of interlaminar connections including the projection from layer 4 to layers 2 and 3, from the superficial layers to layer 5, from layer 5 to layer 6 and from layer 6 to layer 4 (Gilbert and Wiesel, 1979).

In this chapter we will discuss the relationship between the property of end-inhibition and cortical circuitry. Even in layer 4, the initial stage in the cortical circuit, cells are end-inhibited. They respond optimally to a relatively short bar (1°, for example), and as the bar length is increased further, the cells' response is reduced. This reduction in response is progressive, and requires long bars for maximal effect. From experiments in which we correlated receptive field structure with the intrinsic projection pattern, it seemed possible for this property to be generated by a projection from layer 6 to layer 4, an idea that grew out of experiments involving intracellular injection of cortical cells with the enzyme, horseradish peroxidase (HRP). The technique of intracellular recording and dye injection makes it possible to correlate the morphology and projection pattern of an injected cell with its receptive field properties (Gilbert and Wiesel, 1979; Martin and Whitteridge, 1984). An example of a layer 6 cell with a simple receptive field is shown in Fig. 5.1. It showed summation for the increasing length of the stimulating bar up to 4° of visual angle. Cells in layer 6 typically have long receptive fields, showing a progressive enhancement in their response as the stimulating bar is lengthened, often up to 16° in length (Gilbert, 1977). Their receptive fields are therefore much longer than the receptive fields of cells in layer 4 (which generally run from 0.5 to 1° at this eccentricity). A comparison of the length-summation properties of layer 6 and layer 4 cells suggests a possible function for the connection between the two layers, illustrated schematically in Fig. 5.2. As shown on the right, a layer 6 cell contacts an inhibitory interneurone in layer 4, which in turn contacts an excitatory cell in layer 4. This produces a reciprocal relationship in the firing of the layer 6 cell and the second stage layer 4 cell to short and long bar stimuli, as shown in the left side of the figure. The layer 4 cell therefore has a long

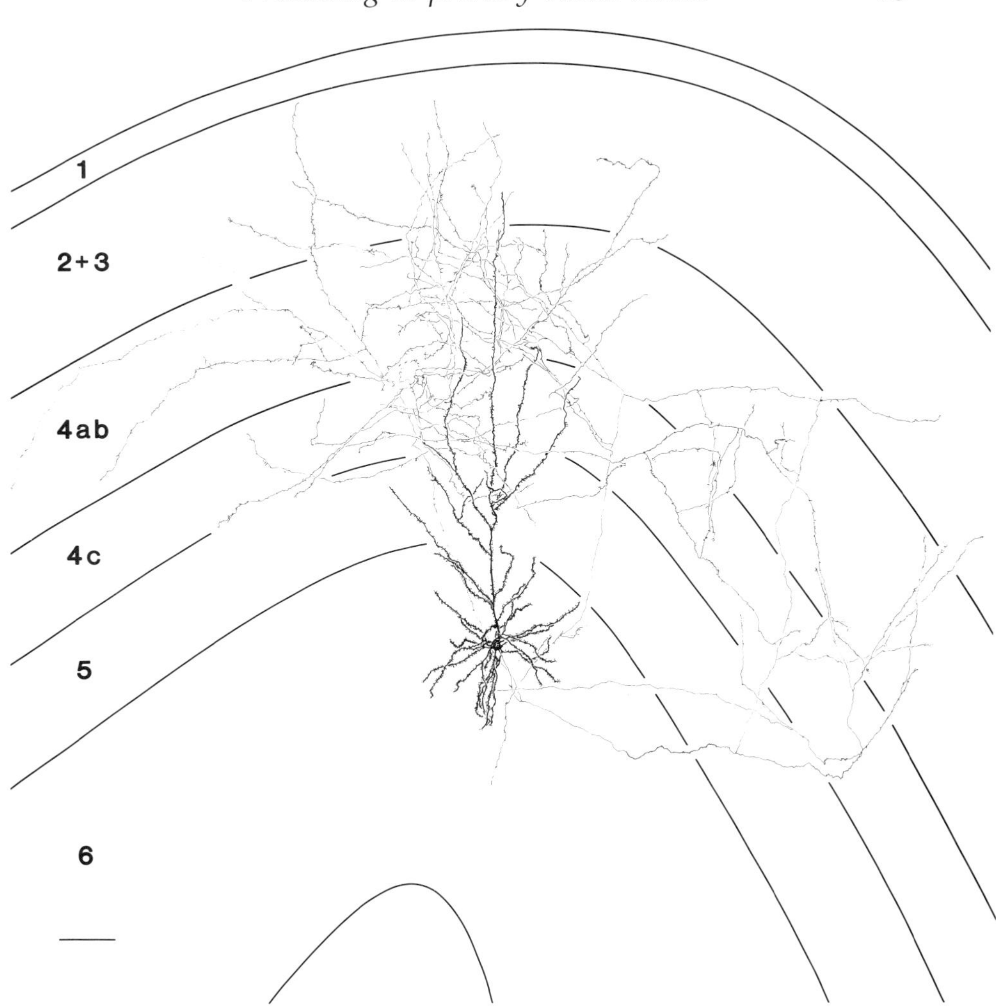

Fig. 5.1 Layer 6 pyramidal cell. The axon arborized primarily within layer 4. The cell had a simple receptive field, and showed summation for the increasing length of the stimulating bar up to 4°. Scale marker = 100 μm.

inhibitory flank, equivalent in size to the field of the layer 6 cell. The excitatory input to the layer 4 cell comes from the LGN, forming the central excitatory region, which is of the simple receptive field type.

The model shows the inhibitory effect from layer 6 to be mediated by an inhibitory interneurone, rather than direct inhibition from layer 6 cells, for the following reasons. Layer 6 pyramidal cells are themselves likely to

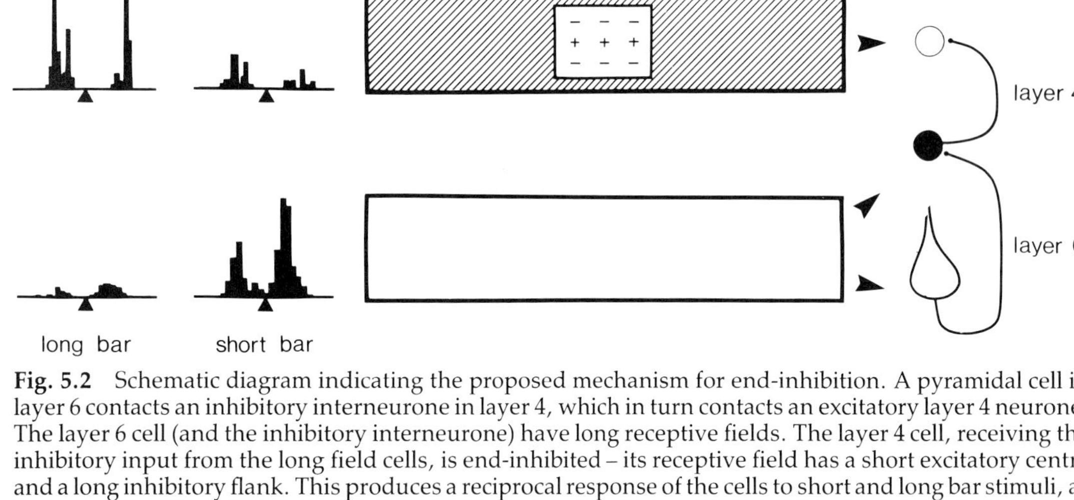

Fig. 5.2 Schematic diagram indicating the proposed mechanism for end-inhibition. A pyramidal cell in layer 6 contacts an inhibitory interneurone in layer 4, which in turn contacts an excitatory layer 4 neurone. The layer 6 cell (and the inhibitory interneurone) have long receptive fields. The layer 4 cell, receiving the inhibitory input from the long field cells, is end-inhibited – its receptive field has a short excitatory centre and a long inhibitory flank. This produces a reciprocal response of the cells to short and long bar stimuli, as shown on the left.

be excitatory. Spiny cells form type I synapses, which are associated with excitatory connections, whereas cells with smooth dendrites form type II synapses, which are thought to be inhibitory. Moreover, layer 6 pyramidal cells show high affinity uptake and transport of aspartic acid, a putative neurotransmitter (Baughman and Gilbert, 1981). The acidic amino acids, including aspartate and glutamate, are excitatory. Finally, electrical stimulation experiments show the existence of an excitatory connection between layer 6 and layer 4 (Ferster and Lindstrom, 1985). Therefore, if the layer 6 to layer 4 pathway is to be inhibitory, it must use an inhibitory interneurone in the connection. To explore this possibility, we examined the cells that were postsynaptic to cells injected intracellularly with HRP at the ultrastructural level. Using serial EM reconstruction of the postsynaptic dendrites, we found that the majority were smooth or sparsely spiny, and therefore belonged to the general class of inhibitory neurones (McGuire *et al.*, 1984), a finding consistent with the idea that the net effect of the layer 6 to layer 4 pathways is inhibitory.

The final step in ascertaining the role of the layer 6 to layer 4 pathway involved a pharmacological approach. By removing the layer 6 cells from the circuit we hoped to obtain evidence for their functional role. The method we used was local application of the inhibitory transmitter, γ-aminobutyric acid (GABA). We restricted the size of the injection to include only layer 6. The effect is reversible, so we could test the effect of layer 6 inactivation on individual cells in layer 4, monitoring their receptive field properties before injection, immediately after injection, and after the layer 6 cells recovered from the injection. An example of this experiment is shown in Fig. 5.3. Before injection the cell showed substantial end-inhibition, such that its response to a long bar was 46% of its response to a bar of optimal length. Immediately after injection the response of the cell to the long bar increased, and the end-inhibition was completely eliminated. After 3 minutes, the cell recovered the end-inhibition it had originally. Other properties, such as directional selectivity and orientation tuning, were unaffected (Bolz and Gilbert, 1986).

Our first choice for the pathway responsible for generating end-inhibition is the direct projection from layer 6 to layer 4, but there are two other indirect pathways between the two layers that should be taken into account. A subcortical nucleus, the claustrum, receives a direct projection from layer 6 and projects in turn to layer 4 (Carey, Bear and Diamond, 1980; Olson and Graybiel, 1980; Sherk and LeVay, 1981). It was found that killing cells in the claustrum, which have long receptive fields similar to layer 6 cells, also reduced the amount of end-inhibition seen in layer 4 (Sherk and LeVay, 1983). Since the input to the claustrum originates from layer 6, our injections potentially blocked both the direct input to layer 4 from layer 6 and the indirect input via the claustrum. The fact that layer 6

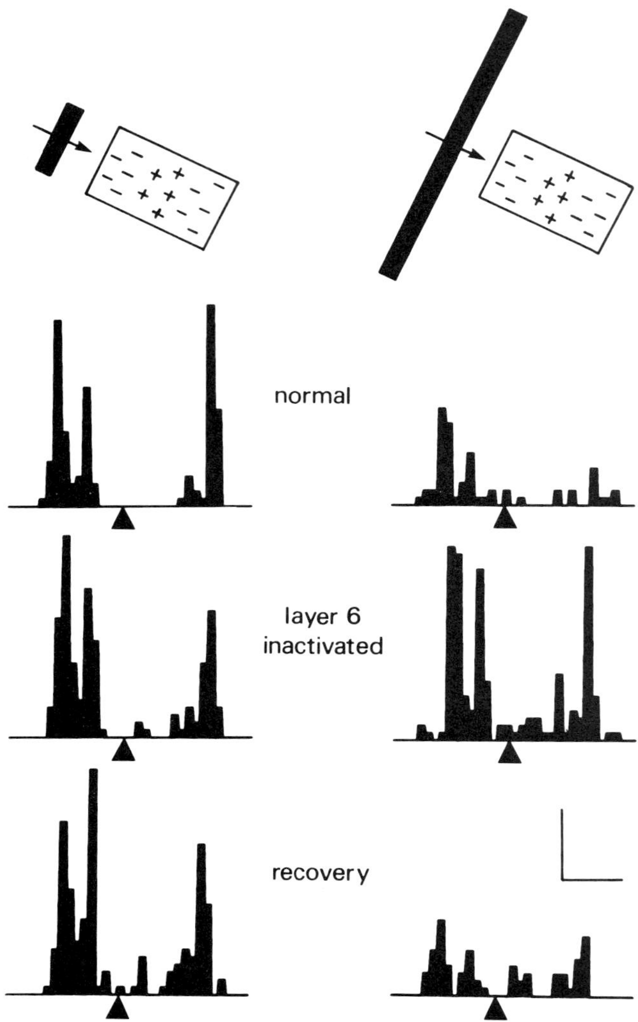

Fig. 5.3 Effect of inactivation of layer 6 on a simple cell in layer 4. The cell's receptive field was 1°×1.75° and had antagonistic on (+) and off (−) subfields when tested with a stationary flashing bar. Layer 6 was inactivated by pressure injection of GABA. Response histograms from 10 stimulus presentations each were made before (top), immediately after (middle) and 3 min after (bottom) GABA injection in layer 6. The triangles under each histogram indicated the point at which the bar reversed direction. The cell was end-inhibited, such that its response to a long bar (8°) was 46% of its response to a bar optimum length (1°). This inhibition was eliminated by inactivation of layer 6 (right column), whereas the cell's response to a short bar was unchanged. Calibration: vertical mark, 10 spikes per bin; horizontal mark, 1 s. (From Bolz and Gilbert (1986).)

inactivation produced a larger effect than claustrum inactivation alone suggests that the direct pathway does play a role in producing end-inhibition. A second indirect pathway involves the LGN, since layer 6 cells are responsible for the major recurrent pathway from cortex to thalamus. It has been shown that LGN cells do show a form of end-inhibition which is reduced by cortical ablation (Sillito, personal communication) but, using our technique of local inactivation, we were unable to show any effect on the LGN end-inhibition. Thus we conclude that layer 6 cells are responsible for end-inhibition, and that a large part of this role is played by the direct connection from layer 6 to layer 4.

Relating individual cortical cells to particular functional properties is an invaluable approach to studying the cortical mechanisms of vision. It is likely to show the connections underlying known functional properties, as shown in the above example. Furthermore, it may also be a useful tool in revealing properties that have not yet been described. The intracellular injections revealed patterns of connections that were unexpected, suggesting communication between cells with non-overlapping receptive fields. These connections are therefore likely to be related to contextual influences on the firing properties of cells. For example, cells in a visual area specializing in motion may play a role in figure–ground discrimination by their sensitivity to relative movement between objects inside and outside their receptive fields (Allman, Miezin and McGuinness, 1985). In an area specializing in colour, the perceptual phenomenon of colour constancy has been observed at the single cell level (Zeki, 1983), a property likely to involve the comparison of reflectance from different parts of the visual field. Cells in the primary visual cortex also may have more complex receptive field properties than those studied up to now. Because of the stereotyped nature of cortical connections, it may be possible to generalize the findings in primary visual cortex to other visual cortical areas and ultimately to regions of cortex serving other functional modalities.

References

Allman, J., Miezin, F. and McGuinness, E. (1985) Stimulus specific responses from beyond the classical receptive field: neurophysiological mechanisms for local–global comparisons in visual neurons. *Ann. Rev. Neurosci.*, **8**, 407–30.

Baughman, R.W. and Gilbert, C.D. (1981) Aspartate and glutamate as possible neurotransmitters in the visual cortex. *J. Neurosci.*, **1**, 427–39.

Bolz, J. and Gilbert, C.D. (1986) Generation of end-inhibition in the visual cortex via interlaminar connections. *Nature*, **320**, 362–5.

Carey, R.G., Bear, M.F. and Diamond, I.T. (1980) The laminar organization of the reciprocal projections between the claustrum and striate cortex in the tree shrew, *Tupaia glis*. *Brain Res.*, **184**, 193–8.

Ferster, D. and Lindstrom, S. (1985) Synaptic excitation of neurones in area 17 of the cat by intracortical axon collaterals of cortico-geniculate cells. *J. Physiol.*, **367**, 233–52.

Gilbert, C.D. (1977) Laminar differences in receptive field properties in cat primary visual cortex. *J. Physiol.*, **268**, 391–421.

Gilbert, C.D. and Wiesel, T.N. (1979) Morphology and intracortical projections of functionally identified neurons in cat visual cortex. *Nature*, **380**, 120–5.

Hubel, D.H. and Wiesel, T.N. (1962) Receptive fields, binocular interactions and functional architecture in the cat's visual cortex. *J. Physiol.*, **160**, 106–54.

Martin, K.A.C. and Whitteridge, D. (1984) Form, function, and intracortical projections of spiny neurones in the striate cortex of the cat. *J. Physiol.*, **353**, 463–504.

McGuire, B.A., Hornung, J.-P., Gilbert, C.D. and Wiesel, T.N. (1984) Patterns of synaptic input to layer 4 of cat striate cortex. *J. Neurosci.*, **4**, 3021–33.

Olson, C.R. and Graybiel, A.M. (1980) Sensory maps in the claustrum of the cat. *Nature*, **288**, 479–81.

Sherk, H. and LeVay, S. (1981) The visual claustrum of the cat. *J. Neurosci.*, **1**, 956–1002.

Sherk, H. and LeVay, S. (1983) Contribution of the cortico-claustral loop to the receptive field properties in area 17 of the cat. *J. Neurosci.*, **3**, 2121–7.

Zeki, S.M. (1983) Colour coding in the cerebral cortex: the reaction of cells in monkey visual cortex to wavelengths and colours. *Neuroscience*, **9**, 741–65.

CHAPTER 6

Functional specialization in the visual cortex and its relation to visual agnosias

SEMIR ZEKI

6.1 Introduction

If one had to summarize the history of cerebral physiology in a few words, one would say that it has consisted largely of an attempt to chart histologically distinct parts of the cerebral cortex and to assign specific functions to each, a theme in which clinical neurologists have had a powerful precedence. Indeed the first unequivocal demonstration of functional localization in the cerebral cortex came from the studies by Broca (1861) who showed that one faculty, that of producing language, was dependent upon the integrity of the third convolution of the left temporal lobe. The years that followed saw a strong emphasis on the relationship of structure to function in the motor cortex, particularly after the epoch-making discoveries of Fritsch and Hitzig (1870) who localized motor activity to a cytoarchitectonically distinct region of the cortex, the excitable motor cortex. This ushered in an era of 'feverish map making' (Sholl, 1956) where each and every cytoarchitectonic difference was used, uncritically (Lashley and Clark, 1946), to subdivide the cortex into a large number of cortical fields, often without assigning functions to them, and culminating in the elaborate cytoarchitectonic maps of the Vogts who divided the cerebral cortex into more than 200 areas, a subdivision which appeared 'fantastic' to some (Sholl, 1956). Attempts to provide elaborate subdivisions of the visual cortex were not lacking, especially in the work of Beck (1934) who was impatient with Filiminoff's (1936) more modest subdivisions, and retorted angrily 'nur hat Filiminoff vergessen mich zu zitieren' (Beck, 1934). But, in general, it was difficult to subdivide either the striate cortex (V1) or the prestriate cortex into anything like the number of cytoarchitectonic subdivisions that clinicians, on the basis of evidence available to them, would have liked. Hence Brodmann (1905), along with von Economo and Koskinas (1925), essentially subdivided the prestriate cortex into two fields (18 and 19; 0A and 0B), a subdivision disputed later by Lashley and Clark (1946) who considered the whole of areas 18 and 19, together with area 7, to form a 'single functional unit' (Lashley and Clark, 1946). This created a problem for the clinicians because the clinical evidence had suggested distinctive perceptual visual afflictions following what, according to the best evidence available at a time antedating brain scans and computerized tomography, appeared to be lesions in prestriate cortex. Thus, von Economo and Koskinas (1925) were forced to provide a functional, as opposed to a cytoarchitectonic, map (Fig. 6.1) in which they entered specific visual functions, but with a question mark, in the

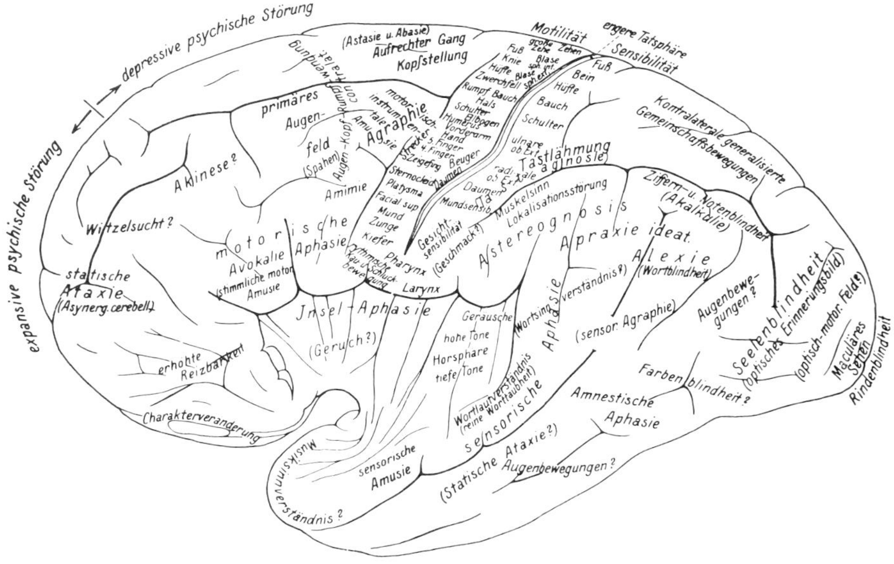

Fig. 6.1 A functional map of the human cerebral cortex, prepared by von Economo and Koskinas (1925).

prestriate cortex: 'Farbenblindheit?', 'Augenbewegungen?' 'Seelenblindheit' (a vague term, derived from Munk (1881)) and were forced to the conclusion: 'Man wird sich auch nicht Forstellen, dürfen; dass eine einzige area immer nur eine einzige Funktion hat', the reference to an area being to a cytoarchitectonic area. With the generally hostile attitude towards localization created by Lashley's work, and the general imprecision of clinical evidence, the notion of submodality localization within the visual system came rapidly to be disregarded, even though occasional, but not compelling, evidence for localization of colour vision in the cortex was produced, notably by Kleist (1937). Also at work against the doctrine of separation of functions was the powerful hierarchical concept, which supposed that all the visual information would be analysed in every visual area, but at a more complex level than the antecedent area (see Zeki, 1984, 1985, for review), of which the most powerful physiological exponent was the work of Hubel and Wiesel (1962, 1965). Another conceptual difficulty, which is what Lashley tried to tackle, is how information that is fractionated can then be reassembled to give us our unitary percept of the visual world, a problem rendered acute by an inadequate anatomy which led to the belief that there were only sparse, one-way anatomical connections between striate and prestriate cortex (see Zeki, 1969a, for review). Thus, by the 1960s there was little solid evidence left to favour the view that different visual functions may be processed in different visual areas.

6.2 The evidence for functional specialization in the visual cortex

A critical twist in this came about with an improvement in anatomical techniques. The use of the relatively much improved Fink-Heimer method allowed the visualization of the projections from primary visual cortex in much greater detail than had previously been possible. An initial first study by Kuypers *et al.* (1965) using this method showed that V1 projects to what was termed the 'circumstriate cortical belt', a large cortical region which includes areas 18 and 19 of Brodmann (1905). This circumstriate cortical belt, in turn, was found to project to inferotemporal cortex (Kuypers *et al.*, 1965), an apparently serial connection in conformity with the hierarchical doctrine. It was only with later anatomical studies, employing small lesions made in V1 (Cragg, 1969; Zeki, 1969b), that it became evident that each part of V1, which represents a particular retinal region, and therefore a corresponding region of the field of view, has independent, and parallel, outputs to differing prestriate regions (Fig. 6.2).

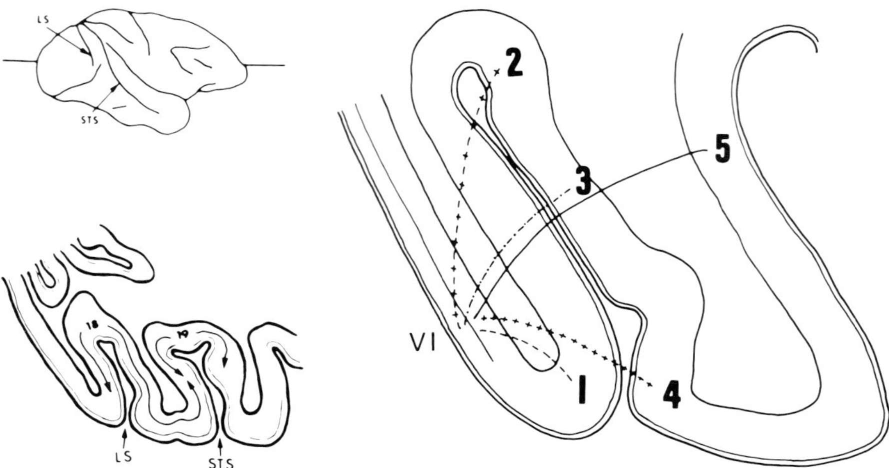

Fig. 6.2 A schematized diagram of the cortical projections from the striate cortex (V1) to the prestriate cortex on a section taken from the level indicated in the insert (upper left). Such a pattern of projections, in which each part of the striate cortex was found to have independent outputs to different parts of the prestriate cortex, forms the basis of the subdivision of prestriate cortex into separate, functionally specialized, visual areas. The inset to lower left shows the disposition of the cytoarchitectonic divisions 18 and 19 of the visual cortex. (From Zeki, S. (1975) *Cold Spring Harbor Symp. Quant. Biol.*, **40**.)

On the basis of this evidence, together with detailed anatomical evidence relating to the callosal connections of prestriate cortex, the latter was subdivided into distinct areas (Zeki, 1969, 1971), thus leading to the demonstration of a multiplicity of distinct visual areas in prestriate cortex. Parallel physiological studies showed that different groups of visual areas execute different tasks, not the same task at ever more complex levels, a finding which led to the concept of functional specialization in the visual cortex (Zeki, 1974, 1978).

A pivotal point in the demonstration of functional specialization in the visual cortex was, in fact, the observation of the projections from V1 to prestriate cortex. Since it would be difficult to imagine that V1 sends the same information to these different visual areas of the prestriate cortex in these independent and parallel pathways, it becomes much more logical to suppose that it sends different kinds of information, a logic that inevitably led to the suggestion that '. . . another of [the major functions of V1] might be to segregate out the information coming over the retino-geniculo-cortical pathways and parcel this information out to different cortical areas for further analysis' (Zeki, 1975). This was not a readily acceptable suggestion at the time, because the most detailed studies of the functional architecture of V1 (Hubel and Wiesel, 1977) had shown it to be largely uniform, with all cells outside layer IVC being orientation selective, one preferred orientation following another in a remarkable sequence tangentially. However, the most recent evidence is compelling in suggesting that there is indeed a profound functional segregation within V1.

One of the visual areas to which V1 projects is V5, the motion area lying in the posterior bank of the superior temporal sulcus. Detailed physiological studies (Zeki, 1974; Gattass and Gross, 1981; Van Essen, Maunsell and Bixby, 1981) have shown that the cells of this area are directionally selective and the recent, elegant, studies of Movshon *et al.* (1984) have shown that cells here respond to the real motion of objects. Equally, the studies of Wurtz and his colleagues in the awake, behaving, monkey show that V5 is specifically concerned with motion in the field of the view (Newsome *et al.*, 1985). An early finding that none of the cells of the motion area (V5) are selective for the colour or wavelength of a stimulus (Zeki, 1974), a finding that was of crucial significance in elaborating the doctrine of functional specialization (Zeki, 1974, 1978), has been amply confirmed (Gattass and Gross, 1981; Van Essen, Maunsell and Bixby, 1981). The development of more sensitive anatomical tracers, such as the method of labelling projecting cells with the enzyme horseradish peroxidase (HRP), has permitted a more detailed visualization of the distribution, within V1, of cells projecting to V5. The first such evidence was obtained by Lund *et al.* (1975) who showed that cells projecting to V5 are segregated within layer 4B and upper layer 6 (the solitary cells of Meynert) (see Fig. 6.3). Recent, more detailed, studies which I have performed with Stewart Shipp have shown that, even within these two layers, not every cell is labelled after massive injections into V5. Thus, within layer 4B, cells projecting to V5 occur in a single row and are separated from each other by unlabelled cells, hence cells likely to be projecting elsewhere, almost certainly to V3 (Burkhalter *et al.*, 1986; Zeki and Shipp, unpublished results), and also to V2 (Rockland and Pandya, 1979; Lund *et al.*, 1981). A similar segregation, but even more striking, is found in upper layer 6, where labelled cells, projecting to V5, occur usually singly and are even more widely separated from each other. A better picture of the remarkable segregation in layer 4B of cells projecting to V5 can be obtained by injecting HRP label into V5, taking tangential sections through layer 4B of V1 and reacting the sections for HRP label. Labelled material appears in discrete clusters, separated from one another by regions without labelled cells (Fig. 6.4). Hence the anatomical evidence shows that cells in V1 projecting to V5 are not only segregated into separate layers but that, within each layer, they are separated from cells projecting elsewhere.

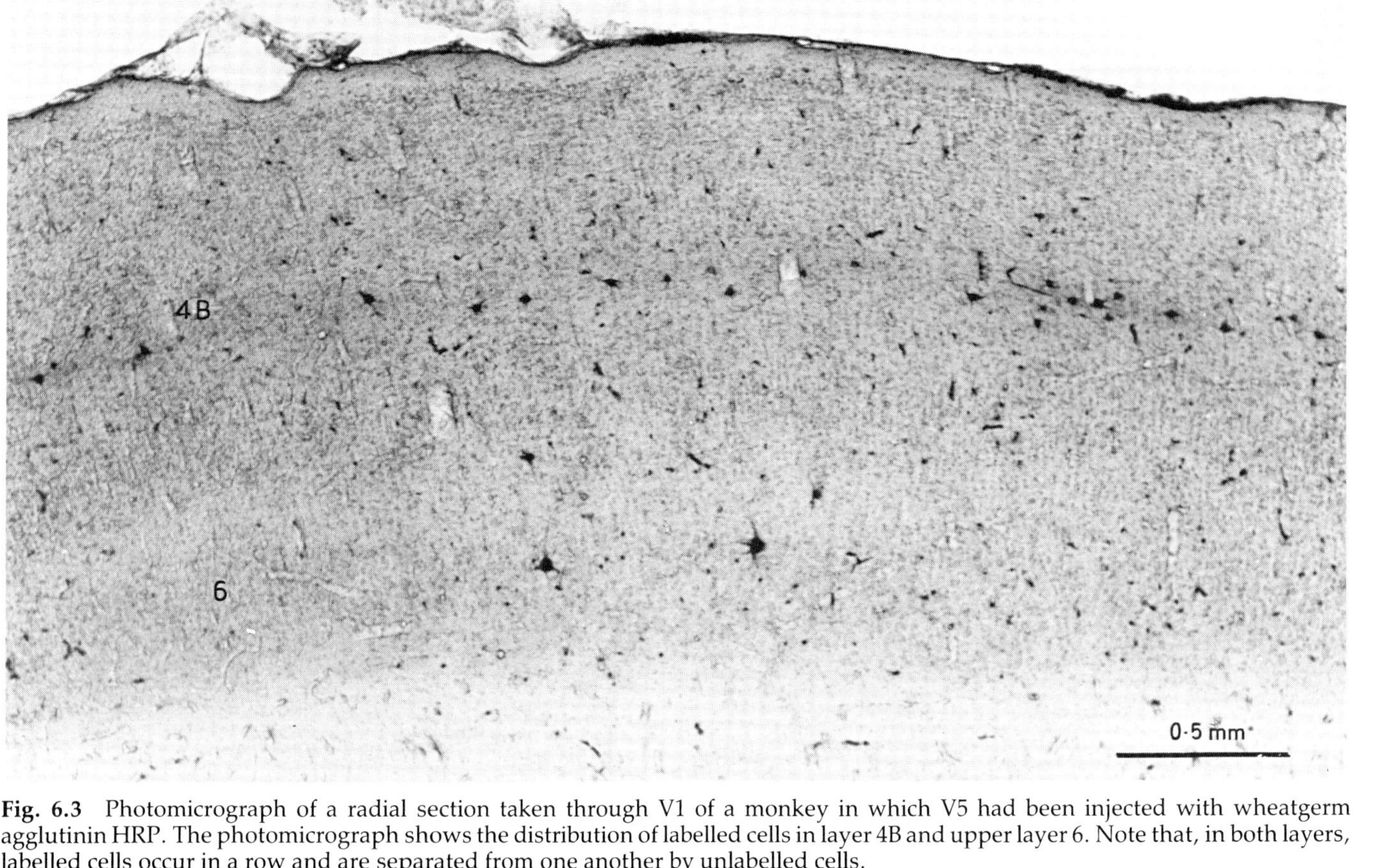

Fig. 6.3 Photomicrograph of a radial section taken through V1 of a monkey in which V5 had been injected with wheatgerm agglutinin HRP. The photomicrograph shows the distribution of labelled cells in layer 4B and upper layer 6. Note that, in both layers, labelled cells occur in a row and are separated from one another by unlabelled cells.

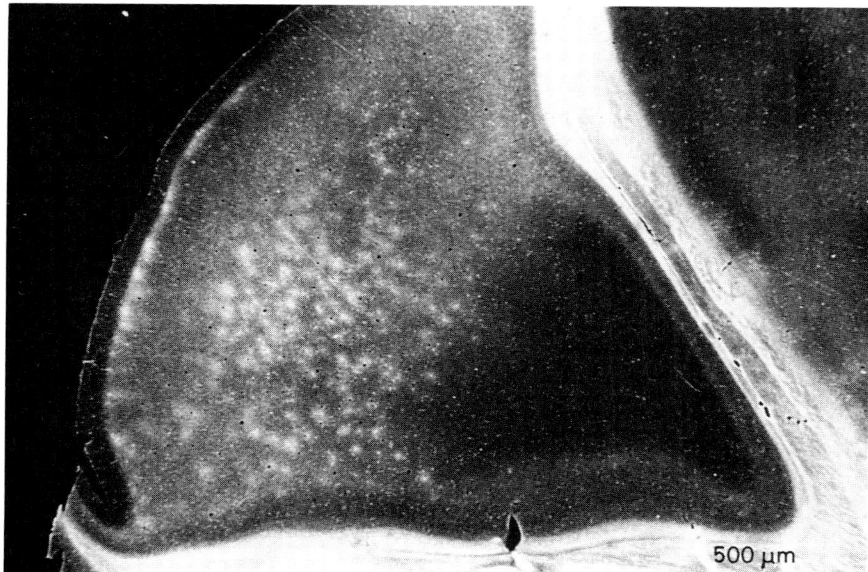

Fig. 6.4 Dark-field photomicrograph of a tangential section taken through layer 4B of a monkey in which V5 had been injected with wheatgerm agglutinin HRP. The photomicrograph gives a better picture of the clustered distribution of labelled material in V1.

Another striking example of the segregation within V1 occurs in layers 2 and 3. When V1 is stained for the metabolic enzyme cytochrome oxidase, the distribution of enzyme activity in layers 2 and 3 is not uniform but occurs in discrete, repetitive clusters which, when viewed in tangential sections, take on the appearance of blobs (Fig. 6.5). Confirming other evidence (Poggio *et al.*, 1975; Zeki, 1983a) which shows that wavelength-sensitive cells are not orientation selective and orientation-selective cells are not wavelength selective, the most recent evidence, combining electrophysiology and cytochrome oxidase histochemistry, shows that these two functional types of cells are segregated in layers 2 and 3 of V1 and that this segregation bears a definite relationship to the pattern of distribution of cytochrome oxidase activity. Thus, wavelength-selective cells are concentrated in the cytochrome oxidase blobs whereas orientation- (but not wavelength-) selective cells are concentrated in the interblob zones (Livingstone and Hubel, 1984). The specific reason for this link between different kinds of function and different levels of metabolic activity remains unknown, but the picture so generated is different from the earlier model of the functional architecture of V1

A

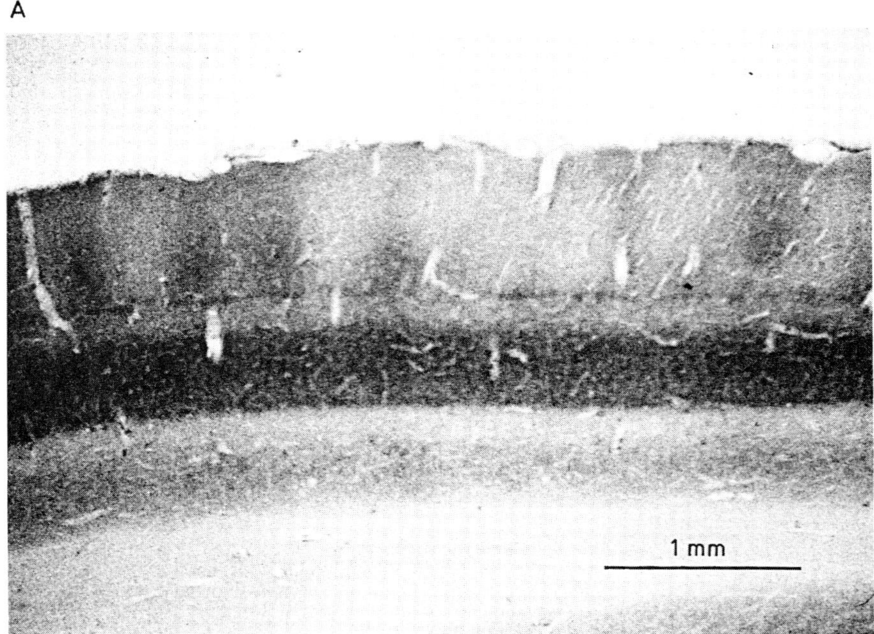

B

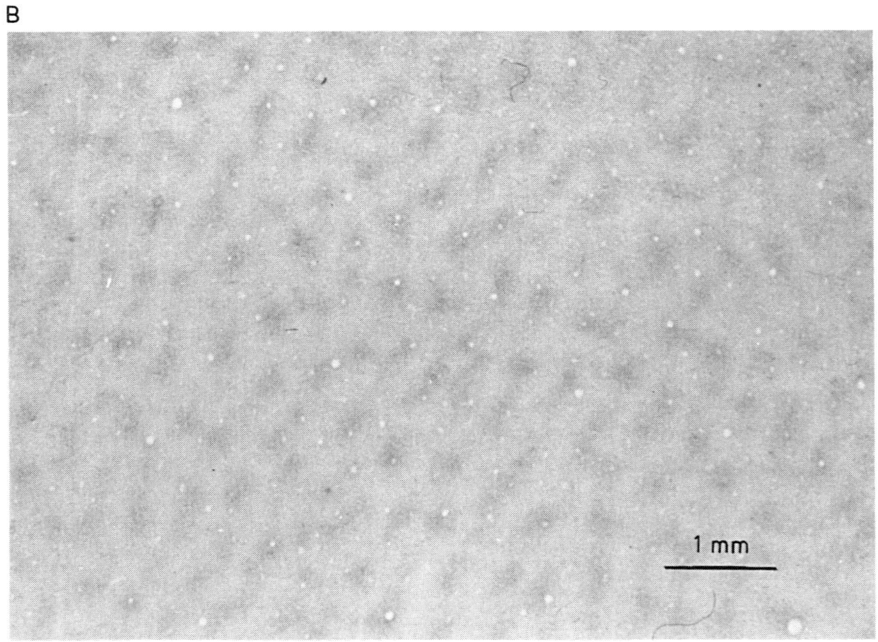

Fig. 6.5 (A) Photomicrograph of a radial section through V1, stained for the mitochondrial enzyme cytochrome oxidase. Among the prominent features are the more densely staining, repetitively occurring, blobs in layers 2 and 3. When a tangential section is taken through the latter layers and stained for cytochrome oxidase (as in B), the remarkable regularity in the distribution of the blobs is seen.

(Hubel and Wiesel, 1977) and would seem to offer powerful support for the segregatory function of V1. This kind of correlation between functional grouping and anatomically demonstrable subdivisions of cortex, revealed in this instance by enzyme histochemistry, takes the ineluctable historical tendency of subdividing the cortex into ever smaller functionally related anatomical units several orders of magnitude further.

Nor is the functional segregation restricted to V1. It also occurs in area V2, which surrounds V1 and receives a systematic, and topographically organized, input from it (Cragg, 1969; Zeki, 1969). When stained for the enzyme cytochrome oxidase, V2 also displays a characteristic distribution pattern, consisting of dark stripes extending from surface to white matter and arranged perpendicular to the border of V2 with V1. These are separated from each other by more lightly staining interstripe zones, containing lower metabolic activity. The dark stripes are of two kinds, thick and thin, although the distinction between the two is not always achieved without difficulty (Fig. 6.6). Earlier physiological recordings in V2 (Baizer, Robinson and Dow, 1977; Zeki, 1978) showed that V2, like V1, has a variety of functional cell types, including orientation-, direction- and wavelength-selective cells. In more recent recordings from V2 in which we tried to study the relationship between the distribution of functional cell groups and the cytochrome oxidase architecture, we found that wavelength-selective cells occur only in thin stripes and never in thick stripes or interstripes. And although not all cells in thin stripes were wavelength selective, some being broad-band, almost none were orientation selective. The latter were found mainly in the thick stripes and the interstripes, but none of these was found to be wavelength sensitive. Moreover, directionally selective cells were found only in the thick stripes, although they were in a minority in terms of the total number of cells sampled in thick stripes (DeYoe and Van Essen, 1985; Shipp and Zeki, 1985). These results suggest that the information that is kept separate in V1 is maintained segregated in V2 and shows, too, from the viewpoint of the localizationist tendency in the history of cerebral physiology, how V2, like V1, can be subdivided into discrete functional groupings with clear anatomical landmarks, a subdivision beyond the dreams of the most ardent localizationist.

The functional groupings in V2 are also highly interesting because of the specificity of connections that obviously confers upon cells in the different stripes the properties they possess. Thus the thin stripes of V2, which contain the wavelength-sensitive cells, are interconnected with the blobs of layers 2 and 3 of V1, which also contain wavelength-sensitive cells (Livingstone and Hubel, 1984), but have no interconnections with interblob regions, which contain orientation-selective cells. The interblobs are, instead, connected with the interstripes of V2 (Livingstone and

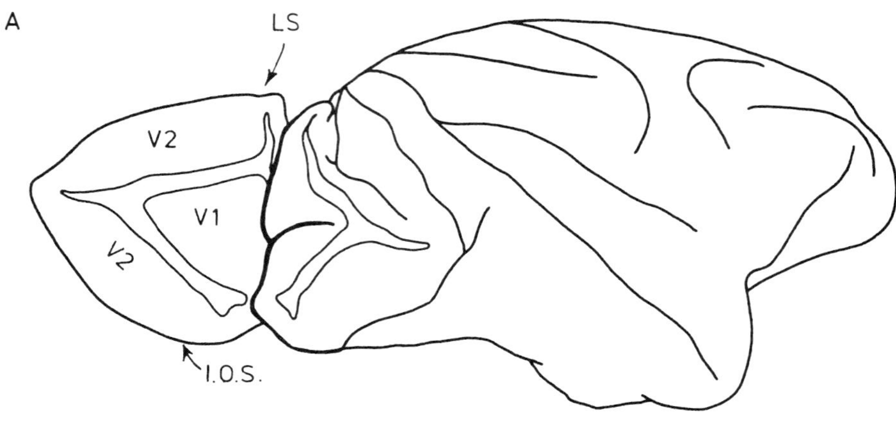

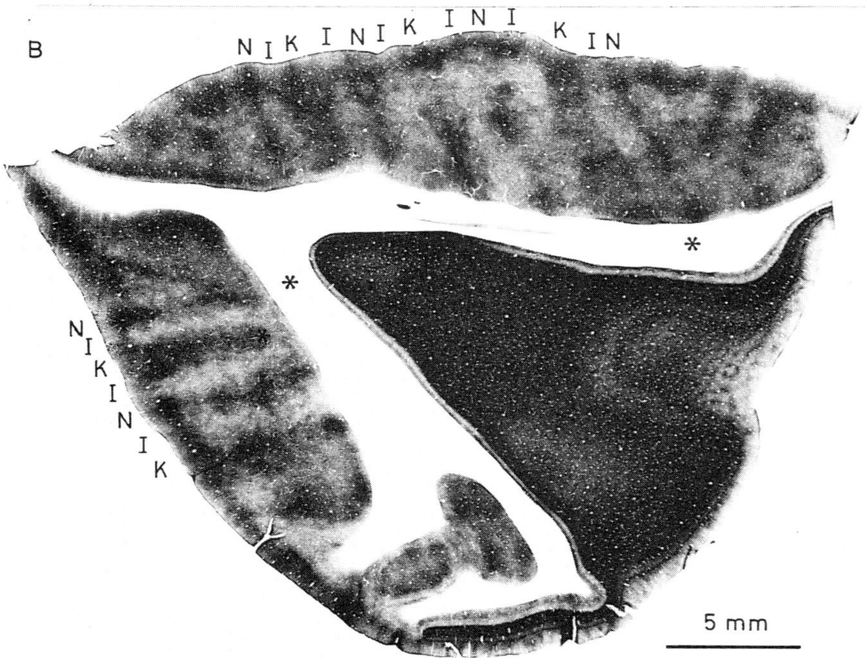

Fig. 6.6 Surface view of the right hemisphere of the brain of a macaque monkey (A) with the occipital operculum removed to reveal the portions of V2 buried in the lunate sulcus (LS) and inferior occipital sulcus (IOS). The occipital operculum so removed is flattened and sectioned in the plane of the paper and stained for the enzyme cytochrome oxidase (B) to show the pattern of thick (K) and thin (N) cytochrome oxidase stripes and the interstripe (I). (Note, stripes can occasionally be seen to bifurcate such as those indicated by the asterisk.)

Hubel, 1984). It is not, unfortunately, clear what the connections of the thick stripes may be.

Early anatomical evidence showed that, like V1, each part of V2 projects to a number of prestriate areas. Among these are its projections to V3 and V4 (Zeki, 1971) and to V5 (Zeki, 1971, 1976). Using the same argument as applied to V1, one could say that since it would be difficult to imagine that V2 sends the same information to these areas in these independent and parallel pathways, it is easier to suppose that it sends different kinds of information. As a corollary to this, it follows that V2 also segregates the information it receives or, more precisely, that the information is maintained segregated in it. Powerful evidence for this supposition has recently been obtained by using a combination of anatomical and histochemical techniques. Thus, when HRP is injected into V5, a functionally specialized visual area, and alternate sections through V2 are stained for HRP label and cytochrome oxidase activity, it is found that labelled cells are confined almost exclusively to the territory of the thick stripes, the very ones that physiological recordings show to contain the directionally selective cells (see Fig. 6.7). By contrast, when the label is injected into the V4 complex, label is found in thin stripes, which contain the wavelength-sensitive cells, as well as in the interstripes, which contain orientation-selective cells (DeYoe and Van Essen, 1985; Shipp and Zeki, 1985). Thus, to a first approximation, with many details left to be settled, the functional segregation in V2, demonstrated by physiological studies, is mirrored by a remarkable specificity of anatomical connections.

6.3 Specific defects in motion and colour perception

Present anatomical and physiological evidence suggests that, to a large extent, information relating to form, colour and motion is maintained separate, at least at early stages of the visual cortical pathways, a finding that provides insights for an understanding of the neurological basis of the visual agnosias in man. Lesions in striate cortex above a certain size (i.e. greater than 1 mm in diameter) would lead to a global scotoma affecting all visual submodalities and referable to a particular region in visual space, since such lesions would affect all the functional subgroupings in that part of the striate cortex. The greater the lesion, the more extensive the scotoma. Similarly, lesions in V2 beyond a certain size, in this case 4 mm (since this is the extent of a complete cycle of a thick stripe, a thin stripe and 2 interstripes), should also affect all visual submodalities, but lesions specific to V2 have never been reported and it is possible that

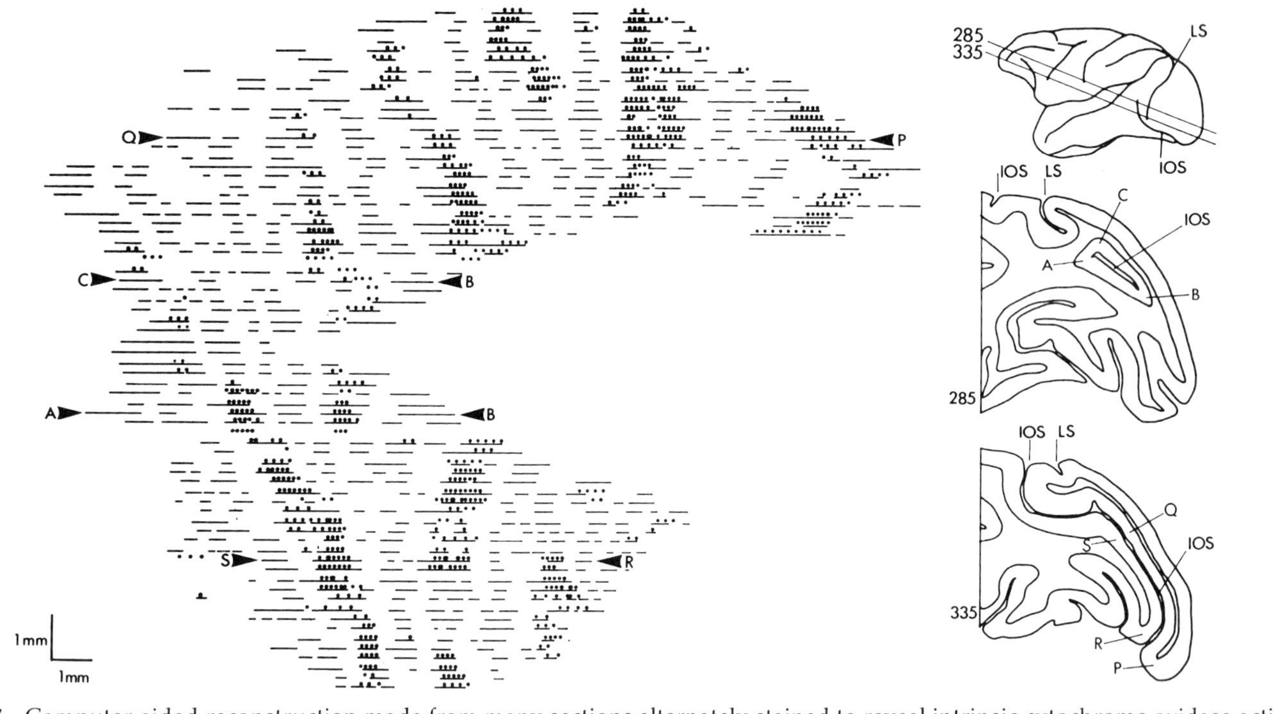

Fig. 6.7 Computer-aided reconstruction made from many sections alternately stained to reveal intrinsic cytochrome oxidase activity and the presence of HRP following an injection into V5. The information from each section was digitized and entered into a computer which could align and straighten each section according to specific landmarks. The distribution of cells is shown as dots and regions densely stained for cytochrome oxidase as broken lines. The reconstruction is symmetrical about the fundus of the inferior occipital sulcus; each line represents one horizontal section, and the diagrams of sections 285 and 338 with the marked points A,B,C,P,Q,R, and S indicate how the overall configuration relates to the anatomy of the cortex. The regions of labelled cells are predominantly centred over the thick cytochrome oxidase stripes. Conventions as in previous figures. Scale bar 1 mm for both axes. (From Shipp and Zeki (1985).)

scotomas resulting from such (theoretical) lesions will be less severe than those affecting V1, since some of the information (e.g. that destined to V5) partially bypasses V2. Among the perceptual agnosias, perhaps the simplest to understand are disturbances of motion perception. The motion pathways appear to be segregated from other pathways at the level of the striate cortex and beyond. Motion-related information, from the cells of layer 4B and upper layer 6 in V1 and from cells in the thick stripes of V2, are relayed to V5. Why V5 should receive information from both V1 and V2, which itself also receives an input from V1, remains unknown. But V5 appears to be a sort of 'motion funnel', through which all information related to motion is relayed, presumably after some kind of transformation, to other motion-related areas of the cerebral cortex, including V5A and V6 (Van Essen, Maunsell and Bixby, 1981; Maunsell and Van Essen, 1983; Zeki, 1986) and to the frontal eye fields (Barbas and Mesulam, 1981). This is the broad motion pathway, but it must not be supposed that V5 does not have other connections with areas which are not obviously motion related in character, and the significance of which is briefly discussed below. Indeed, it has connections with both V3 and V4, though these connections are not as extensive as the ones with V1 and V2. It is obvious, then, that such a system could be specifically disturbed or disrupted and that such disruption should lead to afflictions of motion perception, a specific disturbance that has been well documented by Zihl, von Cramon and Mai (1983) in a patient with a bilateral lesion in the region of the superior temporal sulcus, presumed to include the homologue of V5 in man. That lesions in V5 in monkeys lead specifically to disturbances in motion perception is less certain. While the early work of Cowey (Collin and Cowey, 1980) showed that lesions in V5 had no demonstrable effects, the later studies of Wurtz (Newsome *et al.*, 1985) showed that, after chemical lesions in V5, monkeys were impaired in their initiation of pursuit eye movements to track targets moving within the relevant part of the field of view. Since other eye movements were not affected, the authors concluded that this disability was due to interference with the animals' capacity to see exactly how the stimulus was moving. Recovery from these small, chemical, lesions was, however, rapid in onset. It seems likely that, with more extensive lesions, and ones which involve V5A, more pronounced and long-lasting defects will be produced.

The situation is a little more complex with colour vision, although perceptual defects restricted to colour vision following lesions not involving striate cortex have been described (Damasio *et al.*, 1980). All the available evidence at present shows that information relating to colour is maintained separate from that relating to form and motion in V1 and in V2. In the V4 complex, to which V2 and the foveolar part of V1 project

(Zeki, 1971, 1978; DeYoe and Van Essen, 1985; Shipp and Zeki, 1985), there are regions of high concentrations of colour-coded and wavelength-sensitive cells, separated from each other by regions having higher concentrations of orientation- but not wavelength-sensitive cells (Zeki, 1977). In addition, one subdivision of the V4 complex, V4A, contains a higher proportion of orientation-selective cells than V4 proper, in which there is a higher concentration of wavelength and colour-specific cells (Zeki, 1983a,b,c). There seems little doubt that the V4 complex is heavily involved in the analysis of colour, and lesions there in the macaque monkey have produced significant impairments in monkeys' abilities to discriminate the colour of objects when these are viewed in illuminants of different wavelength composition (Wild *et al.*, 1985). However, the recent evidence of Heywood and Cowey (personal communication) has shown that, after extensive lesions of V4, going beyond the defined boundaries and invading the inferior temporal cortex, there is, in addition to difficulties in hue discrimination, a further difficulty in form discrimination. This, together with the evidence that there are both colour and orientation-selective cells in V4 (Zeki, 1975, 1983a; Desimone *et al.*, 1985), has been taken to show that, whereas motion analysis is separate from the analysis of other attributes of the visual scene, as we suggested earlier (Zeki, 1974), the analysis of form and colour is inextricably linked.

That is certainly one conclusion that may be drawn, but it does have to face several problems. The first is that there are well-documented examples in the clinical literature of defects in colour perception without an attendant defect in the perception of form (see Meadows, 1974; Damasio *et al.*, 1980). Presumably this is due to a set of conditions in which colour pathways are specifically compromised. Secondly, with the exception of Michael's results (Michael, 1978a,b), all others show that wavelength-sensitive cells are not usually orientation selective and vice versa and, moreover, recent evidence (reviewed above) shows that the two types of cell are segregated into different, and histochemically identifiable, parts of areas V1 and V2 (Livingstone and Hubel, 1984; DeYoe and Van Essen, 1985; Hubel and Livingstone, 1985; Shipp and Zeki, 1985). Thirdly, electrophysiological evidence shows that there are many orientation-selective cells in V3 and V3A, but wavelength-sensitive cells are notably absent in these two areas (Van Essen and Zeki, 1978; Zeki, 1978; Baizer, 1982). Thus, the information on form relayed to V3 and V3A must be in some way different from that relayed to the V4 complex and used differently from the way in which it is used in the latter. Finally, it is interesting to reflect that every form has a colour (be that colour grey, or white or black) and every colour has a form, in that it is contained within a certain, definable, space. There seems little that is surprising, therefore, in having an association between form and colour, but this does not mean that the same form cannot have different colours, a fact for which there must be an underlying neurological basis. In summary, while a very strong case has now been made for the association of the V4 complex with colour vision, the case that it may be involved in the analysis of form, *independently of colour*, has yet to be made. This leaves out of account many other interesting defects, the neurological pathways for which remain only poorly understood. It is likely that prosopagnosic defects would result from lesions corresponding to that part of the cortex where so-called 'face' units have been discovered (Perret *et al.*, 1984), but the precise pathways leading to that region of the superior temporal sulcus remain to be elucidated. Equally, the losses of visual spatial orientation are likely to result from lesions in the parietal sulcus (Mountcastle *et al.*, 1984), but the precise pathways leading to that region of the cortex are only sketchily understood.

6.4 The re-entrant systems in the cortex

The demonstration of functionally specialized pathways and areas in the cerebral cortex, even when taken beyond what only a few years ago seemed 'fantastic', still leaves us with the fundamental problem of 'how the specialized parts of the cerebral cortex interact to provide the integration evident in thought and behaviour' (Lashley, 1936). The problem can be made more manageable by restriction to the visual system. A primary prerequisite is to understand the nature of anatomical connections between these different regions and subregions, subserving different submodalities of vision. There are, in theory, several ways in which cortical areas undertaking different tasks can communicate with each other. One would be for all of them to send their outputs to a common area X. In fact there are visual areas, such as the one in the intraparietal sulcus (V7), which receive inputs from more than one area, in this instance from V4 and V5 (Zeki, 1977, and unpublished results; Seltzer and Pandya, 1980; Maunsell and Van Essen, 1983), but there is no known visual area which receives information from all the prestriate areas, and hence this mode of communication seems to be an unlikely one. Another mode might be for two areas to communicate directly with each other. This is common, e.g. between V3 and V4, V4 and V5, V5 and V6 and so on. There are subvarieties of this mode of communication (see Zeki, 1987, for review), which is normally a reciprocal one. A third method would be the re-entrant system (which we distinguish from the reciprocal system) (Edelman and Finkel, 1984). A good example of a re-entrant system is provided by the connections between V1 and V5. The output from V1 to V5 is from layer 4B and layer 6, and is segregated, in the sense that cells projecting to V5 are separated from each other by cells projecting elsewhere (see Fig. 6.3). But the reverse projection, from V5 to V1, is continuous throughout layer 4B and layer 6, and thus invades the territory of cells projecting to V5 *and* elsewhere. This can be shown by injecting V5 with a cocktail of [^{3}H] proline and [^{3}H] leucine and examining the distribution of label in V1, which is then found not to be patchy or clustered in distribution, but continuous (see Fig. 6.8). Thus the back projection from V5 to layer 4B could inform cells projecting to, say V3, of the activity in V5 and hence could modify the nature of the output from layer 4B to V3. There is no evidence that it does so, and the proposition has yet to be tested, but it would be difficult to imagine that the projection from V5 does not carry some information back to V1. In a similar way, the projection from V5 back to layer 6 of V1 is not patchy or clustered around cells projecting to V5, but continuous, and it is thus not difficult to see that the anatomical machinery exists for informing cells projecting to areas outside V5 of the activity in V5.

A similar re-entrant system is in operation between V5 and V2. As shown above, only cells in thick cytochrome oxidase stripes of V2 project to V5, but the re-entrant projection from V5 to V2 is not similarly selective for the thick stripes. Instead it distributes over the interstripes and the thin stripes, the latter of which contain heavy concentrations of wavelength-sensitive cells and project to V4. Here again, we can see that there is an anatomical machinery for informing the colour system of the activity in the motion system, but how this system operates no one knows.

In summary, then, modern evidence lends powerful support to the theory of functional specialization in the visual cortex and within this lie the rudiments of an explanation for the observation of occasional very specific deficits in human visual perception. The functional localization demonstrated with modern techniques continues the historical tendency of subdividing the cortex into even smaller regions and units. Equally, however, these very same techniques provide some evidence for the way in which visual information, once fractionated, can be re-integrated to give us our unitary perception of the visual world.

Acknowledgement

The author's work reported here was supported by grants from the SERC and the Wellcome Trust.

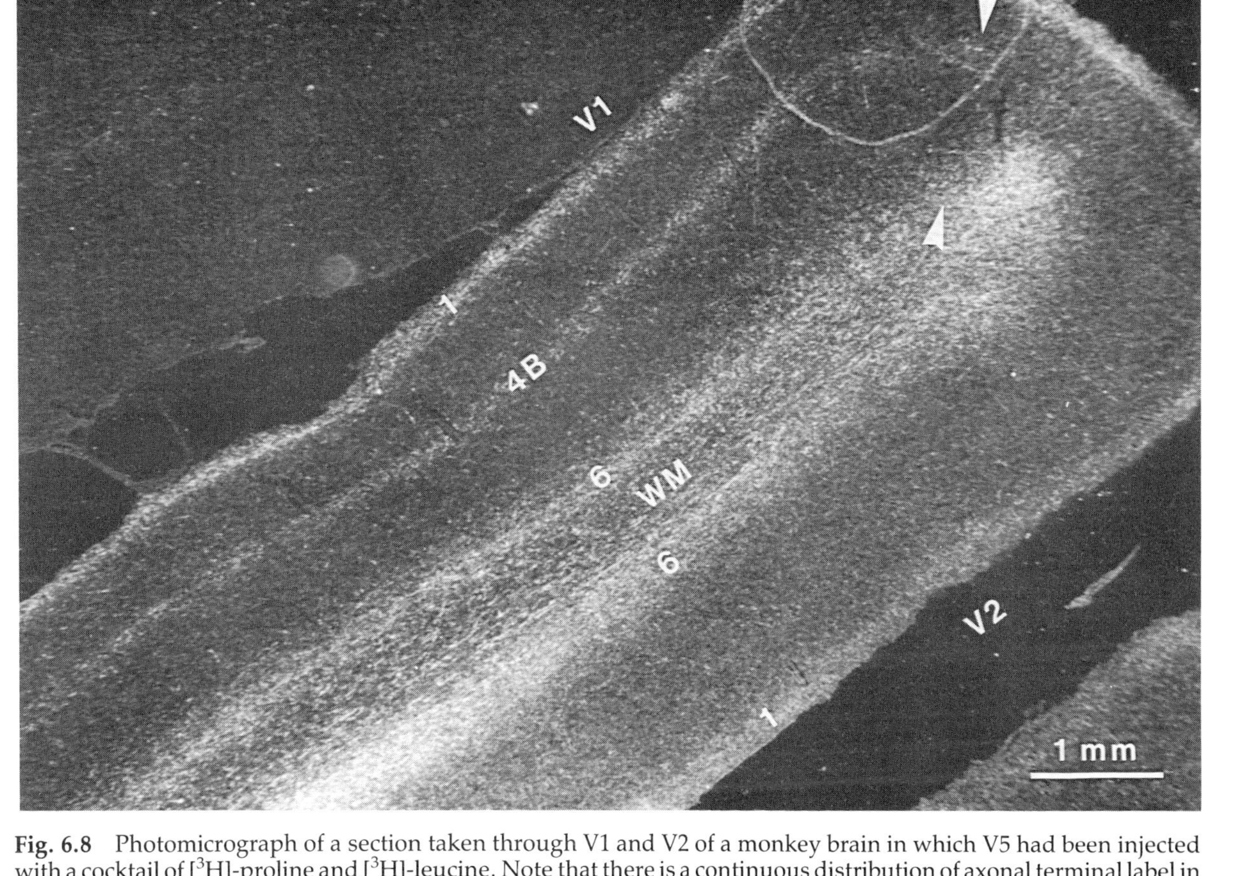

Fig. 6.8 Photomicrograph of a section taken through V1 and V2 of a monkey brain in which V5 had been injected with a cocktail of [^{3}H]-proline and [^{3}H]-leucine. Note that there is a continuous distribution of axonal terminal label in layers 1,4B and 6 of V1 and layers 1 and 6 of V2. In contrast the distributions of labelled cells (revealed by retrograde HRP transport, see Figs 6.3 and 6.7) are more clustered in both V1 and V2. WM = white matter. The V1/V2 boundary lies between the two arrowheads. Scale bar = 1 mm. The slide from which this photomicrograph was prepared was kindly supplied by Professors Galetti and Squattrito.

References

Baizer, J.S. (1982) Receptive field properties of V3 neurons in monkey. *Invest. Ophthalmol.*, **23**, 87–95.

Baizer, J.S., Robinson, D.L. and Dow, B.M. (1977) Visual responses of area 18 neurons in awake behaving monkey. *J. Neurophysiol.*, **40**, 1024–37.

Barbas, H. and Mesulam, M.M. (1981) Organization of afferent input to subdivisions of area 8 in the rhesus monkey. *J. Comp. Neurol.*, **200**, 407–31.

Beck, E. (1934) Der Occipitallen des Affen (*Macacus rhesus*) und des Menschen in seiner cytoarchitektonischen Struktur. I. Teil *Macacus rhesus. J. Psychol. Neurol., Leipzig*, **4b**, 193–323.

Broca, P. (1861) Remarques sur le siege de la faculté de language articulé suivies d'une observation d'aphemie. *Bull. Soc. Anat. Paris*, **6**, 330–57.

Brodmann, K. (1905) Beiträge zur histologischen lokalisation der grosshirnrinde. *J. Psychol. Neurol.*, **4**, 176–226.

Burkhalter, A., Felleman, D.J., Newsome, W.T. and Van Essen, D.C. (1986) Anatomical and physiological asymmetries related to visual areas V3 and VP in macaque ultrastriate cortex. *Vision Res.*, **26**, 63–80.

Collin, N.G. and Cowey, A. (1980) The effect of ablation of frontal eye fields and superior colliculi on visual stability and movement discrimination in rhesus monkeys. *Exp. Brain Res.*, **40**, 251–60.

Cragg, B.G. (1969) The topography of the afferent projections in the circumstriate visual cortex of the monkey studied by the Nauta method. *Vision Res.*, **9**, 733–47.

Damasio, A., Yamada, T., Damasio, H., Corbett, J. and McKee, J. (1980) Central achromatopsia: behavioural anatomic and physiologic aspects. *Neurology*, **30**, 1064–71.

Desimone, R., Schein, S.J., Moran, J. and Ungerleider, L.G. (1985) Contour, colour and shape analysis beyond the striate cortex. *Vision Res.*, **25**, 441–52.

DeYoe, E.A. and Van Essen, D.C. (1985) Segregation of efferent connections and receptive field properties in visual area V2 of the macaque. *Nature*, **317**, 58–61.

Economo, C. von and Koskinas, G.N. (1925) *Cytoarchitektonic der Grosshirnrinde des Erwachsen Menschen*. Springer, Berlin u. Wien.

Edelman, G.M. and Finkel, L.H. (1984) Neuronal group selection in the cerebral cortex, in *Dynamic Aspects of Neocortical Function* (eds G. M. Edelman, W. E. Gall and W. M. Cowan), Wiley, New York, pp. 653–95.

Filiminoff, N.I. (1936) Über die variabilitat der Grosshirnrindenstruktur Mitteilung III Regio occipitalis bei den höheren und niederen Affen. *J. Psychol. Neurol.*, **45**, 69–137.

Fritsch, G. and Hitzig, E. (1870) Ueber die elektrische Erregbarkeit des Grosshirns. *Arch. Anat., Physiol. wissensch. Med.* (Reichert and Du Bois-Reymond), p. 300.

Gattass, R. and Gross, C.G. (1981) Visual topography of striate projection zone (MT) in posterior superior temporal sulcus of the macaque. *J. Neurophysiol.*, **46**, 621–38.

Hubel, D.H. and Livingstone, M.S. (1985) Complex-unoriented cells in a subregion of primate area 18. *Nature*, **315**, 325–7.

Hubel, D.H. and Wiesel, T.N. (1962) Receptive fields, binocular interaction and functional architecture in the cat's visual cortex. *J. Physiol.*, **160**, 106–54.

Hubel, D.H. and Wiesel, T.N. (1965) Receptive fields and functional architecture in two non-striate visual areas (18 and 19) of the cat. *J. Neurophysiol.*, **28**, 229–89.

Hubel, D.H. and Wiesel, T.B. (1977) Functional architecture of macaque monkey visual cortex. *Proc. R. Soc. Lond. B*, **198**, 1–59.

Kleist, K. (1937) Bericht uber die Gehimpathologie in ihrer Bedentung fur Neurologie und Psychiatrie. *Z. ges. Neurol.*, **158**, 159–93.

Kuypers, H.G.J.M., Szwarcbart, M.K., Mishkin, M. and Rosvold, H.E. (1965) Occipitotemporal corticocortical connections in the rhesus monkey. *Exp. Neurol.*, **11**, 245–62.

Lashley, K.S. (1936) *Mass Action in Cerebral Function.* Harvey Lecture Series 26, p. 46.

Lashley, K.S. and Clark, G. (1946) The cytoarchitecture of the cerebral cortex of Ateles: a critical examination of architectonic studies. *J. Comp. Neurol.*, **85**, 223–305.

Livingstone, M.S. and Hubel, D.H. (1984) Anatomy and physiology of a colour system in the primate visual cortex. *J. Neurosci.*, **4**, 309–56.

Lund, J.S., Hendrickson, A.E., Ogren, M.P. and Tobin, E.A. (1981) Anatomical organization of primate visual cortex area VII. *J. Comp. Neurol.*, **202**, 14–45.

Lund, J.S., Lund, R.D., Hendrickson, A.E., Bunt, A.H. and Fuchs, A.F. (1975) The origin of efferent pathways from the primary visual cortex (area 17) of the macaque monkey as shown by retrograde transport of horseradish peroxidase. *J. Comp. Neurol.*, **164**, 287–304.

Maunsell, J.H.R. and Van Essen, D.C. (1983) The connections of the middle temporal visual area (MT) and their relationship to a cortical hierarchy in the macaque monkey. *J. Neurosci.*, **3**, 2563–86.

Meadows, J.C. (1974) Disturbed perception of colours associated with localized cerebral lesions. *Brain*, **97**, 615–32.

Michael, C.R. (1978a) Colour vision mechanisms in monkey striate cortex: simple cells with dual opponent-color receptive fields. *J. Neurophysiol.*, **41**, 1233–49.

Michael, C.R. (1978b) Colour-sensitive complex cells in monkey striate cortex. *J. Neurophysiol.*, **41**, 1250–66.

Mountcastle, V.B., Motter, B.C., Skeinmetz, M.A. and Duffy, C.J. (1984) Looking and Seeing: The visual functions of the parietal lobe, in *Dynamic Aspects of Neocortical Function* (eds G.M. Edelman, W.E. Gall and W.M. Cowan). Wiley, New York, pp. 159–93.

Movshon, J.A., Adelson, E.H., Gizzi, M.S. and Newsome, W.T. (1984) The analysis of moving visual patterns, in *Pattern Recognition Mechanisms* (eds C. Chagass, R. Gattass and C.G. Gross). Pontf. Ac. Sc. Scripta Varia 54, pp. 117–51.

Munk, H. (1881) *Ueber die Funktionen der Grosshirnrinde*, Berlin.

Newsome, W.T., Wurtz, R.H., Dursteler, M.R. and Mikami, A. (1985) Deficits in visual motion processing following ibotenic acid lesions of the middle temporal visual area of the macaque monkey. *J. Neurosci.*, **5**, 825–40.

Perret, D.I., Smith, P.A.J., Potter, D.D., Mistlen, A.J., Head, A.S., Milner, A.D.

and Joeves, M.A. (1984) Neurones responsive to faces in the temporal cortex: studies of functional organisation, sensitivity to identity and relation to perception. *Human Neurobiol.*, **3**, 197–208.

Poggio, G.F., Baker, F.H., Mansfield, R.J.W., Sillito, A. and Grigg, P. (1975) Spatial and chromatic properties of neurons subserving foveal and parafoveal vision in rhesus monkey. *Brain Res.*, **100**, 25–59.

Rockland, K.S. and Pandya, D.N. (1979) Laminar origins and terminations of cortical connections of the occipital lobe in the rhesus monkey. *Brain Res.*, **179**, 3–20.

Seltzer, B. and Pandya, D.N. (1980) Converging visual and somatic sensory cortical input to the intraparietal sulcus of the rhesus monkey. *Brain Res.*, **192**, 339–51.

Shipp, S. and Zeki, S. (1985) Segregation of pathways leading from area V2 to areas V4 and V5 of macaque monkey visual cortex. *Nature*, **315**, 322–5.

Sholl, D.A. (1956) *The Organization of the Cerebral Cortex.* Mathew, London.

Van Essen, D.C. and Zeki, S. (1978) The topographic organization of rhesus monkey prestriate cortex. *J. Physiol.*, **277**, 193–226.

Van Essen, D.C., Maunsell, J.H.R. and Bixby, J.L. (1981) The middle temporal visual area in the macaque: Myeloarchitecture, connections, functional properties and topographic organisation. *J. Comp. Neurol.*, **199**, 293–326.

Wild, H.M., Butler, D., Carden, D. and Kulikowski, J.J. (1985) Primate cortical area V4 important for colour constancy but not wavelength discrimination. *Nature*, **313**, 133–5.

Zeki, S. (1969a) The secondary visual areas of the monkey. *Brain Res.*, **13**, 197–226.

Zeki, S. (1969b) Representation of central fields in prestriate cortex of monkey. *Brain Res.*, **19**, 63–75.

Zeki, S. (1970) Interhemispheric connections of prestriate cortex in monkey. *Brain Res.*, **19**, 63–75.

Zeki, S. (1971) Cortical projections from two prestriate areas in the monkey. *Brain Res.*, **34**, 19–35.

Zeki, S. (1974) Functional organization of a visual area in the posterior bank of the superior temporal sulcus of the rhesus monkey. *J. Physiol.*, **236**, 549–73.

Zeki, S. (1975) The functional organization of projections from striate to prestriate visual cortex in the rhesus monkey. *Cold Spring Harbor Symp. Quant. Biol.*, **15**, 591–600.

Zeki, S. (1976) The projections to the superior temporal sulcus from areas 17 and 18 in the rhesus monkey. *Proc. R. Soc. Lond. B*, **193**, 199–207.

Zeki, S. (1977) Colour coding in the superior temporal sulcus of rhesus monkey visual cortex. *Proc. R. Soc. B*, **197**, 195–223.

Zeki, S. (1978) Uniformity and diversity of structure and function in rhesus monkey prestriate visual cortex. *J. Physiol.*, **277**, 273–90.

Zeki, S. (1983a) The distribution of wavelength and orientation selective cells in different areas of monkey visual cortex. *Proc. R. Soc. Lond. B*, **217**, 449–70.

Zeki, S. (1983b) Colour coding in the cerebral cortex: the reaction of cells in monkey visual cortex to wavelengths and colours. *Neuroscience*, **9**, 741–65.

Zeki, S. (1983c) Colour coding in the cerebral cortex: the responses of wavelength-selective and colour-coded cells in monkey visual cortex to changes in wavelength composition. *Neuroscience*, **9**, 767–81.

Zeki, S. (1984) Looking and seeing, in *The Scientific Basis of Clinical Neurology* (eds C. Kennard and M. Swash). Churchill-Livingstone, Edinburgh, pp. 172–87.

Zeki, S. (1985) Colour pathways and hierarchies in the cerebral cortex, in *Central and Peripheral Mechanisms of Colour Vision* (Wenner-Gren Center International Symposium Series, Vol. 43) (eds D. Ottoson and S. Zeki). Macmillan, London, pp. 19–44.

Zeki, S. (1986) The anatomy and physiology of area V6 of macaque monkey visual cortex. *J. Physiol.*, **381**, 62P.

Zeki, S. (1987) The functional logic of anatomical connections in the cerebral cortex (in preparation).

Zihl, J., von Cramon, D. and Mai, N. (1983) Selective disturbance of movement vision after bilateral brain damage. *Brain*, **106**, 313–40.

CHAPTER 7

Residual vision following lesions of the retrogeniculate visual pathways

CHRISTOPHER KENNARD

7.1 Introduction

Lesions of the retrogeniculate visual pathways, particularly the striate cortex in man, have traditionally been considered to result in complete and permanent visual field loss in an area topographically related to the area damaged (Holmes, 1918). Although some limited return of function occasionally took place, such as movement (Riddoch, 1917) or colour perception (Hine, 1918), Holmes attributed this to degraded vision resulting from incomplete damage to the striate cortex, a view held despite observations (Munk, 1881; Luciani and Seppilli, 1886) that total removal of the striate cortex in monkeys left some degree of visual function (cited in Weiskrantz, 1980). These animal results were confirmed by Kluver (1942), and subsequent clinical observations in humans with occipital lobe lesions did indicate the presence of some residual vision, but this was of only the most primitive visual functions such as the control of pupil size (Magoun, Ranson and Mayer, 1935), the presence of the blink reflex (Edinger and Fischer, 1913; Levinsohn, 1913) and a preserved sensitivity to changes in illumination (Brindley, Gautier-Smith and Lewin, 1969). Unfortunately, most of these observations were based on crude uncontrolled clinical observations, and it is only in the past 15 years or so that there has been renewed interest in the concept of residual visual capabilities in both non-human primates and man. In this chapter these studies will be reviewed with the following aims: to describe the extent and limits of visual recovery in monkeys following ablation of the striate cortex and the likely visual areas subserving this function; similarly in man, to describe experiments on residual vision, often termed 'blind-sight' (Weiskrantz *et al.*, 1974), after lesions of the occipital lobe; and finally, the functional significance of this residual vision and the possible effect of systematic training techniques for enhancing recovery will be reviewed.

7.2 Primate studies

7.2.1 EXTENT OF VISUAL CAPACITIES

The studies of Kluver (1941, 1942), in which he completely removed bilaterally the striate cortex of monkeys, revealed a residual ability to discriminate stimuli differing in total luminous flux, but an inability to see visual properties such as brightness, colour, shape and to judge the dimensions of space. There was then a 20-year hiatus in this line of investigation until Gross and Weiskrantz (1959) and Pasik, Pasik and Bender (1961) challenged these findings, leading to an extensive reinvestigation of the visual capacities of destriate monkeys. Humphrey (1970), in a single case study of a monkey with bilateral striate cortex ablations, showed that she was capable of avoiding obstacles and was sensitive to small objects. Subsequent studies revealed that such monkeys retain the capacity for spatial localization shown by their ability to localize accurately light spots by reaching (Weiskrantz, Cowey and Passingham, 1977; Keating, 1980), and recovered reactions to differences in total luminous flux (Schilder, Pasik and Pasik, 1971). They could also be trained to discriminate a variety of flux-equated figures utilizing brightness and shape (Schilder, Pasik and Pasik, 1971), lines of different orientation (Pasik *et al.*, 1976), spatial frequency (Miller, Pasik and Pasik, 1980) and wavelength cues (Schilder, Pasik and Pasik, 1972; Keating, 1979), but the sensitivity of these attributes was greatly reduced, although an estimate of the visual acuity placed it no worse than the 20/80 level on the Snellen chart (Pasik and Pasik, 1982).

7.2.2 NEURAL CENTRES RESPONSIBLE FOR RESIDUAL VISION

There are a number of non-striate retinal projections which could mediate the residual visual function found in destriate monkeys. These include projections to the accessory optic nucleus and the superior colliculus, the latter projecting indirectly via the pulvinar to the prestriate cortex. In addition the prestriate cortex itself receives a sparse, but direct, visual projection from the dorsal lateral geniculate nucleus (Fries, 1981; Yukie and Iwai, 1981).

Early studies suggested that one reason why Kluver's destriate monkeys had so little return of visual function was that his lesions included the prestriate regions (areas 18 and 19). When such lesions were reproduced, the monkeys were able to make visual discriminations solely on the basis of the flux differences (Pasik and Pasik, 1971), and could not then be trained to achieve the visual discriminations found in animals with ablations of only the striate cortex. The same impairment of residual visual function was found in destriate monkeys in whom aspiration of the superior colliculi or pulvinar was added, indicating that it is the retino-collicular–pulvinar–prestriate cortex pathway which enables retention of the ability to discriminate figures equated for flux. An important function of the superior colliculus, independent of the visual cortex, is shown by monkeys with extensive striate and prestriate cortical ablations who are still able to locate light spots by pointing (Keating, 1980; Solomon, Pasik and Pasik, 1981), a task which requires both stimulus detection and then spatial localization. The monkey loses this ability when bilateral ablation of the striate cortex and superior colliculi are combined (Solomon, Pasik and Pasik, 1981). Using a different means of spatial localization, the accuracy of saccadic eye movements to a target, Mohler and Wurtz (1977) showed the effect of partial lesions to corresponding (in terms of visual field co-ordinate position) regions of the striate cortex and superior colliculus. If either was damaged there was a recovery of spatial localization which did not occur when both lesions were made. These experiments are of additional interest since it was shown that, following a partial striate cortex ablation, systematic training of light sensitivity produced a recovery of the ability to detect and localize targets within the scotoma. When this training was given to only one part of the scotoma, visual function returned to a greater extent in that part compared with the unpractised part of the scotoma (see Section 7.3.4).

The results of the experiments so far discussed suggest a dichotomy of function in the visual pathways. The retino-geniculo-striate pathway is concerned with pattern discrimination ('what things are') and the retino-collicular pathway with spatial localization ('where things are'). This 'two visual systems' hypothesis, as originally proposed by Schneider (1969) on the basis of lesion studies in the hamster, and Trevarthen (1968), has dominated interpretations of experiments in this field, despite those experiments already described which show that, following collicular ablation alone, the cortical visual areas are capable of good spatial as well as pattern vision. It would appear that there is a more complex relationship between these various visual functions and the anatomical connections. Ungerleider and Mishkin (1982) have argued for a 'two cortical systems' hypothesis in primates, in which there is a dorsal striate–prestriate–parietal system serving spatial vision and a ventral, striate–prestriate–inferior temporal system serving pattern vision. In view of the considerable reciprocal connections between the colliculus and the striate and prestriate cortical visual areas, some direct and others indirect, it appears that in the intact animal there are additional interactions between both of these cortical visual systems and the superior colliculus.

7.3 Human studies

7.3.1 RESIDUAL VISION AND 'BLINDSIGHT'

Recent interest in the possibility of residual visual function in human patients with lesions of the retrogeniculate visual pathways can be said to have originated with the first properly controlled study by Poppel, Held and Frost (1973). They introduced the technique of forced choice guessing in which four patients with lesions of the occipital lobe were briefly presented with a moving visual stimulus in their blind visual field. The subjects were instructed to move their eyes towards the target and although totally unaware of its presence they showed a significant correlation between target positions and the amplitudes of the corresponding saccades, at least for eccentricities out to about 25°. In an extensive investigation of patient DB, who had had an almost complete resection of the right calcarine cortex, Weiskrantz *et al.* (1974) found a remarkable degree of residual visual function in his blind homonymous hemianopia. This not only included accurate spatial localization by finger pointing and eye movements to targets presented in the 'blind' field, but also an ability to discriminate between horizontal, vertical and diagonal lines, and between shapes, e.g. 'x' and 'o', and to detect fine sine-wave gratings. They called this residual visual function 'blindsight' to indicate that it was not consciously perceived. Since then the extent of 'blindsight' has been investigated in numerous studies. It is important to recognize that this visual function is present in a scotoma as defined by conventional perimetric testing resulting from a retrogeniculate lesion. It is often stated that patients with 'blindsight' totally lack awareness of the stimuli presented in the scotoma (see Campion, Latto and Smith, 1983) but, in a number of studies (Barbur, Ruddock and Waterfield, 1980; Weiskrantz, 1980; Ross Russell and Bharucha, 1984; Blythe, Kennard and Ruddock, 1987), patients with lesions of the striate cortex have been reported to be consciously aware of the onset of a bright, sometimes moving, target presented in the scotoma, although they are unable to give an adequate description of what it is they have 'seen'. It is only by performing objective measurements using forced choice techniques that the true extent of their residual vision can be determined. It seems probable, however, that the residual visual function found following retrogeniculate lesions in subjects, both with and without conscious awareness of the stimuli, is an expression of similar neural activity and merely represent differences in the degree of responsiveness, although the possibility that they represent completely independent neuronal activities cannot be excluded.

A number of different experimental paradigms have demonstrated a variety of residual visual capacities. The results of Poppel, Held and Frost (1973) using saccadic localization have been confirmed (Perenin and Jeannerod, 1978; Zihl, 1981; Zihl and Werth, 1984; Blythe, Kennard and Ruddock, 1987), as has similar accurate manual localization by finger pointing to 'unseen' targets (Bender and Krieger, 1951; Weiskrantz *et al.*, 1974; Perenin and Jeannerod, 1975, 1978; Perenin, Ruel and Hecaen, 1980; Bridgeman and Staggs, 1982; Blythe, Kennard and Ruddock, 1987). In comparison with the frequency with which spatial localization has been reported, forced-choice form and orientation discrimination has been convincingly shown in only a few patients (Weiskrantz *et al.*, 1974; Perenin, 1978). Other experiments have shown an ability to complete figures presented across the vertical meridian (the completion effect) (Warrington, 1962; Williams and Gassel, 1962), the identification of figures (full and half circles) presented in, outside and across hemianopic areas (Torjussen, 1976), a primitive form of stereopsis (Richards, 1973), the tilt after-effect (Pizzamiglio, Antonuccia and Francia, 1984) and an ability to discriminate displacements of targets when two lights are flashed sequentially (Blythe *et al.*, 1986).

Although it has been argued (Campion, Latto and Smith, 1983) that many of the positive results in studies on residual vision are due to scattered light being perceived by the 'seeing' visual field, a number of experiments have shown this cannot explain the results obtained (Barbur, Ruddock and Waterfield, 1980; Barbur and Ruddock, 1983; Weiskrantz, 1983; Zihl and Werth, 1984; Stoerig, Hubner and Poppel, 1985).

7.3.2 NEURAL CENTRES RESPONSIBLE FOR RESIDUAL VISION

Whereas in animal experiments well-defined regions of the striate and prestriate cortex can be ablated, with subsequent histological verification of the extent of the lesion, this is obviously not possible in man. In man, both infarction and trauma, the commonest aetiologies, result in varying degrees of damage not only to the visual cortex (striate and extrastriate) but also to geniculostriate fibres in the optic radiation. Assessments of the extent of the lesion in cases of residual vision are often underestimated by computerized tomographic (CT) X-ray brain scans and post-mortem verification has not, as yet, become available in the cases so far studied. It needs to be stated from the outset, therefore, that the centres responsible for residual vision in man are hypothetically based and largely dependent on comparison with experiments in subhuman primates.

In man three neural pathways have been suggested as capable of mediating residual vision:

1. residual primary visual projection, either striate cortex or optic radiation;
2. the projection from the lateral geniculate nucleus to the extrastriate cortex;
3. the retino-collicular pathways, with or without projections from the colliculus to the extrastriate cortex via the pulvinar.

The possibility that the spontaneous recovery of hemianopias is due to the presence of a residue of the primary visual pathways was originally proposed by Holmes (1918), and a similar hypothesis has been proposed to explain residual vision (Brindley, Gautier-Smith and Lewin, 1969; Poppel, Held and Frost, 1973; Weiskrantz *et al.*, 1974). This is particularly hard to refute because of the inadequate delineation of lesions in man, as already mentioned, but also the fact that in monkeys the presence of as little as 5% of the geniculostriate projection is adequate for the animals to make quite complex visual discriminations (Keating, 1980). It is only in cases of hemidecortication (Perenin, 1978; Perenin and Jeannerod, 1978), or surgical ablation of the striate cortex (Weiskrantz *et al.*, 1974), that residual vision is known to be mediated without the retino-geniculostriate pathways. In a study of six patients with infantile hemiplegia, who were hemidecorticated in early life for intractable epileptic seizures, Perenin and Jeannerod (1978) found a significant correlation between the position of bright targets within the hemianopic field and the position of corresponding hand pointings. In addition they found significant coarse pattern discrimination (e.g. triangles vs circles; horizontal vs vertical lines), also reported in the patient of Weiskrantz *et al.* (1974). It is perhaps worth considering that all but one of the hemidecorticated patients were less than 10 years old at the time of their operation, and it is possible that a part at least of their residual visual capacity was associated with adaptive mechanisms in other visual pathways only available in the developing brain.

The second neural pathway considered a candidate for mediating residual vision is that from the lateral geniculate nucleus to the extrastriate cortex. This has been shown to be sparse in monkeys (Benevento and

Yoshida, 1981; Fries, 1981; Yukie and Iwai, 1981; Bullier and Kennedy, 1983), and is presumed to exist in man without any direct evidence for its presence. The precise role of this pathway in visual processing even in monkeys is still unclear, as is the extent to which it might degenerate following a lesion of the optic radiation or striate cortex. As a consequence of these uncertainties the role of the geniculo-extrastriate pathway in residual visual function is extremely hypothetical.

The third neural pathway which may be involved in mediating residual visual function is the retino-collicular projection on which most attention has been focused. It has already been mentioned that the superior colliculus projects to the extrastriate cortex via the pulvinar, in this way bringing visual information via the retino-collicular projection to the cortical level. Following lesions of the striate cortex this pathway might be crucial for visual information to be 'consciously' perceived. It is still unknown whether or not the presence of this indirect pathway to the cortex is essential for residual visual function, although in the hemidecorticated patients (Perenin and Jeannerod, 1978) residual function is presumably mediated in the colliculi alone, since following such a lesion in monkeys there is degeneration of the pulvinar nucleus (Van Buren, 1963). If, however, all residual visual function found in human subjects is solely due to collicular function it is somewhat surprising that saccadic localization, considered to be one of its main roles in normal primates (Schiller and Sandell, 1983), is rather poorly performed in a number of human studies (Weiskrantz *et al.*, 1974), despite excellent saccadic localization in monkeys after ablations of the striate cortex (Mohler and Wurtz, 1977). Poppel (1977) has suggested that the reason for such a poor response is analogous to the Sprague effect found in cats (Sprague, 1966). The superior colliculus receives both a facilitory and inhibitory input from the ipsilateral striate cortex and contralateral colliculus respectively. Damage to the striate cortex would, therefore, result in reduced facilitation on the ipsilateral superior colliculus so reducing its inhibitory input on the contralateral colliculus. This in turn results in increased activity in the contralateral colliculus thereby increasing its inhibitory drive on the ipsilateral colliculus which reduces its functional capacity.

7.3.3 FACTORS DETERMINING THE PRESENCE OR ABSENCE OF RESIDUAL VISION

In the previous section the presence or destruction of various neural pathways and connections was discussed in relation to the possible anatomical substrate for residual vision.

From a review of the literature the presence of residual vision, whether it be saccadic or finger pointing localization or pattern discrimination, appears to be an infrequent finding judging from the small number of cases reported. Weiskrantz (1980), in the largest reported series, found only 14 out of 69 with retrogeniculate lesions who showed clear evidence of residual vision. Unfortunately, no attempt was made to correlate the presence or absence of residual vision with patient variables such as age, sex and the aetiology or extent of the lesion in the occipital lobe. In an attempt to study the role of these possible factors Blythe, Kennard and Ruddock (1987) examined 25 consecutive patients suffering from occipital lobe damage resulting in dense (as perimetrically determined) homonymous hemianopias or quadrantanopias. Of these patients only five were able consciously to perceive, albeit vaguely, the onset of a bright moving target in their 'blind' visual field, and it was only in these patients that evidence of residual function was found. These patients were able to make accurate saccades and point to targets, and showed sensitivity in the detection of movement which although reduced did increase as the target speed was increased. Neither the extent of the occipital lobe lesion, as determined by CT scan, or its aetiology (vascular, infarction or trauma) correlated with the presence or absence of the residual vision, but analysis of the age of these five patients at the time of occurrence of their occipital lesion showed that three were less than 10 years of age, one was 23 years and the fifth was unknown. This is in comparison with the other 20 patients in whom the lesion occurred at 20 years of age or over. This, in association with the residual visual function in the hemidecorticate patients previously mentioned (Perenin and Jeannerod, 1978), suggests that if the cortical lesion occurs in the early years, when the brain shows evidence of considerable plasticity, residual vision is more likely to be found. Despite this possibility it must be remembered that a number of cases of residual vision reported in the literature are subjects in whom the lesion occurred at a later age.

7.3.4 THE EFFECT OF TRAINING PROCEDURES ON IMPROVING VISUAL FUNCTION

It has been known for some time that following lesions of the geniculostriate pathway there may be some recovery of visual function (Pöppelreuter, 1917; Riddoch, 1917; Hine, 1918). The aetiology of the lesion to some degree determines the extent of this recovery. Following vascular infarction there may be some initial recovery within the first 7–14 days but subsequently there is a poor prognosis for further recovery (Gloning, Gloning and Tschabitscher, 1962; Haerer, 1973), whereas traumatic damage (mostly due to gunshot wounds) is often followed by considerable recovery (Hine, 1918; Teuber, Battersby and Bender, 1960).

Although several studies of natural recovery have been carried out, systematic attempts to restore visual function after occipital lobe lesions have rarely been reported until recently. Pöppelreuter (1917) trained hemianopic patients mainly in reading, a visual function often causing difficulty to such patients, and found a markedly improved reading performance. Using similar training techniques Preobrazhenskaya (cited by Luria, 1963) reported an enlargement of the perifoveal visual field, again resulting in an improved reading performance. It was the animal experiments of Cowey (1967) and Mohler and Wurtz (1977), described earlier, which showed that, in primates after striate cortex lesions, systematic training resulted in the restoration of detection and localization of light stimuli, which led Zihl and von Cramon (1979, 1985) to study such training techniques in man. Using a psychophysical method in which light difference thresholds were determined repeatedly at the border of the visual field defect in 12 patients, Zihl and von Cramon (1979) showed an improvement in contrast sensitivity and an increase in size of the visual field. The improvement was confined to the trained visual field area and showed interocular transfer indicating its central nature. In further studies (Zihl, 1981; Zihl and von Cramon, 1985) they used a saccadic training technique, in which patients with homonymous visual field defects were forced to make saccadic eye movements to light targets presented briefly in the perimetrically blind regions. This systematic treatment led, in the majority of their 55 patients, to an enlargement of the visual field, an improvement which could not be attributed to spontaneous recovery, since in periods without systematic treatment no spontaneous increase in the visual field was observed. The enlarged visual field, which showed a return of form and colour vision, appeared to remain unchanged even after the treatment had ended. Symptomatically, many of the patients reported improvements in their reading performance and of their avoidance of obstacles located at the affected side. Objective measurement of reading performance confirmed this subjective impression, but part of this improvement in reading may not have been due to enlargement of the visual field but to an improved eye movement strategy. It has been shown that hemianopic patients may develop new and compensatory eye and head movement strategies in order to compensate for their field loss (Gassel and Williams, 1966; Meienberg *et al.*, 1981; Zangemeister *et al.*, 1982).

7.4 Conclusion

There are still many unresolved problems relating to the presence of residual vision in patients with retrogeniculate lesions. It is still unclear why it is that some patients appear to possess residual vision and others do not, despite apparently similar lesions as shown on CT scan (Blythe, Kennard and Ruddock, 1987). This may well be due to an inadequate delineation of cortical damage by CT scanning, and hopefully newer imaging techniques such as nuclear magnetic resonance and positron emission tomography will better define the remaining functional visual areas.

The possible importance of the patient's age at the occurrence of the lesion in determining the extent of residual vision needs further evaluation with larger numbers of patients.

The results of Zihl and von Cramon are very exciting, offering for the first time the possibility of improving visual performance (visual field or saccadic strategy) in patients who are often disabled by the persistence of their hemianopia. There is an urgent need for these results to be reproduced by other centres, especially after the failure of Balliet, Blood and Bach-y-rita (1985) to do so using similar techniques.

References

Balliet, R., Blood, K.M.T. and Bach-y-rita, P. (1985) Visual field rehabilitation in the cortically blind? *J. Neurol. Neurosurg. Psychiat.*, **48**, 1113–24.

Barbur, J.K. and Ruddock, K.H. (1983) The analysis of scattered light effects in hemianopic and normal vision. *Behav. Brain Sci.*, **3**, 448–9.

Barbur, J.L., Ruddock, K.H. and Waterfield, V.A. (1980) Human visual responses in the absence of the geniculo-calcarine tract. *Brain*, **103**, 905–28.

Bender, M.B. and Krieger, H.P. (1951) Visual function in perimetrically blind fields. *Arch. Neurol. Psychiat.*, **65**, 72–9.

Benevento, L.A. and Yoshida, K. (1981) The afferent and efferent organisation of the lateral geniculo-prestriate pathways in the macaque monkey. *J. Comp. Neurol.*, **203**, 455–74.

Blythe, I.M., Bromley, J.M., Kennard, C. and Ruddock, K.H. (1986) Visual discrimination of target displacement remains after damage to the striate cortex. *Nature*, **320**, 619–21.

Blythe, I.M., Kennard, C. and Ruddock, H.H. (1987) Residual vision in patients with retrogeniculate lesions of the visual pathways. *Brain* (in press).

Bridgeman, B. and Staggs, D. (1982) Plasticity in human blindsight. *Vision Res*, **22**, 1199–203.

Brindley, G.S., Gautier-Smith, P.C. and Lewin, W. (1969) Cortical blindness and the functions of the non-geniculate fibres of the optic tracts. *J. Neurol. Neurosurg. Psychiat.*, **32**, 259–64.

Bullier, J. and Kennedy, H. (1983) Projection of the lateral geniculate nucleus onto cortical area V2 in the macaque monkey. *Exp. Brain Res.*, **53**, 168–72.

Campion, J., Latto, R. and Smith, Y.M. (1983) Is blindsight an effect of scattered

light, spared cortex and near threshold vision? *Behav. Brain Sci.*, **6**, 423–86.
Cowey, A. (1967) Perimetric study of field defects in monkeys after cortical and retinal ablations. *Quart. J. Exp. Psychol.*, **19**, 232–45.
Edinger, L. and Fischer, B. (1913) Ein mensch ohne Grosshirn. *Pflüg. Arch. Gesamte Physiol. Menschen Tiere*, **152**, 535–61.
Fries, W. (1981) The projection from the lateral geniculate nucleus to the prestriate cortex of the macaque. *Proc. R. Soc. Lond. B*, **213**, 73–80.
Gassel, M.M. and Williams, D. (1966) Visual function in patients with homonymous hemianopia: oculomotor mechanisms. *Brain*, **86**, 1–36.
Gloning, I. Gloning, K. and Tschabitscher, H. (1962) Die occipitale Blindheit auf vascularer Basio. *Albrecht von Graefe's Arch. Ophthalmol.*, **165**, 138–77.
Gross, C.G. and Weiskrantz, L. (1959) Note on luminous flux discrimination in monkey and man. *Quart. J. Exp. Psychol.*, **11**, 49–53.
Haerer, A.F. (1973) Visual field defects and the prognosis of stroke. *Stroke*, **4**, 163–8.
Hine, M.L. (1918) The recovery of fields of vision in concussion injuries of the occipital cortex. *Br. J. Ophthalmol.*, **2**, 12–25.
Holmes, G. (1918) Disturbances of vision by cerebral lesions. *Br. J. Ophthalmol.*, **2**, 353–84.
Humphrey, N.K. (1970) What the frog's eye tells the monkey's brain. *Brain Behav. Evol.*, **3**, 324–447.
Keating, E.G. (1979) Rudimentary colour vision in the monkey after removal of striate and preoccipital cortex. *Brain Res.*, **179**, 379–84.
Keating, E.G. (1980) Residual spatial vision in the monkey after removal of striate and preoccipital cortex. *Brain Res.*, **187**, 271–90.
Kluver, H. (1941) Visual functions after removal of the occipital lobes. *J. Psychol.*, **11**, 23–45.
Kluver, H. (1942) Functional significance of the geniculo-striate system. *Biol. Symp.*, **7**, 253–99.
Levinsohn, G. (1913) Der optische Blinzel-reflex. *Z. Gesamte Neurol. Psychiatr.*, **20**, 377–85.
Luria, A.R. (1963) *Restoration of Function after Brain Injury*. Pergamon Press, Oxford.
Magoun, H.W., Ranson, W.S. and Mayer, L.L. (1935) The pupillary light reflex after lesions of the posterior commissure in the cat. *Am. J. Ophthalmol.*, **18**, 624–30.
Meienberg, O., Zangemeister, W.H., Rosenberg, M., Hoyt, W.F. and Stark, L. (1981) Saccadic eye movement strategies in patients with homonymous hemianopia. *Ann. Neurol.*, **9**, 537–44.
Miller, M., Pasik, P. and Pasik, T. (1980) Extrageniculostriate vision in the monkey. VII Contrast sensitivity functions. *J. Neurophysiol.*, **43**, 1510–26.
Mohler, C.W. and Wurtz, R.E. (1977) Role of striate cortex and superior colliculus in visual guidance of saccadic eye-movements in monkeys. *J. Neurophys.*, **40**, 74–94.
Pasik, P., Pasik, T. and Bender, M.B. (1961) Light discrimination after additional brain damage in monkeys with bilateral striatectomy. *Fed. Proc. Fed. Am. Soc. Exp. Biol.*, **20**, 328.

Pasik, P., Pasik, T., Nolan, J.T. and Solomon, S.J. (1976) Bar orientation discrimination in normal and destriated monkeys. *Neurosci. Abstr.*, **2**, 1130.

Pasik, T. and Pasik, P. (1971) The visual world of monkeys deprived of striate cortex: effective stimulus parameters and the importance of the accessory optic system. *Vision Res. Suppl.*, **3**, 419–35.

Pasik, T. and Pasik, P. (1982) Visual function in monkeys after total removal of visual cerebral cortex, in *Contributions to Sensory Physiology* (ed. W.D. Neff), Vol. 7. Academic Press, New York, pp. 147–200.

Perenin, M.T. (1978) Visual function within the hemianopic field following early cerebral hemidecortication in man. II Pattern discrimination. *Neuropsychologia*, **16**, 696–708.

Perenin, M.T. and Jeannerod, M. (1975) Residual vision in cortically blind hemifields. *Neuropsychologia*, **13**, 1–7.

Perenin, M.T. and Jeannerod, M. (1978) Visual function within the hemianopic field following early cerebral hemidecortication in man. I Spatial localisation. *Neuropsychologia*, **16**, 1–13.

Perenin, M.T., Ruel, J. and Hecaen, K. (1980) Residual visual capacities in a case of cortical blindness. *Cortex*, **16**, 605–12.

Pizzamiglio, L., Antonucci, G. and Francia, A. (1984) Response of the cortically blind hemifields to a moving visual scene. *Cortex*, **20**, 89–99.

Poppel, E. (1977) Midbrain mechanisms in human vision, in *Neurosciences Research Program Bulletin*, Vol. 15, *Neuronal Mechanisms in Visual Perception* (eds E. Poppel, R. Held and J.E. Dowling). MIT Press, Boston, MA, pp. 335–45.

Poppel, E., Held, R. and Frost, D. (1973) Residual visual function after brain wounds including the central visual pathways in man. *Nature* (*Lond.*), **243**, 295–6.

Poppelreuter, W. (1917) Die Psychischen Schadigungen durch Kopfschreb im Kriege 1914–16, Bard 1: Die Stornugen der Niederen und Hoheren Sehleisturgen durch Verletzugen des Okzipitalhirns. L. Voss, Leipzig.

Richards, W. (1973) Visual processing in scotomata. *Exp. Brain Res.*, **17**, 333–47.

Riddoch, G. (1917) Dissociation of visual perceptions due to occipital injuries with especial reference to appreciation of movement. *Brain*, **40**, 15–57.

Ross Russell, R.W. and Bharucha, N. (1984) Visual localisation in patients with occipital infarction. *J. Neurol. Neurosurg. Psychiat.*, **47**, 153–8.

Schilder, P., Pasik, T. and Pasik, P. (1971) Extrageniculostriate vision in the monkey. II Demonstration of brightness discrimination. *Brain Res.*, **32**, 383–98.

Schilder, P., Pasik, P. and Pasik, T. (1972) Extrageniculostriate vision in the monkey. III Circle vs triangle and 'red vs green' discrimination. *Exp. Brain Res.*, **14**, 436–48.

Schiller, P.H. and Sandell, J.H. (1983) Interactions between visual and electrically elicited saccades before and after superior colliculus and frontal eye field ablations in the rhesus monkey. *Exp. Brain Res.*, **49**, 381–92.

Schneider, G. (1969) Two visual systems. *Science, NY*, **163**, 895–902.

Solomon, S.J., Pasik, T. and Pasik, P. (1981) Extrageniculostriate vision in the monkey. VIII Critical structures for spatial localisation. *Exp. Brain Res.*, **44**, 259–70.

Sprague, J.M. (1966) Interaction of cortex and superior colliculus in mediation of visually guided behaviour in the cat. *Science, NY*, **153**, 1544–7.

Stoerig, P., Hubner, M. and Poppel, E. (1985) Signal detection analysis of residual vision in a field defect due to a post-geniculate lesion. *Neuropsychologia*, **23**, 589–99.

Teuber, H.L., Battersby, W.S. and Bender, M.B. (1960) *Visual Field Defects after Penetrating Missile Wounds of the Brain*. Harvard University Press, Cambridge, MA.

Torjussen, T. (1976) Residual function in cortically blind hemifields. *Scand. J. Psychol.*, **17**, 320–2.

Trevarthen, C.B. (1968) Two mechanisms of vision in primates. *Psychol. Forsch.*, **31**, 299–337.

Ungerleider, L.G. and Mishkin, M. (1982) Two cortical visual systems, in *Analysis of Visual Behaviour* (eds D.J. Ingle, M.A. Goodale and R.J.W. Mansfield). MIT Press, Boston, pp. 549–86.

Van Buren, J.M. (1963) Trans-synaptic retrograde degeneration in the visual system of primates. *J. Neurol. Neurosurg. Psychiat.*, **26**, 402–9.

Warrington, E.K. (1962) The completion of visual forms across hemianopic field defects. *J. Neurol. Neurosurg. Psychiat.*, **25**, 208–17.

Weiskrantz, L. (1980) Varieties of residual experience. *Quart. J. Exp. Psychol.*, **32**, 365–86.

Weiskrantz, L. (1983) Evidence and scotoma. *Behav. Brain Sci.*, **3**, 464–7.

Weiskrantz, L., Cowey, A. and Passingham, C. (1977) Spatial responses to brief stimuli by monkeys with striate cortex ablations. *Brain*, **100**, 655–70.

Weiskrantz, L., Warrington, E.K., Sanders, D.M. and Marshall, J. (1974) Visual capacity in the hemianopic field following a restricted occipital ablation. *Brain*, **97**, 709–28.

Williams, D. and Gassel, M.M. (1962) Visual functions in patients with homonymous hemianopia. *Brain*, **85**, 175–250.

Yukie, M. and Iwai, E. (1981) Direct projection from the dorsal lateral geniculate nucleus to the prestriate cortex in macaque monkeys. *J. Comp. Neurol.*, **201**, 81–97.

Zangemeister, W.H., Meienberg, O., Stark, L. and Hoyt, W.F. (1982) Eye–head coordination in homonymous hemianopia. *J. Neurol.*, **226**, 243–54.

Zihl, J. (1981) Recovery of visual functions in patients with cerebral blindness. *Exp. Brain Res.*, **44**, 159–69.

Zihl, J. and von Cramon, D. (1979) Restitution of visual function in patients with cerebral blindness. *J. Neurol. Neurosurg. Psychiat.*, **42**, 312–22.

Zihl, J. and von Cramon, D. (1985) Visual vield recovery from scotoma in patients with postgeniculate damage: a review of 55 cases. *Brain*, **108**, 335–66.

Zihl, J. and Werth, R. (1984) Contributions to the study of 'blindsight'. I Can stray light account for saccadic localisation in patients with post geniculate field defects. *Neuropsychologia*, **22**, 1–11.

CHAPTER 8

Neuronal mechanisms of face perception and their pathology

D.I. PERRETT, A.J. MISTLIN, A.J. CHITTY
M.H. HARRIES, F. NEWCOMBE AND E. DE HAAN

8.1 The condition of prosopagnosia

Prosopagnosia is an organic condition in which patients are unable to recognize people from their faces (hence the clinical term from Greek; prosopo = face, agnosia = not knowing). The disability includes the faces of highly familiar friends and relatives, and the patients may even fail to recognize pictures of themselves. Despite these impairments patients may come to recognize others by their voices or by the visual appearance of their clothing or postural mannerisms. Such recognition defects cannot be accounted for by simple sensory losses (such as visual field defects or low visual acuity) or general intellectual disturbance (Ettlinger, 1956; Meadows, 1974a; Levin and Peters, 1976).

The nature of the psychological deficits which underlie prosopagnosia has been the focus of debate since the condition first entered the clinical literature (for review of 19th-century descriptions, see Bodamer, 1947). This has been because prosopagnosia often occurs with a number of seemingly unrelated visual and cognitive dysfunctions (Pallis, 1955; Meadows, 1974a; Whiteley and Warrington, 1977; Mollon *et al.*, 1980) including the disturbance of colour vision (achromatopsia), difficulties in route-finding to familiar places and distortions of visual image (metamorphopsia). Each of these disturbances can, however, be dissociated from prosopagnosia since there are reports of individual patients with these latter symptoms but without prosopagnosia and vice versa. Thus Meadows (1974b) described neurological patients with disturbances of colour vision who have no noted face-recognition problems and conversely patients have been studied with deficient face-recognition problems without notable colour-recognition problems (Aptman, Levin and Senelick, 1977; Whiteley and Warrington, 1977, Cases 2 and 3; Damasio, Damasio and Van Hoesen, 1982). The co-occurrence of deficits in particular faculties in some or most patients does not necessarily mean that the different faculties depend on the same neural system. It is more reasonable to assume that face recognition and colour vision involve separate neural mechanisms in different, although possibly neighbouring, brain areas.

It is very unlikely that unintentional brain lesions will result in damage confined entirely to the anatomical boundaries of one brain area destroying all of that area but not affecting adjacent areas. If a brain system is represented in both cerebral hemispheres then it is even more unlikely that damage sufficient to disrupt processing in this system in both hemispheres will not additionally embarrass other systems. The double dissociation between clinical symptoms even in a minority of cases is a strong argument for the existence of distinct neural systems subserving different visual or cognitive capacities.

8.1.1 SPECIFIC VISUAL RECOGNITION LOSSES

The most controversial issue concerning prosopagnosia is whether the visual recognition impairment is confined to faces or extends to other classes of object. Often, examination of patients with prosopagnosia reveals deficits in their recognition of other classes of object where the examples within the class are visually similar, e.g. species of bird (Bornstein, 1963), type of fruit (De Renzi, Faglioni and Spinnler, 1968), articles of clothing, cooking utensils and automobiles (Damasio, Damasio and Van Hoesen, 1982), chairs (Faust, 1955) and buildings (Beyn and Knyazeva, 1962; Cole and Perez-Cruet, 1964; Gloning *et al.*, 1966; Gloning and Quatember, 1966). If the recognition of objects and faces relies on brain systems that are essentially distinct but occur in neighbouring brain areas then, as argued above, one would expect patients to vary in the degree to which they manifest both object and face recognition defects. Most often the symptoms would occur together but occasionally they might occur in isolation (Hecaen and Albert, 1978). Indeed, this is the case: one patient studied by Hecaen *et al.* (1974) was able to recognize famous faces and match faces but was extremely poor in naming or pointing to objects in everyday use; the patient would, for example, mistakenly identify a typewriter as a telephone. Conversely, prosopagnosia has been reported for several patients without such marked object agnosia (e.g. Bornstein and Kidron, 1959; Whiteley and Warrington, 1977; Newcombe, 1979).

Damasio, Damasio and Van Hoesen (1982) have suggested that the underlying deficit lies not in the ability to distinguish between categories of objects (e.g. faces vs cars) but results from 'defective contextual evocation for stimuli belonging to a visually "ambiguous" category'. Thus the patient may be able to recognize a face as being a face but is not able to realize that it is, for example, their spouse's or even their own face. Damasio, Damasio and Van Hoesen (1982) and Damasio (1985) argued that the deficit is not face specific and that when examined appropriately would extend to the discrimination of personal items within other classes of object.

De Renzi (1986) has recently reported evidence against this deficient categorization hypothesis. Patients studied by De Renzi failed to recognize familiar faces but despite this could discriminate between their own personal items (e.g. their wallet or their comb) and equivalent items owned by others.

Perhaps the most bizarre dissociation has come from the study of farmers with prosopagnosia. Bruyer *et al.* (1983) reported one farmer who had no difficulty in recognizing his cows but could not recognize his friends. By contrast, Assal, Faure and Anderes (1984) reported a prosopagnosic patient who recovered his ability to recognize his friends but remained unable to distinguish between his cows!

8.1.2 NEUROPATHOLOGY OF PROSOPAGNOSIA

The locus of brain damage most commonly associated with prosopagnosia is the inferior occipito-temporal region, particularly in the right hemisphere. Meadows (1974a) in his review of available clinical evidence noted the constant factor of a left upper quadrantanopia in reported case histories. He reasoned that the cortex at the junction of the occipital and temporal lobes on the ventral surface of the brain could be the critical site for face processing. Alternatively the critical site might be more anterior in the cortex of the temporal lobe. Damage in the inferior occipito-temporal region is likely to encroach on underlying white matter and could produce its effect on recognition by the destruction of the inferior longitudinal fasciculus, a fibre bundle connecting posterior prestriate areas to anterior temporal areas. Thus Meadows noted that prosopagnosia could arise from the disconnection between critical systems in the temporal cortex and the visual inputs from the posterior visual areas.

8.2 Neurophysiological studies of face processing in monkeys

8.2.1 GENERAL PROPERTIES

Recordings from single neurones in the temporal cortex of macaque monkeys have revealed populations of cells that respond to the sight of faces but not to other stimuli including simple visual stimuli, complex three-dimensional objects, e.g. an alarm clock, or more arousing stimuli such as a snake or banana. The selective responses to faces generalize over variables which are coded in earlier visual processing in striate and prestriate cortex. The cells thus respond to faces irrespective of their retinal position (over very large receptive fields extending at least 20° bilaterally from the fovea), orientation (upright, horizontal, inverted), colour, size (1°–40° of usual angle) and viewing distance (10 cm–5 m). These findings indicate a role for the cells in a very high level of visual representation of information about faces (Bruce, Desimone and Gross, 1981; Perrett, Rolls and Caan, 1982; Desimone *et al.*, 1984; Perrett *et al.*, 1984, 1986a).

8.2.2 VISUAL BASIS OF RESPONSES

Neurophysiological studies have revealed two levels of neuronal encoding of facial information. At the first level the general properties of the face appear to be made explicit. At this level cells respond to many different faces, independent of the species (human or monkey), identity, age or expression.

Covering up different regions of the face (i.e. mouth, eyes) or presenting these regions in isolation revealed that cell responses depend on the presence of facial features. Different cells were selective for different features or combinations of features (some cells preferring the eye region, others the mouth region and/or the hair). Comparison of responses to faces (2D or 3D models) where the features have their normal or symmetrically jumbled positions reveals that many cells are additionally selective for the normal feature configuration and are less responsive to jumbled arrays. Responses to faces thus appear to be based on the visual information arising from individual facial features and their configuration (Perrett, Rolls and Caan, 1982; Perrett and Rolls, 1983).

8.2.3 SENSITIVITY TO HEAD VIEW AND GAZE DIRECTION

Our studies show that while cells responsive to faces respond to many different instances of the face, they are less tolerant to changes in perspective view of the face (Perrett *et al.*, 1985a). Responses to the frontal face decline as it is turned away from the monkey in any direction. Recordings have revealed that there are different populations of cells which are selectively responsive to the other views of the head (Perrett *et al.*, 1985b). In all, we have discovered six populations, each selective for one view (frontal face, left and right profile, back of head, head up and head down). A further population responds to all views of the head.

These findings have suggested a model of visual recognition in which all objects are analysed by reference to a small number of prototypical views of those objects. Outputs from this level of analysis are then fed on to a level which generalizes across all perspective views for that object (Perrett *et al.*, 1984, 1985a, 1986a; cf. Marr and Nishihara, 1978).

Studies of cellular sensitivity to the presence of eyes and the direction of their gaze have revealed that information about head view is integrated with information about the gaze direction in a highly compatible manner (Fig. 8.1). About half the cells tuned to the frontal view of the face were found sensitive to direction of eye gaze and virtually all these cells were found to be selective for the eyes directed towards the monkey (eye contact) over eyes laterally averted. By contrast, cells tuned to the profile view of the head (and sensitive to the gaze direction) were found to be selective for averted gaze compared with eye contact.

The extent of neural encoding of information about where the eyes are

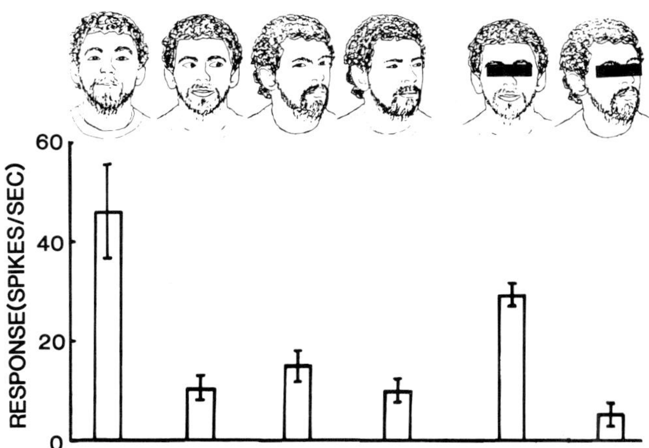

Fig. 8.1 Neuronal sensitivity to head view and gaze direction. Upper: Illustrates the type of stimuli presented to the monkey, full face with eye contact and with eyes averted, half profile face with eye contact and eyes averted, face and half profile with eyes covered. Lower: Illustrates the mean and standard error of responses of one cell to these stimuli. Responses are raised for the face with eye contact and with the eyes covered compared to other conditions.

looking can easily be understood when it is realized how important gaze direction is to communication in social interactions in both human and monkey species (Hinde and Rowell, 1962; Argyle and Cook, 1975; Whiten and Byrne, 1986).

8.2.4 IDENTITY

So far, the description of cells responsive to faces has centred on those sensitive to the general characteristics of faces. We have also found a more abstract level of encoding of facial information. About 10% of cells responsive to the face or other view of the head appear highly selective for additional characteristics of the face. We have studied, for example, a number of cells which give consistently greater responses to the sight of one face known to the monkey than to the sight of other equally familiar faces (e.g. Fig. 8.2). Cells with such selectivity are capable of discriminating between preferred and non-preferred faces over a wide range of viewing conditions including changes in face orientation, viewing distance (Fig. 8.2), facial expression and strength, direction and colour of prevailing illumination (Perrett *et al.*, 1984, 1986a). It is evident from such discrimination in responses that these cells could play an important role in differentiating the identity of familiar faces. It is important to realize that different subpopulations of cells have been found to be selective for other faces familiar to the monkey and that we have found several examples of such selectivity for each individual (see also Rolls, 1984). Thus many cells may contribute to the identification of any one familiar individual, each cell coding slightly different feature characteristics or combination of characteristics.

The coding of identity and expression appears to take place in distinct neuronal populations (Perrett *et al.*, 1984; see also Hay and Young, 1982). Those cells displaying a selectivity amongst individual faces are generally insensitive to the expression of preferred and non-preferred faces. By contrast those cells sensitive to facial expression appear insensitive to identity (or even species). We have thus studied a number of cells selective for open mouth (threat faces) and for grimaces (fearful faces) independent of whether these expressions are displayed either by humans or monkeys.

8.2.5 ANATOMICAL DISTRIBUTION

Reconstructions of cell positions from histology and X-rays of the recording tracks have revealed that the majority of cells in the temporal cortex responsive to faces or to other views of the head are concentrated in two adjacent regions, TPO and PGa (Seltzer and Pandya, 1978), of the

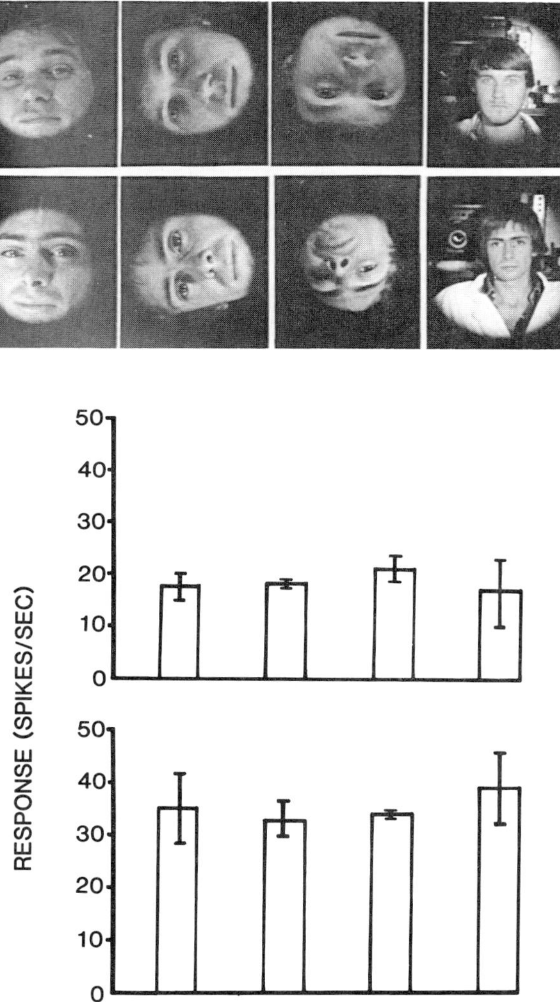

Fig. 8.2 Sensitivity to face identity. Upper: Illustration of two faces under different viewing conditions. Lower: Illustrates the mean and standard error of responses of one cell to the different instances of the two faces.

superior temporal sulcus (STS). These two regions have distinct myelo- and cyto-architecture and run as thin strips along the length of the sulcus.

Even within regions TPO and PGa, cell distribution is not homogeneous. Cells responsive to faces are clumped together both vertically through the thickness of the cortex and in a direction parallel to the surface of the cortex. Clumps containing a high concentration of cells processing faces are separated from each other by clumps of cells processing other types of information. Thus similar principles of functional and structural organization would seem to operate on encoding of visual information in the temporal cortex as have been described elsewhere (Hubel and Wiesel, 1968; Mountcastle, 1978; Szentagothai, 1978). The exact geometry of these clumps is not yet clear, indeed they would seem to range from 0.5 to 4.0 mm across the cortex (Perrett *et al.*, 1984, 1985a, 1986a, 1986b).

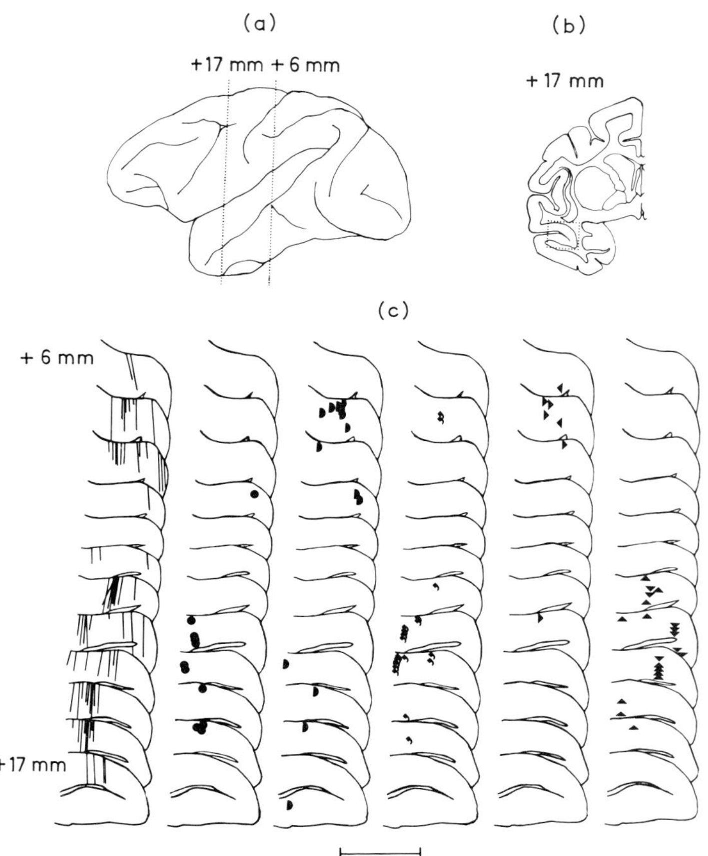

Fig. 8.3 Clumped distribution of cell types within temporal cortex. (a) Lateral view of the monkey brain with the orientation of sections. (b) Outline of brain structures evident in a coronal section through the left hemisphere at +17 mm anterior to the interaural plane. (c) Enlargement of recording area visualized in serial sections (from +6 to +17 mm anterior) from left to right position of cell recording tracks; location of cells selective for faces (●); profiles (◗); rotation of the head (❥); movement left (◀) and right (▶); up (▲) down (▼).

Figure 8.3 illustrates the clumped distribution of one cell population responsive to the face and a different cell population responsive to the profile face. We have found a variety of cell types within the same region of the STS sensitive to visual movement (see Fig. 8.3), in particular head and body movements (Perrett *et al.*, 1985), and to somatosensory and auditory information about unexpected stimuli (Chitty, Mistlin and Perrett, 1985).

The very existence of a clumped distribution of cells selective for particular views of the face indicates that there is a specific anatomical substrate for face processing. This has been suggested but often disputed by studies of prosopagnosia. At the same time the existence of clumps of cells processing other information indicates that this brain area is not face specific.

8.3 Perception of facial attributes in a case of prosopagnosia

If prosopagnosia arises from damage in the human brain to a system equivalent to that studied in the superior temporal sulcus (STS) of the macaque brain, then one expects the sensitivity of STS cells to particular facial attributes to be mirrored by losses in the ability of patients with prosopagnosia to process the same facial attributes. The pathognomonic symptom of prosopagnosic patients is that they cannot recognize faces familiar to them. Such a deficit might be explained by damage to cells in the STS which are selectively responsive to familiar faces but, intermingled with such cells, are a greater percentage of cells sensitive to general attributes of the face. One would, therefore, expect the perception of attributes such as gaze direction and face feature configuration to be impaired in at least some cases of prosopagnosia. The existing literature on prosopagnosia does contain reports of impairments in the perception of general facial characteristics but does not address the specific predictions made above. We have sought to investigate the perception of particular facial attributes in a documented case of prosopagnosia (Newcombe, 1979; Davidoff, Matthews and Newcombe, 1986).

This case (RB) has been described elsewhere (Newcombe, 1979) so only the salient details will be given here. Subject RB has a history of problems in recognizing faces of sudden onset and attributable to vascular disease which have remained evident for over 10 years. He has normal visual acuity and his performance on a variety of spatial tasks (e.g. Hebb's blocks, cube counting, line orientation, tactual maze learning) was average or above. He has an upper left quadrantic field defect and CT scans show a low-density area in the right hemisphere in the occipital temporal region, close to the ventricle and underlying the occipital horn. There is probably a symmetrically placed but smaller lesion in the left hemisphere. In addition, there are two, ill-defined low-density areas around the posterior aspect of the body of the lateral ventricle, underneath the temporo-parieto-occipital junction, and more extensive on the left than on the right.

8.3.1 GAZE DIRECTION SENSITIVITY

Figure 8.4 illustrates the results of a test of sensitivity to gaze direction in which the subjects had to discriminate between pictures of a face looking directly at the camera (eye contact) and pictures where the eyes were averted to the left or right of the camera. (In these pictures the stimulus face was directed at the camera, or 20° to the left, or to the right, of the camera to make the task perceptually more complex). The task was conducted with three levels of difficulty, with the difference between eye contact and averted gaze set at 5°, 10° or 20°.

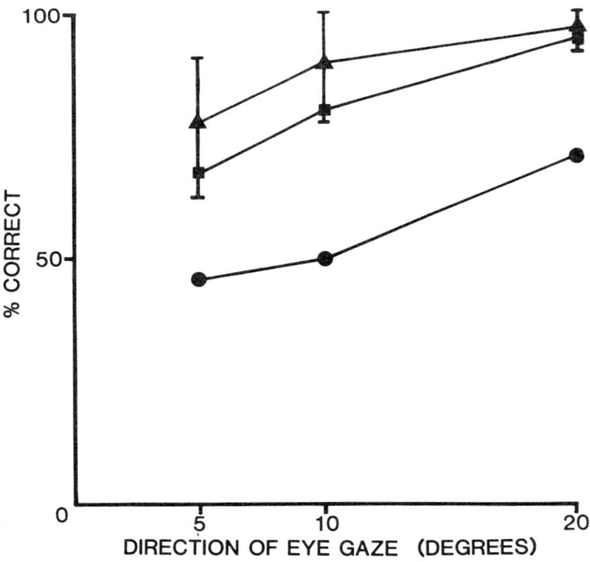

Fig. 8.4 Sensitivity to gaze direction. The mean level of accuracy for discriminating faces with eye contact and with eyes averted is plotted for different degrees of gaze aversion. ▲, performance of normal control subjects (n = 37, mean ± 1 SD); ■, performance of right hemisphere-lesioned group (n = 19); ●, performance of subject with prosopagnosia.

Figure 8.4 compares the performance on this task of a group of patients with long-standing, focal missile injuries in the right cerebral hemisphere, a group of age-matched controls and subject RB. RB's performance is at chance (50%) for 5° and 10° conditions and greater than 3 standard deviations outside the control group range for the 10° and 20° conditions. In contrast, the performance of the group of unselected right hemisphere-lesioned patients (many of whom have visual field defects) does not differ from control subjects on this task.

The marked impairment in RB's perception of gaze direction has been replicated under a variety of experimental conditions over a four-year period. His impairment in this task contrasts with a number of other visual tasks for example line counting, cube counting and judgements of position of a dot within a square boundary (after Warrington and Rabin (1970); Taylor and Warrington (1973)) in which he performs at well above average level. Thus RB's impairment in judging eye gaze cannot be taken as secondary to a more general visuo-spatial disorder. Indeed, he performed normally in a control task specifically designed to match the eye gaze task in difficulty. In this task the subject had to judge the direction of a gun turret on a wooden block model of a tank.

8.3.2 FACE CONFIGURATION

A second task was developed to investigate RB's perception of face configuration. In this task subjects were presented with slides of faces with a normal configuration of facial features or with three different symmetrical jumbled configurations. Faces were presented upright, horizontal (left or right) and inverted. The subjects were given a forced choice discrimination between normal face configurations (irrespective of orientation) and jumbled arrays.

Control subjects are quicker to detect normal configurations than to detect jumbled arrays (Fig. 8.5). This can be interpreted as indicating that these subjects appreciate the gestalt or overall pattern of facial features when they are in the normal order and hence respond quickly.

Subject RB, while able to perform this task, displays the reverse pattern of reaction times; he is quicker to reject jumbled arrays than to accept normal patterns (Fig. 8.5). We interpret this very unusual pattern of performance as arising from an impairment in his ability to appreciate the normal configuration of facial features. We postulate that this forces him to adopt a less-efficient strategy whereby he searches each facial feature, serially checking whether it is in the correct position; if it is so, then he proceeds to the next feature; if not, then the search is terminated and he responds 'jumble'. It is only after exhaustively checking every

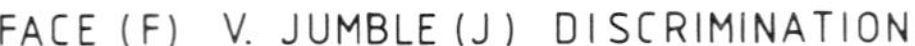

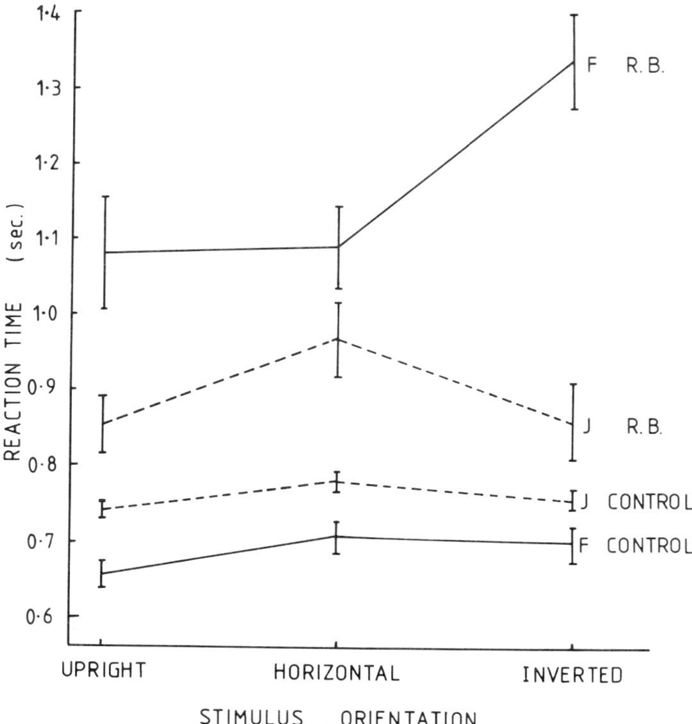

Fig. 8.5 Discrimination of face configuration. The mean reaction time (± 1 SE) is given for faces (——, F) and for jumbled arrays (– – – –, J) presented in upright, horizontal and inverted orientations. CONTROL, performance of normal control group; ——, R.B., performance of subject with prosopagnosia.

feature that he can conclude by default that the configuration must be normal.

These tasks reveal a disturbance in RB's perceptual mechanisms for processing a striking facial feature (eye gaze) and also a configuration of facial features. These disturbances could well arise from damage to neuronal mechanisms homologous to those that we have studied in the macaque temporal cortex which process gaze direction and facial configuration.

8.4 The bearing of neuropsychological studies on prosopagnosia

Data from studies of neurones responsive to faces have a bearing on three issues that recur in the neuropsychological literature on patients with face-recognition deficits (prosopagnosia). These concern the material specificity of the disorder, whether the condition arises from unilateral or bilateral brain damage and whether the deficit is perceptual or mnemonic in nature.

8.4.1 SPECIFICITY

The finding of an anatomically definable subsystem that processes faces within the macaque STS is in accordance with the view that prosopagnosia involves a selective disturbance of a face processing system. But if prosopagnosia were hypothesized to arise from damage to a brain area homologous with the STS of the macaque then it would be unlikely that prosopagnosia could occur in the complete absence of any other visual processing deficit. Since there are other types of visual cell in the STS sensitive to the sight of actions and particular types of body movement, one would expect damage to a human brain system equivalent to the macaque STS to result in additional recognition losses for particular classes of animate objects and movements, though the perception and recognition of arbitrary inanimate objects should not necessarily be affected.

8.4.2 LATERALITY

There is considerable debate concerning the lateralization of face processing in the adult human brain and the extent to which a unilateral lesion can ever produce prosopagnosia (Meadows, 1974a, Lhermitte and Pillon, 1975; Whiteley and Warrington, 1977; Damasio, Damasio and Van Hoesen, 1982; Damasio, 1985; De Renzi, 1986). In the monkey, cells that respond to faces can be found in both the left and right temporal cortex. Our recent analysis of the distribution in five monkeys does indicate a hemispheric difference with a significantly greater number in the left cerebral hemisphere (Perrett *et al.*, 1986b). It remains to be determined whether this difference will hold up over a larger sample. Behavioural studies of monkeys with sectioned corpus callosum also suggest hemispheric lateralization of face processing in monkeys (Hamilton and Vermeire, 1982). In contrast, humans appear to show a right hemisphere dominance for face perception (for discussion, see Perrett *et al.*, 1986b). Though monkey neurophysiology cannot provide a definitive answer concerning human face lateralization, it favours the notion of at least some bilateral processing of facial material and additionally suggests that hemispheric differences could arise simply from a difference in the number of cells devoted to face analysis in the two hemispheres.

8.4.3 PERCEPTION AND MEMORY FOR FACES

Neuropsychological investigations of prosopagnosic patients vary in the emphasis given to the role of deficient perception or deficient memory in producing the symptoms. For some patients the ability to match two simultaneously presented photographs of different views of the same face is impaired (Whiteley and Warrington, 1977; Benton, 1980). Since long-term memory is not needed for this task the deficit of these patients is seen as a problem in perception. The studies of the perception of facial attributes that are described in section 8.3 also point to perceptual deficiencies in one case of prosopagnosia. Given that some patients cannot perceive faces normally it is hardly surprising that they cannot remember them and their problems in face memory can thus be seen as a consequence of face perception deficits. For other patients, face matching is reportedly normal (although latencies are not always systematically measured) and yet recognition of faces is impaired. Here the deficit may not be purely perceptual and is more likely to be mnemonic. The mandatory double dissociation has been reported (Malone *et al.*, 1982; De Renzi, 1986).

Two lines of neurophysiological data suggest a role for the STS cells in face perception. The spectrum of cell types sensitive to the basic features of the face (presence of eyes, facial features, etc.) could be involved in the perception of these facial qualities, the perceptual categorization of a stimulus as a face and the matching of face pictures.

There are many visual transformations (such as changes in image position, viewing distance, strength, direction and colour of ambient illumination) which alter the local values of elementary visual dimensions in the image (brightness, orientation, size and colour of local elements). These visual transformations do not, however, affect a subject's ability to perceive a face in the retinal image, nor do they affect the responses of STS neurones to faces. Other visual transformations (such as contrast reversal, image rotation, coarse quantization and schematization) of an image can leave the majority of local image characteristics unchanged, but yet can dramatically reduce the ease of perceiving a face in the image. These transformations are found to decrease or delay the firing of STS neurones to faces. This presents correlative evidence that the tuning of STS cells relates more closely with face perception than with the sensing of elementary visual dimensions.

On the other hand, the presence of cells which appear selectively tuned for particular faces familiar to the monkey provide evidence for an influence of mnemonic processes on STS cell functioning. It would seem that structural descriptions of known faces could well be stored at the same brain location as structural descriptions of general facial characteristics. In this sense the STS plays a dual role for classifying the basic object category (X is a face) and identifying the exemplar (X is Paul's face).

Disconnection of the visual inputs to the STS would deny all face processing there and would account for the loss of the ability to perceive and match faces in particular cases of prosopagnosia. Disconnection of the STS from memory systems such as the limbic structures might prevent the update of basic descriptions of faces to more specific descriptions of a particular familiar person's face. This could account for intact face perception with impaired face recognition in some cases of prosopagnosia. Indeed, such a disconnection would deny any learning of new faces but might leave intact the recognition of familiar or famous faces since their descriptions as person recognition units would have already been established in the STS prior to its disconnection. Of course, there is more than one set of inputs and outputs from the STS and disconnection of particular projection systems could thus produce a variety of possible syndromes.

Acknowledgements

The neurophysiological work was supported by the MRC and a Royal Society University Fellowship to D.I. Perrett. This work was performed in collaboration with A.S. Head, M.A. Jeeves, A.D. Milner, D.D. Potter and P.A.J. Smith.

References

Aptman, M., Levin, M. and Senelick, R.C. (1977) Alexia without agraphia in a left-handed patient with prosopagnosia. *Neurology*, **27**, 533–6.

Argyle, M. and Cook, M. (1975) *Gaze and Mutual Gaze*. Cambridge University Press, Cambridge.

Assal, G., Faure, C. and Anderes, J.P. (1984) Non-reconnaissance d'animaux familiers chez un paysan: zoo-agnosie ou prosopagnosie pour les animaux. *Rev. Neurol. (Paris)*, **140**, 580–4.

Benton, A.L. (1980) The neuropsychology of face recognition. *Am. Psychol.*, **35**, 176–86.

Beyn, E.S. and Knyazeva, G.R. (1962) The problem of prosopagnosia. *J. Neurol. Neurosurg. Psychiat.*, **25**, 154–8.

Bodamer, J. (1947) Die prosopagnosie. *Arch. Psychiat. Zeitsch. Neur.*, **179**, 6–54.

Bornstein, B. (1963) Prosopagnosia, in *Problems of Dynamic Neurology* (ed. Z. Halpern). Jerusalem Post Press, Jerusalem.

Bornstein, B. and Kidron, D.P. (1959) Prosopagnosia. *J. Neurol. Neurosurg. Psychiat.*, **22**, 124–31.

Bruce, C.J., Desimone, R. and Gross, C.G. (1981) Visual properties of neurones in a polysensory area in superior temporal sulcus of macaque. *J. Neurophysiol.*, **46**, 369–84.

Bruyer, R., Laterre, C., Seron, X., Feyereisen, P., Strypstein, E., Perrard, E. and Redem, D. (1983) A case of prosopagnosia with some preserved covert remembrance of familiar faces. *Brain Cognition*, **2**, 257–84.

Chitty, A.J., Mistlin, A.J. and Perrett, D.I. (1985) Somatosensory and associated visual properties of neurones in a polysensory region of macaque temporal cortex. *J. Physiol.*, **367**, 30p.

Cole, M. and Perez-Cruet, J. (1964) Prosopagnosia. *Neuropsychologia*, **2**, 237–45.

Damasio, A.R. (1985) Prosopagnosia. *Trends Neurosci.*, **8**, 132–5.

Damasio, A.R., Damasio, H. and Van Hoesen, G.W. (1982) Prosopagnosia: Anatomical basis and neurobehavioral mechanism. *Neurology*, **32**, 331–41.

Davidoff, J., Matthews, W.B. and Newcombe, F. (1986) Observations on a case of prosopagnosia, in *Aspects of Face Processing* (*NATO ISI Series*) (eds H. Ellis, M.A. Jeeves, F. Newcombe and A. Young). Martinus Nijoff, Dordrecht, pp. 279–90.

De Renzi, E. (1986) Current issues on prosopagnosia, in *Aspects of Face Processing* (*NATO ISI Series*) (eds H. Ellis, M.A. Jeeves, F. Newcombe and A. Young). Martinus Nijhoff, Dordrecht, pp. 243–52.

De Renzi, E., Faglioni, R. and Spinnler, M. (1968) The performance of patients with unilateral brain damage on face recognition tasks. *Cortex*, **4**, 17–34.

Desimone, R., Albright, T.D. Gross, C.G. and Bruce, C. (1984) Selective properties of inferior temporal neurones in the macaque. *J. Neurosci.*, **4**, 2051–68.

Ettlinger, G. (1956) Sensory deficits in visual agnosia. *J. Neurol. Neurosurg. Psychiat.*, **19**, 297–308.

Faust, C. (1955) *Die zerebralen Herdslorungen bei Hinterhauptsverletzungen und ihre Beurteilung*. G. Thieme Verlag, Stuttgart.

Gloning, L., Gloning, K., Hoff, H. and Tschabitscher, H. (1966) Zur prosopagnosie. *Neuropsychologia*, **4**, 113–32.

Gloning, K. and Quatember, R. (1966) Methodischer beitrag zur untersuchung der prosopagnosie. *Neuropsychologia*, **4**, 133–41.

Hamilton, C.R. and Vermeire, B.A. (1982) Discrimination of monkey faces by split-brain monkeys. *Behav. Brain Res.*, **9**, 263–75.

Hay, D.C. and Young, A.W. (1982) The human face, in *Normality and Pathology in Cognitive Functions*. Academic Press, London, pp. 173–202.

Hecaen, H. and Albert, M.L. (1978) *Human Neuropsychology*. Academic Press, New York.

Hecaen, H., Goldblum, M.C., Masure, M.C. and Ramier, A.M. (1974) Une nouvelle observation d'agnosie d'objet. Déficit de l'association, ou de la categorisation spécifique de la modalité visuelle? *Neuropsychologia*, **12**, 447–64.

Hinde, R.A. and Rowell, T.E. (1962) Communication by posture and facial expression in rhesus monkey (*Macaca mulatta*). *Proc. Zool. Soc. Lond.*, **138**, 1–21.

Hubel, D.H. and Wiesel, T.N. (1968) Receptive fields and functional architecture of monkey striate cortex. *J. Physiol.*, **195**, 215–43.

Levin, M.S. and Peters, B.H. (1976) Neuropsychological testing following head injuries: prosopagnosia without visual field defect. *Dis. Nerv. Syst.*, **32**, 68–71.

Lhermitte, F. and Pillon, B. (1975) La prosopagnosie, rôle de l'hémisphère droit dans la perception visuelle. *Rev. Neurol.*, **131**, 791–812.

Malone, D.R., Morris, H.H., Kay, M.C. and Levin, H.S. (1982) Prosopagnosia: A double dissociation between the recognition of familiar and unfamiliar faces. *J. Neurol. Neurosurg. Psychiat.*, **45**, 820–2.

Marr, D. and Nishihara, H.K. (1978) Representation and recognition of the spatial organization of three dimensional shapes. *Proc. R. Soc. Lond. B*, **200**, 269–94.

McConach, H.R. (1977) Developmental prosopagnosia: a single case report. *Cortex*, **12**, 76–82.

Meadows, J.C. (1974a) The anatomical basis of prosopagnosia. *J. Neurol. Neurosurg. Psychiat.*, **37**, 489–501.

Meadows, J.C. (1974b) Disturbed perception of colours associated with localized cerebral lesions. *Brain*, **97**, 615–32.

Mollon, J.D., Newcombe, F., Polden, P.G. and Radcliffe, E. (1980) On the presence of three core mechanisms in a case of total achromatopsia, in *Colour Vision Deficiencies* (ed. G. Verrest). Hilger, Bristol.

Mountcastle, V.B. (1978) An organizing principle for cerebral function: the unit module and the distributed system, in *The Mindful Brain* (eds G.H. Edelman and V.B. Mountcastle). MIT Press, Cambridge, MA, pp. 7–50.

Newcombe, F. (1979) The processing of visual information in prosopagnosia and acquired dyslexia: functional versus physiological interpretations, in *Research in Psychology and Medicine* (eds D.J. Osbourne, M.M. Grunberg and J.R. Eiser). Academic Press, London.

Pallis, C.A. (1955) Impaired identification of faces and places with agnosia for colours. *J. Neurol. Neurosurg. Psychiat.*, **18**, 218–24.

Perrett, D.I. and Rolls, E.T. (1983) Neural mechanisms underlying the visual analysis of faces, in *Advances in Vertebrate Neuroethology* (eds J.-P. Ewert, R.R. Capranica and D.J. Ingle). Plenum Press, New York, pp. 543–66.

Perrett, D.I., Rolls, E.T. and Caan, W. (1982) Visual neurones responsive to faces in the monkey temporal cortex. *Exp. Brain Res.*, **47**, 329–42.

Perrett, D.I., Smith, P.A.J., Potter, D.D., Mistlin, A.J., Head, A.S., Milner, A.D. and Jeeves, M.A. (1984) Neurones responsive to faces in the temporal cortex: studies of functional organization sensitivity and relation to perception. *Human Neurobiol.*, **3**, 197–208.

Perrett, D.I., Smith, P.A.J., Potter, D.D., Mistlin, A.J., Head, A.S., Milner, A.D.

and Jeeves, M.A. (1985a) Visual cells in the temporal cortex sensitive to face view and gaze direction. *Proc. R. Soc. B.*, **223**, 293–317.

Perrett, D.I., Smith, P.A.J., Mistlin, A.J., Chitty, A.J., Head, A.S., Potter, D.D., Broennimann, R., Milner, A.D. and Jeeves, M.A. (1985b) Visual analysis of body movements by neurones in the temporal cortex of the macaque monkey. A preliminary report. *Behav. Brain Res.*, **16**, 153–70.

Perrett, D.I., Mistlin, A.J., Potter, D.D., Smith, P.A.J., Head, A.S., Chitty, A.J., Broennimann, R., Milner, A.D. and Jeeves, M.A. (1986a) Functional organization of visual neurones processing face identity, in *Aspects of Face Processing* (eds H. Ellis, M.A. Jeeves, F. Newcombe and A. Young). Martinus Nijhoff, Dordrecht, pp. 187–98.

Perrett, D.I., Mistlin, A.J., Chitty, A.J., Smith, P.A.J., Potter, D.D., Broennimann, R. and Harries, M. (1986b) Specialized face processing and hemispheric asymmetry in man and monkey: evidence from single unit and reaction time studies, in *Proceedings of EBBS Conference on Hemispheric Cerebral Asymmetry*, February 1986, *Behav. Brain Res.* (in press).

Rolls, E.T. (1984) Neurones in the cortex of the temporal lobe and in the amygdala of the monkey with responses selective for faces. *Human Neurobiol.*, **3**, 209–22.

Seltzer, B. and Pandya, D.N. (1978) Afferent cortical connections and architectonics of the superior temporal sulcus and surrounding cortex in the rhesus monkey. *Brain Res.*, **149**, 1–24.

Szentagothai, J. (1978) The neurone network of the cerebral cortex: a functional interpretation. The Ferrier Lecture. *Proc. R. Soc. Lond. B*, **201**, 219–48.

Taylor, A.M. and Warrington, E.K. (1973) Visual discrimination in patients with localized cerebral lesions. *Cortex*, **9**, 82–93.

Warrington, E.K. and Rabin, P. (1970) Perceptual moulding in patients with cerebral lesions. *Neuropsychologia*, **8**, 475–87.

Whiteley, A.M. and Warrington, E.K. (1977) Prosopagnosia: a clinical, psychological, and anatomical study of three patients. *J. Neurol. Neurosurg. Psychiat.*, **40**, 394–430.

Whiten, A. and Byrne, R. (1986) The St Andrews catalogue of tactical deception in primates. *St Andrews Psychological Reports*, no. 10.

CHAPTER 9

Visuo-spatial disorders

ENNIO DE RENZI

Long considered a rare event of little consequence for clinical practice, visuo-spatial disorders are now recognized to represent a frequent concomitant of hemispheric disease, having a definite localizing value and affecting everyday activity and rehabilitation. They manifest a wide spectrum of symptoms reflecting impairment of discrete functional stages, and are, therefore, better treated by making reference to the level of space information processing, which has been deranged by cerebral damage. Table 9.1 summarizes the array of symptoms and how they can be organized around the three basic topics of space exploration, perception and memory.

Table 9.1 Synopsis of spatial disorders

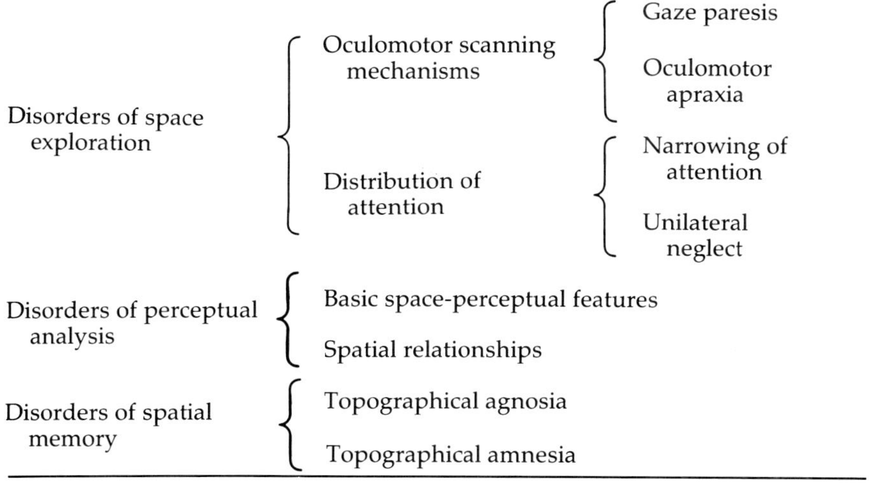

Disorders of space exploration	Oculomotor scanning mechanisms	Gaze paresis
		Oculomotor apraxia
	Distribution of attention	Narrowing of attention
		Unilateral neglect
Disorders of perceptual analysis	Basic space-perceptual features	
	Spatial relationships	
Disorders of spatial memory	Topographical agnosia	
	Topographical amnesia	

9.1 Disorders of space exploration

Preliminary to any type of visuo-perceptual processing of incoming information is a prompt and efficient scanning of the environment: stimuli of interest appearing in the peripheral visual field must first draw the subject's attention and trigger eye movements to ensure their fovealization. The attentional and oculomotor components of this mechanism may be selectively disrupted by focal cerebral lesions, producing different patterns of impaired space exploration.

9.1.1 DISRUPTION OF OCULOMOTOR MECHANISMS

Voluntary and visually elicited saccades are probably monitored by several cortical areas, as suggested by the multiple loci of the cerebral mantle, stimulation of which elicits contraversive eye movements (Wagman *et al.*, 1964), but two areas have acquired a dominant role, the frontal eye field (FEF) or area 8 and the posterior parietal cortex, corresponding to area 7. Both area 8 (Goldberg and Bushnell, 1981) and area 7 (Lynch *et al.*, 1977) contain neurones which fire prior to an eye movement directed to an object of interest for the animal appearing in a given sector of the visual field. Both areas have connections with the cells of the deep layers of the superior colliculus, which also show an enhancement of their discharge contingent on visually elicited saccades (Wurtz and Mohler, 1976). Pathways projecting to the paramedian pontine reticular formation (PPRF), which contains phasic cells activating the oculomotor nuclei, have been traced from area 8 (Leichnetz, 1981) and the superior colliculus. Area 7 has, in addition, neurones discharging (Lynch *et al.*, 1977) when the monkey fixates an object of interest located in a given zone of space (fixation neurones), and neurones discharging before and during smooth pursuit movements of a target moved in a given direction (tracking movements).

Traditionally (Holmes, 1938; Daroff and Hoyt, 1971), the control of saccades has been attributed to area 8 and that of pursuit movements and fixation to the parieto-occipital cortex, but both animal experiments and human studies argue against such a strict segregation of function. In particular, the bulk of clinical evidence speaks in favour of a predominant participation of the posterior parietal cortex in the control of saccades as well as pursuit movements. The two main clinical pictures where both movements are impaired are gaze paresis and oculomotor apraxia.

9.1.2 GAZE PARESIS

Following unilateral hemispheric disease, especially if of abrupt onset, as in a stroke, the patient may be observed to keep his head and eyes turned to the side of lesion and to be unable to move his eyes beyond the midline, either on verbal command or on contralateral presentation of a visual and acoustic stimulus, or when requested to follow a moving target (e.g. the eyes of the examiner who is slowly moving around the bed). Oculo-cephalic movements and vestibular nystagmus are, on the contrary, preserved. This picture is the counterpart of what is observed in the course of adversive seizures, when the head and eyes are forcibly turned towards the side contralateral to lesion. In both cases the reason for the deviation must be sought in a tonic imbalance between the centres in each hemisphere which control contraversive head and eye movements. With the passage of time the patient progressively re-acquires the capacity to move his eyes contralaterally, but for a long time he may find it extremely hard to maintain the extreme position and tends not to look at the examiner when addressed from the contralateral side, although answering his questions.

In spite of the fact that gaze deviation has been known to neurologists since Prévost (1868), and represents a common finding in acute brain-damaged patients, very few studies have been expressly devoted to it. In cases that come to autopsy, the lesion has usually been found to be too large to allow precise anatomico-clinical correlations. Thus the claim, recurrent in the literature (Holmes, 1938; Daroff and Hoyt, 1971; Leigh and Zee, 1983) that it must be ascribed to a lesion of the FEF or its descending pathways rests more on the assumption, derived from animal studies, that these structures are responsible for saccades than on a firm basis of data. To obviate this uncertainty, we (De Renzi *et al.*, 1982) carried out a systematic investigation of the oculomotor behaviour of all patients admitted to our department for a unilateral stroke over a period of 17 months. A total of 436 patients were examined (228 with left brain damage and 208 with right brain damage) and 120 (28%) showed gaze paresis, when tested in the first three days of disease. The sign tended to recover with passage of time, but 24% of the 59 patients who showed it initially and were followed up for two weeks were still markedly impaired. The most interesting and unexpected finding was that gaze paresis occurred with different frequency, severity and duration, depending on which hemisphere was affected. Among right brain-damaged (RBD) patients it was found in 35% of cases, was more marked and lasted on average 14.9 days, whereas in left brain-damaged (LBD) patients, it occurred in 21% of cases, was milder and had a mean duration of 8.6 days; all these differences were significant. These findings were replicated in a second investigation (De Renzi and Colombo, unpublished work) carried out on 227 patients, where again the proportion of patients showing gaze paresis was significantly greater among RBD patients (25%) than LBD patients (16%).

Another element of differentiation between the two hemispheric groups was the pattern of neurological deficits associated with gaze paresis. Among LBD patients the highest occurrence of the deficit was in those who presented with hemiplegia, hemianaesthesia, hemianopia and global aphasia, namely with a massive neurological symptomatology pointing to the involvement of the entire peri-Sylvian territory. In the RBD group, on the contrary, gaze paresis prevailed in patients with signs pointing to a more posterior localization of damage (hemianaesthesia, and/or hemianopia, but not hemiplegia). Eye movement disorders were found in 61% of RBD patients versus only 13% of LBD patients having this cluster of symptoms. We interpreted this finding as evidence that oculomotor control is differently organized in the two hemispheres, being diffusely distributed on the left side and focalized around the parietal lobe on the right side. We argued that this pattern of cortical representation accounts for the prevalence of gaze paresis in RBD patients, because damage to the parietal lobe cannot be easily compensated.

It is noteworthy that oculomotor disorders were seldom seen in patients with hemiplegia without hemianaesthesia and hemianopia, namely with damage not impinging upon the retrorolandic cortex. We have subsequently collected cases with CT evidence of a lesion involving area 8 and none of them showed gaze paresis.

9.1.3 OCULOMOTOR APRAXIA AND BALINT–HOLMES SYNDROME

Patients with gaze paresis cannot explore the contralateral space, because they fail to move their eyes beyond the midline and are forced to look at the ipsilateral space. Patients with the syndrome of oculomotor apraxia, on the contrary, do not have any intrinsic limitation of eye movements and are able to carry out random movements in any direction; yet they are deprived of the ability to control and programme purposeful eye movements. When requested to look at a certain direction, either on verbal command or in response to the appearance of a stimulus, their gaze wanders around aimlessly, at times starting towards the opposite direction and, when arriving by chance on the target, easily loses it. Slow pursuit movements are equally impaired, a sign rarely reported in isolation. Much more frequently it is part of a more complex syndrome of spatial disorientation, where visual inattention and misreaching co-exist. In its most severe expression the former consists of an extreme narrowing of attention permitting the patient to see just one stimulus at a time producing the disappearance of whatever surrounds it. The size of the perceived stimulus is not critical: it may be a large object or drawing as well as a pin but, once it has captured the patient's attention, nothing else is seen. A patient seen in our department (Sorgato, 1976) could not perceive two small dots drawn at a distance of 5 mm. As a consequence, the patient is unable to count objects scattered on a table, to read a text, or to relate the elements of a picture to each other in order to grasp the meaning of the whole. The latter inability is sometimes called simultanagnosia, although this term was introduced into neurological parlance by Wolpert (1924) to designate a disorder of complex picture comprehension not dependent on defective scanning but lying at a level intermediate between intelligence and perception.

Misreaching is the third element of the syndrome. The patient is unable to guide his arm to an object with a single ballistic movement, but gropes for it and reaches out besides the target, under- or over-estimating its distance. Although in the most severe cases the deficit appears when the target is fixated, much more frequently it occurs in peripheral vision and it is indeed crucial to test the patient separately for each visual field and for each hand. The very fact that in some patients errors are confined to one limb is evidence that misreaching cannot be attributed to a deficit of space perception.

The syndrome of global visual disorientation was first reported in detail by Balint (1909) in a patient with a bilateral vascular lesion and rediscovered a few years later by Holmes (1918) in veterans who had sustained missile wounds during the First World War. The eponym of Balint–Holmes syndrome seems appropriate, because the oculomotor disorders were described not by Balint, but by Holmes. There are now more than 10 cases verified at autopsy, and additional cases with CT scan documentation concur in confirming the claim of Balint (1909) and Holmes (1918) that the lesion responsible affects both posterior parietal lobes. Animal experimentation is in good agreement with clinico-pathological evidence in emphasizing the paramount role of this cortical region in monitoring spatial behaviour. In this area, single cell recording has shown the presence not only of neurones discharging before and in the course of saccades, pursuit movements and fixation, as previously mentioned, but also of neurones which enhance their firing in association with visually guided limb movements and neurones active when the animal pays attention to a target appearing in a specific sector of the visual field, also in the absence of any kind of movement. Following bilateral ablation of area 7, the monkey was observed to pay no attention to an object approaching from the periphery, if fixating the examiner (Denny-Brown and Chambers, 1958) and to show gross errors in direction and amplitude of the reaching limb (Faugier-Grimaud, Frenois and Stein, 1978).

Although Balint–Holmes syndrome is characterized by disorientation in the visual space, a severe disruption in guiding eye and hand movements towards a stimulus the position of which is perceived through auditory or proprioceptive modalities has also been occasionally reported. To the few cases mentioned in the literature I now add two further patients.

A few hours after a normal delivery, a 27-year-old woman presented with hypertension, headache, proteinuria and two generalized seizures. She remained drowsy for two days. When consciousness was regained, optic apraxia, misreaching, visual agnosia, memory disorders and a certain degree of anomia were noted. The patient was transferred to our department 20 days later. On examination, she showed no motor and sensory deficit, but missed stimuli in the lower left quadrant on confrontation. She was unable to describe the facial features of a person and complained of seeing shadows in front of her. There was a severe visual agnosia, which contrasted with the correct recognition of handled objects. She was moderately amnesic. The gaze was spontaneously deviated a few degrees to the right and there was limitation in the ability to direct the gaze to the left. Smooth pursuit movements and convergence movements were lost not only when she was requested to follow a moving object, but also when she had to look at her thumb, passively moved by the examiner. Saccades were erratic when elicited by the visual presentation of an object, while they were prompt and precise when directed to an auditory stimulus or to her thumb, displaced by the examiner. She misreached for an object presented in central fixation and even more when it was shown at the periphery of the visual field and she could not look at it. The same difficulty was present when she closed her eyes and tried to grasp her thumb, passively moved by the examiner. CT scan showed bilateral parieto-occipital damage (Fig. 9.1).

The second patient was a 33-year-old man with a history of Wegener's granulomatosis dating back 7 years. In the last 20 days his wife had noticed an impairment in writing and reading and a difficulty in reaching out for objects. On the day of admission he became speechless. Clinical examination revealed no motor, sensory or visual field deficit, but he showed global aphasia (permitting, however, the comprehension of simple commands), severe bilateral apraxia and a complete Balint–Holmes syndrome. He could not see more than one object at a time, was totally unable to direct his eyes to a visual target presented in any part of the visual field, or to make slow pursuit movements, although random movements were full in all directions. He patently misreached objects even when free to fixate them. His behaviour did not improve when the information about the spatial position of the target was conveyed through auditory and proprioceptive modalities. He failed to direct his gaze or

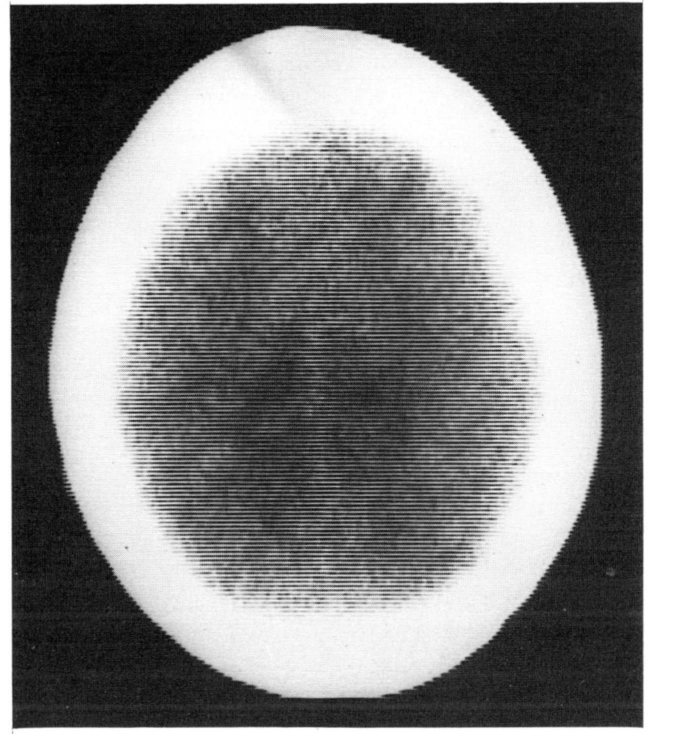

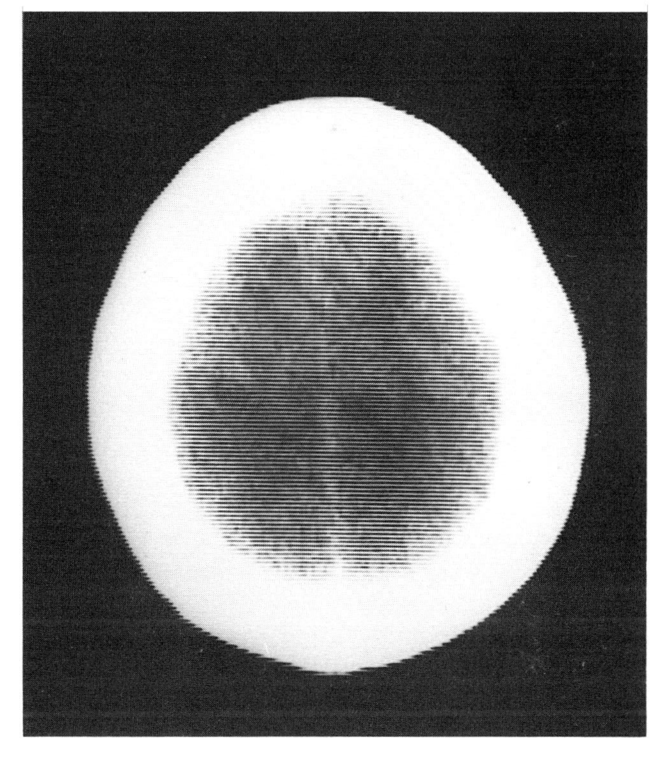

Fig. 9.1 CT scan of a patient with Balint–Holmes syndrome showing biparietal infarction.

limb to a sound or to his thumb and his eyes wandered around helplessly in wrong directions, as if he had no idea of where the target was located. Walking was hindered by his inability to appreciate the distance of objects, which resulted in bumping into obstacles, while when trying to sit down on a chair he failed to orient his body with respect to its plane and fell down ruinously. CT scan showed a left superior temporal and parietal softening but, surprisingly, no sign of right posterior disease, although its presence can be predicated on clinical grounds. This patient shows a strong similarity with the patient reported by Kase and co-workers (1977), and emphasizes that the spatial disorders of the Balint–Holmes syndrome may in some cases involve all modalities, deserving the label of global spatial disorientation.

9.1.4 UNILATERAL NEGLECT

Extreme focalization of attention to the point of ignoring anything else but what the patient is fixating, as seen in Balint–Holmes syndrome, is a rare phenomenon. Much more frequent is the neglect of the contralateral space, resulting from unilateral brain damage, especially of the right hemisphere. The patient behaves as if the space would stop at the midline and fails to direct his attention beyond it, even when task instructions demand the scanning of environment. For instance, when requested to look for an object that the examiner claims is present on the table, the patient keeps on lingering his gaze to the right, never looking to the left; asked to draw a face the left ear and eye is omitted; on eating the food lying on the left half of the dish is not picked up and on shaving the left cheek is ignored. Many types of searching tasks have been devised to provide an objective, standardized measure of this deficit, e.g. crossing out lines scattered on a sheet, match-to-sample tasks, line bisection, etc., but probably the easiest clinical demonstration is to have the patient reading a newspaper headline. Depending on the severity of neglect he may omit a few of the first words of the sentence, or start from the word at the midline, or from the extreme right or even from its last syllables, apparently unconcerned that what he is reading does not make sense. Scrutiny of the patient's oculomotor behaviour sometimes reveals that as soon as the stimulus is presented, he shifts his gaze to the right end of the headline, as if it were magnetically attracted by stimuli on the extreme right; he may then, or may not, progressively regain part of the left space.

The frequency with which hemispheric damage produces neglect depends on the side and site of lesion, the time post-onset of disease and the assessment criteria used. The most remarkable aspect of neglect is its close association with right brain disease. When systematically assessed in consecutive series of patients, its frequency has ranged from 2 to 12%

in LBD patients and 31 to 46% in RBD patients (Hécaen and Angelergues, 1963; Gainotti, 1968; Gloning, Gloning and Hoff, 1968; Faglioni, Scotti and Spinnler, 1971). On the basis of CT scan data, right parietal damage has been found to be the most frequent, although not the exclusive, pathological correlate of neglect (Bisiach, Luzzatti and Perani, 1979; Heilman *et al.*, 1983; Vallar and Perani, 1986), and it has also been reported following frontal (Heilman and Valenstein, 1972), lenticular (Heir *et al.*, 1977) and thalamic (Watson and Heilman, 1979) disease. In the most thorough investigation of the anatomical correlates of neglect in RBD patients (Vallar and Perani, 1986), the deficit was found in 58% of cases with post-Rolandic damage, mainly clustered around the inferior parietal lobule, as opposed to 8% of cases with frontal damage. Neglect after basal ganglia lesions was also found, but inconsistently, occurring in 50% of cases with lesions confined to the thalamus and in 30% of cases with damage limited to the lenticular nucleus.

Follow-up studies have shown that neglect tends to recover, yet it has been reported by Colombo, De Renzi and Gentilini (1982) to be still present 8 to 12 months post-stroke in one-third of the cases initially severely impaired. Interestingly, in this study, the patient with the most persistent and dramatic impairment had two lesions, one involving the parieto-occipital junction and the other the thalamus. Several patients who no longer exhibited neglect, when assessed with classical tests, showed a significant increase in their searching time of the contralateral space on a matching-to-sample test.

Neglect can also affect the personal space, making the patient ignorant of, or indifferent to, the disability affecting the right side of his own body. He denies being hemiplegic (anosognosia), is unconcerned about his motor impairment and claims to be able to carry out activities, such as walking, knitting, playing cards, etc., which require the integrity of both limbs. The relationship of corporeal to extracorporeal neglect is variable (Bisiach *et al.*, 1986), but both aspects are likely to be responsible for the less marked improvement of activities of daily living found six months after a stroke in patients with left hemiplegia as compared to those with right hemiplegia (Denes *et al.*, 1982).

The pathophysiology of neglect and of its asymmetrical occurrence following damage to either hemisphere has not been completely clarified and is likely to involve more than one mechanism. Most authorities consider it a consequence of the disruption of a hemispheric loop subserving direction of attention to the contralateral space, which would involve both cortical and subcortical interconnecting structures, the parietal lobe and frontal lobes, and the basal ganglia including the thalamus. A lesion at any point of this circuit would leave the contralateral space unattended (Heilman, Valenstein and Watson, 1985;

Mesulam, 1985) but, as previously mentioned, there is clear-cut evidence that this loop is hierarchically organized, with the interior parietal lobe playing a pivotal role and the frontal lobe being only marginally implicated. To account for the hemispheric asymmetry of neglect, it has been assumed that while the left brain mediates the deployment of attention to the right space, the right brain surveys both the right and the left space, which would permit a much better compensation following left than right hemisphere damage.

The hypothesis that what happens in the right hemispace activates the two hemispheres while what happens in the left hemispace activates only the right brain gives rise to some problems. If true, normal subjects should show differential accuracy and proficiency in monitoring the two hemispaces, since the right side is attended by left brain neurones plus a part of right brain neurones, while the left side is attended only by a fraction of right brain cells. No evidence of an imbalance in directed attention has ever been shown in normal subjects and it is also hard to imagine how an animal whose attention is biased to one side could have survived in the struggle for existence. I am, therefore, inclined to attribute the different occurrence of neglect not to a predominant role played by the right brain for attention, but to a differential hemispheric organization of attentive functions, which would be more diffusely represented on the left and more focalized on the right, as suggested by the findings of gaze paresis.

9.2 Disorders of space perception

Space perception refers to the processing of sensory data defining the position an object has with respect to the observer or environment, e.g. the identification of its position, orientation, configuration and of its relationships with other objects. It is exceptional that the impairment produced at this functional level gives rise to disorders as disruptive of behaviour as those seen with a deficit of space exploration. A few patients have been reported to collide with objects when walking, to fall to the floor when trying to take a seat because of an inability to estimate distances or to complain that the environment looks all flat, as in a picture or photograph. They usually suffer from bilateral damage and present with Balint–Holmes syndrome. Unilateral damage results in a less dramatic impairment of space perception and requires appropriate tests to be elicited but, if properly assessed, the deficit may be quite clear and is usually associated with right hemisphere disease. Errors of localization on a plane (Faglioni, Scotti and Spinnler, 1971; Hannay, Varney and Benton, 1976), of depth perception in the absence of the aids provided by form cues (Carmon and Bechtoldt, 1969; Hamsher, 1978), of line orientation in a tridimensional or bidimensional space (De Renzi, Faglioni and Scotti, 1971; Benton, Varney and Hamsher, 1978) were all found to be significantly increased in an unselected RBD population, while LBD patients performed no differently from control subjects.

A more complex pattern emerges (De Renzi, 1982) when the patient's task is not confined to localizing or matching simple stimuli, but involves 'spatial thinking', namely mental operations requiring the integration of spatial data in order to build up an internal representation or to infer rules. This is the kind of performance involved in several spatial tasks of intelligence tests (e.g. block designs, picture arrangement, Raven Progressive Matrices, etc.) and has been repeatedly used by psychologists to contrast RBD patients with LBD patients; the results, however, have been partially disappointing. These tests have been found sensitive to brain damage, but do not distinguish whether it is located to the right or left half of the brain, probably because they involve not a single, but several, discrete abilities, spatial as well as non-spatial. A better differentiation between the two hemispheric groups has been achieved with tests requiring the mental rotation of a picture (De Renzi and Faglioni, 1967) or the ability to imagine how it looks when viewed from different perspectives (Butters, Barton and Brody, 1970; Ratcliff, 1979), or a perceptual maze test, in which finding a path on a dot lattice is required (Benton *et al.*, 1963; Colonna and Faglioni, 1966; Archibald, 1978). RBD patients have been consistently reported to score more poorly, attesting to the specialization of this side of the brain in the processing of spatial information.

9.3 Constructional apraxia

It is appropriate to mention at this point constructional apraxia (CA), a disorder that enjoys popularity among clinicians for its ease of ascertainment at the bedside and for its relationship to visuo-spatial perception. It covers activities aimed at assembling the component parts of a whole, under the guidance of a visual or mental model, faithfully respecting their spatial relationships. In clinical practice it is basically assessed by requiring the patient to copy drawings of increasing difficulty or, more rarely, three-dimensional block buildings. Drawing from memory provides a less reliable estimate of constructional performance, because it calls for additional abilities, such as understanding the name of the target and conjuring up its mental representation, and these may be impaired for reasons unrelated to constructional activity *per se*.

Copying drawings implies two stages, the perceptual analysis of the lines composing the model, which must be reproduced one at a time, and the programme and execution of the manual performance. In principle, either of these levels can be responsible for defective copies and there is indeed a trend, recurring in the literature, to contrast two forms of CA, one due to visuo-spatial impairment and linked with right brain damage, and the other due to executive impairment and linked with left brain damage. The basis for this dichotomy is partly found in the qualitative differences observed in the designs produced by the two hemispheric groups, but probably more in the well-established specialization of the right hemisphere for spatial abilities and of the left hemisphere for praxic ones. Considered in this perspective, CA would basically be an agnosia when associated with right brain damage and a true apraxia only when associated with left brain damage.

However, the evidence that can be marshalled in support of this thesis is weak and contradictory. One would expect a deficit of space perception to be associated with RBD patients with CA only, and LBD patients with CA to evince signs of limb apraxia, but no impairment in visuo-spatial analysis. Neither of these predictions are borne out. The correlation of constructional performance with space perception tests has been found to be high and of the same magnitude in both RBD and LBD patients and constructional apraxics of either group scored more poorly than patients without CA (Piercy and Smyth, 1962; De Renzi and Faglioni, 1967; Arena and Gainotti, 1978). A defective analysis of spatial relations would, therefore, appear to play the same role in determining CA, independently of the injured side. As to executive deficit, the assumption that the drawing disability of LBD patients reflects a movement organization disorder is undermined by the finding that there are patients with ideo-motor apraxia who do not manifest CA (Ajuriaguerra, Hécaen and Angelergues, 1960). Much emphasis has been given (Warrington, 1969) to the qualitative differences found in the designs of the two hemispheric groups, which would attest the heterogeneity of the underlying mechanisms but the distinguishing features pointed out by the various studies have been hard to replicate (De Renzi, 1982), apart from the prevalence of signs of left-sided neglect in right hemisphere apraxics. Although the question is not definitively settled (Mack and Levine (1981) did find hemispheric differences), it seems safe to conclude that CA of both hemispheric patients measures to a large extent the same basic disorder in analysing the spatial orientation of the lines constituting a design. It affects about one-third of unselected patients with unilateral brain damage and in RBD patients is frequently associated with parietal lesion. In LBD patients this link is less close, probably because multiple factors may play a role in the genesis of CA (spatial disorders, intellectual deterioration, motor clumsiness, aphasia, etc.).

9.4 Topographical amnesia

The inability to take one's bearing in a familiar environment by a patient with clear consciousness and preservation of general memory probably constitutes the most easily distinguishable type of spatial disorder and it was in fact the first to draw the attention of neurologists and be described in detail (Foerster, 1890; Jackson, 1931). When, as usually happens, it follows a stroke, the patient suddenly discovers that he is no longer able to find his way about in familiar surroundings and may even make mistakes at home trying to go to a given room. A patient of mine confessed that when he was in the corridor of his apartment he had to open a door to know what room was behind it. In hospital the patient desperately looks for the bed number or some landmark (e.g. a clock hanging on the wall of the corridor next to his ward) to find where his room is, and when eventually there, seeks confirmation in personal belongings laid on the night-table. Most patients are equally impaired if requested to draw the spatial arrangement of their home, verbally describe a familiar path and its turns, or locate the main cities on a blank map of their country. As the deficit subsides, the patient regains the ability to take his bearings in surroundings well known before the disease, but still meets with remarkable difficulty in learning a new path (e.g. in the hospital) and helps himself by memorizing cues provided by ward numbers, specific visual signs, written names, etc. (Whitty and Newcombe, 1973).

Close analysis of the patient's behaviour suggests that losing his way may be the consequence of two discrete disabilities, which sometimes co-exist, topographical agnosia and topographical amnesia (Paterson and Zangwill, 1945). A few patients have a deficit in recognizing places, and cannot, therefore, aid themselves with landmarks on the route, e.g. by remembering that when a given building is reached, a right turn must be taken. I saw a patient who long roved the street in which he lived, knowing that his house was there, but remained unable to identify it from among other cottages. When present in its pure form (Pallis, 1955; Whiteley and Warrington, 1978), place agnosia is distinguishable from topographical amnesia, because the patient is able carefully to describe a route and even to draw a plan of it, specifying where and in which direction turns are to be made, but then gets lost when walking in the real surroundings. The patient has no trouble in recognizing that a church is a church or a cottage is a cottage, but fails to identify the specific church or cottage. The question of whether the basic defect is perceptual or amnestic, and if it is indeed specific for places, is still a matter of debate.

A different clinical pattern occurs when failure to find the way is contingent upon the inability to learn or recall the spatial schema of a route (topographical amnesia). Landmarks are recognized but, being devoid of directional value, cannot assist the patient in deciding whether, on arriving at a given point, he has to walk straight forward, or to turn left or right. Understandably, verbal description from memory and drawing a path on a map are equally impaired. In a few severe cases the deficit involves the memory of simpler spatial relationships, e.g. the patient is unable to point to the furniture of his room when he is blindfolded, or to retrace the position of an article he is reading in the newspaper, if this has been removed for a while (De Renzi and Faglioni, 1962; Scotti, 1968). This kind of patient may find it impossible to learn a path on a visually guided maze, despite innumerable trials (De Renzi, Faglioni and Villa, 1977).

There is evidence for an ascendancy of the right hemisphere in memorizing spatial relations and for a critical role played by the hippocampus and the posterior parieto-temporal region of the lateral cerebral mantle. Extensive right hippocampus ablation, carried out for the relief of epilepsy, resulted in a poor performance on tests requiring to learn a path on a maze (Corkin, 1965; Milner, 1965) and to remember the location of a stimulus on an array (Smith and Milner, 1981). Patients with posterior right brain damage have also been reported to be impaired on the maze test (Ratcliff and Newcombe, 1973; De Renzi, Faglioni and Villa, 1977), while patients with a comparable lesion of the left hemisphere performed no differently from normal controls. Although the subjects of these studies did not show manifestations of route-finding disability, their results are in good agreement with those of patients with clinical evidence of topographical disorientation, some of whom had damage to the temporo-parieto-occipital junction on the lateral convexity of the right hemisphere, and others in the territory of the right posterior cerebral artery, which supplies the hippocampus and hippocampal gyrus.

References

Ajuriaguerra, J., Hécaen, H. and Angelergues, R. (1960) Les apraxies: varietés cliniques et latéralisation lésionelle. *Rev. Neurol.*, **102**, 566–94.

Archibald, Y.M. (1978) Time as a variable in the performance of hemisphere-damaged patients on the Elithorn Perceptual Maze Test. *Cortex*, **14**, 22–31.

Arena, R. and Gainotti, G. (1978) Constructional apraxia and visuoperceptive disabilities in relation to laterality of cerebral lesions. *Cortex*, **14**, 463–73.

Balint, R. (1909) Seelenlähmung des Schauens, optische Ataxie, raumliche Stoerung der Aufmerksamkeit. *Monatschrift Psychiat. Neurol.*, **25**, 51–81.

Benton, A.L., Elithorn, A., Fogel, M.L. and Kerr, M. (1963) A perceptual maze test sensitive to brain damage. *J. Neurol. Neurosurg. Psychiat.*, **26**, 540–4.

Benton, A.L., Varney, N.R. and Hamsher, K. de S. (1978) Visuospatial judgment: a clinical test. *Arch. Neurol.*, **35**, 364–7.

Bisiach, E., Luzzatti, C. and Perani, D. (1979) Unilateral neglect, representational

schema and consciousness. *Brain*, **102**, 609–18.
Bisiach, E., Vallar, G., Perani, D., Papagno, C. and Berti, A. (1986) Unawareness of disease following lesions of the right hemisphere: anosognosia for hemiplegia and anosognosia for hemianopia. *Neuropsychologia*, **24**, 471–82.
Butters, N., Barton, M. and Brody, B.A. (1970) Role of the right parietal lobe in the mediation of cross-modal associations and reversible operations in space. *Cortex*, **6**, 174–90.
Carmon, A. and Bechtoldt, H.P. (1969) Dominance of the right cerebral hemisphere for stereopsis. *Neuropsychologia*, **7**, 29–40.
Colombo, A., De Renzi, E. and Gentilini, M. (1982) The time course of visual hemi-inattention. *Arch. Psychiat. Nervenkrankheit.*, **231**, 539–46.
Colonna, A. and Faglioni, P. (1966) The performance of hemisphere-damaged patients on spatial intelligence tests. *Cortex*, **2**, 293–307.
Corkin, S. (1965) Tactually-guided maze learning in man: effects of unilateral cortical excisions and bilateral hippocampal lesions. *Neuropsychologia*, **3**, 339–51.
Daroff, R.B. and Hoyt, W.F. (1971) Supranuclear disorders of ocular control systems in man: clinical, anatomical and physiological correlations, in *The Control of Eye Movements* (eds. P. Bach-y-Rita, C.C. Collins and J.E. Hyde). Academic Press, New York, pp. 176–84.
Denes, G., Semenza, C., Stoppa, E. and Lis, A. (1982) Unilateral spatial neglect and recovery from hemiplegia: a follow-up study. *Brain*, **105**, 543–52.
Denny-Brown, D. and Chambers, R.A. (1958) The parietal lobe and behavior, in *The Brain and Human Behavior*, vol. 36. *Proc. Assoc. Res. Nerv. Ment. Dis.* Wilkins, Baltimore, pp. 35–117.
De Renzi, E. and Faglioni, P. (1962) Il disorientamento spaziale de lesione cerebrale. *Sistema Nervosa*, **14**, 409–36.
De Renzi, E. (1982) *Disorders of Space Exploration and Cognition*. Wiley, Chichester.
De Renzi, E. and Faglioni, P. (1967) The relationship between visuo-spatial impairment and constructional apraxia. *Cortex*, **3**, 327–42.
De Renzi, E., Colombo, A., Faglioni, P. and Gibertoni, M. (1982) Conjugate gaze paresis in stroke patients with unilateral brain damage. *Arch. Neurol.*, **39**, 482–6.
De Renzi, E., Faglioni, P. and Scotti, G. (1971) Judgment of spatial orientation in patients with focal brain damage. *J. Neurol. Neurosurg. Psychiat.*, **34**, 489–95.
De Renzi, E., Faglioni, P. and Villa, P. (1977) Topographical amnesia. *J. Neurol. Neurosurg. Psychiat.*, **40**, 498–505.
Eidelberg, D. and Galaburda, A.M. (1984) Inferior parietal lobule. Divergent architectonic asymmetries in the human brain. *Arch. Neurol.*, **41**, 843–52.
Faglioni, P., Scotti, G. and Spinnler, H. (1971) The performance of brain-damaged patients in spatial localization of visual and tactile stimuli. *Brain*, **94**, 443–54.
Faugier-Grimaud, S., Frenois, C. and Stein, D.G. (1978) Effects of posterior parietal lesions on visually guided behavior in monkeys. *Neuropsychologia*, **16**, 151–68.
Foerster, R. (1890) Uber Rindenblinheit. *Albrecht von Graefe's Arch. Ophthalmol.*, **36**, 94–108.
Gainotti, G. (1968) Les manifestations de négligence et d'inattention pour l'hémispace. *Cortex*, **4**, 64–91.
Gloning, I., Gloning, K. and Hoff, H. (1968) *Neuropsychological Symptoms and*

Syndromes in Lesions of the Occipital Lobe and the Adjacent Areas. Gauthier-Villars, Paris.

Goldberg, M.E. and Bushnell, M.C. (1981) Behavioral enhancement of visual responses in monkey cerebral cortex: II. Modulation in frontal eye fields specifically related to saccades. *J. Neurophysiol.*, **46**, 773–87.

Hamsher, K. de S. (1978) Stereopsis and unilateral brain disease. *Invest. Ophthalmol.*, **17**, 336–42.

Hannay, H.J., Varney, N.R. and Benton, A.L. (1976) Visual localization in patients with unilateral brain disease. *J. Neurol. Neurosurg. Psychiat.*, **39**, 307–13.

Hécaen, H. and Angelergues, R. (1963) *La Cécité Psychique.* Masson, Paris.

Heilman, K.M. and Valenstein, E. (1972) Frontal lobe neglect in man. *Neurology*, **22**, 660–4.

Heilman, K.M., Valenstein, E. and Watson, R.T. (1985) The neglect syndrome, in *Clinical Neuropsychology* (eds P.J. Vinken, G.W. Bruyn, H.L. Klawans and J.H.M. Frederiks) (*Handbook of Clinical Neurology*, vol. 45). Elsevier, Amsterdam, pp. 153–84.

Heilman, K.M., Watson, R.T., Valenstein, E. and Damasio, A.R. (1983) Localization of lesions in neglect, in *Localization in Neuropsychology* (ed. A. Kertesz). Academic Press, New York, pp. 471–92.

Heir, D.B., Davis, K.R., Richardson, E.P. and Mohr, J.P. (1977) Hypertensive putaminal haemorrhage. *Ann. Neurol.*, **1**, 152–9.

Holmes, G. (1918) Disturbances of visual orientation. *Br. J. Ophthalmol.*, **2**, 449–68, 506–18.

Holmes, G. (1938) The cerebral integration of the ocular movements. *Br. Med. J.*, **2**, 107–12.

Jackson, J.H. (1931) Case of large cerebral tumour without optic neuritis and with hemiplegia and imperception. Reprinted in *Selected Writings of John Hughlings Jackson* (ed. J. Taylor). Hodder and Stoughton, London, pp. 146–52.

Kase, C.S., Troncoso, J.F., Court, J.E., Tapia, J.F. and Mohr, J.P. (1977) Global spatial disorientation. *J. Neurol. Sci.*, **34**, 267–78.

Leichnetz, G.R. (1981) The prefrontal cortico-oculomotor trajectories in the monkey. *J. Neurol. Sci.*, **49**, 387–96.

Leigh, R.J. and Zee, D.S. (1983) *The Neurology of Eye Movements.* Davies, Philadelphia.

Lynch, J.C., Mountcastle, V.B., Talbot, W.H. and Yin, T.C.T. (1977) Parietal lobe mechanisms for directed visual attention. *J. Neurophysiol.*, **40**, 362–88.

Mack, J.L. and Levine, R.N. (1981) The basis of visual constructional disability in patients with unilateral cerebral lesions. *Cortex*, **17**, 512–31.

Mesulam, M.M. (1985) Attention, confusional states and neglect, in *Principles of Behavioral Neurology* (ed. M.M. Mesulam). Davies, Philadelphia, pp. 125–68.

Milner, B. (1965) Visually-guided maze learning in man: effects of bilateral hippocampal, bilateral frontal, and unilateral cerebral lesions. *Neuropsychologia*, **3**, 317–88.

Pallis, C.A. (1955) Impaired identification of faces and places with agnosia for colours. *J. Neurol. Neurosurg. Psychiat.*, **18**, 218–24.

Paterson, A. and Zangwill, O.L. (1945) A case of topographical disorientation associated with a unilateral cerebral lesion. *Brain*, **68**, 188–211.

Piercy, M. and Smyth, V.O.G. (1962) Right hemisphere dominance for certain nonverbal intellectual skills. *Brain*, **85**, 775–90.

Prévost, J.L. (1868) De la déviation conjuguée des yeux et de la rotation de la tête dans certains cas d'hémiplégie. Thèse de Paris.

Ratcliff, G. (1979) Spatial thought, mental rotation and the right cerebral hemisphere. *Neuropsychologia*, **17**, 49–54.

Ratcliff, G. and Newcombe, F. (1973) Spatial orientation in man: effects of left, right, and bilateral posterior cerebral lesions. *J. Neurol. Neurosurg. Psychiat.*, **36**, 448–54.

Scotti, G. (1968) La perdita della memoria topografica: descrizione di un caso. *Sistema Nervoso*, **20**, 352–61.

Smith, M.L. and Milner, B. (1981) The role of the right hippocampus in the recall of spatial location. *Neuropsychologia*, **19**, 781–93.

Sorgato, P. (1976) Analisi neuropsicologica delle complicanze cerebrali a lungo termine dell'eclampsia. *Riv. Patol. Nerv. Ment.*, **97**, 371–84.

Vallar, G. and Perani, D. (1986) The anatomy of unilateral neglect after right hemisphere stroke lesions. A clinical/CT scan correlation study in man. *Neuropsychologia*, **24**, 609–22.

Wagman, I.H. (1964) Eye movements induced by electric stimulation of cerebrum in monkeys and their relationship to bodily movements, in *The Oculomotor System* (ed. M.B. Bender). Harper and Row, New York, pp. 18–34.

Warrington, E.K. (1969) Constructional apraxia, in *Handbook of Clinical Neurology*, vol. 4 (eds P.J. Vinken and G.W. Bruyn). North Holland, Amsterdam, pp. 67–83.

Watson, R.T. and Heilman, K.M. (1979) Thalamic neglect. *Neurology*, **29**, 690–4.

Whiteley, A.M. and Warrington, E.K. (1978) Selective impairment of topographical memory: a single case study. *J. Neurol. Neurosurg. Psychiat.*, **41**, 575–8.

Whitty, C.W.M. and Newcombe, F. (1973) R.C. Oldfield's study of visual and topographical disturbances in a right occipito-parietal lesion of 30 years' duration. *Neuropsychologia*, **11**, 471–5.

Wolpert, I. (1924) Die Simultanagnosie. Stoerung der Gesamtauffasssung. *Z. Ges. Neurol. Psychiat.*, **93**, 397–415.

Wurtz, R.H. and Mohler, C.W. (1976) Organization of monkey superior colliculus: enhanced visual response of superficial layer cells. *J. Neurophysiol.*, **39**, 745–65.

CHAPTER 10

Visual agnosia: anatomical and functional accounts

M.J. RIDDOCH AND G.W. HUMPHREYS

10.1 Introduction: deficits in visual recognition

Visual object agnosia may be defined as a loss of the function of recognition of visually presented items (Nielsen, 1946). One of the earliest accounts of this disorder is that of Munk (1881), who observed that destruction of the occipital lobes of the cerebral hemispheres of the dog led to a strange disorder. The dog retained its ability to see and avoid objects but it ceased to 'recognize' them; for example, it would eat soap but not food, it would fail to act in the way it had done pre-lesion when in the vicinity of its bed, its chair or its master, etc. This phenomenon was not restricted to animals since similar deficits were described in the clinical field, i.e. patients with circumscribed lesions were identified as having a particular difficulty in the visual recognition of objects although elementary vision was preserved. Such patients were able to copy the outlines of objects correctly, and could describe their individual parts, but they were quite unable to recognize the object as a whole (Jackson, 1876; Freud, 1891; Charcot, 1886–7; Lissauer, 1890).

Particular issues of concern were whether specific functions were localized in the brain (compare Broca, 1861 with Marie, 1906) and, in cases where correlations obtained between lesion sites and behavioural deficits, whether these correlations were attributable to the hierarchical organization of function (cf. Jackson, 1876). That is, the issues concerned both the relation between the site of damage and the impaired function, and the nature of the impaired function.

Following in the steps of the early neurologists, many attempts were made to attribute particular functions to particular areas of the cortex, but it soon became clear that object recognition difficulties could result from lesions in quite different cortical areas. One way to deal with this problem is to fractionate visual agnosia both in terms of locus of site of lesion and of a description of the resulting deficit. In this chapter we discuss attempts to do this, and hope to illustrate how functional descriptions of deficits (i.e. descriptions which stress the loss of perceptual functions) and anatomical descriptions (i.e. descriptions which stress the lesion site and the functions served by those anatomical sites) can complement each other to form a fuller picture of the processes normally subserving a particular behaviour, and of how those processes can be impaired following brain damage.

10.2 Agnosia: an anatomical account

In discussing the attempts to fractionate agnosia, we separate those which broadly stress the nature and type of brain damage from those which broadly stress the nature of the functional loss, though this separation is by no means complete.

10.2.1 NIELSEN'S ACCOUNT

Attempts to link the classification of visual recognition deficits directly onto lesion sites reached their apogee in the work of Nielsen (1946). He put forward 17 different types of visual agnosia (see Table 10.1).

There are a number of points that may be raised with regard to Nielsen's classification. One is that while much effort is expended in naming and describing the lesion site for letters, words, musical symbols and numerals, functionally, little detailed breakdown is made of visual agnosia for objects, i.e. of different types of agnosic deficit. Nevertheless, elsewhere Nielsen separates the following different forms of agnosia: visual animate object agnosia, visual inanimate object agnosia, visual form agnosia, colour agnosia, visual distance agnosia and visual direction agnosia. These different forms of agnosia essentially describe different behavioural deficits, but the classification provides no way of linking the deficits with the perceptual processes normally involved in, say, the visual recognition of either animate or inanimate objects.

A particular problem with Nielsen's lack of detailed functional breakdown of agnosia is that patients with quite different lesions could be

Table 10.1 Classification of visual agnosia according to Nielsen (1946)

Name	*Lesion site*	*Description of deficit*
Visual angular literal agnosia Visual angular verbal agnosia Visual angular musical agnosia	Angular gyrus	Failure to recognize letters Failure to recognize words Failure to recognize musical symbols
Visual frontal literal agnosia Visual frontal verbal agnosia	Frontal lobe	Failure to recognize letters Failure to recognize words
Visual insular literal agnosia Visual insular verbal agnosia	Insular	Failure to recognize letters Failure to recognize words
Visual occipital literal agnosia Visual occipital verbal agnosia Visual occipital musical agnosia Visual occipital numeral agnosia	Subcortical lesions of the occipital lobe (also possibly cortical lesions of the occipital lobe)	Failure to recognize letters Failure to recognize words Failure to recognize musical symbols Failure to recognize mathematical symbols
Visual subcortical angular musical agnosia Visual subcortical angular verbal agnosia	Subcortical region of angular gyrus	Failure to recognize musical symbols Failure to recognize words
Visual temporal literal (and verbal) agnosia	Wernicke's area or area between Wernicke's area and the angular gyrus	Failure to recognize letter (and words)
Visual parietal numeral agnosia	Interparietal sulcus or subcortical to it	Failure to recognize mathematical symbols
Visual parietal-occipital finger agnosia	Parieto-occipital	Failure to recognize fingers
Visual occipital agnosia (general)	Area 18 of Brodman of the occipital lobe	Failure to recognize objects or symbols by vision alone in spite of adequate perception

given the same general classification, a result which brings the approach into disrepute.

10.2.2 DISCONNECTION ACCOUNTS

A rather different approach to the relationships between lesion sites and visual object recognition deficits is represented by Geschwind's (1965) argument that visual agnosia is one aspect of a disconnection syndrome which also includes alexia without agraphia, colour anomia and right homonymous hemianopia. A lesion resulting in the separation of the visual area from the dominant language area should not allow the naming of stimuli on visual presentation, while the preservation of the ability to copy drawings or letters which cannot be verbally identified would suggest normal, or at least adequate, primary visual perception. The anatomical lesions in these cases are typically thought to destroy the left calcarine cortex and the fibres of the splenium which carry the callosal fibres of the visual regions. Correspondingly, the left visual cortex is destroyed, and the right visual region has lost its commissural connections so it is cut off from the speech areas of the left hemisphere.

Geschwind's (1965) disconnection account only predicts a modality-specific naming disturbance (i.e. optic aphasia; see Lhermitte and Beauvois, 1973; Beauvois, 1982). In contrast, visual agnosia is, by definition, a disorder of recognition, i.e. agnosic patients are unable to demonstrate the recognition of objects that they fail to name (e.g. by gesturing or by circumlocutions). Thus we need to distinguish between visual agnosia and optic aphasia, a step not taken in at least some recent accounts (see Ferro and Santos, 1984).

Patients with lesions precipitating the disconnections indicated by Geschwind should show intact recognition even in the absence of naming, due to intact pathways to the association areas within the right hemisphere. Indeed, evidence favouring the latter pathways comes from work with commissurectomy patients who are able to extract meaning from concrete words and pictures when visual input is restricted to the right hemisphere (see Ratcliff and Newcombe, 1982).

A further problem with the disconnection hypothesis is that it assumes damage to the posterior part of the left hemisphere including damage to the optic radiation or striate cortex, and interruption of forceps major, which carries information from the right occipital lobe to the left hemisphere via the splenium of the corpus callosum. An accompanying defect should therefore be a right homonymous hemianopia, but a review of the cases of associative visual agnosia shows that this is not inevitably the case. For example, the patients described by Spreen, Benton and Van

Allen (1966), Rubens and Benson (1971) and Wapner, Judd and Gardner (1978) do have a right homonymous hemianopia, whereas the patients described by Levine (1978) and Ratcliff and Newcombe (1982) had a left homonymous hemianopia with macular sparing and the patients described by Mack and Boller (1977) and Riddoch and Humphreys (in press) had bilateral visual field defects.

We suggest that the disconnection account does not readily account for visual agnosia. We also suggest that Nielsen's attempt to classify agnosia according to the site of lesion failed because he did not provide a sufficiently detailed functional account of different types of agnosic deficit to allow an accurate mapping between lesion site and functional impairment. What is needed is more consideration of the perceptual functions impaired in visual agnosia, and of the role of these functions in normal object recognition.

10.3 Agnosia: functional accounts

10.3.1 LISSAUER'S ACCOUNT

The earliest functional account of visual agnosia was given by Lissauer (1890), who proposed two forms: apperceptive and associative. Apperceptive visual agnosia was thought to be characterized by a basic defect in visual perception with the result that patients lost the ability to recognize differences that distinguish two similar objects. Associative agnosia, on the other hand, was thought to be characterized by a defective ability to evoke from vision stored conceptual representations of the object. In effect, Lissauer was proposing that two serially organized components are necessary for object recognition: a perceptual component and a conceptual component, plus connections between the two. Anatomically it may be suggested that apperceptive visual agnosia would occur as a result of lesions of the occipital cortex, while associative visual agnosia would occur as a result of a lesion of subcortical pathways linking the occipital cortex with the association areas of the brain. In the case of associative agnosia, the occipital cortex (or perceptual centre) would remain intact (see Hécaen and Albert, 1978).

The first double dissociation suggesting the functional independence of apperceptive and associative agnosia was reported by De Renzi, Scotti and Spinnler (1969), who showed that, relative to left-hemisphere damaged patients, patients suffering right-hemisphere lesions with concomitant visual field defects were impaired on three tasks requiring discrimination of the visual attributes of stimuli: the Ghent overlapping figures test, a face identification test requiring the matching of front-view and profiles of faces, and the Farnsworth-Munsell 100 hue test. These impairments were not due to the presence of visual field defects alone, since similar effects were not found in left-hemisphere damaged patients with visual field defects. In contrast, left-hemisphere damaged patients were impaired relative to the right-hemisphere group on a task requiring pictures of objects to be matched with functionally equivalent but physically different real objects, all shown from a prototypical viewpoint. Presumably, this task requires access to stored knowledge of object function (see also Warrington and Taylor, 1978). Following Lissauer's terminology, De Renzi, Scotti and Spinnler labelled the deficits in processing the physical properties of objects as apperceptive agnosia and the deficits in accessing stored knowledge of objects as associative agnosia.

We may further differentiate between different subclasses of patients who fall within the general outline of apperceptive and associative agnosia given by Lissauer. For instance, some patients have been described with relatively intact brightness and colour discrimination, and yet are quite unable to recognize even the simplest of forms (e.g. Efron, 1968; Benson and Greenberg, 1969; Campion and Latto, 1985; Campion, 1987). Such patients may be described as apperceptive agnosics in the sense that they appear to have intact elementary perceptual processes but impaired form identification, yet the patients clearly differ from the apperceptive agnosics described by De Renzi, Scotti and Spinnler (1969) who showed relatively good ability to classify prototypical functionally equivalent objects. Thus we may need to distinguish different types of apperceptive agnosia.

A similar argument may be made with regard to associative agnosia. The classification of associative agnosia is typically based on patients showing a poor ability to recognize visually presented objects in the presence of a good ability to copy the object. Good copying is taken as an accurate indicator that the perceptual component of object recognition is intact. Riddoch and Humphreys (1987) recently reported the case of a patient, JB, who was unable to match associatively related objects (i.e. who showed poor conceptual knowledge about the object); yet this patient was able to discriminate between familiar objects and novel objects created by exchanging the parts of common objects. This suggests that the patient could access stored structural knowledge of objects from vision, but not stored conceptual knowledge. In contrast, other agnosic patients with intact copying ability are quite unable to discriminate between familiar and novel objects indicating a deficit prior to the stage of accessing stored structural knowledge (Riddoch and Humphreys, in press). A case can thus be made for further fractionating the functional account of visual agnosia.

10.3.2 LURIA'S ACCOUNT

Luria (1966) extended Lissauer's functional account of apperceptive agnosia by proposing a further stage of perceptual processing involving the identification of object parts, which was thought to occur prior to the identification of an object's form. Thus Lissauer's first stage concerning the identification of form was decomposed into two sequential stages: (1) identification of parts; (2) integration of parts. According to Luria, the essential feature of apperceptive agnosia is the failure, on the part of the patient, to integrate the parts of the form into groups. He indicates that eye movements are particularly important in this respect in that they are responsible for performing orienting and exploratory activity. Disruption to the use and control of eye movements could also occur in conjunction with deficits to elementary perceptual processes, such as brightness discrimination. Thus, 'There can be no doubt, however, that a careful pathophysiological study of patients with this disorder will reveal a number of sensory disorders (rapid fatigue from visual reception, impaired visual adaptation, raising of thresholds etc.) that probably become more pronounced when challenged by the more complex forms of visual perception' (Luria, 1977, p. 141). Luria therefore concludes that agnosia represents a complex perceptuomotor breakdown of the active serial feature-by-feature analysis necessary for processing elements of a visual scene or pattern. In normal vision, the early processing and organization of form information is spatially parallel (e.g. Treisman, 1982), so that it follows that the serial identification process observed in agnosic patients must itself be a symptom of a breakdown in parallel processing.

10.3.3 BAY'S ACCOUNT

Luria's (1966) argument for the presence of elementary perceptual deficits in cases of agnosia is, in some respects, similar to that of Bay (1953). Bay demonstrated disorders of visual function in a variety of brain-damaged patients, including a patient with associative visual agnosia, which had not been apparent on standard perimetric testing. He found the retina in patients with apparently normal visual fields showed abnormal fatigue. The abnormality was greatest in the central retinal region, but affected the periphery more (even with prolonged presentation, visual stimuli would tend to drop out of awareness, in the same way as brief peripheral stimuli may do in non-brain-damaged subjects). Bay suggests that the latter result occurred because the functional level of the central areas is normally so high above the functional level of the peripheral areas that, despite its greater damage, the residual function of the central areas is superior to the periphery.

The proposition put by Bay is that the formation of normal sensory perceptions is impaired by this abnormal fatigue. Thus, the visual field is functionally contracted and does not allow for the simultaneous perception of the whole visual stimulus (we take this to mean that such patients process information less efficiently than normal across the visual field, rather than there being absolute field defects). Details of the stimulus may therefore be seen in succession, but it will not be possible for the patient to obtain a holistic description of the item. The effective contraction of normal vision will also affect the perception of the relations between the object and its environment and will lead to disorders of spatial orientation in such patients.

Bay's (1953) argument extends that of Luria (1966), since it incorporates associative as well as apperceptive agnosia, but there are several problems with the account. For instance, Newcombe and Ratcliff (1974) describe a patient with associative visual agnosia who, despite being extensively tested, appeared to have no visual field defect. Also, non-agnosic patients have been documented with disturbances in tachistoscopic detection times at least as severe as those present in the patient described by Bay (1953), but who, none the less, do not have associative visual agnosia (Ettlinger, 1956; Teuber, Battersby and Bender, 1960; Warrington and Rabin, 1970; Ratcliff and Davies-Jones, 1972).

Further, even if the functional capacity of normal vision were impaired in apperceptive and/or associative agnosic patients, of whatever variety, we still need to know how the perceptual processes normally involved in object recognition are affected, to provide a complete functional account. A simple example helps to illustrate this. If we were to build an object-recognition system into a computer, a prerequisite of this system may be the capacity to process large amounts of information in a spatially parallel manner (e.g. see Hinton and Anderson, 1981). However, even when this capacity is built-in to the system, there may be many alternative processes which could be employed to enable object recognition to occur. To explain how object recognition occurs, we need to specify these processes in addition to the capacity constraints involved. It thus follows that disorders of object recognition are not fully explained by positing deficits in processing capacity, without explaining how the mediating processes are also affected.

10.3.4 WARRINGTON'S ACCOUNT

According to the above argument, we need a yet more detailed functional account of visual agnosia and, in particular, one which relates the deficits to the processes normally mediating object recognition. Also, it seems unlikely that the argument for impaired elementary perceptual deficits could explain all agnosias, such as those where patients may show intact access to structural but not conceptual knowledge about objects (Riddoch and Humphreys, 1987).

One example of a more detailed functional account is provided by Warrington (1985) and Warrington and Taylor (1978), who also present a hierarchical view of visual processing. Two post-sensory processing stages are posited involving first, perceptual categorization, followed by semantic categorization. By perceptual categorization, Warrington refers to the ability of the patient to classify an object as having the same structure when seen from a different viewpoint (i.e. the ability to achieve object constancy). By semantic categorization, she refers to the ability of the patient to classify an object according to its function. It also seems plausible that perceptual categorization is itself contingent on the achievement of a structured visual percept by the patient, i.e. it is contingent on Lissauer's first stage of object recognition. Warrington (1985) suggests that perceptual categorization is lateralized to the right hemisphere and semantic categorization to the left. Patients with right hemisphere damage have been shown to be impaired at identifying anomalies in scenes (Milner, 1958), overlapping figures (De Renzi and Spinnler, 1966; De Renzi, Scotti and Spinnler, 1969), incomplete outline drawings (Warrington and James, 1967) and unusual views of pictures (Warrington and Taylor, 1978; Humphreys and Riddoch, 1984); she therefore suggests that such patients have faulty perceptual categorization. This impairment is thought to be distinct from form perception since, in separate studies using different groups of right brain-damaged patients, Warrington has demonstrated intact shape perception (Taylor and Warrington, 1973) and intact shape detection (Warrington and Taylor, 1973).

Warrington's notion of faulty perceptual categorization cannot be equated with the initial stage of processing in Lissauer's scheme (the process of form identification), since patients with impaired perceptual categorization are thought to have intact input representations of form information. Nevertheless, Warrington proposes that patients with selectively impaired perceptual categorization should be termed apperceptive agnosics. In making this step, Warrington apparently wishes to maintain the distinction between a pre-semantic deficit (apperceptive agnosia) and a deficit specially reflecting impaired access to semantic information from vision (associative agnosia). In so doing, she is forced to classify patients whose primary deficit is prior to the stage of perceptual categorization as 'pseudo-agnosics' (cf. Benson and Greenberg, 1969; Campion, 1987), despite the fact that such patients may have relatively intact elementary perceptual functions such as brightness discrimination. Indeed, the possibility that the identification of 2-D forms could be impaired, whilst other visual functions are intact, is emphasized by two patients (Warrington, 1985) who both had normal corrected visual acuity and were able to read small print at normal or near normal speed, yet failed to discriminate shapes matched for total area (and therefore total brightness, see Efron, 1968).

There are also problems with Warrington's 'failure in perceptual categorization' argument. It is not clear whether this is a global term covering several varieties of apperceptive agnosia, for example, can patients who have difficulties in detecting anomalies in scenes (Milner, 1958), or who are impaired at identifying overlapping figures (De Renzi and Spinnler, 1966), or incomplete outline drawings (Warrington and James, 1967) and impaired perception of photographs of faces (De Renzi and Spinnler, 1966) all be classified as having a common 'failing in perceptual categorization', or are these seen to be as separate varieties of visual agnosia? The latter argument seems to be the more likely as it seems reasonable to infer that different processes are necessary in order to perform the different tasks identified above. For example, the Gollin figures task is a graded difficulty task where patients are required to identify incomplete outline drawings of objects (see Warrington and James, 1967; Warrington and Taylor, 1973). In order to interpret the Gollin figures it may be necessary to apply some form of top-down knowledge (e.g. a frame of reference; cf. Hinton, 1981). The figure, although incomplete, may have a familiar shape description which will allow recognition of the shape to take place. In order to identify overlapping figures (see De Renzi and Spinnler, 1966) a different process may be necessary; namely, the ability to separate figure from ground. Furthermore, it also appears that patients may fail on categorization tasks for different reasons, for example, Humphreys and Riddoch (1984) manipulated the way unusual views of objects are obtained. In one instance, the unusual view was of an object rotated in depth, which had the effect of shortening the principal axis of the object (the foreshortened condition). In the other instance, the unusual view was of the object rotated within the plane so that the saliency of what was rated the distinctive feature of the object was decreased, while the saliency of its principal axis remained relatively unaffected (the mimimal feature condition). Four right-hemisphere damaged patients were impaired in the foreshortened condition relative to the minimal feature condition. Another patient, with bilateral occipital damage, was impaired in the minimal feature condition relative to the foreshortened condition, when compared with the differences present in normal subjects. Humphreys and Riddoch have argued that there are therefore at least two ways of achieving object constancy: (1) by the use of global form characteristics, which is rendered difficult by foreshortening; (2) by the use of salient local features, which is rendered difficult by minimal-feature transformations. Right-hemisphere damaged patients seem to depend primarily on global form information, and are significantly affected by gross changes in form that occur as a result of foreshortening. The patient with occipital lesions, however, appeared to be much more dependent on the presence of salient local features for object identification and matching, and so was primarily affected by transformations to salient features of the objects.

Warrington's approach does begin to provide a more detailed analysis of the processes involved in object recognition, but perceptual functions such as perceptual and semantic categorization remain at rather a macroscopic scale of analysis, as do the descriptions of the brain areas supporting such functions. For this reason, we also consider two other recent functional accounts of agnosia.

10.3.5 KERTESZ'S ACCOUNT

Kertesz (1987) attempts to fractionate visual agnosia further than any of the approaches that we have discussed hitherto, whilst remaining within the broad framework provided by Lissauer. Kertesz proposes a multistage model of object recognition and naming, with six independent stages (see Fig. 10.1).

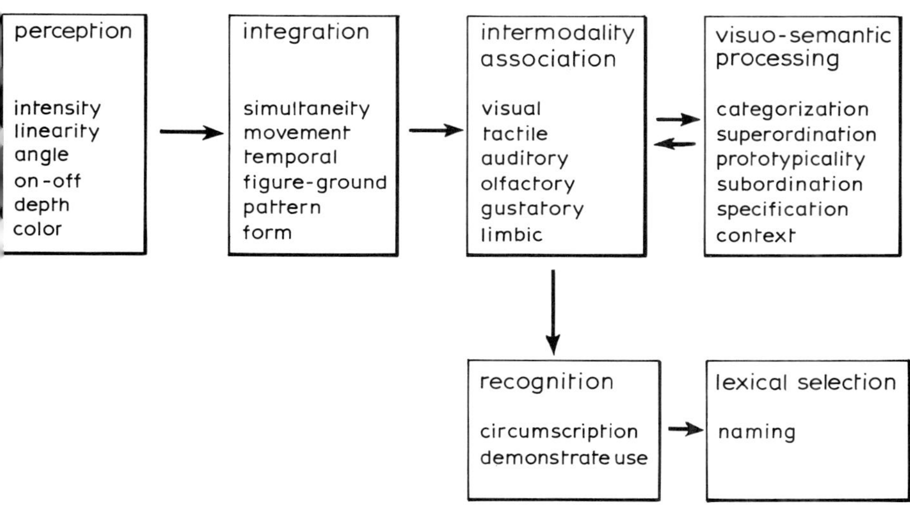

Fig. 10.1 The multistage model of visual object recognition and naming proposed by Kertesz (1987).

1. The first stage concerns perception of the intensity of light, line linearity, angle, depth, colour and the on/off nature of the stimulus.
2. The integration of the elementary aspects of the stimulus (including the simultaneity of features, their temporal relations, possible movement, the spatial pattern, the figure–ground relationship and the overall form).
3. The third stage of intermodality association allows the perceived and visually integrated stimuli to be matched to visual memories and from there to tactile, auditory, olfactory, gustatory and limbic mechanisms that reinforce and selectively influence the visual association.
4. The fourth stage of visuo-semantic processing (concerning categorization, superordination, subordination, specification and context).
5. The stage of recognition (which can be evidenced by circumlocution or by demonstrating the use of an object).
6. Naming.

Kertesz argues that the clinical syndromes of visual agnosia overlap to a considerable extent, and that most syndromes involve at least one, and some all, of the stages. According to Kertesz's model, apperceptive agnosia is characterized by a deficit to Stage 2. Associative agnosia is attributed to impairments to either Stage 3 or 4, although he also states that 'in most cases of predominantly associative agnosia, apperceptive functions are also involved, implying a dual deficit'. Kertesz's model is arranged hierarchically, a deficit at a relatively early stage must have profound consequences on subsequent stages. Thus dual deficits of apperceptive and associative agnosia are difficult to separate from cases where there is a knock-on effect from a deficit at an earlier stage (say in Stage 2).

How does Kertesz's account relate to those we have previously discussed? Stage 2 appears to conform to Luria's stage (2); Stages 4 and 5 appear to conform to Warrington's stage of semantic categorization (though we know of no evidence to support Kertesz's assertion that semantic categorization is independent of recognition). Kertesz's Stage 3 may also be thought to involve access to stored visual knowledge about object structure. If perceptual categorization (i.e. matching objects across viewpoints) involves access to stored visual knowledge about objects, then this stage corresponds to Warrington's stage of perceptual categorization. A problem with this is that patients have been demonstrated to have good categorization ability and yet poor access to stored knowledge of object structure (Riddoch and Humphreys, in press). However, since Kertesz maintains that access to stored structural knowledge is separate from semantic categorization, he can account for patient JB described by Riddoch and Humphreys (1987). JB can be said to have intact processing up to and including Stage 3 (and therefore can judge familiar object structures), but not beyond (and so has poor associative knowledge).

Kertesz makes no attempt to relate his model to the underlying anatomy, other than pointing out that the independent occurrence of apperceptive and associative agnosia in different patients implies that there is some modular arrangement of neural structures paralleling the modular arrangement of visual processing stages in his model.

10.3.6 HUMPHREYS AND RIDDOCH'S ACCOUNT

Another multistage approach to visual object recognition and to visual agnosia has been proposed by Humphreys and Riddoch (1987), an approach based on a background of work with normal non-brain-damaged subjects, which has been strengthened by data obtained from neuropsychological investigations of patients with visual agnosia. An outline of this model is given in Fig. 10.2. Five different levels or stages of processing have been identified:

1. The extraction of form information at different spatial scales including:
   (a) global object shape
   (b) local object features
2. By combining the above information, a retinotopic object description is obtained, i.e. a description that is coded according to the characteristics of the object on the retina.
3. From all the above (1(a), 1(b) and 2) a non-retinotopic description is abstracted. This representation is episodic (i.e. not a permanent representation but a representation that can be derived in a particular instant in time) and also preserves viewpoint.
4. Access to object form knowledge, a permanent memory store specifying object structure coded according to a prototypical viewpoint which is distinct from:
5. Access to semantic knowledge; a permanent memory store concerned with characteristics such as object function.

In addition to these processing stages, Humphreys and Riddoch also posit a set of mapping procedures which set up connections between the non-retinotopic viewpoint-dependent representation of the object. It is via the activation of these mapping procedures that objects in unusual views are recognized (see Hinton, 1981; Humphreys and Quinlan, 1987).

In many respects, the model proposed by Humphreys and Riddoch

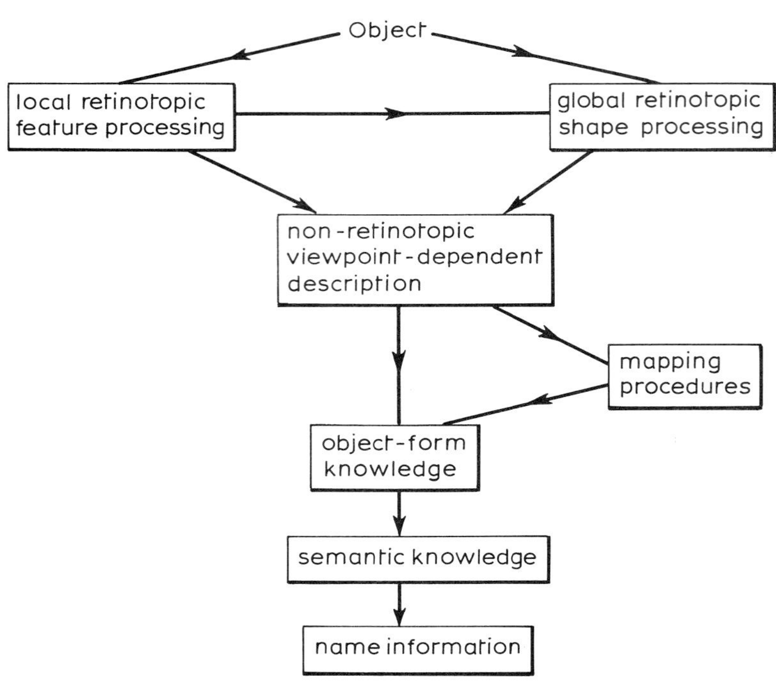

Fig. 10.2 An information processing framework for object recognition and naming, given by Humphreys and Riddoch (in press).

shares characteristics with the earlier models discussed. Like Luria and Kertesz, Humphreys and Riddoch maintain a specific stage of visual integration (Stage 2 above). Warrington's (1985) stage of perceptual categorization is attributed to the activation of mapping procedures from viewpoint-dependent to stored structural representations. Also the distinction between stored structural and semantic knowledge is similar to that made between intermodality visual association and visuo-semantic processing by Kertesz (1987). However, Humphreys and Riddoch's model is somewhat more specific than some of the other approaches discussed, for instance, by specifying form primitives at different spatial scales (see Stage 1 above), it is possible to posit mapping processes at different scales. This can account for the different types of form information used to support object constancy in patients with impaired perceptual categorization (Humphreys and Riddoch, 1984; see Section 10.3.3 above). Also, since object form knowledge is coded to a prototypical viewpoint, patients with impaired mapping procedures may show good recognition of objects in prototypical views (see De Renzi, Scotti and

Spinnler, 1969; Warrington and Taylor, 1978; Humphreys and Riddoch, 1984; Riddoch and Humphreys, 1986; for confirmation of this).

Humphreys and Riddoch (1987) have reconsidered visual agnosia in the light of the above model, and have distinguished five different sorts of agnosia.

(a) Shape agnosia. This terminology refers to those patients with marked difficulties in the processing form (Benson and Greenberg, 1969; Campion and Latto, 1985; Campion, 1987). Such patients may be quite unable to recognize even the simplest of forms while retaining the ability to identify colours and to localize objects by touch. This suggests a deficit in the representation of shape information, which may itself be precipitated by a loss in processing certain form primitives (e.g. Regan, 1982). Interestingly, both Benson and Greenberg's and Campion's patients suffered carbon monoxide poisoning, which likely resulted in disseminated focal atrophy of cortical tissue (Garland and Pearce, 1967). Such a multiplicity of lesions may cause the subjects' visual field to be peppered with minute scotomata (blind spots) which would not necessarily be detected by conventional perimetry (Campion and Latto, 1985; Campion, 1987). The presence of such patchy lesions could impede the formation of boundary contours necessary for form perception, whilst not interfering with the perception of colour, size, brightness and direction.

Since 'shape agnosics' are impaired at an early stage of visual object processing, they will be unable to show normal access to any of the subsequent representations. Clinically this may be demonstrated in a series of simple tests:

1. The patients will be poor at copying visually presented items, suggesting an inability to construct a retinotopic representation.
2. The patients will be deficient at perceptually classifying visual stimuli seen in different views.
3. The patients will be poor at distinguishing between familiar and novel examples of visual stimuli because they are unable to access object form knowledge from vision, but they may be able to access object form knowledge from the semantic system (see Fig. 10.2) and so may be able to draw items from memory.
4. The patients will be poor at demonstrating any knowledge about a visually presented item, such as how it might be used or where it might be found but, if the items are presented via another modality (such as the name of the item, or tactile presentation of the item), such semantic knowledge should be intact.

(b) Integretive agnosia. Boundary formation must occur at different

levels, i.e. not only must the overall shape of the object be identified but also the local boundaries within the object, which help proclaim the uniqueness of the object. For example, features must be separated from the background of a face; and the relationship of such features to each other, together with their relationship to the overall shape of the face, will help specify the unique characteristics of that face. Patients may be impaired at integrating visual information at different spatial scales, and they would be classed as having integretive agnosia. One case has been described by Humphreys, Riddoch and Quinlan (1985) and Riddoch and Humphreys (in press), and the following clinical tests will help in identification:

1. Patients should be able to copy stimulus items because the local and global shape primitives are intact (cf. shape agnosia).
2. They would be impaired at assigning visual stimuli to perceptual categories if the task requires that they relate local aspects of the stimulus item with more global aspects (see Humphreys and Riddoch, 1984, for a discussion of this issue).
3. They would be poor at distinguishing familiar from novel visual stimuli if the task requires the integration of both local and global form information. However, as with patients with shape agnosia, patients with integretive agnosia may be able to access the visual form system from the semantic system and they may, therefore, be able to draw items from memory.
4. They would be poor at demonstrating any semantic knowledge about a visually presented item although such knowledge may be intact.

(c) Transformation agnosia. This term refers to patients who are impaired at perceptually categorizing visually presented items, and cases have been described by Warrington and Taylor (1973, 1978), Humphreys and Riddoch (1984) and Warrington (1985).

The ability perceptually to categorize is important in that it enables normal interaction with the physical environment (allowing objects to be recognized from different angles), but patients with transformation agnosia should not be grossly handicapped perceptually: they should be able to copy visual stimuli, to distinguish between familiar, prototypical objects and novel objects, to draw items from memory and to demonstrate semantic knowledge about objects presented in prototypical views.

(d) Visual form agnosia. Such patients will have difficulty in accessing or using stored information about visual form, and should:

1. Be able to copy visually presented items.
2. Succeed on perceptual classification tasks.
3. Be poor at distinguishing between familiar and novel objects (since this, by definition, requires access to form knowledge).
4. Be poor at demonstrating semantic knowledge about visually presented items.

Patients who only have a problem in accessing form knowledge from vision will be able to draw objects from memory. It is also possible that patients could have a bi-directional deficit, and so have difficulty in accessing form knowledge from a semantic definition (Riddoch and Humphreys, 1987). They would be impaired at drawing from memory.

(e) Semantic agnosia. Patients with semantic agnosia may have impairments within the semantic system itself. They should have no difficulty with visual processing up to this point; thus, they should be able to copy items and perceptually to categorize items. However, they will have difficulty with tasks that require classification on the basis of associative or functional characteristics of the objects (e.g. they will have difficulty in assigning a saw, scissors and a knife to one class on the basis that they all cut). It is quite feasible that not all the semantic system will be impaired, there may just be a localized lesion: this could account for some of the category-specific deficits that have been reported in the literature (e.g. Warrington, 1975; Warrington and Shallice, 1984; although see also Riddoch *et al.*, in press).

Patients with intact structural and semantic representations of objects, but with selective deficits in accessing these objects from vision, would be classified as visual-form access agnosics or as semantic access agnosics (see Riddoch and Humphreys, in press).

10.4 Visual agnosia and anatomy reconsidered

Following the detailed functional account of visual agnosia by Humphreys and Riddoch (1987), it is also possible to give a more precise account of the relations between functional deficits and lesion sites. Thus, Humphreys and Riddoch (1987) argue that the five-part breakdown of agnosia given above maps onto lesion sites in the following way:

1. Multiple minor occipital infarcts may produce shape agnosia (cf. Benson and Greenberg, 1969, and Campion, in press).
2. Right parietal lesions may produce transformational agnosia (see Warrington and Taylor, 1973; 1978; Humphreys and Riddoch, 1984;

Warrington, 1985; Riddoch and Humphreys, 1986).

3. Bilateral occipito-parieto-temporal lesions may produce integretive agnosia (see Albert, Reches and Silverberg, 1975; Mack and Boller, 1977; Wapner, Judd and Gardner, 1978; Ratcliff and Newcombe, 1982; Humphreys and Riddoch, 1984; Humphreys, Riddoch and Quinlan, 1985).
4. Unilateral posterior left hemisphere lesions may produce semantic access agnosia (see Rubens and Benson, 1971; Kertesz, 1979; Davidoff and Wilson, 1985; Riddoch and Humphreys, 1987).
5. Diffuse cerebral atrophy or diffuse bilateral temporal damage may produce semantic agnosia (see Taylor and Warrington, 1971; Warrington, 1975; Warrington and Shallice, 1984).

10.5 Agnosia and its related deficits

In our account of visual agnosia we have concentrated on the deficits which occur in visual object recognition. It is also true that visual agnosia is often accompanied by ancillary deficits, such as prosopagnosia, colour agnosia, topographical agnosia and alexia without agraphia (see, for instance, Kertesz, 1987). The detailed functional account given by Humphreys and Riddoch (1987) predicts different patterns of co-occurrence depending on the form of the agnosia. For instance, impairments to early processes in perceptual organization (as in shape and integretive agnosia) should produce a range of deficits including prosopagnosia, topographical agnosia and alexia without agraphia, since face recognition, the recognition of familiar routes and landmarks, and reading, may all tap similar early visual processes. Such close patterns of co-occurrence may not occur with other forms of agnosia, which may, for instance, reflect the loss of specific types of stored knowledge. In such instances, it is plausible that stored knowledge about visual stimuli other than objects (such as faces or landmarks) could be preserved.

On the other hand, there seems little logical reason to believe that colour information plays a crucial role in object identification given that we recognize without difficulty black and white photographs and line drawings (although it may well complement it; see Ostergaard and Davidoff, 1985). There are thus few functional grounds for believing colour processing to be an integral part of the object recognition system. Cases where colour agnosia co-occurs with visual object agnosia may therefore be most easily attributed to the anatomical proximity of the visual areas concerned respectively with object and colour processing.

10.6 From anatomy to function

We have suggested that a detailed functional account of visual agnosia can help impose order on the seemingly unprincipled set of lesion sites and types which give rise to visual object recognition deficits. In this respect, it is also interesting to note that neurophysiological accounts of behaviour can themselves inform functional accounts. For instance, Humphreys and Riddoch's (1987) model of visual object processing supposes that constancy occurs by mapping viewpoint-dependent representations of objects onto stored representations of object form. Thus, there may be a role for stored form knowledge in object constancy. Some support for this view comes from Weiskrantz and his colleagues on the effects of lesions to the foveal prestriate cortex and to the inferior temporal cortex on object constancy in the monkey. Weiskrantz and Saunders (1984) showed that monkeys with inferior temporal lesions were impaired at both the initial learning of discrimination responses and their generalization to objects transformed in orientation or size. Monkeys with lesions to the foveal prestriate cortex were less impaired at initial shape learning, though they were also impaired at responding to transformed objects. This suggests that lesions to the foveal prestriate cortex of the monkey disrupt the processes used to access stored knowledge about objects when the objects are placed in new views, rather than the storage process itself. In contrast, lesions to the inferior temporal cortex appear to affect both the initial storage of visual information, and the ability to generalize across transformations. That inferior temporal lesions affect object constancy as well as the storage of form information indicates a role for stored knowledge in constancy (see also Humphrey and Weiskrantz, 1969).

Humphreys and Riddoch's (1987) model also maintains that stored knowledge of object form is coded to a specific, prototypical viewpoint. Here, the work of Perrett and his associates is of interest (Perrett *et al.*, 1984, 1985), in that they have identified cells in the superior temporal sulcus of the monkey which respond to particular faces. Furthermore, these cells show a preference for a limited number of different viewpoints. Such results suggest that the stored representations of object form are indeed viewpoint specific.

We have outlined how functional accounts have helped to organize the data on different types of agnosia and sites of lesion, and of how neurophysiological data itself constrains functional accounts of visual object processing. Thus the two approaches can be seen to be adding to our knowledge of visual object recognition and its disorders in a complementary way: a conclusion which we hope would have met the approval of at least some of our predecessors in the field.

Acknowledgements

This work was supported by a grant from the MRC awarded to both authors.

References

Albert, M.L., Reches, D. and Silverberg, R. (1975) Associative visual agnosia without alexia. *Neurology*, **25**, 322–6.

Bay, E. (1953) Disturbances of visual perception and their examination. *Brain*, **76**, 515–50.

Beauvois, M.F. (1982) Optic aphasia: a process of interaction between vision and language. *Phil. Trans. R. Soc. Lond.*, **B298**, 35–47.

Benson, D.F. and Greenberg, J.P. (1969) Visual form agnosia. *Arch. Neurol.*, **20**, 82–9.

Broca, P. (1861) Remarks on the seat of the faculty of articulate language, followed by an observation of aphemia, in *Some Papers on the Cerebral Cortex* (ed. D. Von Bonin, 1960). Thomas, Springfield, IL.

Campion, J. (1987) Apperceptive agnosia: frameworks, models and paradigms, in *Visual Object Processing: A Cognitive Neuropsychological Approach* (eds G.W. Humphreys and M.J. Riddoch). Lawrence Erlbaum, Hillsdale, NJ.

Campion, J. and Latto, R. (1985) Apperceptive agnosia due to carbon monoxide poisoning. An interpretation based on critical band masking from disseminated lesions. *Behav. Brain Res.*, **15**, 227–40.

Charcot, P. (1886–7) *Oeuvres complets.* 9 vols. Bureau du Progrès Medical, Paris.

Davidoff, J. and Wilson, B. (1985) A case of visual agnosia showing a disorder of pre-semantic visual classification. *Cortex*, **21**, 121–34.

De Renzi, E. and Spinnler, H. (1966) Impaired performance on colour tasks in patients with hemispheric damage. *Cortex*, **3**, 194–217.

De Renzi, E., Scotti, G. and Spinnler, H. (1969) Perceptual and associative disorders of visual recognition. *Neurology*, **19**, 634–41.

Efron, R. (1968) What is perception?, in *Boston Studies of the Philosophy of Science*, vol. 4. Humanities Press, New York.

Ettlinger, G. (1956) Sensory deficits in visual agnosia. *J. Neurol. Neurosurg. Psychiat.*, **19**, 297–307.

Ferro, J.M. and Santos, M.E. (1984) Associative visual agnosia: a case study. *Cortex*, **20**, 121–34.

Freud, S. (1891) *Zur auffassung der aphasien.* Deuticke, Leipzig und Wein.

Garland, H. and Pearce, J. (1967) Neurological complications of carbon monoxide poisoning. *Quart. J. Med.*, **144**, 445–55.

Geschwind, N. (1965) Disconnection syndromes in animal and man. *Brain*, **88**, 237–94, 585–644.

Hécaen, H. and Albert, M. (1978) *Human Neuropsychology.* Wiley, New York.

Hinton, G.E. (1981) A parallel computation that assigns canonical object based frames of reference, in *Proceedings of the Seventh International Joint Conference on Artificial Intelligence.* Vancouver, BC, Canada.

Hinton, G.E. and Anderson, J.A. (1981) *Parallel Models of Associative Memory*. Lawrence Erlbaum, Hillsdale, NJ.

Humphrey, N.K. and Weiskrantz, L. (1969) Size constancy in monkeys with infero-temporal lesions. *Quart. J. Exp. Psychol.*, **21**, 225–38.

Humphreys, G.W. and Quinlan, P.T. (1987) Normal and pathological processes in visual object constancy, in *Visual Object Processing: A Cognitive Neuropsychological Approach* (eds G.W. Humphreys and M.J. Riddoch). Lawrence Erlbaum, Hillsdale, NJ, pp. 43–105.

Humphreys, G.W. and Riddoch, M.J. (1984) Routes to object constancy: implications from neurological impairments of object constancy. *Quart. J. Exp. Psychol.*, **36A**, 385–415.

Humphreys, G.W., Riddoch, M.J. and Quinlan, P.T. (1985) Interactive processes in perceptual organisation: evidence from visual agnosia, in *Attention and Performance XI* (eds M.I. Posner and O.S.M. Marin). Lawrence Erlbaum, Hillsdale, NJ.

Humphreys, G.W. and Riddoch, M.J. (1987) The fractionation of visual agnosia, in *Visual Object Processing: A Cognitive Neuropsychological Approach* (eds G.W. Humphreys and M.J. Riddoch). Lawrence Erlbaum, Hillsdale, NJ, pp. 281–306.

Jackson, H. (1876) Case of a large cerebral tumour without optic neuritis and with left hemiplegia and imperception. *Selected Writings*, vol. 2. (Basic Books, New York City, 1958.)

Kertesz, A. (1979) Visual agnosia: the dual deficit of perception and recognition. *Cortex*, **15**, 403–19.

Kertesz, A. (1987) The clinical spectrum and localisation of visual agnosia, in *Visual Object Processing: A Cognitive Neuropsychological Approach* (eds G.W. Humphreys and M.J. Riddoch). Lawrence Erlbaum, Hillsdale, NJ.

Levine, D. (1978) Prosopagnosia and visual object agnosia: a behavioural study. *Brain Lang.*, **5**, 341–65.

Lhermitte, F. and Beauvois, M.F. (1973) A visual-speech disconnection syndrome. Report of a case with optic aphasia, agnosic alexia and colour agnosia. *Brain*, **96**, 695–714.

Lissauer, H. (1890) Ein fall von seelenblindheit nebst einem beitrage zur theorie derselben. *Arch. Psychiat. Nervenkrankheit.*, **21**, 222–70.

Luria, A.R. (1966) *Higher Cortical Functions in Man*. Basic Books, New York.

Luria, A.R. (1977) *The Working Brain*. Penguin Books, London.

Mack, J.L. and Boller, F. (1977) Associative visual agnosia and its related deficits: the role of the minor hemisphere in assigning meaning to visual perceptions. *Neuropsychologia*, **15**, 345–51.

Marie, P. (1906) Revision de la question de l'aphasie. *Semaine Med.*, **21**, 241–7.

Milner, B. (1958) Psychological defects produced by temporal lobe excision. *Proc. Assoc. Res. Nervous and Mental Dis.*, **36**, 244–57.

Munk, H. (1881) *Ueber die Functionen der Grosshirnrinde. Gesammelte Mittheilungen aus den Jahren 1887–1880*. Hirschwald, Berlin.

Newcombe, F. and Ratcliff, G. (1974) Agnosia: a disorder of object recognition, in *Les Syndromes de Disconnexion Calleuse chez l'Homme* (eds F. Michel and B. Schott). Colloque International de Lyon, pp. 317–41.

Nielsen, J.M. (1946) *Agnosia, Apraxia, Aphasia*, 2nd edn. P.B. Hoeber, New York.

Ostergaard, A.L. and Davidoff, J.B. (1985) Some effects of colour on naming and the recognition of objects. *J. Exp. Psychol.: Learning, Memory, and Cognition*, **3**, 579–87.

Perrett, D.I., Smith, P.A.J., Potter, D.D., Mistlin, A.J., Head, A.S., Milner, A.D. and Jeeves, M.A. (1984) Neurones responsive to faces in the temporal cortex: studies of functional organisation, sensitivity to identity and relation to perception. *Human Neurobiol.*, **3**, 197–208.

Perrett, D.I., Smith, P.A.J., Potter, D.D., Mistlin, A.J., Head, A.S., Milner, A.D. and Jeeves, M.A. (1985) Visual cells in the temporal cortex sensitive to face view and gaze direction. *Proc. R. Soc. Lond., B*, **223**, 293–317.

Ratcliff, G. and Davies-Jones, G.A.B. (1972) Defective localisation in focal brain wounds. *Brain*, **95**, 49–60.

Ratcliff, G. and Newcombe, F. (1982) Object recognition: some deductions from the clinical evidence, in *Normality and Pathology in Cognitive Functions* (ed. A.W. Ellis). Academic Press, London, pp. 147–71.

Regan, D. (1982) Visual information channelling in normal and disordered vision. *Psychol. Rev.*, **89**, 407–44.

Riddoch, M.J. and Humphreys, G.W. (1986) Neurological impairments of object constancy: the effects of orientation and size disparities. *Cog. Neuropsychol.*, **3**, 207–24.

Riddoch, M.J. and Humphreys, G.W. (1987) Visual object processing in optic aphasia: a case of semantic access agnosia. *Cog. Neuropsychol.*, **4**, 131–185.

Riddoch, M.J. and Humphreys, G.W. (1987) Deficits in object perception in a case of visual agnosia. *Brain* (in press).

Riddoch, M.J., Humphreys, G.W., Coltheart, M. and Funnell, E. (1988) Semantic systems or system: neurological evidence re-examined. *Cog. Neuropsychol.* (in press).

Rubens, A. and Benson, D. (1971) Associative visual agnosia. *Arch. Neurol. (Chicago)*, **24**, 305–16.

Spreen, O., Benton, A.L. and Van Allan, M.W. (1966) Dissociation of visual and tactile naming in amnesic patients. *Arch. Neurol.*, **13**, 84.

Taylor, A. and Warrington, E.K. (1973) Visual discrimination in patients with localised cerebral lesions. *Cortex*, **9**, 82–93.

Taylor, A. and Warrington, E.K. (1971) Visual agnosia: a single case report. *Cortex*, **7**, 152–61.

Teuber, H.L., Battersby, W.S. and Bender, M.B. (1960) *Somatic Sensory Changes after Penetrating Brain Wounds in Man.* Harvard University Press, Harvard, MA.

Treisman, A. (1982) Perceptual grouping and attention in visual search for features and for objects. *J. Exp. Psychol.: Human Perception and Performance*, **8**, 194–214.

Wapner, W., Judd, T. and Gardner, H. (1978) Visual agnosia in an artist. *Cortex*, **7**, 152–61.

Warrington, E.K. (1975) The selective impairment of semantic memory. *Quart. J. Exp. Psychol.*, **27**, 635–57.

Warrington, E.K. (1985) Agnosia: the impairment of object recognition, in *Handbook of Clinical Neurology*, vol. 1. *Clinical Neuropsychology* (ed. J.A.M. Fredericks). Elsevier Science, Amsterdam, pp. 333–49.

Warrington, E.K. and James, M. (1967) Disorders of visual perception in patients with cerebral lesions. *Cortex*, **9**, 82–93.
Warrington, E.K. and Rabin, P. (1970) Perceptual matching in patients with localised cerebral lesions. *Neuropsychologica*, **8**, 475–87.
Warrington, E.K. and Shallice, T. (1984) Category specific semantic impairments. *Brain*, **107**, 829–54.
Warrington, E.K. and Taylor, A.M. (1973) The contribution of the right parietal lobe to object recognition. *Cortex*, **9**, 152–64.
Warrington, E.K. and Taylor, A.M. (1978) Two categorical stages of object recognition. *Perception*, **7**, 695–705.
Weiskrantz, L. and Saunders, R.C. (1984) Impairments of visual object transforms in monkeys. *Brain*, **107**, 1033–72.

Part II

The Ocular Motor System

CHAPTER 11

Anatomy of the ocular motor nuclei

J.A. BÜTTNER-ENNEVER

All vertebrates, from primitive fish up to primates, have six eye muscles which are controlled by three groups of motoneurones lying in the brainstem: the oculomotor nucleus (III), the trochlear nucleus (IV) and the abducens nucleus (VI). Different animals use different types of eye movement, but there are at least five basic types. (1) *Saccades*, i.e. rapid conjugate eye movements, move the eyes from one fixation point to another, and the term includes voluntary saccades as well as the fast phases of vestibular and optokinetic nystagmus (Fuchs, Kaneko and Scudder, 1985). (2) *Vestibulo-ocular reflexes* and (3) *optokinetic responses* are slow compensatory movements used to stabilize the retinal image during head or visual-surround movements (Precht, 1978; Simpson, 1984). (4) *Smooth pursuit* movements are used to follow a small moving visual object (Büttner, Boyle and Markert, 1986). (5) *Convergence* is a very slow disconjugate movement of the eyes used by frontal-eyed foveate animals for stereoscopic vision.

Over the last 20 years it has become clear from the results of lesion experiments and single unit recordings from the brainstem of awake animals that each type of eye movement is controlled by a relatively independent premotor network and these networks converge generally at the level of the motoneurone (Robinson, 1968). This is an important feature of the oculomotor system since it simplifies the analysis of eye movements considerably (Fig. 11.1). In this chapter we describe first the localization of motoneurones of the extraocular eye muscles and then show how this map can be used to interpret the function of the inputs to the motoneurones from the various separate premotor networks, in particular those from the saccadic system.

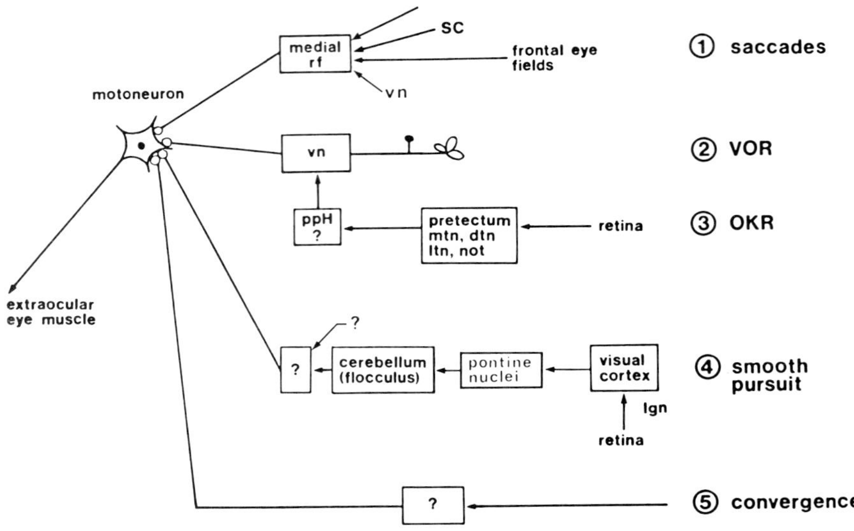

Fig. 11.1 A simplified diagram of the premotor networks subserving five different eye movement types. These networks mostly converge at the level of the motoneurone. Abbreviations: dtn, dorsal terminal nucleus; lgn, lateral geniculate nucleus; ltn, lateral terminal nucleus; mtn, medial terminal nucleus; not, nucleus of the optic tract; OKR, optokinetic response; pph, nucleus prepositus hypoglossi; rf, reticular formation; sc, superior colliculus; vn, vestibular nuclei; VOR, vestibulo-ocular reflex.

11.1 Organization of motoneurones in the oculomotor nucleus (III)

There are several neuroanatomical tracer substances such as horseradish peroxidase (HRP), wheat germ agglutinin (WGA) or the conjugate of WGA and HRP (WGA.HRP) that, when injected into a region containing axon terminals, are internalized and subsequently transported along the axon back to the parent cell body (retrograde transport) where the substances accumulate and can be visualized by standard staining procedures (Büttner-Ennever, Streit and Horn, in press). These methods are simpler and more sensitive than the older degeneration tracing techniques. A map of the location of the motoneurone pools in the oculomotor nucleus was constructed after injections of HRP, WGA or WGA.HRP into the extraocular eye muscles of monkeys (Fig. 11.2). The most significant differences between the old (Warwick, 1953) and new schemes are: (1) the medial rectus has a multifocal representation (Büttner-Ennever and Akert, 1981), (2) large and small diameter motoneurones are not inter-

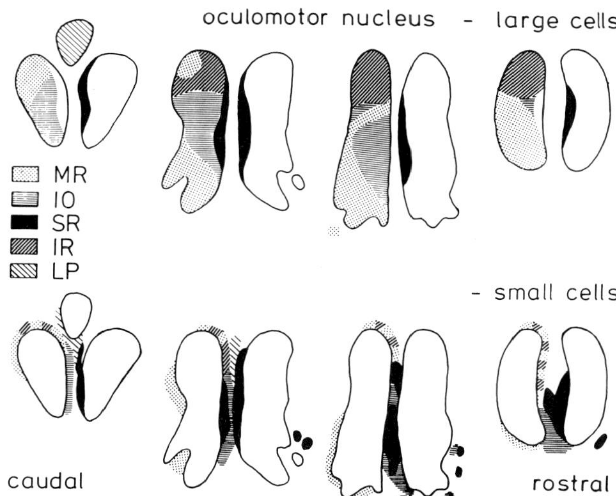

Fig. 11.2 Drawing of four levels of the monkey oculomotor nucleus showing the organization of the motoneurone pools of the five muscles (MR, IO, SR, IR and LP). In the upper drawing the organization of the large motoneurones (cell diameter $>22\mu$m) are plotted: the lower drawings show the localization of the small motoneurones (cell diameter $<22\mu$m). The small motoneurones lie around the perimeter of the classical oculomotor nucleus, and are not intermingled with the large motoneurones. Abbreviations: extraocular eye muscles – IO, inferior oblique; IR, inferior rectus; LP, levator palpebrae; LR, lateral rectus; MR, medial rectus; SO, superior oblique; SR, superior rectus.

mingled but tend to lie separately, large motoneurones within the classical oculomotor nucleus and small motoneurones lying around the border of the nucleus (Büttner-Ennever, d'Ascanio and Gysin, 1982b), (3) the small motoneurones are organized so that those of medial rectus (MR) and inferior rectus (IR) lie together dorsomedially (called subgroup C in Büttner-Ennever and Akert, 1981), whereas superior rectus (SR) and inferior oblique (IO) motoneurones are found along the midline (Fig. 11.2).

The orbital layer of the extraocular eye muscles, which lies against the bony orbit, contains muscle fibre types with high mitochondrial content and a rich capillary blood supply (Spencer and Porter, 1981), which makes them more suited for continuous or tonic activity (i.e. maintaining eye position) than the inner or global layer. The global layer, lying against the eye-ball, contains muscle fibres which are more suited for phasic activity. The orbital muscle fibres of the medial rectus muscle are innervated mainly by the small motoneurones of the subgroup C (Büttner-Ennever and Akert, 1981). It is a general principle, although not a rule, that small motoneurones have a lower threshold than large motoneurones, i.e. they tend to be tonically active (Henneman, Somojen and Carpenter, 1965). According to this, it might be expected that the small motoneurones would innervate the orbital muscle layer and participate more in maintaining eye position, rather than the fast components of eye movements, and this has been found to be the case in the human (Scott and Collins, 1973).

Convergence is a slow type of eye movement which involves predominantly the activation of MR and IR and it seems likely that premotor inputs to the small motoneurones of subgroup C could arise from areas of the brain involved in the generation of convergence eye movements (Mays, 1984). An input to the small neurones of the oculomotor nucleus lying in the midline (Fig. 11.2) should lead to a slow tonic activation of SR and IO, which would generate a slow upward deviation of the eye. Thus the small motoneurones lying around the perimeter of III appear to possess a functional organization which could provide the basis for slow tonic eye movements.

This map of the organization of motoneurones in the oculomotor nucleus can be used to interpret which eye muscles are activated by the various inputs terminating in III in the monkey. As shown in Fig. 11.1 the motoneurones receive afferents from the vestibular nuclei, mediating the vestibulo-ocular reflexes and also the optokinetic responses. The anatomy of the premotor inputs from the smooth pursuit and convergence network is not as well understood as the organization of the premotor network for saccades, which has been the subject of many recent studies. The saccadic premotor network lies in the medial reticular formation of the mesencephalon, pons and medulla (Fig. 11.3), and its connectivity and organization will be described in the following sections (see review by Fuchs, Kaneko and Scudder, 1985).

11.2 Inputs to the oculomotor nuclei involved in saccades

Clinical, lesion and single unit studies of the paramedian pontine reticular formation (PPRF) (Fig. 11.3) all indicate its importance in the generation of rapid eye movements. Lesions of PPRF lead to ipsilateral horizontal conjugate gaze paralysis, and no rapid eye movements, whether voluntary saccades or the quick phase of optokinetic or vestibular nystagmus, can be made towards the lesioned side (Henn *et al.*, 1984). Single unit studies of PPRF showed that there are two main saccade-related cell types: burst neurones and pause neurones. The burst cells are subdivided into longlead and shortlead burst neurones depending on the latency of

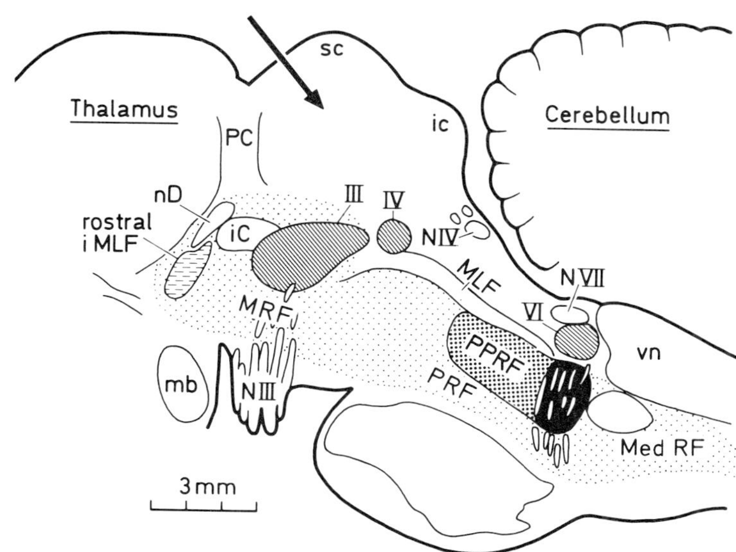

Fig. 11.3 A schematic sagittal view of the brain stem reticular formation in monkey, to demonstrate the anatomical localization of some structures involved in the generation of saccades. Omnipause neurones are located at the level of the abducens rootlets, in caudal PPRF in the black area; the white region just caudal to this in the medullary reticular formation marks the location of the horizontal inhibitory burst units. Abbreviations: III, oculomotor nucleus; IV, trochlear nucleus; VI, abducens nucleus; iC, interstitial nucleus of Cajal; ic, inferior colliculus; iMLF, (rostral) interstitial nucleus of MLF; mb, mammillary body; medRF, medullary reticular formation; MLF, medial longitudinal fasciculus; MRF, mesencephalic reticular formation; NIII, oculomotor nerve; NIV, trochlear nerve; NVII, facial nerve; nD, nucleus Darkschewitsch; PC, posterior commissure; PPRF, paramedian pontine reticular formation; PRF, pontine reticular formation; sc, superior colliculus; vn, vestibular nuclei.

their activity *before* the onset of the saccade. Several studies showed that from an analysis of the burst of activity in the shortlead burst neurones, the size, direction and timing of the saccade could be accurately predicted. These findings emphasize the exact nature of the premotor network for saccades and an equally exact set of anatomical projections have been found in the reticular formation subserving this function. Using more recent neuroanatomical techniques it was shown that neurones in caudal PPRF projected directly to the abducens nucleus, where two distinct populations of neurones are known to exist: lateral rectus motoneurones (LR), and abducens internuclear neurones (Büttner-Ennever and Henn, 1976). The axons of the abducens internuclear neurones cross the midline and ascend in the contralateral medial longitudinal fasciculus (MLF) to

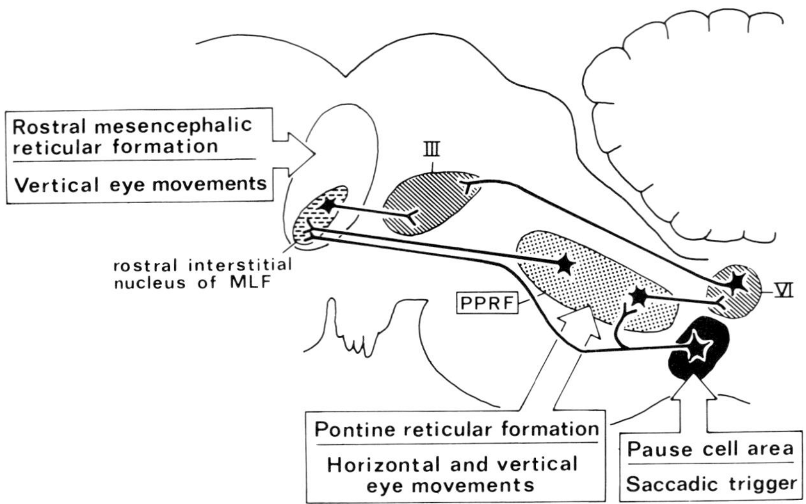

Fig. 11.4 A view of the brainstem similar to Fig. 11.3 showing some of the basic connections involved in the generation of the horizontal and vertical components of saccades. For the sake of simplicity only the oculomotor (III) and abducens nuclei (VI) are drawn.

terminate in the oculomotor nucleus. Using the revised map of the motoneurone pools in the oculomotor nucleus it was shown that this pathway contacted all groups of medial rectus motoneurones (Büttner-Ennever and Akert, 1981). It is via this internuclear pathway that PPRF, the premotor centre for horizontal saccades, activates the medial rectus (MR) motoneurones (Fig. 11.4). Thus a lesion of the MLF will lead among other symptoms to a paralysis of MR for all rapid eye movements, i.e. internuclear ophthalmoplegia (Leigh and Zee, 1983), but will leave convergence eye movements intact. A lesion of the abducens nucleus 'alone' will lead to a paralysis of not only LR but also all rapid eye movements of the contralateral MR (Henn and Büttner, 1982) (parts of this network are shown in Fig. 11.4).

11.3 The rostral mesencephalic reticular formation – vertical saccadic component

The premotor neurones for the horizontal saccadic component lie in PPRF close to the abducens nucleus. Similarly, the premotor network for the vertical saccadic component lies near the motoneurones for the vertical extraocular eye muscles in the rostral mesencephalic reticular formation (MRF) (Fig. 11.3). This anatomical separation of the vertical and horizontal premotor network means that lesions of the MRF can result in the occurrence of an isolated vertical gaze paralysis, leaving horizontal gaze intact. The exact location of the vertical premotor network has recently been studied (Büttner-Ennever *et al.*, 1982a). Physiological and anatomical studies of this area show that one part of the MRF, the rostral interstitial nucleus of the MLF (rostral iMLF), contains vertical shortlead bursters, and that these neurones project directly to the vertical motoneurone pools of the oculomotor nucleus (Figs 11.3 and 11.4). The role of the interstitial nucleus of Cajal (iC) which lies immediately caudal to rostral iMLF is still not clear.

Vertical longlead burst neurones are only found in rostral PPRF. Since these are considered to take part in the initial stages of the saccadic-processing, it appears that PPRF is involved in the early stages of both horizontal and vertical saccade generation. The vertical longlead bursters in PPRF are thought to project to the vertical shortlead burst neurones lying in the rostral iMLF, which in turn activate the vertical motoneurones (Fig. 11.4).

11.4 The dorsomedullary reticular formation

A group of inhibitory premotor burst neurones, which serve to relax the horizontal antagonistic eye muscles during a saccade, has been located close to the midline just caudal to the abducens nucleus. These cells have been shown to project directly to the contralateral abducens nucleus where they inhibit both the lateral rectus motoneurones and, via the internuclear neurones, the medial rectus motoneurones on the other side (Hikosaka *et al.*, 1978; Yoshida *et al.*, 1981). Like the other burst neurone regions these cells receive an input from PPRF (Langer and Kaneko, 1983). Similar sets of inhibitory burst neurones for the vertical motoneurones are to be expected, and, although they probably lie somewhere in the medial reticular formation, their location is as yet unknown.

A saccade can occur in any direction so that vertical and horizontal saccadic components must be co-ordinated, which is achieved by a type of trigger system which has been studied a great deal over the past 10 years. It is interesting to speculate whether such a trigger mechanism exists in other motor systems.

11.5 Omnipause neurones – the saccadic trigger

Omnipause neurones are one highly specific type of pause neurone found close to the midline in caudal PPRF. Their high level of spontaneous activity is interrupted shortly before every rapid eye movement (saccade), independent of its size or direction, hence the name 'omnipause neurones'. They have axons which contact all known shortlead burst neurones, i.e. the horizontal shortlead bursters in caudal PPRF, the vertical shortlead bursters in rostral iMLF (Fig. 11.4) and the inhibitory horizontal burst neurones in the rostral medullary reticular formation. Stimulation of the omnipause region blocked or interrupted saccades in midflight (see Fuchs, Kaneko and Scudder, 1985). These studies support the original suggestion that the omnipause neurones operate as a trigger system for the saccade (Keller, 1974; Robinson, 1975) and exert a tonic inhibition on the shortlead burst cells; when the activity is interrupted shortly before the saccade, the inhibition is removed and this enables the shortlead bursters to activate the motoneurones and bring about the appropriate saccade. The omnipause neurones form a compact cell group which lies close to the midline at the level of the abducens rootlets. They can be recognized in monkey and man on the basis of cytoarchitecture alone (Büttner-Ennever *et al.*, in press) and the cell group has been called nucleus raphe interpositus (rip) to distinguish it from the adjacent nucleus raphe pontis. The omnipause cell group (rip) receives direct inputs from structures such as the superior colliculus, and frontal eye fields (Stanton, Goldberg and Bruce, in press) – structures which are both involved in the generation of saccadic eye movements. A projection to rip would enable the parent cell group to control the triggering, i.e. timing, of the saccadic event. Disorders of the saccadic trigger could lead to conditions such as opsoclonus and ocular bobbing, and oculomotor apraxia (Leigh and Zee, 1983). It may be possible in the future to reveal some neuroanatomical basis for these deficits.

In summary: the medial mesencephalic, pontine and medullary reticular formation is involved in the elaboration of horizontal and vertical premotor signals for saccade generation, and all have direct inputs onto the oculomotor nuclei. Omnipause neurones normally inhibit the output of the saccadic premotor network, but shortly before a saccade they themselves are inhibited, which allows the premotor network to activate the motoneurones of the oculomotor nuclei (III, IV, VI) and generate a saccade.

Acknowledgement

This work was supported by the Deutsche Forschungsgemeinschaft SFB 220/D8.

References

Büttner, U., Boyle, R. and Markert, G. (1986) Cerebellar control of eye movements, in *The Oculomotor and Skeletalmotor System* (eds H.-J. Freund, U. Büttner, B. Cohen and J. Noth). *Prog. Brain Res.*, **64**, 225–33.

Büttner-Ennever, J.A. and Akert, K. (1981) Medial rectus subgroups of the oculomotor nucleus and their abducens internuclear input in the monkey. *J. Comp. Neurol.*, **197**, 17–27.

Büttner-Ennever, J.A. and Henn, V. (1976) An autoradiographic study of the pathways from the pontine reticular formation involved in horizontal eye movements. *Brain Res.*, **108**, 155–64.

Büttner-Ennever, J.A., Büttner, U., Cohen, B. and Baumgartner, G. (1982a) Vertical gaze paralysis and the rostral interstitial nucleus of the medial longitudinal fasciculus. *Brain*, **105**, 125–49.

Büttner-Ennever, J., d'Ascanio, P. and Gysin, R. (1982b) The arrangement of large and small motoneurons in the oculomotor nucleus of the monkey, in *Physiological and Pathological Aspects of Eye Movements* (eds A. Roucoux and M. Crommelinick). Junk Publ., The Hague, pp. 345–9.

Büttner-Ennever, J.A., Cohen, B. Pause, M. and Fries, W. (in press) A raphe nucleus of the pons containing omnipause neurons of the oculomotor system of the monkey. *J. Comp. Neurol.*

Büttner-Ennever, J.A., Streit, W. and Horn, A. (in press) Lectins as neuroanatomical tracers. *Acta Histochem.*

Fuchs, A.F., Kaneko, C.R.S. and Scudder, C.A. (1985) Brainstem control of saccadic eye movement. *Ann. Rev. Neurosci.*, **8**, 307–37.

Henn, V. and Büttner, U. (1982) Disorders of horizontal gaze, in *Functional Basis of Ocular Motility* (eds G. Lennerstrand, D. Zee and E. Keller). Pergamon Press, Oxford, pp. 239–55.

Henn, V., Lang, W., Hepp, K. and Reisine, H. (1984) Experimental gaze palsies in monkeys and their relation to human pathology. *Brain*, **107**, 619–36.

Henneman, E., Somojen, G. and Carpenter, D.O. (1965) Excitability and inhibitability of motoneurons of different sizes. *J. Neurophysiol.*, **28**, 599–620.

Hikosaka, O., Igusa, Y., Nakao, S. and Shimazu, H. (1978) Direct inhibitory synaptic linkage of pontomedullary reticular burst neurons with abducens motoneurons in the cat. *Exp. Brain Res.*, **33**, 337–52.

Keller, E.L. (1974) Participation of medial pontine reticular formation in eye movement generation in the monkey. *J. Neurophysiol.*, **37**, 316–32.

Langer, T. and Kaneko, C.R.S. (1983) Efferent projections of the cat oculomotor reticular omnipause neuron region: an autoradiographic study. *J. Comp. Neurol.*, **217**, 288–306.

Leigh, R.J. and Zee, D. (1983) *The Neurology of Eye Movement*. F.A. Davis Co., Philadelphia.

Mays, L.M. (1984) Neural control of vergence eye movements: convergence and divergence neurons in midbrain. *J. Neurophysiol.*, **51**, 1091–108.

Precht, W. (1978) *Neuronal Operation in the Vestibular System.* Springer-Verlag, Berlin.
Raybourn, M.S. and Keller, E.L. (1977) Colliculoreticular organization in primate oculomotor system. *J. Neurophysiol.*, **40**, 861–78.
Robinson, D.A. (1968) Eye movement control in primates. *Science*, **16**, 1219–24.
Robinson, D.A. (1975) Oculomotor control signals, in *Basic Mechanisms of Oculomotor Motility and their Clinical Implications* (eds G. Lennerstrand and P. Bach-y-Rita). Pergamon, Oxford, pp. 337–74.
Scott, A.B. and Collins, C.C. (1973) Division of labor in the human extraocular muscle. *Arch. Ophthalmol.*, **90**, 319–22.
Simpson, J.I. (1984) The accessory optic system. *Ann. Rev. Neurosci.*, **7**, 13–41.
Spencer, R.F. and Porter, J.D. (1981) The innervation and structure of extraocular muscles of the monkey in comparison to the cat. *J. Comp. Neurol.*, **198**, 649–65.
Stanton, G.B., Goldberg, M.E. and Bruce, C.J. (in press) Cortical projections from saccadic eye movement sites in the macaque's frontal eye fields (FEF). *J. Comp. Neurol.*
Warwick, R. (1953) Representation of the extraocular muscles in the oculomotor nuclei of the monkey. *J. Comp. Neurol.*, **98**, 449–504.
Yoshida, K., McCrea, R., Berthoz, A. and Vidal, P.P. (1981) Properties of immediate inhibitory burst neurons controlling horizontal rapid eye movements in the cat, in *Progress in Oculomotor Research Dev. Neurosci.* (eds A. Fuchs and W. Becker), vol. 12. Elsevier/North-Holland, New York, pp. 71–80.

CHAPTER 12

Brainstem control of horizontal gaze: effect of lesions

CHARLES PIERROT-DESEILLIGNY

12.1 Introduction

For the last 12 years, much precise morphological and electrophysiological experimental research, as well as clinical studies using eye movement recordings, have greatly improved our knowledge of horizontal gaze organization in the brainstem. Both types of data will be summarized here, with special reference to the clinical characteristics useful in the topographical diagnosis of oculomotor syndromes resulting from focal lesions. The final common neural pathway for lateral eye movements and the different supranuclear structures located in the brainstem will be successively reviewed, including a special mention of those involved in saccades and foveal smooth pursuit, since the other eye movements are reviewed elsewhere in this volume.

12.2 Final common pathway of lateral eye movements

12.2.1 EXPERIMENTAL DATA

It has now been fully demonstrated by morphological studies in the cat and monkey that the abducens nucleus contains two intermingled types of neurones (Graybiel and Hartwieg, 1974; Graybiel, 1977; Bienfang, 1978;

Steiger and Büttner-Ennever, 1979; Carpenter and Batton, 1980; Büttner-Ennever and Akert, 1981; Langer *et al.*, 1986; McCrea, Strassman and Highstein, 1986): (1) the abducens motoneurones that innervate the lateral rectus muscle and (2) the internuclear neurones which decussate at the level of the abducens nucleus, run through the medial longitudinal fasciculus (MLF) and project on to the medial rectus muscle motoneurones in the contralateral oculomotor nucleus. Electrophysiological studies in the cat and monkey have shown that internuclear neurones receive the same afferents as motoneurones (Baker and Highstein 1975; Highstein *et al.*, 1976) and, like them, carry a horizontal gaze signal correlated both with eye position and velocity and are consequently involved in all types of lateral eye movements (King, Lisberger and Fuchs, 1976; Pola and Robinson, 1978; Delgado-Garcia, Del Pozo and Baker, 1986). Lesions in the monkey confined to the abducens nucleus (Carpenter, McMasters and Hanna, 1963) or to the MLF (Carpenter and McMasters, 1963; Evinger, Fuchs and Baker, 1977) have respectively induced a complete paralysis of ipsilateral conjugate eye movements and an adduction paralysis in the ipsilateral eye only (with convergence conserved in both cases).

Two points concerning the afferents to the medial rectus muscle motoneurones have not yet been completely cleared up. First, what is the functional role of the excitatory ascending tract of Deiters described in the cat (Gacek, 1971; Baker and Highstein, 1978; Reisine, Strassman and Highstein, 1981) and monkey (Lang, Büttner-Ennever and Büttner, 1979)? This tract connects the lateral vestibular nucleus with the ipsilateral medial rectus muscle motoneurones monosynaptically and courses laterally to the MLF in the posterior tegmentum. It carries an eye position and head velocity signal, which appears redundant given the signal mediated by the internuclear neurones. However, it has been suggested that its action in man could be either insignificant or inoperative since no lateral conjugate adductive movement beyond the midline is possible after a selective lesion of the internuclear neurones (Pierrot-Deseilligny, 1985). Second, are the medial rectus muscle motoneurones inhibited by inhibitory neurones during contralateral eye movements? In the cat, inhibition of these motoneurones has been considered as either absent or weak (Baker and Highstein, 1978; Uchino *et al.*, 1979; Grantyn *et al.*, 1980; Hikosaka, Igusa and Imai, 1980; Nakao and Sasaki, 1980), for rapid as well as for slow eye movements. Furthermore, no inhibitory tract terminating at this level has as yet been identified. In man, it has also been suggested on electromyographical grounds that an inhibition of medial rectus muscle motoneurones is unlikely (Pierrot-Deseilligny and Chain, 1979). Thus, the decrease of activity in these motoneurones could essentially be controlled by the disfacilitation arising from the internuclear neurones.

Accordingly, besides a complete control of the lateral rectus muscle motoneurones, it appears that the abducens nucleus also controls almost all (if not all!) the activity of the medial rectus muscle motoneurones during all lateral conjugate eye movements in both horizontal directions through its internuclear neurones. It may therefore be considered, at least in binocular species, as the final common pathway of these movements.

12.2.2 LESIONS IN MAN

The motoneurones, the internuclear neurones and the abducens nucleus, forming the different parts of the final common pathway are described successively.

(a) Motoneurones. A selective clinical lesion of the abducens motoneurones in the pons, sparing the other oculomotor structures, is infrequent. As such a lesion is necessarily located in the basis pontis (Figs 12.1, 12.2 and 12.5, syndrome 1), the adjacent pyramidal tract is also generally damaged, resulting in the classic Millard–Gubler syndrome with a sixth nerve paralysis on the side of the lesion (with usually a peripheral facial paralysis on the same side) and a motor deficit (sparing the face) on the opposite side. This syndrome was observed in the patient whose oculomotor characteristics are shown in Fig. 12.3A. The lesion, visible on CT scan, involved only the right part of the basis pontis. The patient exhibited a complete abduction paralysis in the right eye for all lateral eye movements, including reflex vestibular oculocephalic movements. It may further be observed in recordings (direct current electro-oculography) that the peak velocity of the paralysed eye returning from the medial position to the midline was almost twice as slow as that of the normal eye, for saccades as well as for oculocephalic movements (Fig. 12.3Aa and c). This is easily explained by the fact that a normal velocity results from the concomitant actions of the contracting agonist muscle and the relaxing antagonist muscle, whereas in this case the latter was acting alone. Lastly, when the lateral rectus muscle is totally paralysed, a noticeable tonic deviation of the eye in its internal hemifield of movement is usual. However, the complete relaxation of the antagonist medial rectus muscle during return movements allows the eye to reach the midline transitorily. This line cannot be crossed since, for all eye movement performed beyond it, the agonist muscle contraction is indispensable. All these phenomena are exactly reversed when the medial rectus muscle motoneurones are damaged in the oculomotor nucleus and/or in their peduncular course (see below, syndrome 6 and Fig. 12.6).

(b) Internuclear neurones. When one MLF is damaged between the abdu-

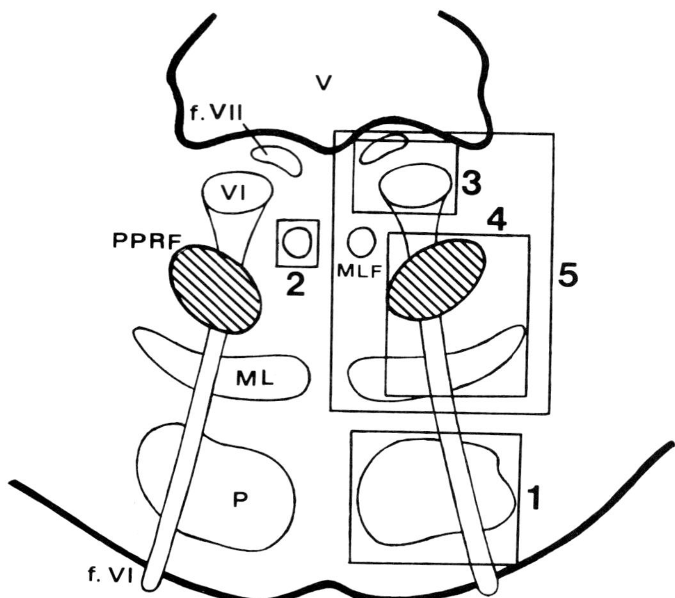

Fig. 12.1 Horizontal section of the lower pons. C, cerebellum; f. III, fibres of the oculomotor nucleus; f. VI, fibres of the abducens nucleus; f. VII, facial fibres; ML, medial lemniscus; MLF, medial longitudinal fasciculus; NRTP, nucleus reticularis tegmenti pontis; P, pyramidal tract; PH, nucleus prepositus hypoglossi; PN, pontine nuclei; PPRF, paramedian pontine reticular formation; SC, superior colliculus; SRF, supragigantocellular reticular formation; V, fourth ventricle; VN, vestibular nuclei; III, oculomotor nucleus; IV, trochlear nucleus; VI, abducens nucleus; 1, basis pontis syndrome; 2, internuclear ophthalmoplegia; 3, abducens nucleus syndrome; 4, caudal PPRF syndrome; 5, one-and-a-half syndrome; 6, paramedian midbrain syndrome.

cens nucleus and the oculomotor nucleus (Figs 12.1, 12.2 and 12.5, syndrome 2) the axons of the internuclear neurones are interrupted and a unilateral internuclear ophthalmoplegia results, which includes: (1) complete paralysis of adduction in the ipsilateral eye for all conjugate lateral eye movements (Pierrot-Deseilligny and Chain, 1979, Case 1) (Fig. 12.3Bb and c, left eye), usually with preservation of convergence; (2) monocular, or predominantly monocular, nystagmus in the contralateral eye, when this eye is in abduction. As the MLF is located very near the midline, both fasciculi are often damaged simultaneously leading to bilateral internuclear ophthalmoplegia, in which both of the above signs are found in each eye. If the MLF is partially damaged, only an adduction paresis is observed, at times subtle and recognized only from recordings by a slight slowing of saccade velocity (Crane *et al.*, 1983). When a complete adduc-

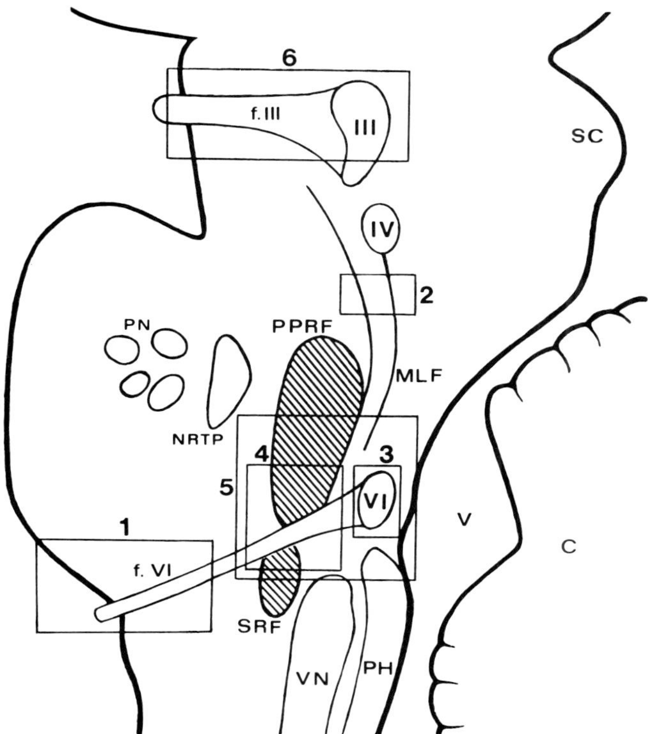

Fig. 12.2 Sagittal view of the brainstem. Abbreviations: see Fig. 12.1.

tion paralysis exists in one eye, there is in this eye a clear slowing of saccades returning to the midline, as in the case shown here (Fig. 12.3Ba, left eye). On the other hand, it must be noted that the peak velocity of the same eye returning to the midline with oculocephalic movement (Fig. 12.3Bc, left eye) is not apparently decreased (contrary to the observation with damage to the abducens motoneurones previously described). The absence of clear impairment of this velocity may be due to the contribution of a permanent tonic activity of the medial rectus muscle motoneurones in slow eye movements directed towards adduction. This residual activity, probably related to the convergence system, is well known in internuclear ophthalmoplegia (Pierrot-Deseilligny and Chain, 1979) and could also exist in abducens nucleus lesions. Alternatively, some action of the ascending tract of Deiters, perhaps existing in a vestigial form in man (Pierrot-Deseilligny, 1985), is also possible in this movement.

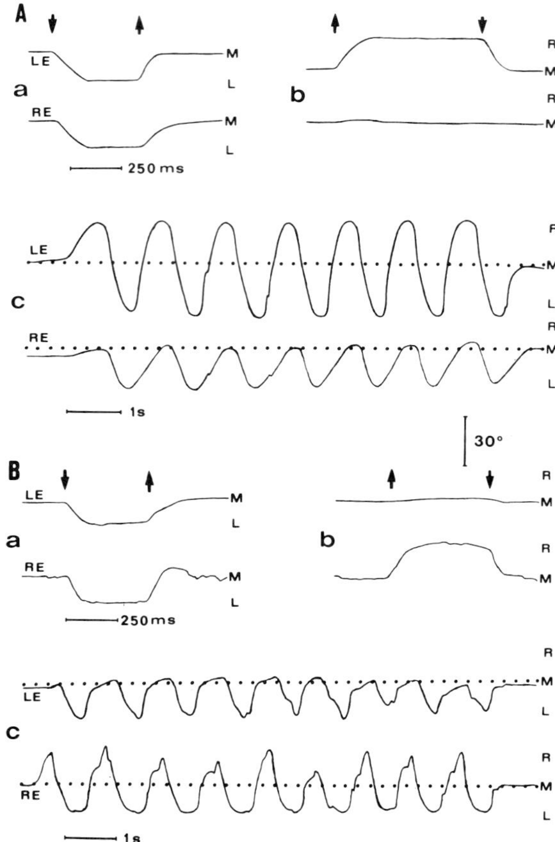

Fig. 12.3 Cases with lesions of the abducens nucleus motoneurones and of the internuclear neurones. A: Patient with lesion of the right abducens motoneurones; a, leftward saccades; b, rightward saccades; c, oculocephalic movement. B: Patient with left internuclear ophthalmoplegia; a, leftward saccades; b, rightward saccades; c, oculocephalic movement. See the text for the description of oculomotor disorders. L = left; LE = left eye; M = midline; R = right; RE = right eye. Arrows indicate the beginning of saccades.

If the pathophysiology of adduction paralysis in internuclear ophthalmoplegia is not in doubt, that of abduction nystagmus of the contralateral eye is still not yet clear. Many interpretations have been proposed (for review, see Leigh and Zee, 1983), but none is really satisfactory. As fixation and certain slow eye movements, such as foveal smooth pursuit, are somewhat defective in the eye moving towards abduction, damage to a pathway involved in these functions has been suspected (Pierrot-Deseilligny and Chain, 1979). The authors suggested that damage to the descending internuclear neurones of the oculomotor nucleus, described in the cat and monkey (Maciewicz and Phipps, 1983; Langer *et al.*, 1986), could be responsible for these disorders. These neurones seem to be controlled by the medial rectus muscle motoneurones and project on to the abducens nucleus (mainly contralaterally) by passing through the periphery of the MLF. However, it now appears more probable (although not yet demonstrated) that these internuclear neurones of the oculomotor nucleus are involved in inhibition of the abducens motoneurones by the convergence system. Their variable impairment in MLF lesions could perhaps explain the variable preservation of convergence in internuclear ophthalmoplegia. As an alternative to the previous hypothesis, damage to the afferents to the interstitial nucleus of the MLF or to this nucleus itself, lying in the portion of the MLF located above the abducens nucleus, could account for the disorders of fixation and slow eye movements: (1) in the monkey, the interstitial nucleus of the MLF projects on to the flocculus (Langer *et al.*, 1985b), a structure obviously involved in fixation and foveal smooth pursuit in both man and monkey (Zee *et al.*, 1981; Büttner and Waespe, 1984; Baloh, Yee and Honrubia, 1986); (2) the disorders actually concern both eyes (Pierrot-Deseilligny and Chain, 1979), but appear exclusively or predominantly on the eye opposite to the lesion because of the adduction paralysis of the ipsilateral eye. The afferents of this nucleus are not well known, although it has been reported in the monkey that the internuclear neurones themselves send collaterals to it (McCrea, Strassman and Highstein, 1986). Accordingly, a pathway carrying an important eye position signal from the abducens nucleus (but perhaps also from other structures) to the flocculus could be interrupted by the MLF lesion, at the level of (or before the relay in) the interstitial nucleus of the MLF. All the connections and the precise physiological role of this nucleus, however, are still to be determined.

Internuclear opthalmoplegia is also characterized by a hypermetry of all saccades directed towards abduction in the eye opposite to the lesion (Baloh, Yee and Honrubia, 1978; Zee, Hain and Carl, 1987). To understand this anomaly, it is helpful to review briefly the neural signals driving motoneurones and eye muscles during saccades, namely the pulse-step change in innervation (Robinson, 1964, 1981; Leigh and Zee, 1983; Zee, 1986). The pulse, proportional to eye velocity, corresponds to a high-frequency burst of phasic activity observed in the motoneurones as well as electromyographically in the agonist muscle. It generates the force overcoming orbital viscous drag and allows the eye to move quickly to another position. The step, proportional to eye position, corresponds to the appropriate change of the tonic activity at the end of the saccade necessary to hold the eye in its new position against orbital elastic-restoring forces. Normally, the pulse and the step, controlled by distinct structures in the brainstem (see below, the premotor structures) are appropriately matched in order to prevent any post-saccadic drift. In internuclear ophthalmoplegia, saccades directed towards abduction are hypermetric and immediately followed by a rapid post-saccadic drift in the opposite direction. The quick phases of the abduction nystagmus are also hypermetric, with at the end of the saccade a movement directed towards adduction which may be divided into two parts: first, an extremely rapid post-saccadic drift, corresponding to the overshoot of saccade, followed by the slow phase, properly so-called, of the abduction nystagmus. The overshoot of saccades could be due to an adaptive central mechanism attempting to overcome the adduction paralysis by an increase of the pulse (Baloh, Yee and Honrubia, 1978). The initial rapid post-saccadic drift could be explained by a mismatch in this case between the pulse and the step, the latter not being increased proportionally. Lastly, the second only really slow component of the slow phase of the abduction nystagmus could be due to combined damage to a pathway involved in horizontal position maintenance (see above).

(c) Abducens nucleus. A selective lesion of the abducens nucleus (Figs 12.1, 12.2 and 12.5, syndrome 5) induces a complete ipsilateral paralysis of all conjugate lateral eye movements (Pierrot-Deseilligny and Goasguen, 1984) (Fig. 12.4Ab and c). As the fibres of the facial nerve are in the immediate vicinity, there is usually an ipsilateral peripheral facial paralysis also. Return saccades from the contralateral (here left) position persist, slightly slowed by the absence of the agonist muscle action (Fig. 12.4Aa). Persistence of vestibular saccades (quick phases of nystagmus) directed ipsilaterally in the hemifield of movement contralateral to a selective lesion of the abducens nucleus has furthermore been reported in the monkey (Carpenter, McMasters and Hanna, 1963). The mechanisms explaining the presence of these different saccades will be discussed below. The peak velocities of oculocephalic movements of the eyes returning to the midline were different for each eye, those of the right eye in this case being clearly slower than those of the left eye (Fig. 12.4Ac). The paralysed agonist muscles were respectively the lateral rectus and the medial rectus and hypotheses about these distinct peak velocities have been proposed above in discussion of the selective lesions of abducens motoneurones and of the internuclear neurones. Finally, these different clinical features confirm that the abducens nucleus syndrome is the sum of both syndromes resulting from the individual impairments of abducens motoneurones and of the internuclear neurones, and consequently supports the fact that the final common pathway of lateral eye move-

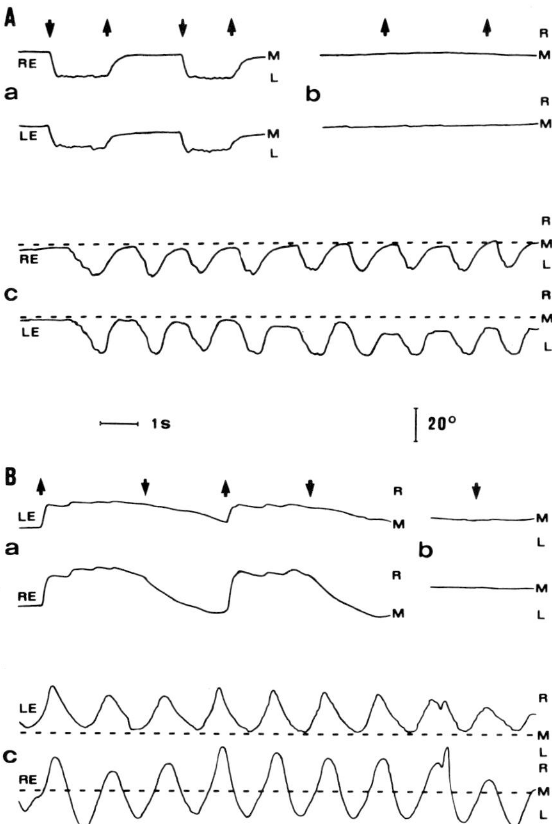

Fig. 12.4 Cases with lesions of the abducens nucleus and of the caudal PPRF. A: Patient with lesion of the right abducens nucleus; a, leftward saccades; b, rightward saccades; c, oculocephalic movement. B: Patient with lesion of the left caudal PPRF; a, rightward saccades; b, leftward saccades; c, oculocephalic movement. See the text for the description of oculomotor disorders. Abbreviations: see Fig. 12.3

ments does begin in the abducens nucleus. However, this nucleus could also perform other functions as yet barely known (Langer *et al.*, 1986). In particular, it could transmit the signal of the real eye position to certain supranuclear structures (see below) such as the nucleus prepositus hypoglossi (McCrea and Baker, 1985) and the flocculus, on to which it projects directly (Langer *et al.*, 1985b) and possibly also indirectly via the interstitial nucleus of the MLF (see above).

12.3 Immediate premotor structures

The immediate premotor structures are the last relays of the different pathways terminating in the abducens nucleus. The pontine reticular formations are the final common pathway of all rapid eye movements.

12.3.1 PONTINE RETICULAR FORMATIONS

(a) Experimental data. Electrophysiological studies in the monkey and cat have shown that the paramedian pontine reticular formation (PPRF) – extending from the rostral pole of the abducens nucleus to the ponto-peduncular junction, ventral to the MLF – contains excitatory burst neurones active just prior to and during all types of ipsilateral saccades (Sparks and Travis, 1971; Luschei and Fuchs, 1972; Keller, 1974; Henn and Cohen, 1976; Lestienne, Whittington and Bizzi, 1981; Hepp and Henn, 1983; Fuchs, Kaneko and Scudder, 1985). These neurones constitute the generator of the saccadic pulse and remain silent during fixation and slow eye movements. Their discharge patterns depend on eye velocity which is proportional to the movement amplitude. The step integrating the new position of the eye after the saccade could originate either from the nucleus prepositus hypoglossi or from the medial vestibular nucleus or from these two structures at the same time (Cannon and Robinson, 1986). Except for saccades, the excitatory burst neurones are permanently inhibited by the omnipause neurones, located rostral to the abducens nucleus, very near the midline (Fig. 12.5), and whose tonic activity ceases just prior to and during saccades (Keller, 1974; King, Precht and Dieringer, 1980; Evinger, Kaneko and Fuchs, 1982; Kaneko and Fuchs, 1982; Langer and Kaneko, 1983; Curthoys, Markham and Furuya, 1984). In the monkey and cat, the PPRF projects directly on to the ipsilateral abducens nucleus (Büttner-Ennever and Henn, 1976; Graybiel 1977; Langer *et al.*, 1986).

Fig. 12.5 Clinical characteristics and physiological interpretation of horizontal oculomotor syndromes. 1, basis pontis syndrome; 2, internuclear ophthalmoplegia; 3, abducens nucleus syndrome; 4, caudal PPRF syndrome; 5, one-and-a-half syndrome; 6, paramedian midbrain syndrome (the side of syndromes 4 and 6 is reversed with regard to that of syndromes shown in Figs 12.4B and 12.6). EBN, excitatory burst neurone; EVN, excitatory vestibular neurone; IBN, inhibitory burst neurone; IN, internuclear neurone; IVN, inhibitory vestibular neurone; L, left; LE, left eye; LR, lateral rectus muscle; M, midline; MLF, medial longitudinal fasciculus; MN, motoneurone; MR, medial rectus muscle; MVN, medial vestibular nucleus; P, pause neurone; PPRF, paramedian pontine reticular formation; R, right, RE, right eye; SRF, supragigantocellular reticular formation; STLS, suprareticular tracts of lateral saccades; III, oculomotor nucleus; VI, abducens nucleus; VIII, vestibular nerve.

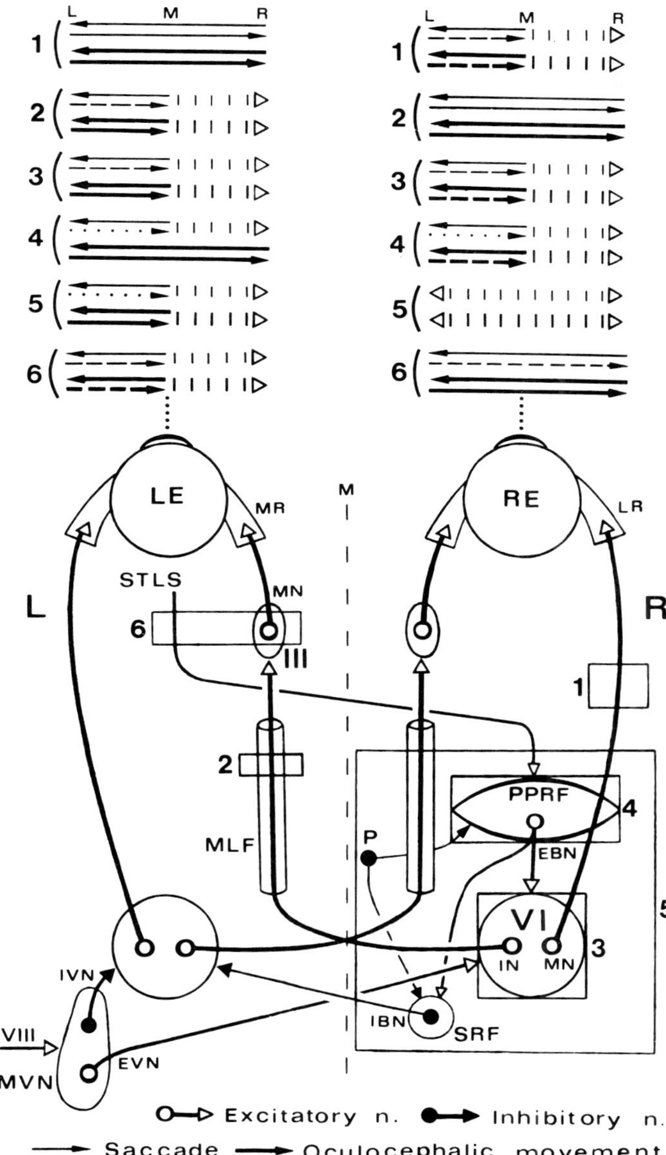

L
M
R
1
2
3
4
5
6
LE
RE
MR
LR
M
STLS
MN
III
L
R
PPRF
EBN
P
MLF
VI
IN
MN
IVN
VIII
MVN
EVN
IBN
SRF
Excitatory n.
Inhibitory n.
Saccade
Oculocephalic movement
&
Slightly slowed movement
Very slow movement
No movement

The inhibitory burst neurones are also active just prior to and during all types of ipsilateral saccades. They lie in the dorsal reticular formation of the pontomedullary junction in the cat (Hikosaka and Kawakami, 1977; Yoshida *et al.*, 1982), but appear to be located a little more rostrally in the monkey, in the supragigantocellular reticular formation (SRF) lying in the caudal part of the pontine tegmentum just ventrally and caudally to the abducens nucleus (Porter, Guthrie and Sparks, 1985; Langer *et al.*, 1986). They project monosynaptically on to the contralateral abducens nucleus (Fig. 12.5) which they phasically inhibit during ipsilateral saccades. Inactive during fixation and slow eye movements, being inhibited by the omnipause neurones which project on to them directly (Nakao, Curthoys and Markham, 1980; Furuya and Markham, 1982; Langer and Kaneko, 1983), their activity could be driven both by the cessation of the omnipause neurones inhibition and by an excitatory command arising from the excitatory burst neurones (Sasaki and Shimazu, 1981; Yoshida *et al.*, 1982).

Unilateral acute lesions of the PPRF in the monkey have induced a contralateral tonic deviation of both eyes, a complete ipsilateral paralysis of all saccades (including those which should occur in the contralateral hemifield of movement) and a paralysis of ipsilateral reflex movements (Cohen, Komatsuzaki and Bender, 1968). However, ipsilateral reflex movements were again possible beyond the midline as soon as the contralateral tonic deviation (observed during several days or weeks) had regressed. More recently, bilateral lesions of the caudal PPRF with kainic acid (damaging the cellular bodies but sparing the axons of neurones) have led to a complete paralysis of horizontal saccades with preservation of horizontal vestibular reflex movements and the smooth pursuit component of optokinetic nystagmus (Henn *et al.*, 1984).

(b) Lesions in man. Unilateral damage to the caudal PPRF in man (Figs 12.1, 12.2 and 12.5, syndrome 4) induces a contralateral tonic deviation and an impairment of all ipsilateral eye movements (including vestibular reflex ones) only when the lesion has an acute onset (Pierrot-Deseilligny, unpublished cases). When the lesion is progressive (e.g. in tumours) the tonic deviation is either absent or weak and the oculomotor syndrome then has four main characteristics (Pierrot-Deseilligny *et al.*, 1979): (1) absence of all saccades (including the quick phase of nystagmus) directed ipsilaterally, namely in the whole field of eye movement, with an extremely slow voluntary eye movement (10 to 20°/s) replacing voluntary saccades from the contralateral position to the midline, which cannot be crossed voluntarily (Pierrot-Deseilligny, Chain and Lhermitte, 1982) (Fig. 12.4Bab); (2) absence or persistence (Kommerell *et al.*, 1987; Pierrot-Deseilligny, unpublished data) of ipsilateral pursuit movements beyond the midline, these movements persisting in the contralateral hemifield of

movement, although usually partly saccadic contralaterally to the lesion; (3) persistence of ipsilateral vestibular reflex eye movements for the eye contralateral to the lesion (Fig. 12.4Bc, right eye); (4) absence of these movements in the ipsilateral hemifield of movement for the eye ipsilateral to the lesion, with some slowing of the return movement to the midline (Fig. 12.4Bc, left eye).

Experimental data (see above) allow us to account for the disorders of saccades and oculocephalic movements. The absence of ipsilateral saccades (beyond the midline) is explained by damage to the excitatory burst neurones of the PPRF controlling the phasic excitation of the agonist muscles. The absence of all saccades directed ipsilaterally in the contralateral hemifield of movement is due to the lack of inhibitory burst neurone activity (in the SRF), either damaged by the lesion (the caudal PPRF being very close to the SRF) or only disconnected from the PPRF (see Figs 12.2 and 5). The pathophysiology of the very slow movement replacing voluntary saccade returning to the midline is not totally clear. It could be a rather passive movement occurring when the contraction of the antagonist muscles ceases, the eyes returning to the midline, partly at least, by the orbital visco-elastic forces. In the abducens nucleus lesion seen previously, ipsilateral saccades persisted in the contralateral hemifield of movement since both premotor structures necessary to the phasic inhibition of the antagonist muscles (namely the PPRF and the SRF, both ventral to the lesion) were spared (Fig. 12.5). These saccades were slightly slowed simply by the absence of concomitant phasic excitation of the agonist muscles.

The persistence of an ipsilateral oculocephalic movement in the contralateral eye after a caudal PPRF lesion is explained by the preservation of the whole pathway mediating the essential vestibular input to the medial rectus muscle motoneurones, namely the contralateral medial vestibular nucleus, the ipsilateral abducens nucleus and the contralateral MLF (Pierrot-Deseilligny *et al.*, 1979) (Fig. 12.5). The absence of ipsilateral oculocephalic movement in the ipsilateral eye is due to the combined damage to the motoneurones of the abducens nucleus (Pierrot-Deseilligny *et al.*, 1979; Leigh and Zee, 1983), passing through the caudal part of the PPRF and the rostral part of the SRF before reaching the basis pontis (Fig. 12.2). Therefore, in this caudal PPRF syndrome, both a supranuclear paralysis of conjugate eye movements (for saccades) and a complete infranuclear abduction paralysis are associated. It must be noted that in this case, as in the other lesions of the abducens nucleus motoneurones (either in the basis pontis or in the nucleus itself), the peak velocity of the oculocephalic movement directed towards the midline in the eye with the abduction paralysis is slowed (see above). In a PPRF lesion a little more rostrally located, the abducens nucleus motoneurones are preserved and ipsilateral oculocephalic movements persist for both eyes (Leigh and Zee, 1983).

Some other clinical aspects deserve to be mentioned. In bilateral PPRF lesions all horizontal saccades are absent, but some horizontal vestibular and pursuit eye movements persist (Pierrot-Deseilligny *et al.*, 1984; Baloh, Furman and Yee, 1985). In partial PPRF damage (Büttner-Ennever *et al.*, 1985; Hanson *et al.*, 1986), horizontal saccades are more or less slowed. As the PPRF is just dorsal to the medial lemniscus (Fig. 12.1), this fasciculus is also usually impaired in a PPRF lesion, with a consequent sensory deficit on the side contralateral to the lesion. When the lesion extends dorsally to the abducens nucleus (syndrome 3 + syndrome 4), the characteristics of the abducens nucleus syndrome and those of the PPRF syndrome are combined, resulting in both a complete ipsilateral paralysis of all conjugate lateral eye movements (specific to the former) and the absence of ipsilateral saccades in the contralateral hemifield of movement (specific to the latter). In the case described by Foville (1858), without pathological study, there was a complete conjugate lateral eye movement paralysis on one side and a sensory and motor deficit of the limbs on the opposite side: it may be (in this probable vascular case) that the lesion involved all the paramedian part of the pons (Fig. 12.1, syndromes 1, 4 and 3). Lastly, when a tegmental lesion damaging the PPRF and the abducens nucleus extends to the MLF located on the same side, a one-and-a-half syndrome appears (Fisher, 1967; Pierrot-Deseilligny *et al.*, 1981a; Boggouslavsky *et al.*, 1984): with (1) a paralysis of all conjugate lateral eye movements ('one') ipsilateral to the lesion; and (2) an ipsilateral internuclear ophthalmoplegia ('and-a-half'), including (a) an adduction paralysis in the ipsilateral eye and (b) an abduction nystagmus in the contralateral eye (Figs 12.1, 2 and 5, syndrome 5). Thus, in this syndrome, the eye ipsilateral to the lesion remains fixed on the midline during all conjugate lateral eye movements (but it can converge), and the opposite eye can only move from the midline to the contralateral position. Variations of this syndrome exist when, for example, MLF damage is combined with damage either to the abducens nucleus only or to the PPRF only (Pierrot-Deseilligny *et al.*, 1981a).

12.3.2 OTHER PREMOTOR STRUCTURES

Among the other premotor structures projecting monosynaptically on to the abducens nucleus, only the role of the vestibular nuclei is at all known. The medial vestibular nucleus is the premotor relay for all horizontal reflex eye movements induced by head movement (vestibulo-ocular reflex), neck movement (cervico-ocular reflex) and visual full-field movement (visuo-ocular reflex). Each medial vestibular nucleus contains an excitatory neurone projecting on to the contralateral abducens nucleus (Fig. 12.5) and an inhibitory neurone projecting on to the ipsilateral abducens nucleus (Hikosaka *et al.*, 1977; McCrea *et al.*, 1980). Head velocity as well as *eye position* are encoded in the activity of these neurones, called 'vestibular plus position neurones'. They may be considered as the final common pathway of almost all, if not all (see below, foveal smooth pursuit), slow eye movements. In the medial vestibular nucleus there are other neurones, apparently more numerous than the previous ones, active during head movement ('vestibular only neurones') or during both head movement and saccades ('vestibular plus saccade neurones') (Fuchs and Kimm, 1975) but these neurones do not project directly on to the abducens nucleus (McCrea *et al.*, 1980). Lastly, it must be noticed that, at least in the cat, the axons of the excitatory vestibular neurones projecting on to the abducens nucleus pass through or very close to the ipsilateral abducens nucleus before reaching the contralateral abducens nucleus (McCrea *et al.*, 1981).

Each of the two nuclei prepositus hypoglossi, located caudally to the abducens nucleus and medially to the vestibular nuclei, also project monosynaptically on to both abducens nuclei, with a predominantly contralateral projection (McCrea and Baker, 1985). In the cat, the nucleus prepositus hypoglossi neurones are primarily (although not exclusively) involved in ipsilateral eye movements, their activity encoding mainly eye position or both eye position and velocity equally (Lopez-Barneo *et al.*, 1982). Their connections are particularly abundant and complex since they both receive afferents from and send efferents to the contralateral nucleus prepositus hypoglossi, the extraocular motor nuclei (abducens and oculomotor nuclei), the PPRF and the region of the reticular formations containing the inhibitory burst neurones, the vestibular nuclei, the superior colliculus and the flocculus (McCrea and Baker, 1985). Although surely fundamental to horizontal gaze control, the role of the nucleus prepositus hypoglossi is still hypothetical. The characteristics of its electrophysiological activity and of its connections suggest (1) that it could construct an efferent copy of oculomotor activity and distribute it to the other brainstem areas controlling gaze, and/or (2) that it could be a premotor relay participating in eye position integration and essential for mediation of certain slow eye movements such as foveal smooth pursuit. If the premotor relay of foveal smooth pursuit is not the nucleus prepositus hypoglossi, it could be formed by those neurones of the vestibular nuclei encoding eye position, or by a cellular group lying ventrally to the abducens nucleus and specifically involved in ipsilateral smooth pursuit (Eckmiller and Bauswein, 1986) but as yet barely known. The absence of smooth pursuit in certain clinical lesions located in the region of the PPRF could simply result from impairment of fibres passing in the vicinity of the PPRF, either near the abducens nucleus or in the dorsal part of the basis pontis (see below). Lastly, besides the region of the oculomotor nucleus (see above), some other areas of the brainstem – such as the superior colliculus, the interstitial nucleus of Cajal and the nucleus reticularis tegmenti pontis – project directly on to the abducens nucleus in the monkey (Langer *et al.*, 1986). These afferents are scarce compared to all those which have been previously discussed and their physiological roles are not yet clear.

12.4 Afferent pathways

12.4.1 SACCADES

(a) Experimental data. The role of the different afferents to the PPRF is still somewhat uncertain. In the cat, one afferent, originating from the medial vestibular nucleus (type II neurone) and projecting on to the contralateral omnipause neurones (located near the PPRF), could be inhibitory and involved in the triggering of quick phases of vestibular nystagmus (Ito, Markham and Curthoys, 1986). Other afferents in the monkey, probably acting complementarily in the triggering of voluntary and visually guided saccades (Schiller *et al.*, 1980), arise directly from the superior colliculus (Harting, 1977; Raybourn and Keller, 1977; Schnyder *et al.*, 1985) and the frontal eye fields (Brucher, 1964; Leichnetz, Smith and Spencer, 1984; Schnyder *et al.*, 1985), which both contain cells active just prior to these movements (Wurtz and Albano, 1980; Bruce and Goldberg, 1985). The superior colliculus receives cortical afferents from the frontal eye fields and the posterior parietal cortex (see, for review, Pierrot-Deseilligny *et al.*, 1987). In the upper brainstem, the frontal afferents could pass through the internal part of the pyramidal tract and decussate near the pontopeduncular junction (Brucher, 1964). The collicular afferents decussate in the dorsal tegmentum (decussation of Meynert) and pass through the predorsal bundle, located just ventrally to the MLF (Harting, 1977). Some parallel colliculo-reticular fibres relay in the central mesencephalic reticular formation before joining the direct colliculo-reticular tract (Cohen and Büttner-Ennever, 1984).

Other tracts originating from the frontal eye fields (Leichnetz, Smith and Spencer, 1984) and the superior colliculus (Harting, 1977) relay in the monkey in the nucleus reticularis tegmenti pontis, located medially in the ventral tegmentum of the midpons (Fig. 12.2). The nucleus reticularis tegmenti pontis essentially projects on to the cerebellar vermis in the monkey and cat (Brodal, 1980, 1982; Gerrits and Voogd, 1986). In the monkey, this pathway is involved in saccades (Crandall and Keller, 1985), probably especially in their calibration (Ritchie, 1976; Optican and Robinson, 1980; Leigh and Zee, 1983). The efferent side of this cerebellar pathway could reach the abducens nucleus by passing through the fastigial nuclei and then either through the nucleus prepositus hypoglossi (McCrea and Baker, 1985) or through the PPRF (Carpenter, 1959; Schnyder *et al.*, 1985), or through both.

(b) Lesions in man. Unilateral paramedian impairment of the midbrain tegmentum (Figs. 12.2 and 12.5, syndrome 6) causes monocular adduction paralysis in the ipsilateral eye and paresis of contralateral saccades in the opposite eye (Zackon and Sharpe, 1984). Oculomotor recordings in such a case, in which a vascular paramedian lesion probably damaged the right oculomotor nucleus (Pierrot-Deseilligny *et al.*, 1981b, Case 2), are shown in Fig. 12.6. Visually guided saccades to the right were almost normal, although slightly hypometric (Fig. 12.6Aa). Visually guided saccades to the left were absent beyond the midline in the right eye because of the complete adduction paralysis (Fig. 12.6Ab). They were defective in the left eye: their amplitude and peak velocity were clearly decreased, and their latencies were significantly increased (compared to those of saccades to the right, using the Student's paired *t*-test, with right latencies = 226 ± 40 ms and left latencies = 275 ± 36 ms). These different defects of contralateral saccades may be explained by damage to the suprareticular tracts involved in these movements before their decussation. Indeed, they course in the paramedian part of the midbrain tegmentum and in the internal portion of the pyramidal tract (see above). On the other hand, oculocephalic movement of the left eye was bilaterally normal in this case and that of the right eye was limited to its external hemifield of movement (Fig. 12.6B), as was expected.

12.4.2 FOVEAL SMOOTH PURSUIT

Foveal smooth pursuit movement was also impaired in the previous case. It was partly saccadic bilaterally, but especially to the right (Fig. 12.6C), namely ipsilaterally to the lesion, as in one of the two cases reported by Zackon and Sharpe (1984). The final tracts of foveal smooth pursuit are little known and its premotor relay (medial vestibular nucleus, or nucleus prepositus hypoglossi, . . .) has not yet been identified with certainty. Before the premotor relay, the cerebellum (particularly the flocculus) is surely involved in this movement and, although not indispensable for its existence, participates, in the monkey, to a great part of its gain (eye velocity on target velocity) (Zee *et al.*, 1981; Eckmiller and Westheimer, 1983). In the monkey, one of the few floccular efferents project on to the

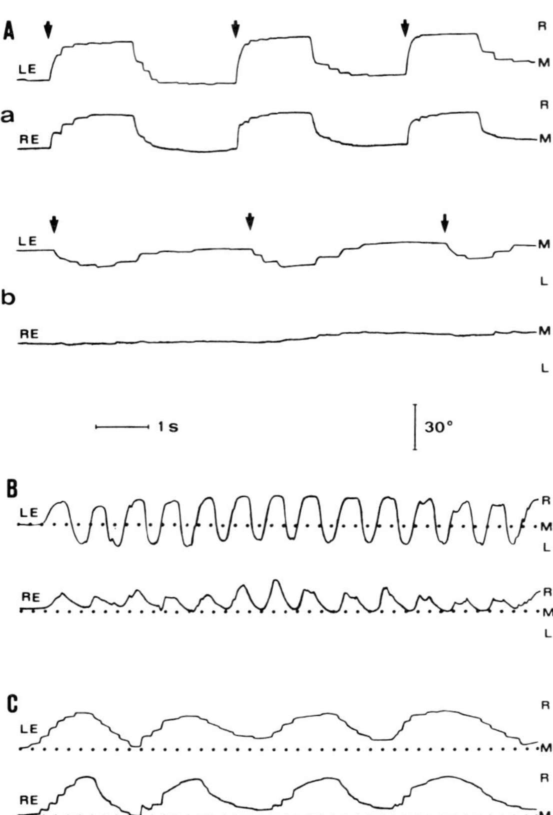

Fig. 12.6 Case with right paramedian lesion of the midbrain. A, Saccades; (a) rightwards; (b) leftwards. B, oculocephalic movement. C, foveal smooth pursuit (in the right hemifield of movement). Abbreviations: see Fig. 12.3.

ipsilateral medial vestibular nucleus (Langer *et al.*, 1985a) (Fig. 12.7). As the 'vestibular only' neurones are not obviously influenced by lesions of the flocculus (Waespe and Henn, 1985), it may be deduced that the floccular action could be exerted on the 'vestibular plus position' neurones (projecting on to both abducens nuclei, see above), which now appears to be confirmed in the monkey (Lisberger and Pavelko, 1984; Büttner, Boyle and Markert, 1986). Given that besides the medial vestibular nucleus there is apparently no other floccular projection on to structures involved in lateral eye movements, the medial vestibular nucleus could be a necessary relay in smooth pursuit movements and even perhaps their immediate premotor relay (if the nucleus prepositus

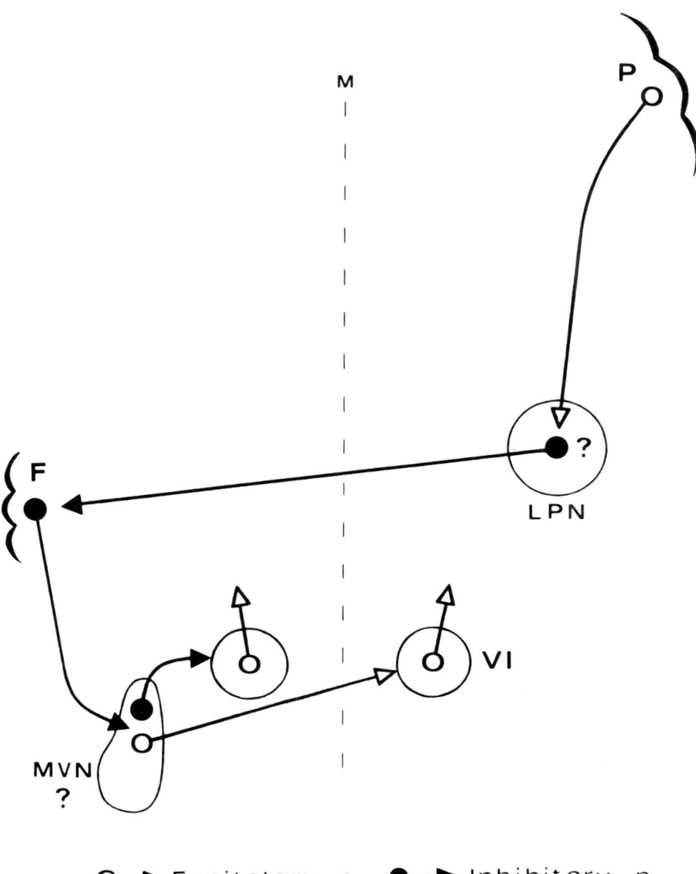

Fig. 12.7 Hypothetical circuitry of foveal smooth pursuit. F, flocculus; LPN, lateral pontine nuclei; M, midline; MVN, medial vestibular nucleus; P, posterior cerebral cortex; VI, abducens nucleus; ?, the inhibitory nature of the ponto-floccular neurone and a relay in the MVN are still uncertain.

hypoglossi is not an indispensable relay between the medial vestibular nucleus and the abducens nucleus).

The floccular afferents involved in smooth pursuit could originate in the monkey from the contralateral dorso-lateral pontine nuclei (Suzuki and Keller, 1984; Langer *et al.*, 1985b), which receive an ipsilateral projection from the posterior parietal cortex (Leichnetz, Smith and Spencer, 1984; Weber and Yin, 1984) (Fig. 12.7). This cortical region probably controls foveal smooth pursuit in both lateral directions both in the monkey (Lynch *et al.*, 1977; Lynch and McLaren, 1982; Kawano, Sasaki and Yamashita, 1984) and in man (Baloh, Yee and Honrubia, 1980; Pierrot-Deseilligny, Gray and Brunet, 1986), with a clear predominance (at least in man) for ipsilateral movement. The parieto-pontine projection being ipsilateral, it follows that unilateral midbrain lesions (Zackon and Sharpe, 1984; our case) induce a predominantly ipsilateral impairment of foveal smooth pursuit, as do unilateral cortical or capsular posterior lesions (Pierrot-Deseilligny, unpublished cases). If all the tonic neurones forming this parieto-ponto-cerebello-vestibulo-nuclear pathway were excitatory, unilateral cerebellar lesions would induce a contralateral foveal smooth pursuit disorder but, in the monkey (Westheimer and Blair, 1974; Eckmiller and Westheimer, 1983) as well as in man (Avanzini *et al.*, 1979), unilateral cerebellar lesions actually induce an ipsilateral foveal smooth pursuit disorder. Furthermore, the Purkinje cell activity in the flocculus increases with ipsilateral foveal smooth pursuit and decreases with contralateral pursuit movement (Miles and Fuller, 1975; Büttner and Waespe, 1984). Consequently, if the parieto-nuclear pathway as indicated by morphological studies does include a double decussation (pontofloccular and vestibulo-nuclear), it may be hypothesized that at least two of its neurones are inhibitory. As it has been already suggested on electrophysiological grounds that the flocculo-vestibular neurone is inhibitory (Ito, Highstein and Fukuda, 1970; Shimazu and Smith, 1971; Miles *et al.*, 1980) the other inhibitory neurone could be the pontofloccular neurone (or the cortico-pontine one). This arrangement (Fig. 12.7) continues to imply an ipsilateral foveal smooth pursuit disorder in cases of parietal lesion. Moreover, it would also imply an ipsilateral foveal smooth pursuit disorder in cases of floccular lesion. Indeed, with the impairment of such an inhibitory flocculo-vestibular neurone, the tonic activity of the excitatory neurones of the ipsilateral medial vestibular nucleus would increase as would that of the contralateral abducens nucleus, leading to a contralateral drift of gaze along with a foveal smooth pursuit deficit ipsilateral to the cerebellar lesion. However, such a theoretical organization, which consolidates the main experimental and clinical data known so far, has to be confirmed by further research.

12.5 Conclusions

Although the concept of a final common pathway of horizontal gaze beginning in the abducens nucleus is now adequately supported in binocular species, further study in the different species (including lateral-eyed ones) of the possible excitatory and inhibitory afferents to the medial rectus muscle motoneurones avoiding the abducens nucleus remains to be done. The physiological role and the anatomical connections of certain supranuclear structures – such as the nuclei prepositus hypoglossi, the tonic cells of the PPRF, the nucleus reticularis tegmenti pontis, the different pontine nuclei and the interstitial nucleus of the MLF – are not yet clearly established and need much more experimental and clinical research. Lastly, the mechanisms and location(s) of eye position integration as well as the terminal circuitry involved in foveal smooth pursuit are still very theoretical.

References

Avanzini, G., Girotti, F., Crenna, P. and Negri, S. (1979) Alterations of ocular motility in cerebellar pathology. *Arch. Neurol.*, **36**, 274–80.

Baker, R. and Highstein, S.M. (1975) Physiological identification of interneurons and motoneurons in the abducens nucleus. *Brain Res.*, **91**, 292–8.

Baker, R. and Highstein, S.M. (1978) Vestibular projections to medial rectus subdivision of oculomotor nucleus. *J. Neurophysiol.*, **41**, 1629–46.

Baloh, R.W., Furman, J. and Yee, R.D. (1985) Eye movements in patients with absent voluntary horizontal gaze. *Ann. Neurol.*, **17**, 283–6.

Baloh, R.W., Yee, R.D. and Honrubia, V. (1978) Internuclear ophthalmoplegia. I. Saccades and dissociated nystagmus. *Arch. Neurol.*, **35**, 484–9.

Baloh, R.W., Yee, R.D. and Honrubia, V. (1980) Optokinetic nystagmus and parietal lobe lesions. *Ann. Neurol.*, **7**, 269–76.

Baloh, R.W., Yee, R.D. and Honrubia, V. (1986) Late cortical cerebellar atrophy. Clinical and oculographic features. *Brain*, **109**, 159–80.

Bienfang, D.C. (1978) The course of direct projections from the abducens nucleus to the contralateral medial rectus subdivision of the oculomotor nucleus in the cat. *Brain Res.*, **145**, 277–89.

Bogousslavsky, J., Miklossy, J., Regli, F., Deruaz, J.P. and Despland, P.A. (1984) One-and-a-half syndrome in ischaemic locked-in state: a clinico-pathological study. *J. Neurol. Neurosurg. Psychiat.*, **47**, 927–35.

Brodal, P. (1980) The projection from the nucleus reticularis tegmenti pontis to the cerebellum in the rhesus monkey. *Exp. Brain Res.*, **38**, 29–36.

Brodal, P. (1982) Further observations on the cerebellar projections from the pontine nuclei and the nucleus reticularis tegmenti pontis in the rhesus monkey. *J. Comp. Neurol.*, **204**, 44–55.

Bruce, C.J. and Goldberg, M.E. (1985) Primate frontal eye fields. I. Single neurons discharging before saccades. *J. Neurophysiol.*, **53**, 603–35.

Brucher, J.M. (1964) *L'aire oculogyre frontale du singe. Ses fonctions et ses voies efférentes.* Arscia, Bruxelles.

Büttner, U., Boyle, R. and Markert, G. (1986) Cerebellar control of eye movements, in *Progress in Brain Research* (eds H.J. Freund, U. Büttner, B. Cohen and J. Noth), vol. 64. Elsevier, Amsterdam, pp. 225–33.

Büttner, U. and Waespe, W. (1984) Purkinje cell activity in the primate flocculus during optokinetic stimulation, smooth pursuit eye movements and VOR-suppression. *Exp. Brain Res.*, **55**, 97–104.

Büttner-Ennever, J.A. and Akert, K. (1981) Medial rectus subgroups of the oculomotor nucleus and their abducens internuclear input in the monkey. *J. Comp. Neurol.*, **197**, 17–27.

Büttner-Ennever, J.A. and Henn, V. (1976) An autoradiographic study of the pathways from the pontine reticular formation involved in horizontal eye movements. *Brain Res.*, **108**, 155–64.

Büttner-Ennever, J.A., Wadia, N.H., Sakai, H. and Schendemann, G. (1985) Neuroanatomy of oculomotor structures in olivopontocerebellar atrophy (OPCA) patients with slow saccades. *J. Neurol.*, **232** (suppl), 285.

Cannon, S.C. and Robinson, D.A. (1986) The final common integrator is in the prepositus and the vestibular nuclei, in *Adaptive Processes in Visual and Oculomotor Systems* (eds E.L. Keller and D.S. Zee). Pergamon Press, Oxford, pp. 307–12.

Carpenter, M.B. (1959) Lesions of the fastigial nuclei in the rhesus monkey. *Am. J. Anat.*, **104**, 1–34.

Carpenter, M.B. and Batton, R.R. (1980) Abducens internuclear neurons and their role in conjugate horizontal gaze. *J. Comp. Neurol.*, **189**, 191–209.

Carpenter, M.B. and McMasters, R.E. (1963) Disturbances of conjugate horizontal eye movements in the monkey. II. Physiological effects and anatomical degeneration resulting from lesions in the medial longitudinal fasciculus. *Arch. Neurol.*, **8**, 347–68.

Carpenter, M.B., McMasters, R.E. and Hanna, C.R. (1963) Disturbances of conjugate horizontal eye movements in the monkey. I. Physiological effects and anatomical degeneration resulting from lesions of the abducens nucleus and nerve. *Arch. Neurol.*, **8**, 231–47.

Cohen, B. and Büttner-Ennever, J.A. (1984) Projections from the superior colliculus to a region of the central mesencephalic reticular formation (cMRF) associated with horizontal saccadic eye movements. *Exp. Brain Res.*, **57**, 167–76.

Cohen, B., Komatsuzaki, A. and Bender, M.B. (1968) Electro-oculographic syndrome in monkeys after pontine reticular formation lesions. *Arch. Neurol.*, **18**, 78–92.

Crandall, W.F. and Keller, E.L. (1985) Visual and oculomotor signals in nucleus reticularis tegmenti pontis in alert monkey. *J. Neurophysiol.*, **54**, 1326–45.

Crane, T.B., Yee, R.D., Baloh, R.W. and Hepler, R.S. (1983) Analysis of characteristic eye movement abnormalities in internuclear ophthalmoplegia. *Arch. Ophthalmol.*, **101**, 206–11.

Curthoys, I.S., Markham, C.H. and Furuya, N. (1984) Direct projection of pause neurons to nystagmus-related excitatory burst neurons in the cat pontine reticular formation. *Exp. Neurol.*, **83**, 414–22.

Delgado-Garcia, J.M., Del Pozo, F. and Baker, R. (1986) Behavior of neurons in the abducens nucleus of the alert cat. II. Internuclear neurons. *Neuroscience*, **17**, 953–73.

Eckmiller, R. and Bauswein, E. (1986) Smooth pursuit eye movements, in *Progress in Brain Research* (eds H.J. Freund, U. Büttner, B. Cohen and J. Noth), vol. 64. Elsevier, Amsterdam, pp. 313–23.

Eckmiller, R. and Westheimer, G. (1983) Compensation of oculomotor deficits in monkeys with neonatal cerebellar ablations. *Exp. Brain Res.*, **49**, 315–26.

Evinger, C., Fuchs, A.F. and Baker, R. (1977) Bilateral lesions of the MLF in monkeys. Effect on the horizontal and vertical components of voluntary and vestibular induced eye movements. *Exp. Brain Res.*, **20**, 1–20.

Evinger, C., Kaneko, C.R.S. and Fuchs, A.F. (1982) Activity of omnipause neurons in alert cats during saccadic eye movements and visual stimuli. *J. Neurophysiol.*, **47**, 827–44.

Fisher, C.M. (1967) Some neuro-ophthalmological observations. *J. Neurol. Neurosurg. Psychiat.*, **30**, 383–92.

Foville, A. (1858) Note sur une paralysie peu connue de certains muscles de l'œil et sa liaison avec quelques points de l'anatomie et la physiologie de la protubérance annulaire. *Gaz. Heb. Méd. Chir.*, **3**, 146–51.

Fuchs, A.F. and Kimm, P. (1975) Unit activity in vestibular nucleus of the alert monkey during horizontal angular acceleration and eye movement. *J. Neurophysiol.*, **38**, 1140–61.

Fuchs, A.F., Kaneko, C.R.S. and Scudder, C.A. (1985) Brainstem control of saccadic eye movements. *Ann. Rev. Neurosci.*, **8**, 307–37.

Furuya, N. and Markham, C.H. (1982) Direct inhibitory synaptic linkage of pause neurons with burst inhibitory neurons. *Brain Res.*, **245**, 139–43.

Gacek, R.R. (1971) Anatomical demonstration of the vestibulo-ocular projections in the cat. *Acta Otolayrngol., Stockholm, Suppl.*, **293**, 1–63.

Gerrits, N.M. and Voogd, J. (1986) The nucleus reticularis tegmenti pontis and the adjacent rostral paramedian reticular formation: differential projections to the cerebellum and the caudal brain stem. *Exp. Brain Res.*, **62**, 29–45.

Grantyn, A., Grantyn, R., Gaunitz, U. and Robiné, K.P. (1980) Sources of direct excitatory and inhibitory inputs from the medial rhombencephalic tegmentum to lateral and medial rectus motoneurons in the cat. *Exp. Brain Res.*, **39**, 49–61.

Graybiel, A.M. (1977) Direct and indirect preoculomotor pathways in brainstem: an autoradiographic study of the pontine reticular formation in the cat. *J. Comp. Neurol.*, **175**, 37–78.

Graybiel, A.M. and Hartwieg, A. (1974) Some afferent connections of the oculomotor complex in the cat: an experimental study with tracer techniques. *Brain Res.*, **81**, 543–9.

Hanson, M.R., Hamid, M.A., Tomsak, R.L., Chou, S.S. and Leigh, R.J. (1986) Selective saccadic palsy caused by pontine lesions; clinical, physiological and pathological correlations. *Ann. Neurol.*, **20**, 209–17.

Harting, J.D. (1977) Descending pathways from the superior colliculus: an autoradiographic analysis in the Rhesus Monkey. *J. Comp. Neurol.*, **173**, 585–612.

Henn, V. and Cohen, B. (1976) Coding of information about rapid eye movements in the pontine reticular formation of alert monkey. *Brain Res.*, **108**, 307–25.

Henn, V., Lang, W., Hepp, K. and Reisine, H. (1984) Experimental gaze palsies in monkeys and their relation to human pathology. *Brain*, **107**, 619–36.

Hepp, K. and Henn, V. (1983) Spatio-temporal recoding of rapid eye movement signals in the monkey paramedian pontine reticular formation (PPRF). *Exp. Brain Res.*, **52**, 105–20.

Highstein, S.M., Maekawa, K., Steinacker, A. and Cohen, B. (1976) Synaptic input from the pontine reticular nuclei to abducens motoneurons and internuclear neurons in the cat. *Brain Res.*, **112**, 162–7.

Hikosaka, O. and Kawakami, T. (1977) Inhibitory reticular neurons related to the quick phase of vestibular nystagmus. Their location and projection. *Exp. Brain Res.*, **27**, 377–96.

Hikosaka, O., Igusa, Y. and Imai, H. (1980) Inhibitory connections of nystagmus-related reticular burst neurons in the abducens, prepositus hypoglossi and vestibular nuclei in the cat. *Exp. Brain Res.*, **39**, 301–11.

Hikosaka, O., Maeda, M., Nakao, S., Shimazu, H. and Shinoda, Y. (1977) Presynaptic impulses in the abducens nucleus and their relation to postsynaptic potentials in motoneurons during vestibular nystagmus. *Exp. Brain Res.*, **27**, 355–76.

Ito, M., Highstein, S.M. and Fukuda, J. (1970) Cerebellar inhibition of the vestibulo-ocular reflex in rabbit and cat and its blockage by picrotoxin. *Brain Res.*, **17**, 524–6.

Ito, J., Markham, C.H. and Curthoys, I.S. (1986) Direct projection of Type II vestibular neurons to eye movement-related pause neurons in the cat pontine reticular formation. *Exp. Neurol.*, **91**, 331–42.

Kaneko, C.R.S. and Fuchs, A.F. (1982) Connections of cat omnipause neurons. *Brain Res.*, **241**, 166–70.

Kawano, K., Sasaki, M. and Yamashita, M. (1984) Response properties of neurons in posterior parietal cortex of monkey during visual-vestibular stimulation. I. Visual tracking neurons. *J. Neurophysiol.*, **51**, 340–51.

Keller, E.L. (1974) Participation of medial reticular formation in eye movement generation in monkey. *J. Neurophysiol.*, **37**, 316–32.

King, W.M., Lisberger, S.G. and Fuchs, A.F. (1976) Responses of fibres in medial longitudinal fasciculus of alert monkeys during horizontal and vertical conjugate eye movements evoked by vestibular or visual stimuli. *J. Neurophysiol.*, **39**, 1135–49.

King, W.M., Precht, W. and Dieringer, N. (1980) Afferent and efferent connections of cat omnipause neurons. *Exp. Brain Res.*, **38**, 395–403.

Kommerell, G., Henn, V., Bach, M. and Lücking, C.H. (1987) Unilateral lesion of the paramedian pontine reticular formation. *Neuro-ophthalmology*, **7**, 93–8.

Lang, W., Büttner-Ennever, J.A. and Büttner, U. (1979) Vestibular projections to the monkey thalamus: an autoradiographic study. *Brain Res.*, **177**, 3–17.

Langer, T., Fuchs, A.F., Chubb, M.C., Scudder, C.A. and Lisberger, S.G. (1985a) Floccular efferents in the rhesus macaque as revealed by autoradiographic and horseradish peroxidase. *J. Comp. Neurol.*, **235**, 26–37.

Langer, T., Fuchs, A.F., Scudder, C.A. and Chubb, M.C. (1985b) Afferents to the flocculus of the cerebellum in rhesus macaque as revealed by retrograde transport of horseradish peroxidase. *J. Comp. Neurol.*, **235**, 1–25.

Langer, T.P. and Kaneko, C.R.S. (1983) Efferent projections of the cat oculomotor reticular omnipause neuron region: an autoradiographic study. *J. Comp. Neurol.*, **217**, 288–306.

Langer, T., Kaneko, C.R.S., Scudder, C.A. and Fuchs, A.F. (1986) Afferents to the abducens nucleus in the monkey and cat. *J. Comp. Neurol.*, **245**, 379–400.

Leichnetz, G.R., Smith, D.J. and Spencer, R.F. (1984) Cortical projections to the paramedian tegmental and basilar pons in the monkey. *J. Comp. Neurol.*, **228**, 388–408.

Leigh, R.J. and Zee, D.S. (1983) *The Neurology of Eye Movements*. Davis, Philadelphia.

Lestienne, F., Whittington, D.A. and Bizzi, E. (1981) Single cell recording from the pontine reticular formation in monkey: behavior of preoculomotor neurons during eye–head coordination, in *Progress in Oculomotor Research* (eds A.F. Fuchs and W. Becker). Elsevier, Amsterdam, pp. 325–33.

Lisberger, S.G. and Pavelko, T.A. (1984) Functional properties of brainstem cells inhibited from the cerebellar flocculus in monkey. *Soc. Neurosci., Abstr.*, **10**, 988.

Lopez-Barneo, J., Darlot, C., Berthoz, A. and Baker, R. (1982) Neuronal activity in prepositus nucleus correlated with eye movement in the alert cat. *J. Neurophysiol.*, **47**, 329–52.

Luschei, E.S. and Fuchs, A.F. (1972) Activity of brainstem neurons during eye movements of alert monkeys. *J. Neurophysiol.*, **35**, 455–61.

Lynch, J.C. and McLaren, J.W. (1982) The contribution of parieto-occipital association cortex to the control of slow eye movements, in *Functional Basis of Ocular Motility Disorders* (eds G. Lennestrand, D.S. Zee and E.L. Keller). Pergamon Press, Oxford, pp. 501–10.

Lynch, J.C., Mountcastle, V.B., Talbot, W.H. and Yin, T.C.T. (1977) Parietal lobe mechanisms for directed visual attention. *J. Neurophysiol.*, **40**, 362–88.

Maciewicz, R. and Phipps, B.S. (1983) The oculomotor internuclear pathways: a double retrograde labeling study. *Brain Res.*, **262**, 1–8.

McCrea, R.A. and Baker, R. (1985) Anatomical connections of the nucleus prepositus of the cat. *J. Comp. Neurol.*, **237**, 377–407.

McCrea, R.A., Strassman, A. and Highstein, S.M. (1986) Morphology and physiology of abducens motoneurons and internuclear neurons intracellularly injected with horseradish peroxidase in alert squirrel monkeys. *J. Comp. Neurol.*, **243**, 293–308.

McCrea, R.A., Yoshida, K., Berthoz, A. and Baker, R. (1980) Eye movement related activity and morphology of second order vestibular neurons terminating in the cat abducens nucleus. *Exp. Brain Res.*, **40**, 468–73.

McCrea, R.A., Yoshida, K., Evinger, C. and Berthoz, A. (1981) The location axonal arborization and termination sites of eye-movement-related secondary vestibular neurons demonstrated by intra-axonal H.R.P. injection in the cat, in *Progress in Oculomotor Research* (eds A.F. Fuchs and W. Becker). Elsevier, Amsterdam, pp. 379–86.

Miles, F.A. and Fuller, J.H. (1975) Visual tracking in the primate flocculus. *Science*, **189**, 1000–5.

Miles, F.A., Fuller, J.H., Braitman, D.J. and Dow, B.M. (1980) Long-term adaptive changes in primate vestibuloocular reflex. III. Electro-physiological observations in flocculus of normal monkey. *J. Neurophysiol.*, **43**, 1437–76.

Nakao, S. and Sasaki, S. (1980) Excitatory input from interneurons in the abducens nucleus to medial rectus motoneurons mediating conjugate horizontal nystagmus in the cat. *Exp. Brain Res.*, **39**, 23–32.

Nakao, S., Curthoys, I.S. and Markham, C.H. (1980) Direct inhibitory projection of pause neurons to nystagmus-related pontomedullary reticular burst neurons in the cat. *Exp. Brain Res.*, **40**, 283–93.

Optican, L.M. and Robinson, D.A. (1980) Cerebellar-dependent adaptive control of primate saccadic system. *J. Neurophysiol.*, **44**, 1058–76.

Pierrot-Deseilligny, C. (1985) Circuits oculomoteurs centraux. *Rev. Neurol.*, **141**, 349–70.

Pierrot-Deseilligny, C. and Chain, F. (1979) L'ophtalmoplégie internucléaire. *Rev. Neurol.*, **135**, 485–513.

Pierrot-Deseilligny, C. and Goasguen, J. (1984) Isolated abducens nucleus damage due to histocytosis X. Electro-oculographic analysis and physiological deductions. *Brain*, **107**, 1019–32.

Pierrot-Deseilligny, C., Chain, F. and Lhermitte, F. (1982) Syndrome de la formation réticulaire pontique. Précisions physiopathologiques sur les anomalies des mouvements oculaires volontaires. *Rev. Neurol.*, **138**, 517–32.

Pierrot-Deseilligny, C., Chain, F., Gray, F., Escourolle, R. and Castaigne, P. (1979) Paralysies supranucléaires de la latéralité d'origine protubérantielle. A propos de deux observations anatomo-cliniques avec enregistrements électro-oculographiques et électromyographiques. *Rev. Neurol.*, **135**, 741–62.

Pierrot-Deseilligny, C., Chain, F., Serdaru, M., Gray, F. and Lhermitte, F. (1981a) The 'one-and-a-half' syndrome. Electro-oculographic analyses of five cases with deductions about the physiologic mechanisms of lateral gaze. *Brain*, **104**, 665–99.

Pierrot-Deseilligny, C., Goasguen, J., Chain, F. and Lapresle, J. (1984) Pontine metastatis with dissociated bilateral horizontal gaze paralysis. *J. Neurol. Neurosurg. Psychiat.*, **47**, 159–64.

Pierrot-Deseilligny, C., Gray, F. and Brunet, P. (1986) Infarcts of both inferior parietal lobules with impairment of visually guided eye movements, peripheral visual inattention and optic ataxia. *Brain*, **109**, 81–97.

Pierrot-Deseilligny, C., Rivaud, S., Penet, C. and Rigolet, M.H. (1987) Latencies of visually guided saccades in unilateral hemispheric cerebral lesions. *Ann. Neurol.*, **21**, 138–48.

Pierrot-Deseilligny, C., Schaison, M., Bousser, M.G. and Brunet, P. (1981b) Syndrome nucléaire du nerf moteur oculaire commun. A propos de deux observations cliniques. *Rev. Neurol.*, **137**, 217–22.

Pola, J. and Robinson, D.A. (1978) Oculomotor signals in medial longitudinal fasciculus of the monkey. *J. Neurophysiol.*, **41**, 245–59.

Porter, J.D., Guthrie, B.L. and Sparks, D.L. (1985) Selective retrograde transneural transport of wheat germ agglutinin-conjugated horseradish peroxidase in the oculomotor system. *Exp. Brain Res.*, **57**, 411–16.

Raybourn, M.S. and Keller, E.L. (1977) Colliculoreticular organization in primate oculomotor system. *J. Neurophysiol.*, **40**, 861–78.

Reisine, H., Strassman, A. and Highstein, S.M. (1981) Eye position and head velocity signals are conveyed to medial rectus motoneurons in the alert cat by the ascending tract of Deiters'. *Brain Res.*, **211**, 153–7.

Ritchie, L. (1976) Effects of cerebellar lesions on saccadic eye movements. *J. Neurophysiol.*, **39**, 1246–56.

Robinson, D.A. (1964) The mechanics of human saccadic eye movement. *J. Physiol.*, **174**, 245–64.
Robinson, D.A. (1981) Control of eye movements, in *Handbook of Physiology* (ed. V.B. Brooks). American Physiological Society, Bethesda, pp. 1275–320.
Sasaki, S. and Shimazu, H. (1981) Reticulovestibular organization participating in generation of horizontal fast eye movement. *Ann. NY Acad. Sci.*, **374**, 130–43.
Schiller, P.H., True, S.D. and Conway, J.L. (1980) Deficits in eye movements following frontal eye-field and superior colliculus ablations. *J. Neurophysiol.*, **44**, 1175–89.
Schnyder, H., Reisine, H., Hepp, K. and Henn, V. (1985) Frontal eye field projection to the paramedian pontine reticular formation traced with wheat germ agglutinin in the monkey. *Brain Res.*, **329**, 151–60.
Shimazu, H. and Smith, C. (1971) Cerebellar and labyrinthine influences on single vestibular neurons identified by natural stimuli. *J. Neurophysiol.*, **34**, 493–508.
Sparks, D.L. and Travis, R.P. (1971) Firing patterns of reticular formation neurons during horizontal eye movements. *Brain Res.*, **33**, 477–81.
Steiger, H.J. and Büttner-Ennever, J.A. (1979) Oculomotor nucleus afferents in the monkey demonstrated with horseradish peroxidase. *Brain Res.*, **160**, 1–15.
Suzuki, D.A. and Keller, E.L. (1984) Visual signals in the dorsolateral pontine nucleus of the alert monkey: their relationship to smooth-pursuit eye movement. *Exp. Brain Res.*, **53**, 473–8.
Uchino, Y., Suzuki, S., Mitazawa, T. and Watanabe, S. (1979) Horizontal canal input to cat extraocular motoneurons. *Brain Res.*, **177**, 231–40.
Waespe, W. and Henn, V. (1985) Cooperative functions of vestibular nuclei neurons and floccular Purkinje cells in the control of nystagmus slow phase velocity: single cell recordings and lesion studies in the monkey, in *Adaptive Mechanisms in Gaze Control* (eds A. Berthoz and G. Melvill Jones). Elsevier, Amsterdam, pp. 233–50.
Weber, J.T. and Yin, T.C.T. (1984) Subcortical projections at the inferior parietal cortex (area 7) in the stump-tailed monkey. *J. Comp. Neurol.*, **224**, 206–30.
Westheimer, G. and Blair, S.M. (1974) Functional organization of primate oculomotor system revealed by cerebellectomy. *Exp. Brain Res.*, **21**, 463–72.
Wurtz, R.H. and Albano, J.E. (1980) Visual-motor function of the primate superior colliculus. *Ann. Rev. Neurosci.*, **3**, 189–226.
Yoshida, K., McCrea, R., Berthoz, A. and Vidal, P.P. (1982) Morphological and physiological characteristics of inhibitory burst neurons controlling horizontal rapid eye movements in the alert cat. *J. Neurophysiol.*, **48**, 761–84.
Zackon, D.H. and Sharpe, J.A. (1984) Midbrain paresis of horizontal gaze. *Ann. Neurol.*, **16**, 495–504.
Zee, D.S. (1986) Brain stem and cerebellar deficits in eye movement control. *Trans. Ophthalmol. Soc.*, **105**, 700–4.
Zee, D.S., Hain, T.C. and Carl, J.R. (1987) Abduction nystagmus in internuclear ophthalmoplegia. *Ann. Neurol.*, **21**, 383–8.
Zee, D.S., Yamazaki, A., Butler, P.H. and Gücer, G. (1981) Effects of ablation of flocculus and paraflocculus on eye movements in primate. *J. Neurophysiol.*, **46**, 878–99.

CHAPTER 13

Brainstem control of vertical gaze

R. JOHN LEIGH

13.1 Introduction: new developments in understanding disorders of vertical gaze

Though clinicians have reported on vertical gaze disorders for over a century, understanding of the pathological physiology of these disturbances has been slow to come. This has been partly because of difficulties in mapping the anatomical substrate for vertical gaze and partly because of lack of a reliable clinical method to measure vertical eye movements. Now that the magnetic search coil method is being more widely used in clinical centres, it has been possible to better define disorders of each of the functional classes of vertical eye movements: saccades, smooth pursuit, vestibular-optokinetic, vergence and gaze-holding mechanisms. Although electro-oculography can provide some indication of loss of motility, it cannot be relied upon for quantification of dynamic properties of vertical eye movements (Fig. 13.1). Magnetic resonance imaging (MRI) may help identify brainstem structures that cause specific deficits of vertical gaze and promises to be much superior to computed tomography scanning in localizing brainstem lesions.

In this chapter certain disorders of each functional class of eye movement will be reviewed, relating behavioural deficits to current notions of the anatomy and physiology of vertical gaze.

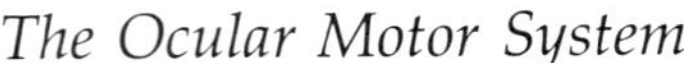

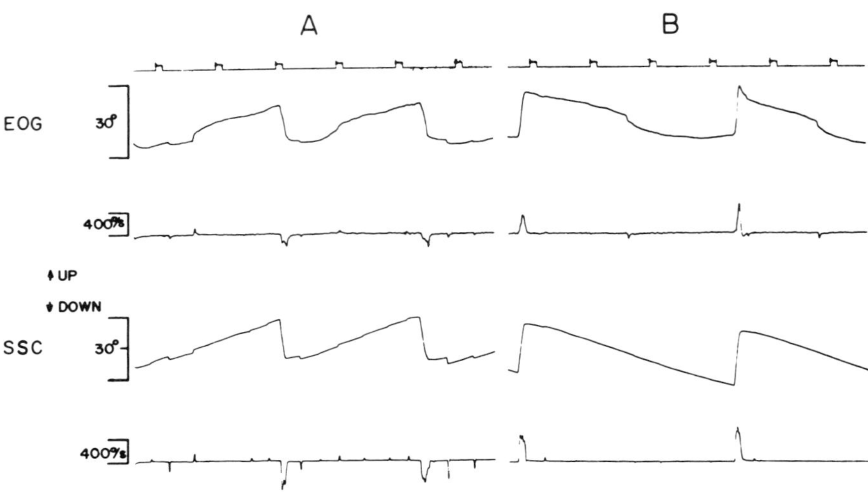

Fig. 13.1 Simultaneous electro-oculography (EOG) and magnetic search coil (SSC) records of vertical nystagmus induced by an 'optokinetic' stimulus. EOG presents a 'nystagmus record', but not the reliable measurements of eye movements that the SSC provides.

13.2 Saccades and quick phases of nystagmus

There is now general agreement that the rostral interstitial nucleus of the medial longitudinal fasciculus (riMLF) houses burst neurones that provide oculomotor neurones with the neural pulse for vertical saccades (Büttner-Ennever and Buettner, 1978). The organization and projections of the riMLF, however, are still debated. Büttner-Ennever *et al.* (1982), on the basis of clinical material and comparative anatomical studies in monkey, have proposed that the lateral portion of the nucleus encodes downward saccades and sends its axons through the medial portion of the riMLF which encodes upward saccades. Thus, bilateral lateral riMLF lesions cause a downward saccadic palsy; bilateral medial riMLF lesions cause a palsy of upward and downward saccades. On the basis of clinicopathological correlation, Pierrot-Deseilligny *et al.* (1982) proposed the converse up–down localization within the riMLF.

Anatomical tracer studies demonstrate that the riMLF projects predominantly *ipsilaterally* to the oculomotor nucleus (Steiger and Büttner-Ennever, 1979), but there is a commissure between the riMLF that runs, in part, through the posterior commissure. In a recent case report, Ranalli, Sharpe and Fletcher (1986) measured the deficits in a patient with an autopsy-proven *unilateral* riMLF lesion, which also involved the rostral tip of the interstitial nucleus of Cajal and the ventral portion of the nucleus of the posterior commissure. Unlike previous case reports of vertical gaze palsy with unilateral lesions, the posterior commissure itself was spared. This patient had a total saccadic palsy above the midline and slowed upward and downward saccades in a 15° range below the midline, which gives support to the view that the commissure of the riMLF is important for upward saccades.

In a study of vertical gaze palsies, Baloh, Furman and Yee (1985) found an interesting discrepancy in the saccadic deficits produced by extrinsic lesions (pressing on the posterior commissure) and intrinsic midbrain lesions. Extrinsic lesions tended to cause restricted range of upward saccades, with hypometria, but normal velocity (a finding that deserves systematic study with the magnetic search coil method). Intrinsic lesions produce slowing of vertical saccades with possible hypometria. Thus, lesions that affect the riMLF produce saccadic slowing, but it seems that slow vertical saccades need not always imply disease of the riMLF *per se*; disruption of inputs to the riMLF may also lead to slow saccades. Evidence for this postulate comes from quantitative morphometric studies of the riMLF in brains of patients with Huntington's disease who demonstrated slow saccades before death; only one out of four such brains showed a significant loss of neurones that might be burst cells (Leigh *et al.*, 1985). Similarly, both experimental and clinical lesions of the paramedian pontine reticular formation (PPRF), besides producing slow or absent horizontal saccades, also caused slow vertical saccades (Henn *et al.*, 1984; Hanson *et al.*, 1986). Thus, lesions of the rostral pons may produce slow vertical saccades.

13.3 Smooth pursuit

Although much has been learnt about the anatomical substrate for smooth pursuit over the past five years, the pathway for vertical smooth pursuit is still uncertain. It seems likely that secondary areas of visual cortex project, via dorsolateral pontine nuclei, to the cerebellum, including the flocculus (Glickstein *et al.*, 1980; Suzuki, May and Keller, 1986) which, in turn, projects to the y-group of the vestibular complex. Here, Chubb and Fuchs (1981) have identified units that discharge during upward smooth pursuit or combined eye–head tracking (cancellation of the vestibulo-ocular reflex). Since the y-group projects directly to oculomotor neurones, this may well be one portion of the vertical pursuit pathway. Downward pursuit may be mediated via other portions of the vestibular nucleus and the medial longitudinal fasciculus (MLF).

Smooth pursuit is often impaired with brainstem lesions; it is the most fragile class of eye movements in humans, and bilateral lesions of the MLF impair vertical smooth pursuit more than saccades, as expected (Leigh, Newman and King, 1982). In contrast, lesions of the riMLF may relatively spare smooth pursuit when compared with saccadic deficits. In diffuse degenerative conditions that cause slow vertical saccades, such as progressive supranuclear palsy, vertical smooth pursuit is often also involved, but to a lesser extent. Deficits of vertical smooth pursuit and combined eye–head tracking are usually commensurate (Fig. 13.2).

Systematic studies of vertical smooth pursuit in normal subjects are presently under way and preliminary results show up–down asymmetries that will have to be taken into account before abnormal pursuit can be clearly defined (Bowman and Hotson, 1986; Pavelko, Lisberger and Vu, 1986).

13.4 Vestibulo-optokinetic responses

A great deal of progress has been made in understanding the vertical vestibulo-ocular and optokinetic responses in recent years. When vestibular nystagmus is induced by sudden acceleration to a sustained angular velocity, in darkness, nystagmus persists longer than can be accounted for by the mechanical properties of the labyrinthine semicircular canals. This perseveration of the raw vestibular signal – called 'velocity storage' by Raphan, Matsuo and Cohen (1979) – is left–right symmetrical in the horizontal plane. In the vertical plane up–down symmetry depends upon otolithic influences. Thus, with the head tilted to one side and rotation about an earth–vertical axis, upward velocity storage exceeds downward velocity storage (Baloh *et al.*, 1983; Matsuo and Cohen, 1984).

With vertical gaze disorders, the vertical vestibulo-ocular reflex (VOR) can often induce a larger range of eye movements than can saccades or smooth pursuit. To some extent this can be attributed to direct projections from the vestibular nuclei to the oculomotor nucleus. Whether clinical disorders produce asymmetrical, vertical velocity storage remains to be seen. One simple clinical test is to ask the patient vigorously to shake his or her head in pitch for 10 to 20 s and then look for post-head-shaking nystagmus which, if present, would indicate asymmetric vertical velocity storage. Quantitative measurement of nystagmus should enable determination of the time constants of upward and downward VOR that can be compared with those of normal subjects (Baloh *et al.*, 1983). Thus, even though the 'elementary vestibulo-ocular reflex' may be preserved, the dynamics of this reflex may be altered so pointing to disturbances in vertical velocity storage. Experimental evidence strongly suggests that

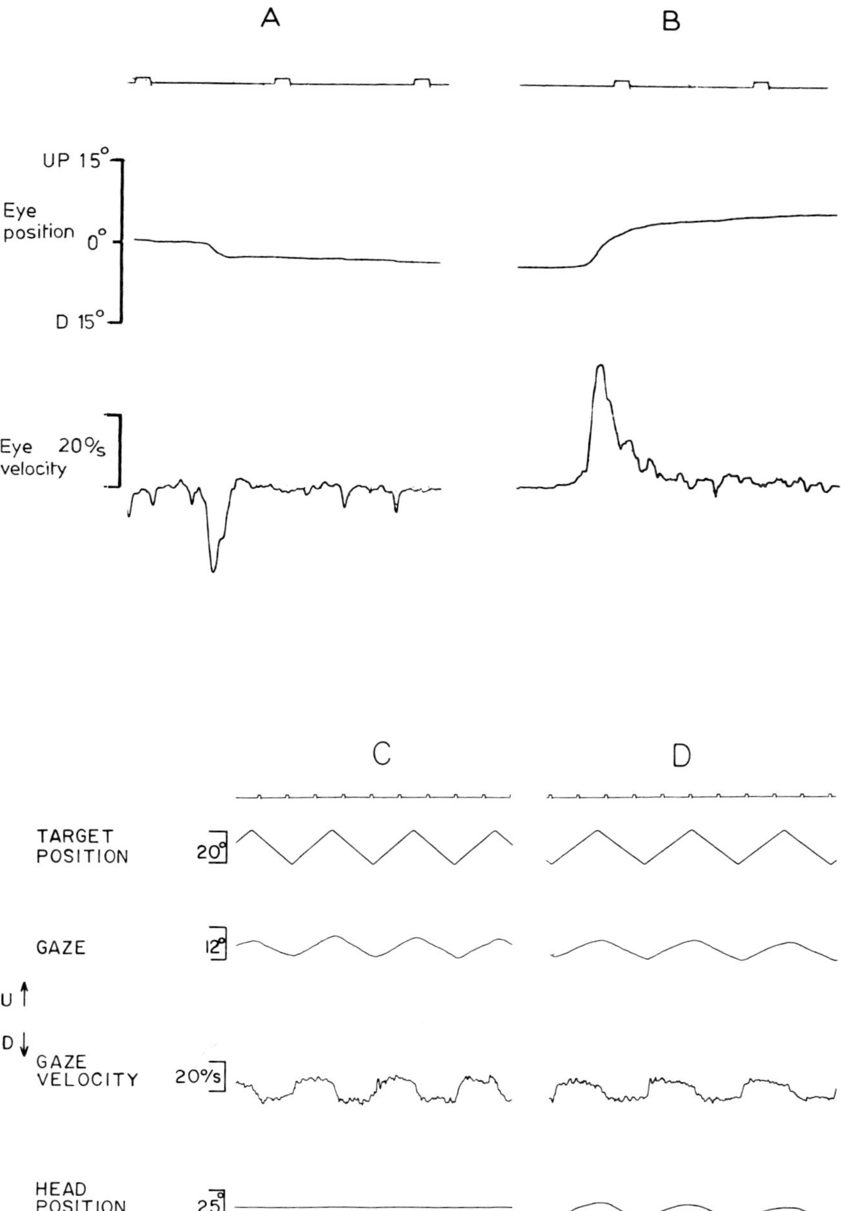

Fig. 13.2 Records from a patient with progressive supranuclear palsy. Saccades were slow both downward (A) and upward (B). Smooth vertical pursuit (C) and combined eye–head tracking (D) were impaired commensurately.

the interstitial nucleus of Cajal is important for vertical velocity storage (Anderson, Precht and Pappas, 1979; King and Leigh, 1982).

Spontaneous nystagmus that is upbeating or downbeating in the primary position has been attributed to an imbalance of vertical smooth pursuit (Zee, Friendlich and Robinson, 1974), an imbalance of central connections of the vertical semicircular canals (Baloh and Spooner, 1981) and, most recently, a disturbance of otolithic connections (Fisher *et al.*, 1983). Evidence accrued for this last view includes the observations that convergence and static head tilt influenced such nystagmus. When direct tests of otolithic function (such as rotation of the head around an axis tilted from the vertical, e.g. barbecue spit rotation) become more generally used, these hypotheses should be amenable to more direct testing.

13.5 Gaze-holding mechanisms (neural integrator)

In order to hold the eyes in an eccentric position in the orbit requires a sustained contraction of the extraocular muscles; otherwise the elastic restoring forces of the orbit will pull back the eye to primary position. To bring about such a sustained muscle contraction requires a step change in activity of the ocular motor neurones. The ocular motor step is a 'position' command but the saccadic, pursuit, vestibular and optokinetic signals are all encoded in terms of eye velocity. Consequently, a mathematical integration of neurally encoded signals is required (Skavenski and Robinson, 1973). The location of the neural circuits responsible for this integration of ocular motor signals has remained unclear until recently. Carpenter (1972) and Robinson (1974) showed that cerebellar connections are important, but cerebellectomy did not abolish the whole integrator. Though it was suspected that the paramedian pontine reticular formation (PPRF) was important for neural integration, Henn *et al.* (1984) demonstrated that chemical lesions of the PPRF did not affect the neural integrator. More recently, Cannon and Robinson (1985) have shown that chemical lesions of the nucleus prepositus hypoglossi and adjacent vestibular nucleus effectively abolish the horizontal neural integrator: after a saccade takes the eye to an eccentric orbital position, the eye drifts back with a time constant of 200 ms – which is that due to orbital elastic restoring forces. Cannon and Robinson also noted that bilateral chemical lesions impaired vertical gaze-holding, but less than for horizontal (mean time constant of drift was 2.5 s). From these results, therefore, it appears that the nucleus prepositus hypoglossi and the adjacent vestibular nuclei make an appreciable contribution to the vertical neural integrator. The nucleus prepositus hypoglossi projects to the oculomotor nucleus (Steiger and Büttner-Ennever, 1979), but more than one pathway is probably important in conveying vertical eye position information to the midbrain. One is the MLF; another pathway is the brachium conjunctivum (King and Leigh, 1982). Bilateral internuclear ophthalmoplegia causes vertical gaze-evoked nystagmus (Fig. 13.3). (It is important to differentiate the 'common neural integrator' from a separate, partial integration of vestibular signals only – so-called 'velocity storage' – which is discussed above.)

What rostral, brainstem structures contribute to the integration of vertical ocular motor signals? Lesions of the posterior commissure impair all classes of upward eye movements, and if partial, may lead to gaze-evoked nystagmus on attempted upward gaze (Baloh, Furman and Yee, 1985). Which connections in the posterior commissure contribute to this remains unknown. Patients with bilateral lesions affecting the riMLF usually have a predominantly downward saccadic palsy; inability to sustain a downward deviation of the eyes has not been reliably measured. Whether the interstitial nucleus of Cajal contributes to vertical neural integration remains unsettled, though it appears to contribute to vertical velocity storage.

It seems likely, therefore, that a number of pathways contribute to the vertical neural integrator. It also seems possible that the neural integrator for upward movements is different from that for downward movements, both anatomically and, perhaps, pharmacologically. One piece of evidence for the latter speculation comes from the clinical condition,

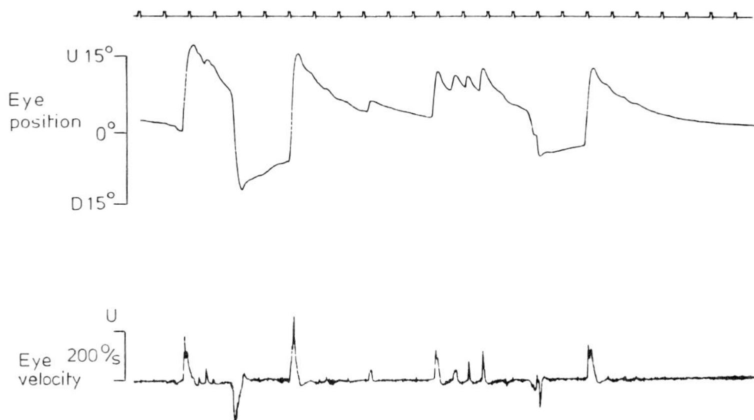

Fig. 13.3 Vertical gaze-evoked nystagmus in a patient with bilateral internuclear ophthalmoplegia. The time constant of centripetal drift of the eyes is greater than 200 ms, indicating that some vertical integrator function still persists.

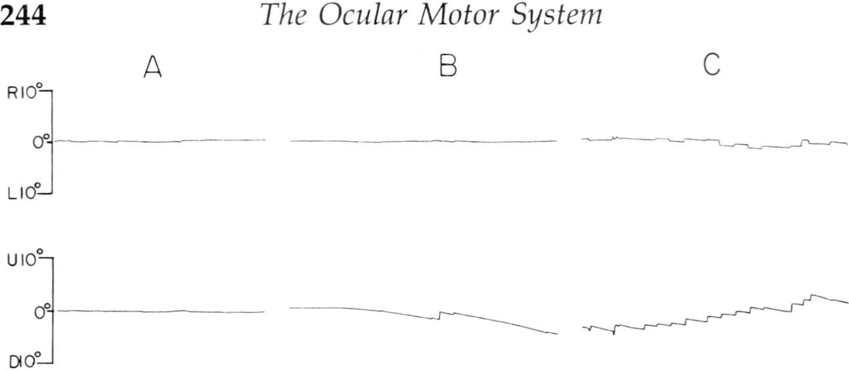

Fig. 13.4 (A) Eye movements of a normal subject before smoking a cigarette. The arrow indicates when a solitary light-emitting diode (LED) was turned off and the subject was then in total darkness. (B) Immediately after four inhalations of a cigarette, fixation of the LED was steady, but when it was turned off (arrow) upbeating nystagmus commenced. (C) Upbeating nystagmus, in darkness, 30 s after smoking a cigarette. Upper trace: horizontal position; lower trace: vertical position.

oculogyric crisis. During an attack, the eyes cannot be brought below the horizontal meridian except during a blink (Foley, Civil and Leigh, 1985). Within the upper field of gaze, however, all eye movements seem to be relatively normal. Hence, the condition seems to be an 'offset' in the vertical integrator. Attacks can usually be terminated by administration of an anticholinergic agent, suggesting that pathways subserving upward and downward gaze utilize different neurotransmitters. Supportive evidence for this notion is the recent study by Sibony, Evinger and Manning (1987), which demonstrated that normal subjects develop upbeat nystagmus, in darkness, after smoking a cigarette (Fig. 13.4). Tobacco-induced nystagmus may well be vestibular in origin and suggests upward–downward pharmacological differences here also.

13.6 Disorders of vertical ocular alignment

Vertical misalignment of the visual axes due to disturbance of pre-nuclear inputs – skew deviation – is a fairly common finding in patients with brainstem lesions. Skew deviation has been attributed to disturbance of otolithic inputs, anywhere from the labyrinth to the midbrain (Keane, 1975). Although skew deviation is generally thought of as a concomitant deviation – a misalignment that is constant for all angles of gaze – in about 10% of patients, this is not the case. Keane (1985) reported on 47 patients with skew deviation in whom the hypertropia alternated on gaze to either side. He was careful to exclude patients who might have a trochlear nerve palsy or childhood squint. Adduction hypotropia was almost as common as adduction hypertropia. Most of Keane's subjects had pretectal lesions, suggesting that the interstitial nucleus of Cajal and the posterior commissure were involved. In another study, Moster *et al.* (1984) reported that alternating skew deviation was often associated with downbeat nystagmus, indicative of a lesion at the cervicomedullary junction.

Slowly alternating skew deviation (during attempted fixation with the eyes near primary position) is a rare disorder in which one eye falls and the other rises; the period of this oscillation is about 2 to 3 min (Corbett *et al.*, 1981). Such patients may have other evidence of pretectal disease and torsional nystagmus. Other reports have described periodic (but not alternating) skew deviation associated with torsional nystagmus and a head tilt (ear to shoulder) on the side opposite to the higher eye (Rabinovitch, Sharpe and Sylvester, 1977; Hedges and Hoyt, 1982; Greenberg and DeWitt, 1983). A similar 'ocular tilt' reaction was produced experimentally in monkeys by Westheimer and Blair (1975) when they stimulated in the region of the interstitial nucleus of Cajal. Thus, these phenomena probably represent imbalance of central otolithic connections. The periodicity of the attacks may be related to vestibular adaptation mechanisms which are thought to be also responsible for periodic alternating nystagmus (Leigh, Robinson and Zee, 1981). Otolithic and semicircular canal afferents converge in the vestibular 'velocity storage element', which depends upon the cerebellar nodulus (Waespe, Cohen and Raphan, 1985). It seems possible, therefore, that when reliable measurements of periodic skew deviation become available (using the torsion search coil) that mathematical descriptions of these phenomena will be possible. It is interesting to note that baclofen (which abolishes acquired period alternating nystagmus) suppressed the attacks of periodic skew deviation when it was tried in one patient (Hedges and Hoyt, 1982).

Another unusual disorder, 'monocular elevation paresis', has been reinterpreted, recently, on the basis of CT findings (Ford *et al.*, 1984). The patient had impaired elevation of the right eye, equal in adduction and abduction. This upward limitation applied for all classes of eye movements. Since the principal elevator of the eye, the superior rectus, receives its innervation from the contralateral oculomotor nucleus, a lesion contralateral to the side of the elevation paresis had been assumed (Jampel and Fells, 1968; Lessel, 1975). The patient described by Ford and colleagues, however, had a CT abnormality in the midbrain on the same side as the elevator weakness. These authors interpret their findings by postulating involvement of the riMLF on the right, which they hypothesize projected to the left oculomotor nucleus via the posterior commissure, but Steiger and Büttner-Ennever (1979) have demonstrated that the riMLF projections to the oculomotor nucleus are mainly ipsilateral. Moreover, involvement of the vertical vestibulo-ocular reflex in this patient indicates a lesion beyond the confines of the riMLF. Thus, further data – accurate measurements of eye movements and reliable anatomical information – are necessary to settle the mechanisms of this rare condition.

13.7 Opportunities for future studies

The trend towards reliable measurement of vertical eye movements will, no doubt, increase the contribution that clinical studies can make towards the understanding of vertical gaze. The availability of a scleral search coil that can sense torsional eye rotations opens up an area that is a natural extension of vertical disorders, for example, conditions such as see-saw nystagmus. Nevertheless, the success of these techniques will always depend on an approach in which specific questions are being asked and hypotheses tested. In this regard, clinicians will need to pay close attention to discoveries made by their neuroscience colleagues.

Acknowledgements

I am grateful to Holly Stevens for editorial assistance. Supported by the Veterans Administration, the Evenor Armington Fund and NASA contract 9-17439.

References

Anderson, J.H., Precht, W. and Pappas, C. (1979) Changes in the vertical vestibulo-ocular reflex due to Kainic acid lesions of the interstitial nucleus of Cajal. *Neurosci. Lett.*, **14**, 259–64.

Baloh, R.W., Furman, J.M. and Yee, R.D. (1985) Dorsal midbrain syndrome: clinical and oculographic findings. *Neurology*, **35**, 54–60.

Baloh, R.W., Richman, L., Yee, R.D. and Honrubia, V. (1983) The dynamics of vertical eye movements in normal human subjects. *Aviat. Space Environ. Med.*, **54**, 32–8.

Baloh, R.W. and Spooner, J.W. (1981) Downbeat nystagmus: a type of central vestibular nystagmus. *Neurology*, **31**, 304–10.

Bowman, D.K. and Hotson, J.R. (1986) Vertical smooth pursuit does not catch-up to horizontal. *Suppl. Invest. Ophthalmol. Vis. Sci.*, **27**, 156.

Büttner-Ennever, J.A. and Büttner, U. (1978) A cell group associated with vertical eye movements in the rostral mesencephalic reticular formation of the monkey. *Brain Res.*, **151**, 31–47.

Büttner-Ennever, J.A., Buettner, U. Cohen, B. and Baumgartner, G. (1982) Vertical gaze paralysis and the rostral interstitial nucleus of the medial longitudinal fasciculus. *Brain*, **105**, 125–49.

Cannon, S.C. and Robinson, D.A. (1985) Neural integrator failure from brain stem lesions in monkey. *Suppl. Invest. Ophthalmol. Vis. Sci.*, **26**, 3–47.

Carpenter, R.H.S. (1972) Cerebellectomy and the transfer function of the vestibulo-ocular reflex in the decerebrate cat. *Proc. R. Soc. Lond. B.*, **181**, 353–74.

Chubb, M.C. and Fuchs, A.F. (1981) The role of dentate nucleus and y-group in the generation of vertical smooth eye movements. *Ann. NY Acad Sci.*, **374**, 446–51.

Corbett, J.J., Schatz, N.J., Shults, W.T., Behrens, M. and Berry, R.G. (1981) Slowly alternating skew deviation: description of a pretectal syndrome in three patients. *Ann. Neurol.*, **10**, 540–6.

Fisher, A., Gresty, M., Chambers, B. and Rudge, P. (1983) Primary position upbeating nystagmus. A variety of central positional nystagmus. *Brain*, **106**, 949–64.

Foley, J.M., Civil, R.H. and Leigh, R.J. (1985) Oculogyric crises. *Ann. Neurol.*, **18**, 138.

Ford, S.C., Schwartze, G.M., Weaver, R.G. and Troost, B.T. (1984) Monocular elevation paresis caused by an ipsilateral lesion. *Neurology*, **34**, 1264–7.

Glickstein, M., Cohen, J.L., Dixon, B., Gibson, A., Hollins, M., Labossiere, E. and Robinson, F. (1980) Corticopontine visual projections in macaque monkeys. *J. Comp. Neurol.*, **190**, 209–29.

Greenberg, H.S. and DeWitt, L.D. (1985) Periodic non-alternating ocular skew deviation accompanied by head tilt and pathologic lid retraction. *J. Clin. Neuro-ophthalmol.*, **3**, 181–4.

Hanson, M.R., Hamid, M.A., Tomsak, R.L., Chou, S.M. and Leigh, R.J. (1986) Selective saccadic palsy due to pontine lesions: clinical, physiological and pathological correlations. *Ann. Neurol.*, **20**, 209–17.

Hedges, T.R. and Hoyt, W.F. (1982) Ocular tilt reaction due to an upper brainstem lesion: paroxysmal skew deviation, torsion and oscillation of the eyes with head tilt. *Ann. Neurol.*, **11**, 537–40.

Henn, V., Lang, W., Hepp, K. and Reisine, H. (1984) Experimental gaze palsies in monkeys and their relation to human pathology. *Brain*, **107**, 619–36.

Jampel, R.S. and Fells, P. (1968) Monocular elevation paresis caused by a central nervous system lesion. *Arch. Ophthalmol.*, **80**, 45–57.

Keane, J.R. (1975) Ocular skew deviation: analysis of 100 cases. *Arch. Neurol.*, **32**, 185–90.

Keane, J.R. (1985) Alternating skew deviation: 47 patients. *Neurology*, **35**, 725–8.

King, W.M. and Leigh, R.J. (1982) Physiology of vertical gaze, in *Functional Basis of Ocular Motility Disorders* (eds G. Lennerstrand, D.S. Zee and E.L. Keller). Pergamon, Oxford, pp. 267–76.

Leigh, R.J., Newman, S.A. and King, W.M. (1982) Vertical gaze disorders, in *Functional Basis of Ocular Motility Disorders* (eds G. Lennerstrand, D.S. Zee and E.L. Keller). Pergamon, Oxford, pp. 257–66.

Leigh, R.J., Parhad, I.M., Clark, A.W., Buettner-Ennever, J.A. and Folstein, S.E. (1985) Brainstem findings in Huntington's disease. Possible mechanisms for slow vertical saccades. *J. Neurological. Sci.*, **71**, 247–56.
Leigh, R.J., Robinson, D.A. and Zee, D.S. (1981) A hypothetical explanation for periodic alternating nystagmus. *Ann. NY Acad. Sci.*, **374**, 619–35.
Lessel, S. (1975) Supranuclear paralysis of monocular elevation. *Neurology*, **25**, 1134–6.
Matsuo, V. and Cohen, B. (1984) Vertical optokinetic nystagmus and effects of gravity. *Exp. Brain Res.*, **53**, 197–216.
Moster, M.L., Schatz, N.J., Bosley, T.M., Savino, P.J., Sergott, R.C. and Harbour, R.C. (1984) Alternating ipsilateral hypotropia on lateral gaze in patients with lower brain stem disorders. *Ann. Neurol.*, **16**, 115.
Pavelko, T.A., Lisberger, S.L. and Vu, T. (1986) Weighting of the visual field for the initiation of horizontal and vertical smooth pursuit eye movements in rhesus monkey. *Suppl. Invest. Ophthalmol. Vis. Sci.*, **27**, 155.
Pierrot-Deseilligny, C., Chain, F., Gray, F., Serdaru, M., Escourolle, R., Lhermitte, F. (1982) Parinaud's syndrome. Electro-oculographic and anatomical analyses of six vascular cases with deductions about vertical gaze organization in the premotor structures. *Brain*, **105**, 667–96.
Rabinovitch, H.E., Sharpe, J.A. and Sylvester, T.O. (1977) The ocular tilt reaction. A paroxysmal dyskinesia associated with elliptical nystagmus. *Arch. Neurol.*, **95**, 1395–8.
Ranalli, P.J., Sharpe, J.A. and Fletcher, W.A. (1986) Vertical saccadic, pursuit and vestibular paresis with a unilateral midbrain lesion: pathophysiological correlations. *Neurology, Suppl.*, **36**, 192.
Raphan, T., Matsuo, V. and Cohen, B. (1979) Velocity storage in the vestibulo-ocular reflex arc (VOR). *Exp. Brain Res.*, **35**, 229–48.
Robinson, D.A. (1974) The effect of cerebellectomy on the cat's vestibuloocular integrator. *Brain Res.*, **71**, 195–207.
Sibony, P.A., Evinger, C. and Manning, K.A. (1987) Tobacco induced primary position upbeat nystagmus. *Ann. Neurol.*, **21**, 53–8.
Skavenski, A.A. and Robinson, D.A. (1973) Role of abducens neurons in vestibulo-ocular reflex. *J. Neurophysiol.*, **36**, 724–38.
Steiger, H.J. and Büttner-Ennever, J.A. (1979) Oculomotor nucleus afferents in the monkey demonstrated with horseradish peroxidase. *Brain Res.*, **160**, 1–15.
Suzuki, D.A., May, J. and Keller, E.L. (1986) Smooth pursuit eye movement deficit with pharmacological lesions in monkey dorsolateral pontine nucleus. *Soc. Neurosci., Abstr.*, **10** (part 1), 58.
Waespe, W., Cohen, B. and Raphan, T. (1985) Dynamic modification of the vestibulo-ocular reflex by the nodulus and uvula. *Science*, **228**, 194–202.
Westheimer, G. and Blair, S.M. (1975) Synkinesis of head and eye movements evoked by brain stem stimulation in the alert monkey. *Exp. Brain Res.*, **24**, 89–95.
Zee, D.S., Friendlich, A.R. and Robinson, D.A. (1974) The mechanism of downbeat nystagmus. *Arch. Neurol.*, **30**, 227–37.

CHAPTER 14

Cortical control of eye movements

RONALD J. TUSA

Our knowledge of the cortical control of eye movements has greatly increased in the past few years based on studies in both patients and non-human primates. The classic concept that the frontal eye fields are responsible for generating contralateral saccades and the parietal cortex is responsible for generating ipsilateral smooth pursuit needs to be modified. Instead, it appears that saccades and smooth pursuit are each mediated by areas in both frontal and parietal cortex. The cortical control of eye movements should be viewed as consisting of at least three separate systems: (1) an *afferent system*, which processes target location and motion; (2) *efferent saccade and smooth pursuit systems*, which transmit the commands for initiating eye movements to the brainstem; and (3) an *attention/spatial map system*, which interfaces between the afferent and efferent systems. This chapter will summarize our current understanding of the anatomy, physiology, and effects of lesions in each of these systems. In addition, we will speculate upon the pathophysiology underlying blindsight, saccade palsies, gaze deviations, ocular motor apraxia, and spasm of fixation in patients with cortical lesions.

14.1 Classification of eye movements

It is important to develop a classification of eye movements since cortical lesions affect eye movements differently depending upon the behavioural condition in which they are generated. A simple classification of saccades affected by cortical lesions is illustrated in Table 14.1. We will refer to these types of saccades throughout the paper.

Table 14.1 Classification of saccades

I. *INTENTIONAL SACCADES*	Volitional saccades made to a predetermined visual target (visually guided saccades) or generated when the goal for the saccade is known but there is no visible target (non-visually guided saccades).
A. *Visually guided saccades*	
B. *Non-visually guided saccades*	
1. *Predictive saccades*	Saccades generated before the target is stepped to a predictable location.
2. *Target-searching*	Saccades generated when the goal is to fixate the target, but the target is not visible and its specific location is unknown. (Saccades generated to a target stepped into a homonymous hemianopsia.)
3. *Remembered target*	Saccades generated to a location in the visual hemifield in which a target has been previously presented.
4. *Anti-saccades*	In this task the subject is to generate a saccade not to the location of a suddenly appearing visual target, but to its mirror location in the opposite direction.
II. *REFLEXIVE SACCADES*	Saccades that draw the eyes to novel stimuli that suddenly occur within the environment.
III. *SPONTANEOUS SACCADES*	Seemingly random saccades generated when the subject is in the dark or facing a featureless Ganzfeld and is not required to perform any particular behavioural task.

14.2 Cortical systems mediating eye movements

The cortical generation of eye movements requires a number of steps that are mediated by at least three systems including an afferent, efferent, and attention/spatial map system. These systems are schematized in Fig. 14.1, and the location of the cortical areas within these systems in the monkey brain are shown in Fig. 14.2. Many of these cortical areas correspond to cytoarchitectonic areas defined by Von Bonin and Bailey (1947). The location of the corresponding cytoarchitectonic areas in the human brain are shown in Fig. 14.3.

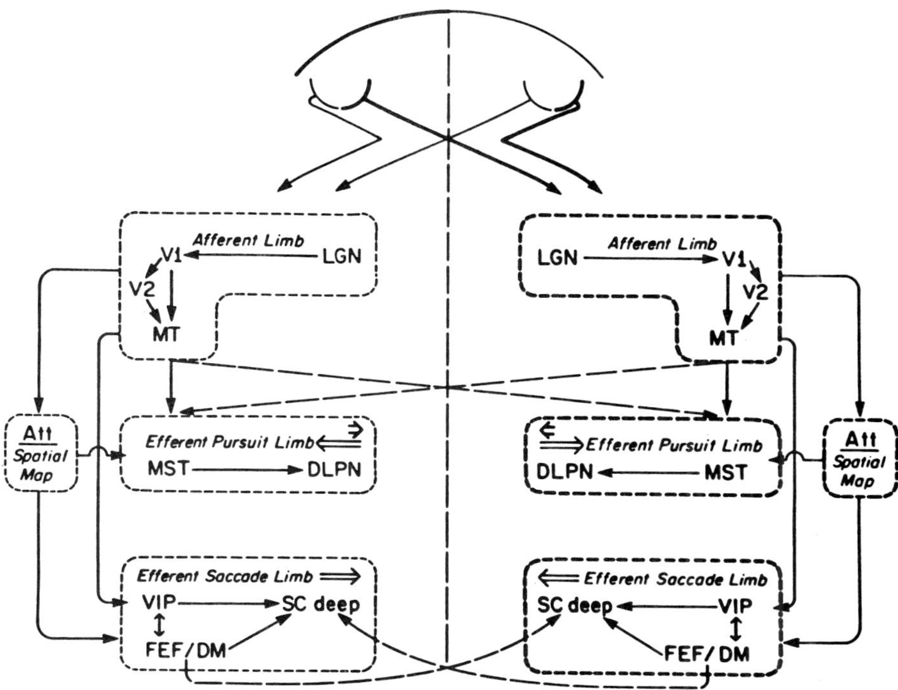

Fig. 14.1 Schematic diagram illustrating some of the afferent and efferent cortical pathways believed to be involved in generating eye movements in monkeys. The double arrows indicate the degree in which the efferent systems mediate ipsilateral versus contralateral eye movements. The cortical systems involved in shifting visual attention and coding an internal map of extrapersonal space (Att/Spatial Map) interface with the cortical afferent and efferent pathways. LGN, lateral geniculate nucleus; V1, striate cortex; V2, prestriate cortex; MT, middle temporal area; MST, medial superior temporal area; DLPN, dorsal lateral pontine nucleus; VIP, ventral intraparietal area; FEF, frontal eye fields; DM, dorsal medial area; SCdeep, deep and intermediate layers of the superior colliculus. See text for details.

14.2.1 AFFERENT SYSTEM

(a) Anatomy and physiology. The geniculo-striate pathway (LGN-V1) in monkeys processes information about target position in the contralateral visual hemifield (Fig. 14.1). This system, along with its projections to an area in occipitotemporal cortex called the middle temporal area (MT), also processes information about target motion in all directions for stimuli in the contralateral visual hemifield (Van Essen and Maunsell, 1983). Area

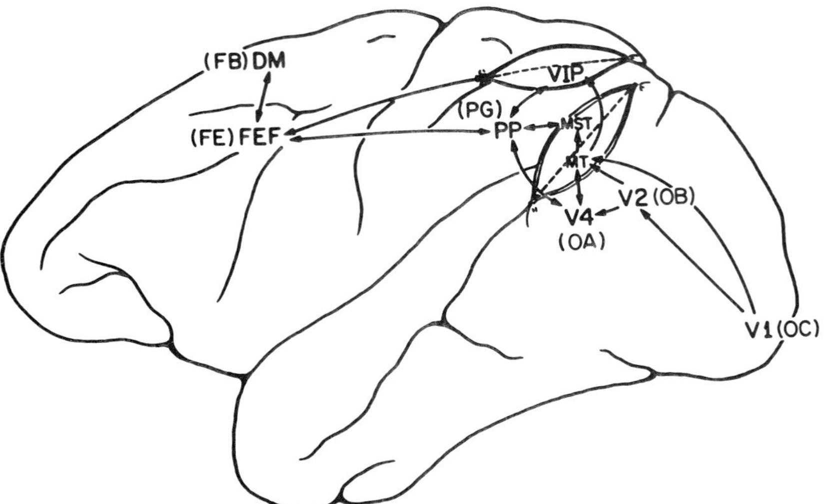

Fig. 14.2 Lateral surface of a monkey brain illustrating the location and connections of cortical areas believed to be involved in the generation of eye movements. The location of the cortical areas are based on electrophysiological studies. The cytoarchitectonically defined areas that roughly correspond to these electrophysiologically defined areas are enclosed in parentheses. Areas VIP and PP lie within cytoarchitectonic area PG. A portion of the superior temporal sulcus (containing MT and MST) and intraparietal sulcus (containing VIP) has been spread apart and the fundi of these sulci are represented as dashed lines.

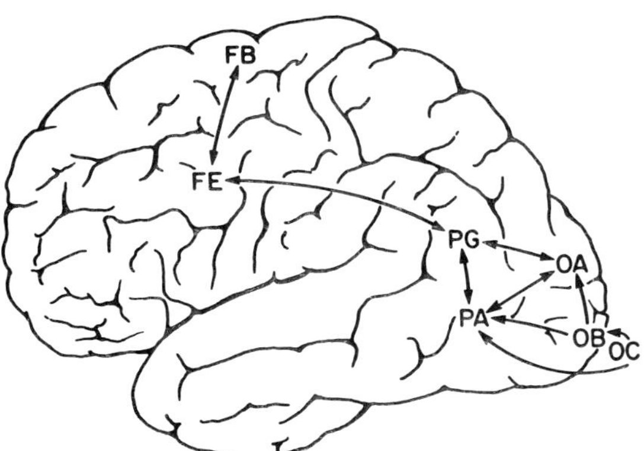

Fig. 14.3 Cytoarchitectonically defined cortical areas in the human brain (Von Economo, 1929) that correspond to the cytoarchitectonically defined areas in the monkey brain shown in Fig. 14.2. Based on the myelination pattern, portions of PA in the human brain may be the homologue to areas MT and MST in the monkey (Allman, 1977). The anatomical connections among the cortical areas in the human brain are based on connections described in the monkey brain.

V1 projects directly to the middle temporal area and indirectly to the middle temporal area via prestriate cortex (V2).

(b) Lesions. A unilateral lesion in area V1 (striate cortex) in monkeys and patients results in a contralateral visual hemifield defect; consequently, visually guided saccades to targets stepped into the contralateral visual hemifield and the initiation of smooth pursuit eye movements to targets stepped into and moved within this visual hemifield do not occur (Mohler and Wurtz, 1977; Newsome *et al.*, 1985; Leigh and Thurston, 1986). Because this is solely a visual afferent defect, there is no impairment in the ability to generate non-visually guided saccades into this hemifield, nor is there a defect in the ability to generate smooth pursuit eye movements in any direction as long as the target is kept in the normal visual hemifield.

A unilateral lesion in the middle temporal area in monkeys does not cause a visual hemifield defect, but does cause a defect in motion analysis in the contralateral visual hemifield (Newsome *et al.*, 1986). Consequently, accurate visually guided saccades are made to stationary targets in the contralateral visual hemifield, but saccades to targets moving in any direction within the contralateral visual hemifield are inaccurate because target speed is not taken into account when the saccade is generated. In addition, smooth pursuit is not initiated for targets moving in any direction in the contralateral visual hemifield. Similar results have been found in patients with occipitotemporal cortical lesions (Zihl, Von Cramon and Mai, 1983).

Following a lesion involving striate cortex, visually guided saccades to stationary targets in the defective visual hemifield eventually recover in monkeys (Mohler and Wurtz, 1977; Zee *et al.*, 1987; Segraves *et al.*, 1987), and possibly in human patients (Zihl and Werth, 1984). This recovery has been termed *blindsight* in patients; they do not actually perceive the target, yet they can accurately guess the location of the target by either pointing or making a saccade to the target.

This recovery of visually guided eye movements in the absence of recovery of visual perception is consistent with physiological studies in monkeys. No visual perceptual capabilities would be expected to recover following a striate cortex lesion since the occipitotemporal projection system, involved in object recognition, is critically dependent on the geniculate–striate pathway (Rocha-Miranda *et al.*, 1975). In contrast, visually guided saccades may recover following striate cortical lesions since neurones in the middle temporal area on the side of the striate cortical lesion can eventually use target location and velocity information mediated by the retina–superior colliculus–pulvinar pathway (Rodman, Gross and Albright, 1985). This pathway to cortex is believed to be crucial for mediating recovery of visually guided saccades as no recovery occurs following unilateral striate combined with superior collicular lesions in monkeys, or extensive unilateral cortical lesions involving the entire cortical afferent pathway (Mohler and Wurtz, 1977; Tusa, Zee and Herdman, 1986a).

14.2.2 EFFERENT SMOOTH PURSUIT SYSTEM

(a) Anatomy and physiology. The cortical efferent pathway for generating the command for smooth pursuit eye movements in the monkey probably includes an area in occipitotemporal cortex called the medial superior temporal area and its projections to subcortical regions including the dorsolateral pontine nucleus and possibly the pretectal/accessory optic system (Sakata, Shibutani and Kawano, 1983; Suzuki and Keller, 1984; Wurtz and Newsome, 1985; Mustari *et al.*, 1986). Unlike the afferent system, the efferent smooth pursuit system in each hemisphere mediates smooth pursuit for targets in either visual hemifield. The majority of neurones in the medial superior temporal area discharge during ipsilateral smooth pursuit eye movements, although a small number of neurones also discharge during contralateral pursuit (Kawano, Sasaki and Yamashita, 1984). The double arrows within the efferent pursuit limb in Fig. 14.1 indicate the degree in which the efferent system mediates ipsilateral versus contralateral eye movements. Since smooth pursuit can be generated in any direction for targets located in either the left or right visual hemifield, the efferent pursuit pathway in each hemisphere must get information from both the ipsilateral and contralateral afferent systems. This could be mediated via the interhemispheric projections between the middle temporal area and medial superior temporal area (dashed lines in Fig. 14.1; Ungerleider and Desimone, 1986).

(b) Lesions. A unilateral lesion in the medial superior temporal area in monkeys results in a smooth pursuit motor defect. Smooth pursuit to targets moving towards the side of the lesion is impaired no matter where the target is located within the ipsilateral or contralateral visual hemifield (Newsome, Dürsteler and Wurtz, 1986; Dürsteler, Wurtz and Newsome, 1987). We have found that large unilateral cortical lesions in monkeys impair smooth pursuit towards the side of the lesion at all target speeds, impair smooth pursuit away from the side of the lesion at high target speeds, and impair vertical smooth pursuit at all target speeds (Tusa, Zee and Herdman, 1986a). Bilateral deficits in smooth pursuit following a unilateral cortical lesion have also been reported in patients (Troost and Abel, 1982). Based on these studies, it appears that the cortical efferent pursuit pathway within one hemisphere can mediate ipsilateral smooth pursuit at low velocities, but that the efferent pursuit pathways in both

hemispheres are required to mediate horizontal smooth pursuit at high velocities and vertical smooth pursuit at all velocities.

Following a unilateral cortical lesion in patients and monkeys, there is also a deficit in the slow-phase component of optokinetic nystagmus that resembles the deficit in smooth pursuit (Baloh, Yee and Honrubia, 1980; Tusa, Zee and Herdman, 1984). During binocular or monocular viewing in monkeys, slow phases directed towards the side of the lesion are impaired at all target speeds, and slow phases directed away from the lesion are impaired at high target speeds. Further quantitative studies of optokinetic nystagmus and pursuit need to be done in patients with unilateral cortical lesions.

Smooth pursuit eye movements and optokinetic nystagmus slowly improve during the first year following a large unilateral cortical lesion in monkeys (Tusa, Zee and Herdman, 1986a). By one year, maximum pursuit eye velocity reaches pre-operative values in all directions except towards the lesioned side, where pursuit only reaches 70–80% of pre-operative values. This recovery in smooth pursuit eye velocity is probably mediated by cortex in the intact hemisphere, as smooth pursuit in patients is persistently impaired following bilateral lesions involving occipitotemporal cortex (Zihl, Von Cramon and Mai, 1983).

Monkeys with a unilateral cortical lesion also have a persistent spontaneous nystagmus that interferes with smooth pursuit. The slow phases of this nystagmus are directed away from the side of the lesion with speeds of 1–2°/s. Consequently, for targets moving away from the lesioned side, eye velocity was higher than target velocity by 1–2°/s requiring small back-up saccades, and for targets moving towards the lesioned side, eye velocity was lower than target velocity by 1–2°/s requiring small catch-up saccades. Similar findings have been reported in human patients following unilateral cortical lesions (Leigh and Thurston, 1986).

Preliminary data suggest that the frontal eye fields may also be involved in generating smooth pursuit eye movements. Neurones in this region discharge during smooth pursuit in the monkey (Bruce and Goldberg, 1985), and frontal lobe lesions involving the frontal eye fields impair smooth pursuit in both monkeys and patients (Pyykko *et al.*, 1984; Keating, Gooley and Kenney, 1985; Lynch and Allison, 1985). It is not clear whether the frontal eye fields and the medial superior temporal area have different roles in the generation of smooth pursuit, but preliminary studies in monkeys suggest that the frontal eye fields may be more involved in generating smooth pursuit to targets moving in a predictable pattern (Keating, Gooley and Kenney, 1985).

14.2.3 EFFERENT SACCADE SYSTEM

(a) Anatomy and physiology. The cortical efferent pathways in the monkey for initiating saccades are not well defined but probably include two parallel pathways (Schiller, True and Conway, 1980; see Fig. 14.1). The first pathway is from frontal cortex, which includes the frontal eye fields and probably the dorsomedial region in the supplementary motor area (Schlag and Schlag-Rey, 1985). These two cortical areas contain neurones that discharge before intentional saccades, and stimulation of these areas results in contralaterally directed saccades (Bruce and Goldberg, 1985; Bruce *et al.*, 1985; Schlag and Schlag-Rey, 1985). The frontal eye fields and the dorsomedial region in turn project to the intermediate and deep layers of the superior colliculus (SCdeep; Fig. 14.1), as well as directly to the paramedian reticular formation (Distel and Fries, 1982; Leichnetz, Spencer and Smith, 1984; Schnyder *et al.*, 1985). In addition, these cortical areas project to SCdeep via the basal ganglia (caudate nucleus–substantia nigra pars reticulata). A second efferent saccade pathway includes cortical area(s) within parieto-occipital cortex (Schiller, 1977; Keating *et al.*, 1983). The specific cortical area(s) involved in this more posterior pathway is not known, but probably includes an area in the ventral bank of the intraparietal sulcus, which has been called several different names including VIP, POa, and LIP (Van Essen and Maunsell, 1983; Lynch, Graybiel and Lobeck, 1985; Gnadt, Andersen and Blatt, 1986). This region contains neurones that discharge before intentional saccades, and stimulation of it results in contralaterally directed saccades (Lynch, 1981; Shibutani, Sakata and Hyvarinen, 1984). This region also has a dense projection to SCdeep (Lynch, Graybiel and Lobeck, 1985). Thus, there appear to be three cortical 'saccade' regions in monkey including frontal eye fields, dorsomedial, and VIP. Based on cerebral blood flow studies in patients there may also be three cortical saccade regions in the human brain. Human subjects generating visually guided intentional saccades show increased blood flow in the frontal eye fields, supplementary motor cortex, and in a more posterior region caudal to the central sulcus (Melamed and Larsen, 1979; Fox *et al.*, 1985).

(b) Lesions. We have found that monkeys with large unilateral cortical lesions involving all the cortical saccade regions are still able to make spontaneous saccades and quick phases of nystagmus in both horizontal directions, but are unable initially to generate any intentional or reflexive saccades away from the lesioned side (Tusa, Zee and Herdman, 1986b). Based on these data, we speculate that the 'saccade' areas within cerebral cortex initiate contralaterally directed intentional and reflexive saccades. The superior colliculus and other subcortical structures probably initiate

contralaterally directed spontaneous saccades and quick phases of nystagmus (Hikosaka and Wurtz, 1985). Patients with unilateral cortical lesions are also unable initially to generate contralaterally directed saccades (Sharpe, 1982). This deficit is often referred to as a *saccade or gaze palsy*, although it is not known what types of saccades are involved in this deficit.

Within several days to weeks following a large unilateral cortical lesion, monkeys and patients recover the ability to initiate saccades away from the side of the lesion. This recovery could be mediated by the frontal eye fields and dorsomedial areas in the intact cerebral hemisphere, as these cortical areas have bilateral projections to SCdeep (indicated by the dashed line in Fig. 14.1; Distel and Fries, 1982).

Very little is known about the effect of cortical lesions on vertical saccades. We have found that monkeys with large unilateral cortical lesions are unable to generate pure vertical visually guided saccades to targets stepped or moved in the vertical direction throughout the 1.5-year post-operative period (Tusa, Zee and Herdman, 1986b). Instead, the animals generate oblique saccades, tilted 10–15° towards the side of the lesion. These oblique saccades are probably due to the unopposed action of cerebral cortex in the intact hemisphere. Thus, cortical areas in both hemispheres are required to generate purely vertical visually guided saccades.

Finally, it appears that different types of intentional saccades are mediated by frontal and parieto-occipital cortex. Frontal lobe lesions in patients and monkeys impair non-visually guided intentional saccades, but not visually guided intentional saccades (Guitton, Buchtel and Douglas, 1985; Deng *et al.*, 1986; Bruce and Borden, 1986). Conversely, parieto-occipital lobe lesions in patients impair visually guided intentional saccades, but not non-visually guided intentional saccades (Tsutsui *et al.*, 1980).

14.2.4 VISUAL ATTENTION/SPATIAL MAP SYSTEM

(a) Anatomy and physiology. Several areas are involved in the development of an internal spatial map of extrapersonal space and shifts in visual attention including posterior parietal, prefrontal, and possibly prestriate cortex (Mesulam, 1981; Moran and Desimone, 1985). These cortical regions in turn interconnect cortical regions within the cortical afferent and efferent pathways described above (Barbas and Mesulam, 1981; Pandya and Seltzer, 1982; Petrides and Pandya, 1984).

(b) Lesions. We have found that monkeys with large unilateral cortical lesions have two major ocular motor deficits that vary with the position of

the eye in the orbit, i.e. are based on a craniotopic (head-centred) co-ordinate system (Tusa, Zee and Herdman, 1986b). We speculate that these deficits are due to dysfunction in directing visual attention and/or in constructing an internal spatial map of extrapersonal space. First, smooth pursuit, optokinetic nystagmus, quick phases of nystagmus in the light, spontaneous saccades in the light, reflexive saccades, and intentional saccades will not initially move the eyes into craniotopic space contralateral to the lesion. Thus, these animals have a *gaze deviation* towards the side of the lesion, which we attribute to a defect in visual attention or in the spatial map of contralateral craniotopic space. Cortically induced gaze deviations in patients may also be due to a defect in visual attention or in an internal spatial map. Patients with parieto-occipital or frontal lobe lesions that result in contralateral hemispatial neglect do not readily generate smooth pursuit, spontaneous, or intentional saccades into the contralateral hemispace (De Renzi *et al.*, 1982; Reeves *et al.*, 1984; Bogousslavsky and Regli, 1986; Meienberg, Harrer and Wehren, 1986). It is not yet known whether these ocular motor deficits in patients are based on a head-centred or body-centred spatial map.

These ocular motor deficits in monkeys and patients eventually recover, which may be mediated by cortical areas in the intact cerebral hemisphere. After recovery of the gaze deviation from a unilateral prefrontal lobe lesion in monkeys or in patients, a subsequent frontal lobe lesion on the intact side results in a prolonged gaze deviation towards the side of the second lesion (Latto and Cowey, 1971; Steiner and Melamed, 1984).

The second craniotopic-related ocular motor defect we found in monkeys involves the destination and latency of intentional saccades. Once contralaterally directed intentional saccades recover into contralateral craniotopic space, they are generated in a staircase pattern, and their amplitude and latency depends on the position of the eye in the orbit before the saccade. Saccades made from the most eccentric orbital position on the side of the lesion have the largest amplitudes and shortest latencies. Saccades generated from positions in the orbit contralateral to the side of the lesion have progressively smaller saccade amplitudes and longer latencies. This defect persisted to 1.5 years post-operatively, which was the duration of the study. Patients with hemispatial neglect from parietal and possibly frontal lobe lesions also generate staircase saccades away from the side of the lesion (Girotti *et al.*, 1983; Meienberg, 1983; Perenin and Vighetto, 1983; Page, Barratt and Gresty, 1984). In addition, the latency of these saccades to visual targets is increased (Sundquist, 1979). It is not yet known whether the amplitude and latency of saccades in patients with unilateral cortical lesions also varies as a function of orbital position.

14.3 Clinical syndromes

14.3.1 ACQUIRED OCULAR MOTOR APRAXIA

Patients with ocular motor apraxia can generate spontaneous saccades and quick phases during vestibular and optokinetic stimulation, but cannot generate intentional saccades or smooth pursuit eye movements (Cogan and Adams, 1953). It is difficult to extract from the clinical literature a clear understanding of the anatomical localization of ocular motor apraxia, but based on the work in monkeys, one might expect that a complete ocular motor apraxia occurs only following a bilateral lesion involving both frontal and parieto-occipital cortex. Only this lesion would eliminate all of the saccade and pursuit efferent cortical pathways. Based on studies in monkeys, a bilateral lesion restricted to the parieto-occipital lobe in patients would be expected to result primarily in a loss of smooth pursuit and possibly visually guided saccades. A bilateral lesion restricted to the frontal lobe would be expected to result primarily in a loss of non-visually guided intentional saccades.

14.3.2 SPASM OF FIXATION

Spasm of fixation is an ocular motor deficit in which patients have great difficulty in eliciting intentional saccades, especially when they are viewing a complex visual scene (Holmes, 1930). If the visual scene is replaced by a homogeneous scene, they are usually able to saccade to a single visual target placed in their peripheral visual field, but they may have difficulty in moving their eyes off the target unless the visual scene is again replaced by a homogeneous white scene. This probably represents a bilateral deficit in shifting visual attention mediated by cortical areas in parieto-occipital and frontal cortex. This is consistent with what is known about the aetiology of Balint's syndrome. Balint (1909) described a complex syndrome consisting of spasm of fixation, optic ataxia, and simultanagnosia. It is currently believed that a complete and persistent Balint's syndrome requires bilateral parieto-occipital and frontal lobe lesions (Hécaen and Ajuriaguerra, 1954; Hausser, Robert and Giard, 1980).

14.4 Future research

It appears that cortical lesions affect saccades and smooth pursuit eye movements differently depending on the behavioural context in which these eye movements are generated. Therefore, saccades and smooth pursuit should be systematically studied under a number of different conditions (e.g. Table 14.1 for saccades). In addition, it appears that different eye movement deficits occur depending upon which cortical subsystem is lesioned. Therefore, eye movement deficits should be examined from the perspective of damage to afferent, efferent, and attention/spatial map systems.

Although our understanding of the cortical control of eye movements in patients and monkeys has significantly increased in the past several years, there are still a number of issues that need further investigation. Does recovery of visually guided saccades in patients with visual cortex damage (blindsight) depend upon the extent of the cortical lesion in extrastriate cortex? Do 'cortically induced saccade or gaze palsies' require damage to both frontal and parietal cortex, and do these 'palsies' include all saccade types or only intentional and reflexive saccades? Does frontal cortex primarily mediate predictive smooth pursuit and non-visually guided intentional saccades while parietal cortex primarily mediates unpredictive smooth pursuit and visually guided saccades? What are the deficits in vertical smooth pursuit and vertical visually guided saccades in patients with cortical lesions? Are eye movement deficits in patients with hemispatial neglect based on a disturbance in contralateral craniotopic space? What are the differences in eye movement deficits in patients with neglect from prefrontal versus posterior parietal cortical damage?

Acknowledgements

Supported by NINCDS Grant NS00804 and by the Sloan Foundation.

References

Allman, J.M. (1977) Evolution of the visual system in the early primates, in *Progress in Psychology, Physiology and Psychiatry* (eds J.M. Sprague and A.N. Epstein). Academic Press, New York, pp. 1–53.

Balint, R. (1909) Seelenlahmung des 'Schauens' optische Ataxia raumliche Storung der Aufmerksamkeit. *Monatsschrift fur Psychiat. Neurol.*, **25**, 51–81.

Baloh, R.W., Yee, R.D. and Honrubia, V. (1980) Optokinetic nystagmus and parietal lobe lesions. *Ann. Neurol.*, **7**, 269–76.

Barbas, H. and Mesulam, M.-M. (1981) Organization of afferent input to subdivisions of area 8 in the rhesus monkey. *J. Comp. Neurol.*, **200**, 407–31.

Bogousslavsky, J. and Regli, F. (1986) Pursuit gaze defects in acute and chronic unilateral parieto-occipital lesions. *Eur. Neurol.*, **25**, 10–18.

Bruce, C.J. and Borden, J.A. (1986) The primate frontal eye fields are necessary for predictive saccadic tracking. *Soc. Neurosci., Abstr.*, **12**, 1086.

Bruce, C.J. and Goldberg, M.E. (1985) Primate frontal eye fields: I. Single neurons discharging before saccades. *J. Neurophysiol.*, **53**, 603–35.

Bruce, C.J., Goldberg, M.E., Bushnell, M.C. and Stanton, G.B. (1985) Primate frontal eye fields: II. Physiological and anatomical correlates of electrically evoked eye movements. *J. Neurophysiol.*, **54**, 714–34.

Cogan, D.G. and Adams, R.D. (1953) A type of paralysis of conjugate gaze (ocular motor apraxia). *Arch. Ophthalmol.*, **50**, 434–42.

Deng, Shu-Yi, Goldberg, M.E., Segraves, M.A., Ungerleider, L.G. and Mishkin, M. (1986) The effect of unilateral ablation of the frontal eye fields on saccadic performance in the monkey, in *Adaptive Processes in Visual and Oculomotor Systems* (eds E.L. Keller and D.S. Zee). Pergamon, Oxford, pp. 201–8.

De Renzi, E., Colombo, A., Faglioni, P. and Gilbertoni, M. (1982) Conjugate gaze paresis in stroke patients with unilateral damage. *Arch. Neurol.*, **39**, 482–6.

Distel, H. and Fries, W. (1982) Contralateral cortical projections to the superior colliculus in the macaque monkey. *Exp. Brain Res.*, **48**, 158–62.

Dürsteler, M.R., Wurtz, R.H. and Newsome, W.T. (1987) Directional pursuit deficits following lesions of the foveal representation within the superior temporal sulcus of the macaque monkey. *J. Neurophysiol.* **57**, 1262–87.

Fox, P.T., Fox, J.M., Raichle, M.E. and Burde, R.M. (1985) The role of cerebral cortex in the generation of voluntary saccades: a positron emission tomographic study. *J. Neurophysiol.*, **54**, 348–69.

Girotti, F., Casazza, M., Musicco, M. and Avanzini, G. (1983) Oculomotor disorders in cortical lesions in man: the role of unilateral neglect. *Neuropsychologia*, **21**, 543–53.

Gnadt, J.W., Andersen, R.A. and Blatt, G.J. (1986) Spatial, memory, and motor-planning properties of saccade-related activity in the lateral intraparietal area (LIP) of macaque. *Soc. Neurosci., Abstr.*, **12**, 458.

Guitton, D., Buchtel, H.A. and Douglas, R.M. (1985) Frontal lobe lesions in man cause difficulties in suppressing reflexive glances and in generating goal-directed saccades. *Exp. Brain Res.*, **58**, 455–72.

Hausser, C.O., Robert, F. and Giard, N. (1980) Balint's syndrome. *Can. J. Neurol Sci.*, **7**, 157–61.

Hécaen, H. and Ajuriaguerra, J. (1954) Balint's syndrome (psychic paralysis of visual fixation) and its minor forms. *Brain*, **77**, 373–400.

Hikosaka, O. and Wurtz, R.H. (1985) Modification of saccadic eye movements by GABA-related substances. II. Effect of muscimol and bicuculline in monkey superior colliculus. *J. Neurophysiol.*, **53**, 266–91.

Holmes, G. (1930) Spasm of fixation. *Trans. Ophthalmol. Soc. UK.*, **50**, 253–62.

Kawano, K., Sasaki, M. and Yamashita, M. (1984) Response properties of neurons in posterior parietal cortex of monkey during visual-vestibular stimulation. I. Visual tracking neurons. *J. Neurophysiol.*, **51**, 340–51.

Keating, E.G., Gooley, S.G. and Kenney, D.V. (1985) Impaired tracking and loss of predictive eye movements after removal of the frontal eye fields. *Soc. Neurosci., Abstr.*, **11**, 472.

Keating, E.G., Gooley, S.G., Pratt, S.W. and Kelsey, J.E. (1983) Removing the superior colliculus silences eye movements normally evoked from stimulation of parietal and occipital eye fields. *Brain Res.*, **269**, 145–8.

Latto, R. and Cowey, A. (1971) Fixation changes after frontal eye-field lesions in monkeys. *Brain Res.*, **30**, 25–36.

Leichnetz, G.R., Spencer, R.F. and Smith, D.J. (1984) Cortical projections to the paramedian tegmental and basilar pons in the monkey. *J. Comp. Neurol.*, **228**, 338–408.

Leigh, R.J. and Thurston, S.E. (1986) Recovery of ocular motor function in humans with cerebral lesions, in *Adaptive Processes in Visual and Oculomotor Systems* (eds E.L. Keller and D.S. Zee). Pergamon, Oxford. pp. 231–8.

Lynch, J.C. (1981) The functional organization and posterior parietal association cortex. *Behav. Brain Sci.*, **3**, 485–534.

Lynch, J.C. and Allison, J.D. (1985) A quantitative study of visual pursuit deficits following lesions of the frontal eye fields in rhesus monkeys. *Soc. Neurosci., Abstr.*, **11**, 473.

Lynch, J.C., Graybiel, A.M. and Lobeck, L.J. (1985) The differential projection of two cytoarchitectonic subregions of the inferior parietal lobule of macaque upon the deep layers of the superior colliculus. *J. Comp. Neurol.*, **235**, 241–54.

Meienberg, O. (1983) Clinical examination of saccadic eye movements in hemianopia. *Neurology*, **33**, 1311–15.

Meienberg, O., Harrer, M. and Wehren, C. (1986) Oculographic diagnosis of hemineglect in patients with homonymous hemianopia. *J. Neurol.*, **233**, 97–101.

Melamed, E. and Larsen, B. (1979) Cortical activation pattern during saccadic eye movements in humans: localization by focal cerebral blood flow increases. *Ann. Neurol.*, **5**, 79–88.

Mesulam, M.-M. (1981) A cortical network for directed attention and unilateral neglect. *Ann. Neurol.*, **10**, 309–25.

Mohler, C.W. and Wurtz, R.H. (1977) Role of striate cortex and superior colliculus in visual guidance of saccadic eye movements in monkeys. *J. Neurophysiol.*, **40**, 74–94.

Moran, J. and Desimone, R. (1985) Selective attention gates visual processing in the extrastriate cortex. *Science, NY*, **229**, 782–4.

Mustari, M.J., Fuchs, A.F., Wallman, J., Langer, T.P. and Kaneko, C.R.S. (1986) Visual and oculomotor response properties of single units in the lateral terminal nucleus (LTN) of the behaving rhesus macaque. *Soc. Neurosci., Abstr.*, **12**, 459.

Newsome, W.T., Dursteler, M.R. and Wurtz, R.H. (1986) The middle temporal visual area and the control of smooth pursuit eye movements, in *Adaptive Processes in Visual and Oculomotor Systems* (eds E.L. Keller and D.S. Zee). Pergamon, Oxford, pp. 223–30.

Newsome, W.T., Wurtz, R.H., Dursteler, M.R. and Mikami, A. (1985) Punctate chemical lesions of striate cortex in the macaque monkeys: effect on visually guided saccades. *Exp. Brain Res.*, **58**, 392–9.

Page, N.G.R., Barratt, H.J. and Gresty, M.A. (1984) Gaze abnormalities with chronic cerebral lesions in man, in *Theoretical and Applied Aspects of Eye Movement Research* (eds A.G. Gale and F.G. Johnson). AG Elsevier Science Publishers, pp. 397–402.

Pandya, D.N. and Seltzer, B. (1982) Intrinsic connections and architectonics of posterior parietal cortex in the rhesus monkey. *J. Comp. Neurol.*, **204**, 196–210.

Perenin, M.T. and Vighetto, A. (1983) Optic ataxia: a specific disorder in visuomotor coordination, in *Spatially Oriented Behavior* (eds A. Hein and M. Jeannerod). Springer-Verlag, New York, pp. 305–26.

Pyykko, I., Dahlen, A.-I., Schalen, L. and Hindfelt, B. (1984) Eye movements in patients with speech dyspraxia. *Acta Otolaryngol.*, **98**, 481–9.

Petrides, M. and Pandya, D.N. (1984) Projections to the frontal cortex from the posterior parietal region in the rhesus monkey. *J. Comp. Neurol.*, **228**, 105–16.

Reeves, A.G., Perret, J., Jenkyn, L.R. and Saint-Hilaire, J.M. (1984) Pursuit gaze and the occipitoparietal region. *Arch. Neurol.*, **41**, 83–4.

Rocha-Miranda, C.E., Bender, D.G., Gross, C.G. and Mishkin, M. (1975) Visual activation of neurons in inferotemporal cortex depends on striate cortex and forebrain commissures. *J. Neurophysiol.*, **38**, 475–91.

Rodman, H.R., Gross, C.G. and Albright, T.D. (1985) Removal of striate cortex does not abolish responsiveness of neurons in visual area MT of the macaque. *Soc. Neurosci., Abstr.*, **11**, 1246.

Sakata, H., Shibutani, H. and Kawano, K. (1983) Functional properties of visual tracking neurons in posterior parietal association cortex of the monkey. *J. Neurophysiol.*, **49**, 1364–80.

Schiller, P.H. (1977) The effect of superior colliculus ablation on saccades elicited by cortical stimulation. *Brain Res.*, **122**, 154–6.

Schiller, P.H., True, S.D. and Conway, J.L. (1980) Deficits in eye movements following frontal eye-field and superior colliculus ablations. *J. Neurophysiol.*, **44**, 1175–89.

Schlag, J. and Schlag-Rey, M. (1985) Unit activity related to spontaneous saccades in frontal dorsomedial cortex of the monkey. *Exp. Brain Res.*, **58**, 208–11.

Schnyder, H., Reisine, H., Hepp, K. and Henn, V. (1985) Frontal eye field projection to the paramedian pontine reticular formation traced with wheat germ agglutinin in the monkey. *Brain Res.*, **329**, 151–60.

Segraves, M.A., Goldberg, M.E., Deng, S.Y., Bruce, C.J., Imgerleider, L.G. and Mishkin, M. (1987) The rate of striate cortex in the guidance of eye movements in the monkey. *J. Neuroscience*, **7**, 3040–50.

Sharpe, J.A. (1982) Cerebral ocular motor deficits, in *Functional Basis of Ocular Motility Disorders* (eds G. Lennerstrand, D.S. Zee and E.L. Keller). Pergamon, Oxford, pp. 479–88.

Shibutani, H., Sakata, H. and Hyvarinen, J. (1984) Saccade and blinking evoked by microstimulation of the posterior parietal association cortex of the monkey. *Exp. Brain Res.*, **55**, 1–8.

Steiner, I. and Melamed, E. (1984) Conjugate eye deviation after acute hemispheric stroke: delayed recovery after previous contralateral frontal lobe damage. *Ann. Neurol.*, **16**, 509–10.

Sundquist, A. (1979) Saccadic reaction-time in parietal-lobe dysfunction. *Lancet*, **i**, 870.

Suzuki, D.A. and Keller, E.L. (1984) Visual signals in the dorsolateral pontine nucleus of the alert monkey: their relationship to smooth-pursuit eye movements. *Exp. Brain Res.*, **53**, 473–8.

Troost, B.T. and Abel, L.A. (1982) Pursuit disorders, in *Functional Basis of Ocular Motility Disorders* (eds. G. Lennerstrand, D.S. Zee and E.L. Keller). Pergamon, Oxford, pp. 511–16.

Tsutsui, J., Takeda, J., Ichihashi, S., Kimura, H. and Shirabe, T. (1980) Ocular motor apraxia and lesions of the visual association area. *Neuro-Ophthalmology*, **1**, 149–54.

Tusa, R.J., Zee, D.S. and Herdman, S.J. (1984) Effects of unilateral cerebral cortex lesions on eye movements in monkeys. *Soc. Neurosci., Abstr.*, **10**, 912.

Tusa, R.J., Zee, D.S. and Herdman S.J. (1986a) Recovery of oculomotor function in monkeys with large unilateral cortical lesions, in *Adaptive Processes in Visual and Oculomotor Systems* (eds E.L. Keller and D.S. Zee). Pergamon, Oxford, pp. 209–16.

Tusa, R.J., Zee, D.S. and Herdman, S.J. (1986b) Effect of unilateral cerebral cortical lesions on ocular motor behavior in monkeys: saccades and quick phases. *J. Neurophysiol.*, **56**, 1590–1625.

Ungerleider, L.G. and Desimone, R. (1986) Cortical connections of visual area MT in the macaque. *J. Comp. Neurol.*, **248**, 190–222.

Van Essen, D.C. and Maunsell, J.H.R. (1983) Hierarchial organization and functional streams in the visual cortex. *Trends Neurosci.*, **6**, 370–5.

Von Bonin, G. and Bailey, P. (1947) *The Neocortex of Macaca*. University of Illinois Press, Urbana, IL.

Von Economo, C.F. (1929) *The Cytoarchitectonics of the Human Cerebral Cortex*. Oxford Medical Publications, London.

Wurtz, R.J. and Newsome, W.T. (1985) Divergent signals encoded by neurons in extrastriate areas MT and MST during smooth pursuit eye movements. *Soc. Neurosci., Abstr.*, **11**, 1246.

Zee, D.S., Tusa, R.J., Herdman, S.J., Butler, P.H. and Gucer, G. (1986) Effects of occipital lobectomy upon eye movements in primate. *J. Neurophysiol.*, **58**, 883–907.

Zihl, J. and Werth, R. (1984) Contributions to the study of 'blindsight'. II. The role of specific practice for saccadic localization in patients with postgeniculate visual field defects. *Neuropsychologia*, **22**, 13–22.

Zihl, J., Von Cramon, D. and Mai, N. (1983) Selective disturbance of movement vision after bilateral brain damage. *Brain*, **106**, 313–40.

CHAPTER 15

Do the basal ganglia have a role in the control of eye movements?

J.M. GIBSON

The primary effects of basal ganglia disease in man are disorders of muscle tone, posture and movement control. Whilst it has long been recognized that subtle eye movement abnormalities occur in basal ganglia disease, these are of but little assistance to the clinician making the diagnosis. Indeed, the presence of a gross disorder in eye movements such as nystagmus or a gaze palsy would point to pathology outside the basal ganglia. Recent interest in the study of eye movements in basal ganglia disease has stemmed from the fact that eye movement control can be separated into well-defined subsystems (saccadic, smooth pursuit, vestibular, vergence and optokinetic) and, using modern accurate non-invasive methods of recording, the motor control of the eye in man can be much more easily studied than is the case for the limbs. It has also been possible to gain some insights into the functions of the basal ganglia through the study of eye movements in experimental animals, in which single cell recordings can be made and neurotransmitters modulated, and by looking at human basal ganglia diseases. In this review I will firstly describe some recent animal experiments which suggest mechanisms by which the basal ganglia might influence eye movements, and then discuss the ocular motor findings in idiopathic Parkinson's disease, MPTP parkinsonism and Huntington's disease. Conditions such as progressive supranuclear palsy and olivopontocerebellar atrophy are not discussed because these have obvious brainstem or cerebellar pathology to explain their ocular motor abnormalities.

Classical accounts of the supranuclear control of eye movements do not include the basal ganglia in the control structure (Bender, 1980). The basal ganglia have no direct anatomical connections with the ocular motor system, but the pars reticulata of the substantia nigra (SN_r) sends axons to the superior colliculus (Jayaraman, Batton and Carpenter, 1977). The major source of input to the SN_r is from the caudate nucleus, which in turn receives afferent input from association and frontal cortical areas (Webster, 1965; Royce, 1982). The frontal eye fields have a well-defined role in the generation of saccades (Bender, 1980).

The bulk of the evidence supporting a role for the basal ganglia in ocular motor control concerns the mechanisms by which the SN_r modulates superior colliculus activity, particularly in relation to saccades. Stimulation of the caudate nucleus inhibits SN_r firing (Yoshida and Precht, 1971), and the nigro-collicular pathway is also inhibitory, using gamma-aminobutyric acid (GABA) as its transmitter (Vincent *et al.*, 1978). In a series of experiments on monkeys, Hikosaka and Wurtz (1983a,b,c,d, 1985a,b, 1986) have greatly elucidated the role played by SN_r in saccadic control and these experiments will be summarized in some detail. The monkeys were trained to fixate a central target and the responses of cells in SN_r studied in the following paradigms: (a) to saccades made in response to a peripheral target appearing immediately after removal of the central fixation spot; (b) to saccades made in response to a peripheral target in addition to the central fixation spot; (c) to a saccade made to the remembered location of a peripheral target which was briefly flashed on; (d) to spontaneous saccades made with no external stimulus. These workers found that cells in the pars compacta of the substantia nigra (SN_c) had low firing rates and tended to fire after the task was begun or a reward given. By contrast, saccade-related cells, located in the lateral part of SN_r had high resting discharge rates and responded to saccades by a sudden decrease in their firing rates. These cells responded to either visual or auditory targets (but not both – no bimodal cells were found) in the contralateral visual field, and their response was enhanced if a saccade occurred. Different classes of cells were found depending upon the visual task. Fixation-related cells decreased their firing rate in response to fixation and not the appearance of a novel peripheral stimulus provided fixation was maintained. They also decreased firing rate when the fixation point was removed. It was felt that such fixation-dependent cells act to signal the initiation or termination of visually guided eye movement. Of great interest was the discovery of cells that only responded to remembered targets. The system did not appear to have any role in the generation of spontaneous saccades. In additional experiments, Hikosaka and Wurtz (1985a,b) demonstrated reciprocal effects from the injection of muscimol, a GABA agonist, in the SN_r, and bicuculline, a GABA antagonist, in the superior colliculus. These produced irrepressible saccades towards the movement field of the injection site and an inability to maintain fixation at a different point. By contrast, muscimol injection of the superior colliculus produced slowed, hypometric saccades with long latencies especially to remembered saccades, whilst the frequency of spontaneous saccades was reduced. This effect of muscimol in reducing saccadic velocity as well as amplitude was unexpected and had not been demonstrated in previous lesioning experiments on the superior colliculus. Hikosaka and Wurtz (1986) produced an identical effect acutely, using lidocaine injection in the superior colliculus and postulated that compensatory mechanisms could rapidly overcome saccadic slowing produced by lesions outside the paramedian pontine reticular formation.

In further studies, Hikosaka and Wurtz (1983d) were able to strengthen the importance of the link between the SN_r and superior colliculus by identifying saccade-related cells in superior colliculus and antidromically stimulating SN_r cells that showed visual and saccade responses. An invariant inverse relationship in the firing rates in SN_r and superior colliculus was always found so that a decrease in SN_r rate always coincided with an increase in superior colliculus activity. This finding suggests that SN_r tonically inhibits the superior colliculus and, when this tonic inhibition is reduced, there is a greater chance of the generation of a burst of firing that will lead to a saccade.

The major difference between responses in SN_r and superior colliculus is that the latter showed identical increases in rate with saccades of a given direction and size, irrespective of the mode of initiation, whereas the SN_r activity was highly contingent upon the behavioural context, whether visual, auditory or memory, but never modulating with spontaneous saccades.

Thus the SN_r only has a role in the modification of the saccadic behaviour of the superior colliculus under specific limited circumstances, and other important pathways, e.g. those from the frontal eye fields to superior colliculus, may generate spontaneous saccades without the participation of SN_r. The possible role of the basal ganglia in the control of other eye movement systems is largely unknown, although Boussaoud and Joseph (1985) demonstrated decreased vestibulo-ocular reflex gain after ipsilateral SN_r muscimol injection in the cat and argue that the basal ganglia might modify the vestibulo-ocular reflex via a pathway from superior colliculus to nucleus prepositus hypoglossi.

15.1 Parkinson's disease

Parkinson's disease is the commonest disease of the basal ganglia. Infrequent blinking is a hallmark of the akinetic facies typical of the disease, but gross ocular motor signs are not a feature. There is no reliable and objective method of measuring akinesia in Parkinson's disease, and indeed the very term akinesia poses considerable problems of definition (Ad Hoc Committee, 1981). Limb motor studies of Parkinson's disease are complicated by variability of performance, learning effects, and deciding exactly which parameters of movements to use (Draper and Johns, 1964; Flowers, 1976, 1978a,b; Evarts, Teravainen and Calne, 1981; Bloxham, Mindel and Frith, 1984), and longitudinal studies of limb function to assess the progress of the disease have not gained wide acceptance. In contrast to limb movements, eye movements are relatively easy to measure and analyse as the 'oculomotor plant' is a constant load system with well-recognized modes of operation (Dodge, 1903). The interest in eye movements in Parkinson's disease is generated by the possibility of quantifying akinesia in such a relatively simple control system.

Corin, Elizan and Bender (1972) in a large qualitative study noted abnormal smooth pursuit and saccades particularly in the vertical plane and also felt that the worst abnormalities were found in those patients with the most severe Parkinson's disease. Prior to the advent of the magnetic search coil technique it was not possible to obtain very accurate recordings of vertical eye movements and so published quantitative accounts have concentrated on the horizontal systems. The first such study (Melvill Jones and De Jong, 1971) of saccades made in response to the random appearance of visual stimuli, showed that whilst the Parkinson's disease patients exhibited an abnormal tendency to make hypometric (undershooting) saccades, the velocities, durations and latencies were normal implying that the brainstem saccade generator was intact. By contrast, Shibasaki, Tsuji and Kuroiwa (1979) and White *et al.* (1983b) reported prolonged latencies and saccadic slowing, particularly in more severely affected patients. The major difficulties in evaluating these studies is the lack of homogeneity of patients, and the absence of controls for drug effects which can cause abnormal eye movements in Parkinson's disease (Shimizu *et al.*, 1977). In addition there was no systematic attempt to correlate eye and limb dysfunction.

In an attempt to clarify this situation we have carried out a study of untreated, mildly affected Parkinson's disease patients using computer analysis of saccadic and smooth pursuit systems. In addition, akinesia in the limbs was measured using manual tracking of similar saccadic or smooth pursuit stimuli (Gibson, Pimlott and Kennard, 1987). This study showed that for the eye, accuracy of initial saccades was significantly impaired, indicating hypometria, but saccadic latencies and peak velocities were normal. Saccadic durations showed a significant increase, however, and the saccadic latency scatter was increased indicating greater variability in Parkinson's disease ocular motor performance. For the manual 'saccadic' tasks, more severe abnormalities in latencies, velocities and durations were found, as would be expected from the clinical examinations.

Successful therapy with dopaminergic drugs resulted in improved saccadic accuracy alone, but no such change was demonstrated in those patients who did not clinically respond to treatment. It seems reasonable to assume that, whilst saccadic slowing may be present in very advanced cases of the disease, variability of performance and inaccuracy characterize the saccadic 'abnormalities' in Parkinson's disease, but that the ocular motor system is much less affected than are the limbs.

15.1.1 SMOOTH PURSUIT FUNCTION IN PARKINSON'S DISEASE

There is less controversy about the presence and nature of the smooth pursuit abnormality in Parkinson's disease described erroneously as 'saccadic' or even worse 'cogwheel' (by analogy with cogwheel rigidity of the limbs). The major quantitative study of smooth pursuit in Parkinson's disease (Melvill Jones and De Jong, 1976) on treated patients demonstrated that impaired smooth pursuit was due to a reduction in velocity gain (i.e. ratio of eye/target velocity) rather than phase lag. In normals a reduction in the smooth pursuit velocity gain will result in compensatory 'catching' up saccades, but in Parkinson's disease this mechanism fails.

Previously untreated Parkinson's disease patients also show a decrease in smooth pursuit velocity gain which improves with successful treatment (Gibson, Pimlott, and Kennard, 1987). Further evidence to support a role for the dopaminergic system in Parkinson's disease ocular motor performance comes from two sources. First, patients with 'on–off' fluctuations in their akinesia show improved saccadic accuracy and smooth pursuit when 'on' (Gibson and Kennard, 1986), although Sharpe *et al.* (1986) reported no change in smooth pursuit. Secondly, a patient with MPTP parkinsonism showed dramatic saccadic hypometria and loss of smooth pursuit gain during a drug 'holiday' when his limb akinesia was very severe, and both the ocular and limb function recovered with the reintroduction of dopaminergic drugs (Hotson, Langston and Langston, 1986).

15.1.2 VESTIBULO-OCULAR REFLEX IN PARKINSON'S DISEASE

White, Saint-Cyr and Sharpe (1983a) found low vestibulo-ocular reflex gains in advanced patients although visual augmentation was preserved and proposed a mechanism involving lack of modulation in a cortical loop controlling the vestibulo-ocular reflex.

15.1.3 HIGHER LEVEL OCULAR MOTOR PROBLEMS IN PARKINSON'S DISEASE

In his tracking studies on limb movements in Parkinson's disease Flowers (1976, 1978a,b) felt that the patients had become slow and inaccurate because they were forced to make continual checks on the outside world to monitor progress rather than use a smooth internally generated command sequence. Abnormal error correction times had previously been documented (Angel, Alston and Garland, 1971). A concomitant of this was an inability to 'predict' future movement requirements in a non-random task (Flowers, 1978b). The question of error correction timing and prediction is relatively easily examined in the ocular motor system, particularly with saccades. De Jong and Melvill Jones (1971) found significant impairment in patients attempting self-paced alternating saccades between two fixed visual targets due to (a) increased fixation times, and (b) hypometria with prolonged correction times between under-shooting saccades. Gibson and Kennard (in preparation) have shown that saccadic hypometria in Parkinson's disease is improved by additional visual inputs which parallels what has been found with regard to limb tracking (Cooke, Brown and Brooks, 1978). With regards to prediction in the ocular motor system Bronstein and Kennard (1984) found impairment of predictive saccadic and smooth pursuit function as well as an inability of patients to improve their performance if the predictive nature of the stimulus was made known to them.

Patients with early untreated disease show variable, often inaccurate and perhaps minimally slowed saccades. Changes occurring with dopaminergic treatment, 'on–off' fluctuations and in MPTP poisoning suggest a role for nigrostriatal dopaminergic pathways in eye movement control. From the animal experiments discussed above, it would be expected that in Parkinson's disease there is defective disinhibition of the superior colliculus because lack of striatal dopamine leads to relative failure of inhibition of SN_r. The experimental equivalent is in the animals with muscimol injection of the superior colliculus, or bicuculline injection of SN_r. These certainly showed inaccurate hypometric saccades, but the most striking finding was saccadic slowing, which is not a feature in early Parkinson's disease. Perhaps this difference is simply due to the extent of striatal dopamine loss, or perhaps the insidious onset of the disease in humans allows time for adaptive mechanisms to develop. If the 'nigro-collicular' theory of saccadic defects is correct, a unilateral saccadic deficit away from the site of the lesion could be predicted in patients with predominantly unilateral Parkinson's disease. Carl and Wurtz (1985) have found asymmetric deficits in the execution of saccades to remembered targets. The explanation for these higher-level defects in saccadic control which lead to failure of predictive mechanisms is unknown at present.

The anatomical pathways involved in smooth pursuit function are not yet well understood, but it is known that they are widespread in the nervous system and that smooth pursuit itself is exquisitely vulnerable to the effects of disease and drugs (Leigh and Zee, 1983). The finding of parallel hand and eye smooth pursuit deficits in Parkinson's disease possibly implies a role for the basal ganglia in velocity matching of effector organ to moving target but the mechanisms are obscure.

15.2 Huntington's disease

In terms of limb motor control, Huntington's disease, in which there is loss of caudate neurones, offers a contrasting model to Parkinson's disease in which nigrostriatal dopamine is deficient (Marsden, 1985). It is, therefore, interesting to look at the ocular motor abnormalities which have been described in Huntington's disease bearing in mind, of course, that pathological changes occurring outside the caudate could be at least partly responsible. In addition, pathognomonic features of Huntington's disease, namely chorea and dementia, make ocular motor studies technically difficult, and workers probably tend to select patients with the minimum of these with the result that perhaps their results cannot be applied as generally as those in Parkinson's disease.

Starr (1967) found ocular motor abnormalities of gross proportions in three out of nine patients with Huntington's disease and pointed to a dissociation of saccadic and smooth pursuit. These subjects had virtual absence of voluntary saccades but preservation of smooth pursuit. In one case where eye movement recordings were done, an interesting blink-saccade facilitation was found, whereby saccades without blinks were excessively slow, but returned to normal if initiated with a blink. (This subject additionally failed to produce saccades with optokinetic or caloric stimuli and showed no saccadic breakdown of smooth pursuit in response to intravenous barbiturate.) Such 'blink-saccade synkinesis' has been reported in patients with cerebellar or brainstem disease, and it has been suggested that blinks could inhibit abnormal pause cell activity in the brainstem and thus allow saccades to occur (Zee *et al.*, 1983).

Saccadic–smooth pursuit dissociation was confirmed by Petit and Milbled (1973) who found most abnormality on upward gaze. Saccadic instability, akin to limb chorea, was described by Avanzini *et al.* (1979) who found that patients would frequently make saccades away from the fixation spot and, during attempted smooth pursuit, the eyes would frequently be sent off course by unwanted saccades.

The largest systematic study of ocular motor function in Huntington's disease (Leigh *et al.*, 1983), on 50 patients with objective measurements in 15, again demonstrated marked fixational difficulties, with the occurrence of very large saccades, often greater than 10°, taking the eyes off target, and saccadic intrusions occurring during smooth pursuit or attempted vergence. It seemed that the Huntington's disease patients were incapable of suppressing a saccade to an extraneous target. By contrast, patients showed great difficulty with voluntary saccadic initiation, often using a head-thrusting strategy reminiscent of congenital ocular motor apraxia (Miller, 1985), or else blinks to initiate saccades. Slow saccades and impaired smooth pursuit gain was found in advanced cases but saccadic–smooth pursuit dissociation was not seen. The vestibulo-ocular reflex was normal.

15.2.1 POSSIBLE PATHOPHYSIOLOGY OF OCULAR MOTOR ABNORMALITIES IN HUNTINGTON'S DISEASE

The most interesting finding is the fixational instability with saccades occurring at rest and during non-saccadic eye movements, because it seems to correspond to limb chorea. Distractibility and inability to suppress saccades have also been reported in man following frontal lobe lesions performed for epilepsy, in the absence of chorea (Guitton, Buchtel and Douglas, 1982). The other common clinical situation in which dopaminergic excess occurs is in Parkinson's disease patients suffering from excess L-dopa who exhibit chorea and frequent blinking. Their abnormal eye movements are, however, in marked contrast to those described in Huntington's disease, consisting of slow to and fro movements worse in darkness and suppressed by fixation (Shimizu *et al.*, 1977).

The data of Hikosaka and Wurtz discussed above show that the superior colliculus will generate unwanted saccades when released from tonic inhibition by lesioning SN_r or by pharmacological manipulation. Such loss of nigral control of the superior colliculus in Huntington's disease could result from loss of striatal gamma-aminobutyric acid. Slowing of saccades from disease within the CNS is usually ascribed to loss of burst cell function in the brainstem (Leigh and Zee, 1983), but the experiments of Hikosaka and Wurtz indicate that disruption of the superior colliculus input into the brainstem can also lead to saccadic slowing, possibly by impaired inhibition of pause cells. Further indirect support for this theory comes from a recent autopsy study on four Huntington's disease patients previously documented to have slowed vertical saccades, who did not show significant loss of cells in the rostral interstitial nucleus of the medial longitudinal fasciculus (Leigh *et al.*, 1985), an area important in the generation of such saccades (Büttner-Ennever *et al.*, 1982).

Further studies of ocular motor function in Huntington's disease are needed, in the light of the new information on the function of the SN_r and, in particular, it would be of great interest to compare subjects with rigid and non-rigid variants of the condition.

15.3 Conclusions

Alexander, De Long and Strick (1986) have proposed five parallel circuits linking the basal ganglia and cerebral cortex including a motor thalamo-cortical, and an ocular motor, circuit. They propose that each circuit is engaged in the reception of 'multiple partially overlapping corticostriate inputs which are progressively integrated in their passage through the pallidum and nigra to restricted parts of the thalamus and then back to a single cortical area'. Lidsky *et al.* (1983) see the basal ganglia acting in a 'sensory gating' capacity in that appropriate motor behaviour can be produced in response to a given set of sensory inputs. I would suggest that the rather complex ocular motor abnormalities observed in Parkinson's and Huntington's disease may demonstrate some of the overlap suggested by Alexander and may be interpreted in the terms of altered behavioural responses to sensory inputs suggested by Lidsky *et al.*

References

Ad Hoc Committee (WFN) (1981) The classification of extrapyramidal disorders. *J. Neurol. Sci.*, **51**, 311–27.

Alexander, G.E., De Long, M.R. and Strick, P.L. (1986) Parallel organisation of functionally separated circuits linking basal ganglia and cortex. *Ann. Rev. Neurosci.*, **9**, 357–81.

Angel, R.W., Alston, W. and Garland, H. (1971) L-dopa and error correction time in Parkinson's disease. *Neurology*, **21**, 1255–60.

Avanzini, G., Girotti, F., Caraceni, T. and Spreafico, R. (1979) Oculomotor disorders in Huntington's chorea. *J. Neurol. Neurosurg. Psychiat.*, **42**, 581–9.

Bender, M.B. (1980) Brain control of conjugate horizontal and vertical eye movements. *Brain*, **103**, 23–69.

Bloxham, C.A., Mindel, T.A. and Frith, C.D. (1984) Initiation and execution of predictable and unpredictable movements in Parkinson's disease. *Brain*, **104**, 371–84.

Boussaoud, D. and Joseph, J.P. (1985) Role of cat substantia nigra pars reticulata in eye and head movements II. Effects of local pharmacological injections. *Exp. Brain Res.*, **57**, 297–304.

Bronstein, A.M. and Kennard, C. (1984) Predictive eye movements in normal subjects and in Parkinson's disease, in *Theoretical and Applied Aspects of Eye Movement Research* (eds A.G. Gale and F. Johnson). Elsevier North-Holland, Amsterdam, pp. 463–72.

Büttner-Ennever, J.A., Büttner, V., Cohen, B. and Baumgartner, G. (1982) Vertical gaze paralysis and the rostral interstitial nucleus of the medial longitudinal fasciculus. *Brain*, **105**, 125–49.

Carl, J.R. and Wurtz, R.H. (1985) Asymmetry of saccadic control in patients with hemi-Parkinson's disease. *Invest. Ophthalmol. Vis. Sci.* (*Suppl.*), **26**, 258.

Cooke, J.D., Brown, J.D. and Brooks, V.B. (1978) Increase dependence of visual information for movement control in patients with Parkinson's disease. *J. Can. Sci. Neurol.*, **5**, 413–15.

Corin, M.S., Elizan, T.S. and Bender, M.B. (1972) Oculomotor dysfunction in patients with Parkinson's disease. *J. Neurol. Sci.*, **15**, 251–65.

De Jong, J.D. and Melvill Jones, G. (1971) Akinesia, hypokinesia and bradykinesia in the oculomotor system of patients with Parkinson's disease. *Exp. Neurol.*, **32**, 58–68.

Dodge, R. (1903) Five types of eye movement in the horizontal meridian plane of the field of regard. *Am. J. Physiol.*, **8**, 307–29.

Draper, I.T. and Johns, R.J. (1964) The disordered movement in Parkinson's disease and the effect of drug treatment. *Bull. Johns Hopkins Hosp.*, **115**, 465–80.

Evarts, E.V., Teravainen, H. and Calne, D.B. (1981) Reaction time in Parkinson's disease. *Brain*, **104**, 167–86.

Flowers, K.A. (1976) Visual 'closed-loop' and 'open-loop' characteristics of voluntary movement in patients with parkinsonism and intention tremor. *Brain*, **99**, 269–310.

Flowers, K.A. (1978a) Lack of prediction in the motor behaviour of Parkinson's disease. *Brain*, **101**, 35–52.

Flowers, K.A. (1978b) Some frequency response characteristics of Parkinsonism on pursuit tracking. *Brain*, **101**, 19–34.

Gibson, J.M. and Kennard, C. (1986) Quantitative study of 'on–off' fluctuations in the ocular motor system in Parkinson's disease, in *Advances in Neurology* (eds M.D. Yahr and K.J. Bergmann), vol. 45. Raven Press, New York, pp. 329–33.

Gibson, J.M., Pimlott, R.M. and Kennard, C. (1987) Oculomotor and manual tracking in Parkinson's disease and the effect of treatment. *J. Neurol. Neurosurg. Psychiat.*, **50**, 853–60.

Guitton, D., Buchtel, H.A. and Douglas, R.M. (1982) Disturbances of voluntary saccadic eye movement following discrete unilateral frontal lobe removals, in *Functional Basis of Ocular Motility Disorders* (eds G. Lennerstrand, D.S. Zee and E.L. Keller), Pergamon, Oxford, pp. 497–9.

Hikosaka, O. and Wurtz, R.H. (1983a) Visual and oculomotor functions of monkey substantia nigra pars reticulata I. Relation of visual and auditory responses to saccades. *J. Neurophysiol.*, **49**, 1230–53.

Hikosaka, O. and Wurtz, R.H. (1983b) Visual and oculomotor functions of monkey substantia nigra pars reticulata II. Visual responses related to fixation of gaze. *J. Neurophysiol.*, **49**, 1254–67.

Hikosaka, O. and Wurtz, R.H. (1983c) Visual and oculomotor functions of monkey substantia nigra pars reticulata III. Memory contingent visual and saccadic responses. *J. Neurophysiol.*, **49**, 1268–84.

Hikosaka, O. and Wurtz, R.H. (1983d) Visual and oculomotor functions of monkey substantia nigra pars reticulata IV. Relation of substantia nigra to superior colliculus. *J. Neurophysiol.*, **49**, 1285–301.

Hikosaka, O. and Wurtz, R.H. (1985a) Modification of saccadic eye movements by GABA related substances I. Effect of muscimol and bicuculline in monkey superior colliculus. *J. Neurophysiol.*, **53**, 266–91.

Hikosaka, O. and Wurtz, R.H. (1985b) Modification of saccadic eye movements by GABA related substances II. Effects of muscimol in monkey substantia nigra pars reticulata. *J. Neurophysiol.*, **53**, 292–308.

Hikosaka, O. and Wurtz, R.H. (1986) Saccadic eye movements following injection of lidocaine into the superior colliculus. *Exp. Brain Res.*, **61**, 531–9.

Hotson, J.R., Langston, E.B. and Langston, J.W. (1986) Saccade responses to dopamine in human MPTP-induced parkinsonism. *Ann. Neurol.*, **20**, 456–63.

Jayaraman, A., Batton, R.R. and Carpenter, M.B. (1977) Nigrotectal projections in the monkey: an autoradiographic study. *Brain Res.*, **135**, 147–52.

Leigh, R.J., Newman, S.A., Folstein, S.E., Lasker, A.G. and Jensen, B.A. (1983) Abnormal ocular motor control in Huntington's chorea. *Neurology*, **33**, 1268–75.

Leigh, R.J., Parhad, I.M., Clark, A.W., Büttner-Ennever, J.A. and Folstein, S.E. (1985) Brainstem findings in Huntington's disease: possible mechanisms for slow vertical saccades. *J. Neurol. Sci.*, **71**, 247–56.

Leigh, R.J. and Zee, D.S. (1983) *The Neurology of Eye Movements.* Davis, Philadelphia.

Lidsky, T.I., Manetto, C. and Schneider, J.S. (1983) A consideration of sensory factors involved in motor functions of the basal ganglia. *Brain Res. Rev.*, **9**, 133–46.

Marsden, C.D. (1985) The basal ganglia, in *Scientific Basis of Clinical Neurology* (eds M. Swash and C. Kennard). Churchill Livingstone, London, pp. 56–76.

Melvill Jones, G. and De Jong, J.D. (1971) Dynamic characteristics of saccadic eye movements in Parkinson's disease. *Exp. Neurol.*, **31**, 17–31.

Melvill Jones, G. and De Jong, J.D. (1976) Visual tracking of sinusoidal target movement in Parkinson's disease. *DRB Aviation Medical Research Unit Reports*: D.R., **225**, 271–87.

Miller, N.R. (1985) *Walsh and Hoyt's Clinical Neuroophthalmology*, 4th edn, vol. 2. Williams and Wilkins, Baltimore, pp. 750–1.

Petit, H. and Milbled, G. (1973) Anomalies of conjugate ocular movements in Huntington's chorea: application to early detection, in *Advances in Neurology* (eds A. Barbeau, T.N. Chase and G.W. Paulson), vol. 1. Raven Press, New York, pp. 287–94.

Royce, G.J. (1982) Laminar origin of cortical neurons which project upon the caudate nucleus: a horseradish peroxidase investigation in the cat. *J. Comp. Neurol.*, **205**, 8–29.

Sharpe, J.A., Fletcher, W.A., Lang, A.E. and Zackon, D.H. (1986) Smooth pursuit during dose-related on–off fluctuations in Parkinson's disease. *Neurology*, **36** (Suppl. 1), 245.

Shibasaki, H., Tsuji, S. and Koroiwa, Y. (1979) Oculomotor abnormalities in Parkinson's disease. *Arch. Neurol.*, **36**, 360–4.

Shimizu, N., Cohen, B., Bala, S.P., Meridoza, M. and Yahr, M.D. (1977) Ocular dyskinesias in patients with Parkinson's disease treated with levadopa. *Ann. Neurol.*, **1**, 167–71.

Starr, A. (1967) A disorder of rapid eye movements in Huntington's chorea. *Brain*, **90**, 545–63.

Vincent, S.R., Hattori, T. and McGeer, E.G. (1978) The nitrotectal projection: a biochemical and ultrastructural characterisation. *Brain Res.*, **151**, 159–64.

Webster, K.E. (1965) The cortico-striatal projection in the cat. *J. Anat.*, **99**, 329–37.

White, O.B., Saint-Cyr, J.A. and Sharpe, J.A. (1983a) Ocular motor deficits in Parkinson's disease. I. The horizontal vestibulo-ocular reflex and its regulation. *Brain*, **106**, 555–70.

White, O.B., Saint-Cyr, J.A., Tomlinson, R.D. and Sharpe, J.A. (1983b) Ocular motor deficits in Parkinson's disease. II. Control of the saccadic and smooth pursuit systems. *Brain*, **106**, 571–8.

Yoshida, M. and Precht, W. (1971) Monosynaptic inhibition of neurons of the substantia nigra by caudato nigral fibers. *Brain Res.*, **32**, 225–8.

Zee, D.S., Chu, P.C., Leigh, R.J., Savino, P.J., Schatz, N.J., Reingold, D.B. and Cogan, D.G. (1983) Blink-saccade synkinesis. *Neurology*, **33**, 1233–6.

CHAPTER 16

Smooth pursuit eye movements, optokinetic nystagmus and vestibulo-ocular reflex suppression

ULRICH BÜTTNER

16.1 Introduction

Smooth pursuit eye movements (SPEM) are used to track small, moving visual objects. They are found only in species with a fovea and permit the maintenance of a clear image of the moving object. Under normal circumstances not only the eyes but also the head is involved in tracking moving objects. The vestibulo-ocular reflex (VOR), which normally drives the eyes in the direction opposite to the head movement, has to be suppressed under these conditions. It appears that the central nervous system actually generates a smooth pursuit signal to cancel the VOR: accordingly, a smooth pursuit deficit is accompanied by disturbed VOR-suppression (VOR-supp.).

There is also a large body of evidence that smooth pursuit mechanisms participate in the generation of optokinetic nystagmus, i.e. the oculomotor response to large moving visual scenes. It is now established that two components contribute to the generation of optokinetic nystagmus (Cohen, Matsuo and Raphan, 1977). One is called the 'direct' component and has been related to smooth pursuit mechanisms, and can be demonstrated best by the rapid increase in slow-phase eye velocity

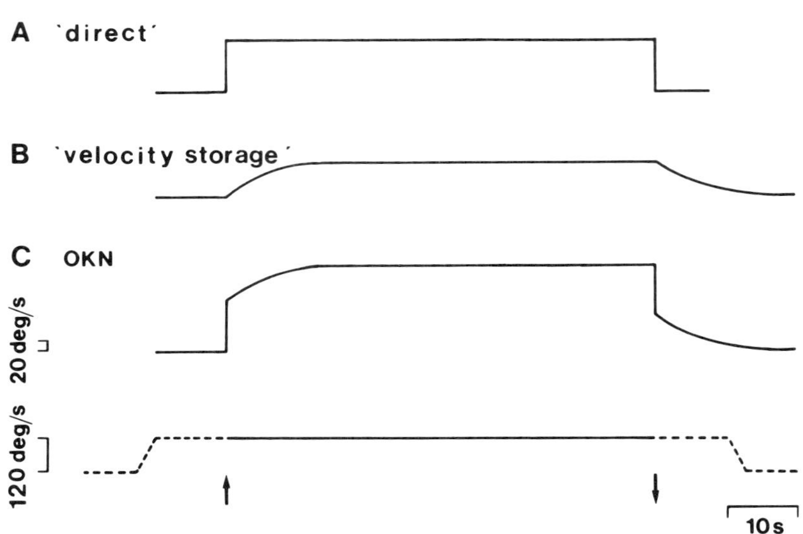

Fig. 16.1 Schematic drawing of the contribution of the 'direct' (A) and 'velocity storage' (B) component to the generation of slow-phase optokinetic nystagmus (OKN) velocity (C) in response to a high-velocity optokinetic stimulus (bottom trace). Arrows indicate light on (up) and off (down). Whereas the 'direct' component leads to rapid increase and decrease in slow-phase eye velocity after light on and off, the changes caused by the 'velocity storage' component are more gradual. The two components summate during high-velocity OKN. The continuation of nystagmus in the dark is called optokinetic after-nystagmus (OKAN). (From Simons and Büttner, 1985.)

after the sudden presentation of a constant velocity optokinetic stimulus (Fig. 16.1). In contrast, the 'indirect' or 'velocity storage' component leads to a more gradual increase in slow-phase eye velocity during continuous stimulation. It expresses itself most clearly during optokinetic after-nystagmus (OKAN) – the nystagmus which continues after the light has been turned off (Fig. 16.1; Cohen, Matsuo and Raphan, 1977; Simons and Büttner, 1985). The 'velocity storage' component can be related to changes in activity in the vestibular nuclei (Waespe and Henn, 1977).

16.2 General properties

Generally SPEM can only occur when a moving object is visible, but it is well known that a number of subjects can track their own outstretched finger in the dark, and a few can do this just by imagining a moving target.

The stimulus velocity on the fovea or perifoveal region is the most important parameter to induce SPEM, but target position is also an important factor, as can be shown by placing an afterimage near the fovea, which induces SPEM (Kommerell and Täumer, 1972). When foveal vision is prevented, SPEM can also be elicited from extra-foveal regions (Winterson and Steinman, 1978).

The latency for the initiation of SPEM is 130 ms (Robinson, 1965), which is shorter than for a saccade. Velocities of more than 100°/s can be achieved (Lisberger *et al.*, 1981; Simons and Büttner, 1985). Eye velocity is usually slightly less than stimulus velocity. The gain (eye velocity/ stimulus velocity) is better when predictable (i.e. sinusoidal) stimuli are used. With sinusoidal stimulation the gain rapidly falls off at frequencies above 1 Hz (Barnes, Benson and Prior, 1978).

An important factor for the clinical evaluation of smooth pursuit deficits is the influence of age. The decrease in performance is considerable and starts noticeably at an early age (Fig. 16.2; Sharpe and Sylvester, 1978; Simons and Büttner, 1985).

Most experimental work on SPEM has been performed in the monkey, which can be easily trained to execute SPEM, its performance being at least equal to that of man, achieving smooth pursuit velocities above 120°/s (Lisberger *et al.*, 1981); during sinusoidal tracking the gain characteristics for monkey and man are also comparable (Fuchs, 1967).

Rabbits have no fovea and hence no SPEM. Cats, with a coarse area centralis, can track small objects only at velocities below 1°/s (Evinger and Fuchs, 1978). With larger stimuli the performance improves, but still only up to 20°/s (Robinson, 1981).

If smooth pursuit signals are used to suppress the VOR, quantitative aspects of smooth pursuit performance and VOR-supp. should be the same. This has indeed been shown for man and monkey (Barnes, Benson and Prior, 1978; Lisberger *et al.*, 1981; Chambers and Gresty, 1983).

As a general rule for clinical examination, optokinetic nystagmus in the horizontal plane should reach 60°/s slow-phase velocity. The maximal response velocity depends on the size of the stimulus (Dichgans, Kolb and Wolpert, 1974). With full-field stimulation, nystagmus velocities above 120°/s can be achieved (Fig. 16.2). In general, maximal optokinetic nystagmus velocities in man are slightly higher than maximal smooth pursuit velocities. As with smooth pursuit, maximal optokinetic nystagmus velocity decreases considerably with age, about 1°/s for every year above the age of 20 (Simons and Büttner, 1985). The decrease of maximal optokinetic nystagmus velocity with age is even more pronounced than that of smooth pursuit velocity, since both components of optokinetic nystagmus, the 'direct' (smooth pursuit) and the 'velocity storage' (OKAN) component are affected by age (Fig. 16.2). With sinusoidal

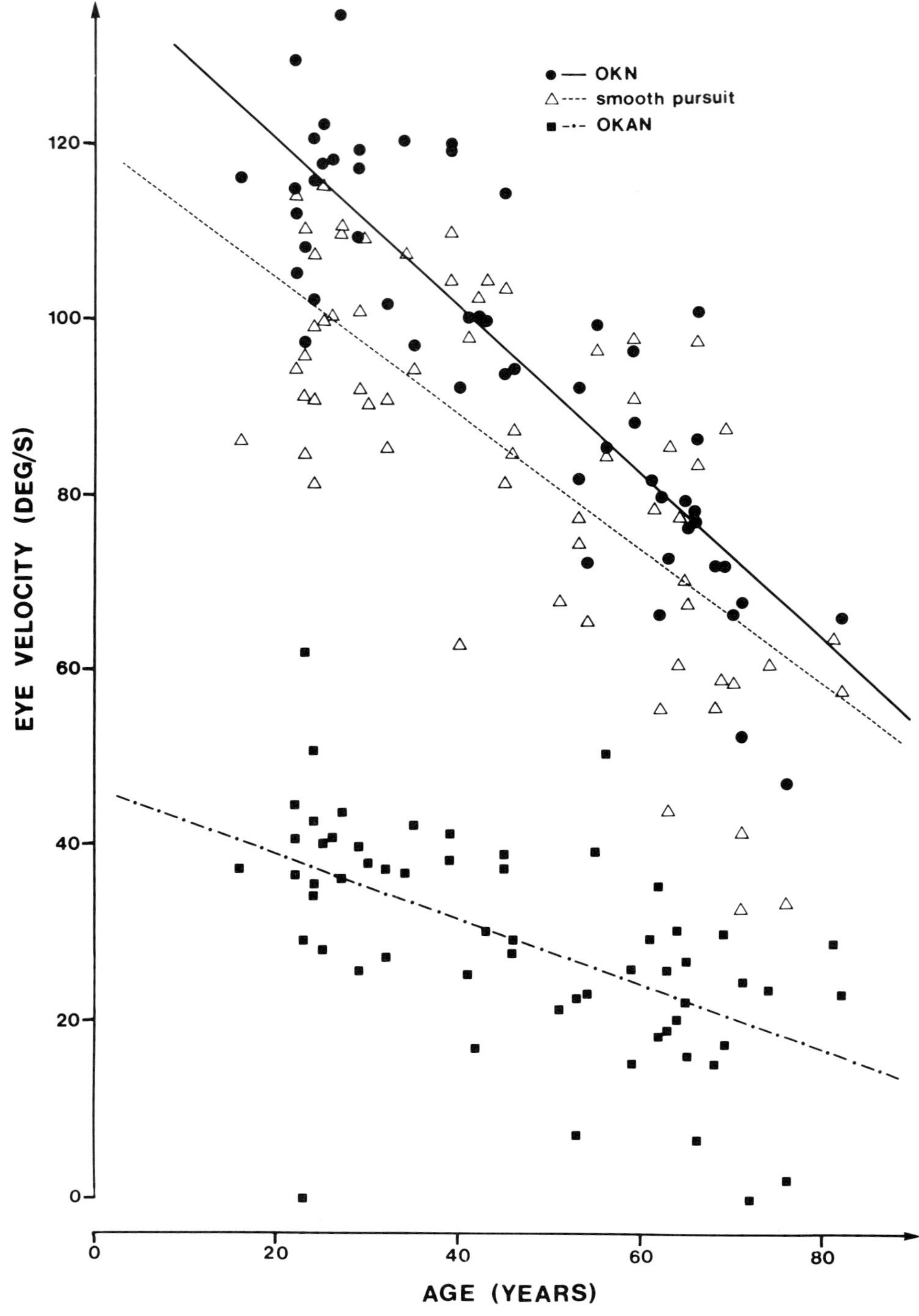

OKN
smooth pursuit
OKAN
EYE VELOCITY (DEG/S)
120
100
80
60
40
20
0
0
20
40
60
80
AGE (YEARS)

stimulation, optokinetic responses in man still can be obtained above 1 Hz (Trincker, Sieber and Bartual, 1961).

Whereas OKAN in humans is often weak, variable and sometimes virtually absent, OKAN in the monkey is much stronger and can reach values up to 80–100°/s (Cohen, Matsuo and Raphan, 1977; Büttner, Meienberg and Schimmelpfennig, 1983). With this in mind it is not surprising that maximal optokinetic nystagmus velocities can reach more than 180°/s in the monkey (Cohen, Matsuo and Raphan, 1977; Büttner, Meienberg and Schimmelpfennig, 1983), values much higher than those found in humans. Sinusoidal stimulation still leads to optokinetic responses at frequencies above 3 Hz (Paige, 1983; Boyle, Büttner and Markert, 1985). In the cat, optokinetic stimulation initially leads to slow-phase velocity of only 7°/s ('direct' component). After prolonged stimulation it reaches 25–30°/s due to the addition of the 'velocity storage' component (Evinger and Fuchs, 1978). In the rabbit, maximal optokinetic nystagmus velocity after prolonged stimulation can reach values above 40°/s (Collewijn, personal communication).

Although basically SPEM depends on an intact fovea, there is also evidence that extra-foveal regions can participate in the generation of SPEM. In both man (Winterson and Steinman, 1978) and cat (Michalski, Kossut and Zernecki, 1977) tracking movements from extra-foveal regions could be elicited, when foveal vision was prevented.

Also in the monkey extra-foveal retinal regions contribute to smooth pursuit mechanisms (Büttner, Meienberg and Schimmelpfennig, 1983). Lesions up to 12° centred on the fovea (diameter 6° in the monkey) have virtually no effect on the 'direct' (smooth pursuit) component. With larger lesions (more than 25–30° diameter) the 'direct' optokinetic nystagmus-response is still about 50% compared to the response of the normal eye (Büttner, Meienberg and Schimmelpfennig, 1983).

16.3 The neural pathway mediating smooth pursuit

Smooth pursuit eye movements are the result of a complex visuo-oculomotor transformation process, which involves many structures at

---

Fig. 16.2 Influence of age on maximal velocity of slow-phase optokinetic nystagmus (OKN), smooth pursuit eye movements (smooth pursuit) and optokinetic after-nystagmus (OKAN). Shown are the data of 63 normal subjects and the linear regression lines. All three parameters decrease with age. Note that the influence of age is even more pronounced for OKN than for smooth pursuit eye movements, which reflects that both, the 'direct' (smooth pursuit) and the 'velocity storage' (OKAN) component of OKN decrease with age. (From Simons and Büttner, 1985.)

the cortical as well as cerebellar and brainstem level. The exact anatomical pathways by which the visual signals eventually reach the oculomotor nuclei is still not fully understood. It is also not clear at which level, and how, the transformation from a visual motion to an oculomotor signal occurs. As described above, optokinetic nystagmus and smooth pursuit performance in humans are practically identical, since the 'velocity storage' component of optokinetic nystagmus is so poorly developed in man. Furthermore, optokinetic nystagmus in patients is only seldom studied in a manner which activates the 'velocity storage' component. Thus, in general, clinical studies on smooth pursuit and optokinetic nystagmus-deficits can be treated as interchangeable. One big advantage of larger optokinetic stimuli is that the selective attention necessary for foveal pursuit is not mandatory, attention being often a major problem in patients. In addition the size of the optokinetic stimuli plays a role, since smaller stimuli allow the detection of unilateral pathological findings more easily (Dichgans, Kolb and Wolpert, 1974).

16.3.1 CORTEX

Visual signals for SPEM generation reach the visual cortex via the lateral geniculate nucleus (LGN). The main processing of moving visual stimuli seems to occur in the extrastriate visual cortex which is composed of several areas. One major pathway involved in visual motion processing related to SPEM projects to the middle temporal area in the superior temporal sulcus (Maunsell and van Essen, 1983). In the monkey, neurones here encode the retinal slip of the visual target during SPEM (Wurtz and Newsome, 1985). The middle temporal area projects to the medial superior temporal area, where neurones which respond specifically during SPEM are found. Thus neurones in the medial superior temporal area encode parameters of eye velocity rather than visual parameters (Wurtz and Newsome, 1985). The medial superior temporal area projects also to the posterior parietal cortex (Maunsell and van Essen, 1983).

At present, it seems reasonable to assume that the signals relevant for SPEM are derived mainly from parietotemporal association cortex (particularly from the middle temporal, medial superior region) and have access to the brainstem and the cerebellum via the projection to the ipsilateral pontine nuclei (Fig. 16.3; Glickstein *et al.*, 1980).

Clinically, it is accepted that a cortical lesion affects SPEM mainly to the ipsilateral side (optokinetic nystagmus to the contralateral side, since nystagmus direction is labelled after the fast phase). The investigations by Davidoff *et al.* (1966) showed that cortical lesions of a variety of locations could lead to an optokinetic nystagmus-deficit, but such lesions are most effective, and occur most frequently, in the parietotemporal region,

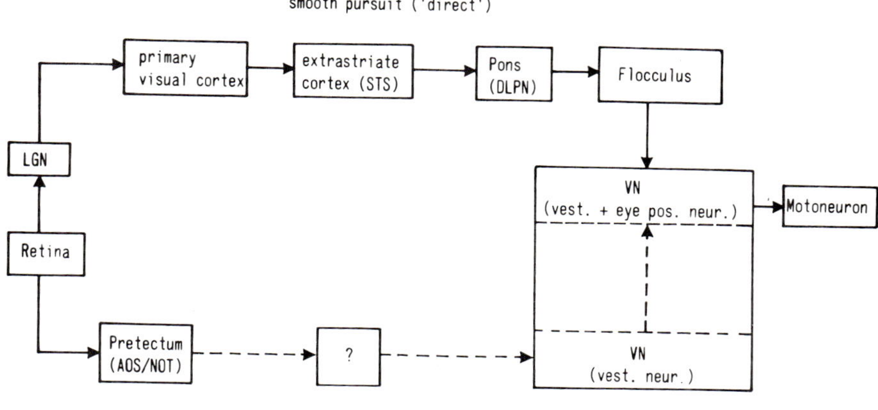

Fig. 16.3 Possible pathways for the transmission of smooth pursuit ('direct' component of OKN) signals and the 'velocity storage' component of OKN. Note that the smooth pursuit signals definitively involve the cortex and the cerebellum, whereas the 'velocity storage' component relies solely on brainstem structures. Both signals may converge at the level of the vestibular + position neurones (vest. + pos. neur.) within the vestibular nuclei, before they reach the motoneurone. Vestibular + position neurones also encode eye position during spontaneous eye movements in contrast to the vestibular only neurones (vest. only neur.). Abbreviations: AOS, nuclei of the accessory optic system; DLPN, dorsolateral pontine nucleus; LGN, lateral geniculate nucleus; STS, superior temporal sulcus; VN, vestibular nuclei.

particularly when deeper structures are involved (Kömpf, 1985). This might correspond with the middle temporal and medial superior temporal areas in the superior temporal sulcus of the monkey. Parietal cortex lesions also affect optokinetic nystagmus (Baloh, Yee and Honrubia, 1980). It is of interest that optokinetic nystagmus can be normal with lesions restricted to the calcarine cortex (Daroff and Hoyt, 1971) and even after bilateral occipital lobe lesions (Baloh, Yee and Honrubia, 1980).

16.3.2 BRAINSTEM

The paramedian pontine reticular formation (PPRF) has been clearly outlined as the immediate premotor structure for saccade generation. Unilateral lesions here lead to a loss of all saccades to the ipsilateral side, leaving SPEM intact (Henn and Büttner, 1982). Such a definitive premotor structure for SPEM has not been outlined in the brainstem. Recent experimental evidence from the monkey suggests that the dorsolateral pontine nucleus (DLPN) plays an important role in the generation of SPEM (Suzuki and Keller, 1984; May, Keller and Crandall, 1985). The DLPN receives an input from the superior temporal sulcus, where middle temporal and medial superior temporal areas are located (Glickstein *et al.*, 1980). It projects to the flocculus (Fig. 16.4; Langer *et al.*, 1985) and to the vermis lobules VI and VII (Brodal, 1979). Both cerebellar structures are involved in the control of SPEM (see below).

The brainstem also contains most of the structures essential for the generation of the 'velocity storage' component of optokinetic nystagmus. Visual signals from the retina initially reach the nuclei of the accessory optic system and the nucleus of the optic tract (Precht, 1982). Via additional, yet unknown, structures the information reaches the vestibular nuclei, where neurones are activated not only during vestibular but also during optokinetic nystagmus and afternystagmus (Waespe and Henn, 1977; Buettner and Büttner, 1979). An involvement of NRTP (nucleus reticularis tegmenti pontis) in the mediation of the 'velocity storage' component of optokinetic nystagmus has been discussed for afoveate animals and the cat, but is not supported by single unit recordings in the alert monkey (Crandall and Keller, 1985). Thus, the pathways by which the visual information for the 'velocity storage' component reaches the vestibular nuclei is still unknown. A role for the cerebellum is unlikely, since cerebellectomy does not abolish the 'velocity storage' component of optokinetic nystagmus (Keller and Precht, 1978).

Besides an involvement of vestibular nuclei in the 'velocity storage' component of optokinetic nystagmus, there is also increasing evidence that certain parts of the vestibular nuclei participate in the generation of SPEM ('direct' component of optokinetic nystagmus); this is partly based on anatomical studies, which demonstrate that the flocculus (an important structure in SPEM generation, see below) sends its efferents almost exclusively to the vestibular nuclei (Fig. 16.3; Langer *et al.*, 1985), and not to the oculomotor nuclei. However, studies in behaving monkeys did not show effects of floccular activity changes on vestibular nuclei neurones (Keller and Daniels, 1975; Buettner and Büttner, 1979), the reason probably being that these results were obtained mainly from group I and II vestibular nuclei neurones, neurones without eye position sensitivity. Lisberger and Pavelko (1984) recently demonstrated that floccular Purkinje cells in the monkey project onto group III (vestibular + position) vestibular nuclei neurones. These neurones encode eye position during spontaneous eye movements, and probably receive a disynaptic input from the vestibular nerve. Thus, functionally these group III neurones are situated between pure vestibular neurones (group I and II) and oculomotor nuclei neurones, but anatomically they lie within the

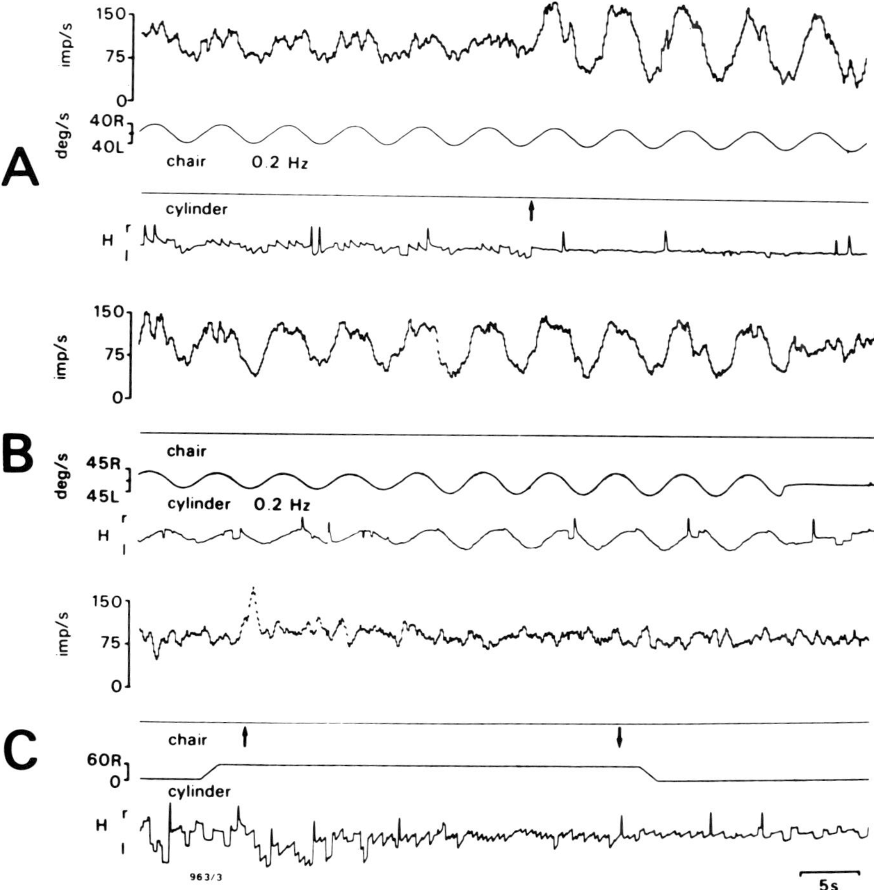

Fig. 16.4 Purkinje cell activity (simple spike) in the flocculus of the alert monkey during VOR, VOR-supp. (A), smooth pursuit eye movements (B) and constant velocity optokinetic nystagmus (C). Traces from above: neuronal activity, stimulus velocity and horizontal eye position. In (A) the monkey is sitting in the dark on a vestibular turntable and is rotated about the vertical axis. At the upward arrow he suppresses his VOR by fixating a small light spot attached to the turntable. There is strong modulation of PC activity during VOR-supp. In (B) the monkey tracks a small light spot attached to a cylinder in an otherwise dark surround. Constant velocity optokinetic stimulation (C) only leads to a transient neuronal activity increase after light on (upward arrow). Downward arrow: light off. Note that there are no activity changes after the initial transient, despite the fact that slow phase OKN-velocity in (C) and SPEM velocity in (B) are similar (Büttner and Waespe, unpublished results).

vestibular nuclei complex, and may relay floccular activity to the oculomotor nuclei (Fig. 16.3).

Clinically very little is known about specific brainstem lesions which cause SPEM or optokinetic nystagmus-deficits. There are even contradictory reports as to whether unilateral deficit arises from an ipsilateral or a contralateral lesion (Dichgans, von Reutern and Römmelt, 1978; Zackon and Sharpe, 1984). In order to distinguish smooth pursuit deficits caused by brainstem or cerebellar lesions it is, in many instances, useful to test for vestibular responses as well. These are often enhanced in cerebellar, and reduced in brainstem lesions (Dichgans and Jung, 1975). If prolonged optokinetic stimulation leads to nearly normal optokinetic nystagmus velocities (Yee *et al.*, 1979), intact brainstem structures are likely, since the 'velocity storage' component of optokinetic nystagmus depends almost exclusively on brainstem structures, in contrast to the 'direct' (smooth pursuit) component, which definitively requires cortical as well as cerebellar structures.

16.3.3 CEREBELLUM

The flocculus, as part of the vestibulo-cerebellum, is the structure most intensively investigated in relation to SPEM. In the monkey, lesions here lead to impaired SPEM, VOR-supp. and optokinetic nystagmus (Zee *et al.*, 1981). A group of Purkinje cells, the only output element of the cerebellum, also responds specifically during these paradigms (Lisberger and Fuchs, 1978; Waespe and Henn, 1981; Büttner and Waespe, 1984).

Specifically, these Purkinje cells respond during SPEM under all conditions but, during constant velocity optokinetic stimulation, only at slow-phase eye velocities above 40–60°/s, i.e. the OKAN saturation velocity (Fig. 16.4). However, the same Purkinje cells respond vigorously during sinusoidal optokinetic stimulation at frequencies above 0.1 Hz over the whole eye velocity range (Büttner, Boyle and Markert, 1986). These findings are considered as evidence that the same neuronal elements encode parameters of SPEM and the 'direct' component of optokinetic nystagmus. They also led to the flocculus/vestibular nuclei complementary hypothesis (Waespe and Henn, 1981) according to which the vestibular nuclei subserve certain, generally more basic, oculomotor functions, like the VOR and low constant-velocity optokinetic nystagmus. In contrast, Purkinje cells in the flocculus are modulated, whenever the vestibular nuclei cannot provide a response pattern, which would allow oculomotor responses with a minimal retinal slip to visual stimuli, as is the case during SPEM, VOR-supp., high constant-velocity and sinusoidal optokinetic nystagmus above 0.1 Hz (Fig. 16.5).

It should be stressed, that lesions of the flocculus do not abolish SPEM

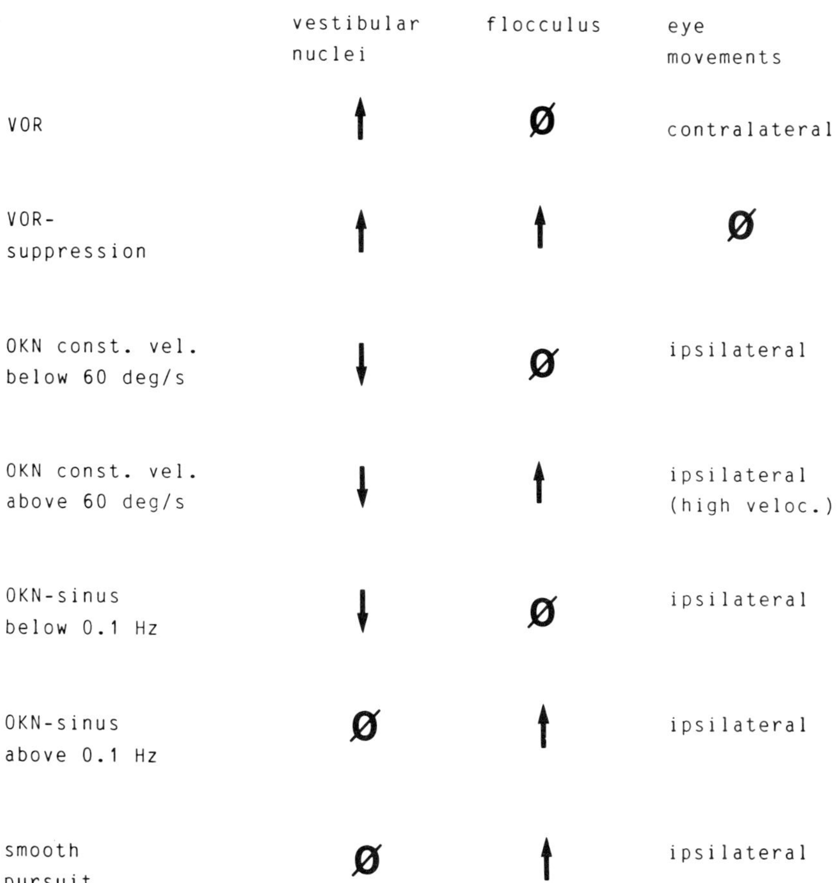

Fig. 16.5 Complementary activity of a vestibular nuclei (vestibular only) neurone and a Purkinje cell in the flocculus during different oculomotor paradigms. The responses to stimuli (vestibular, optokinetic and smooth pursuit) moving ipsilaterally to the recording side are shown qualitatively. This leads to activation (upward arrow) during the VOR for the vestibular nuclei neurone and during smooth pursuit eye movements for the Purkinje cell. Downward arrow: decrease in neuronal activity. Ø: no changes. Direction and occurrence of *slow* eye movement component is shown on the right. Note that it can be predicted from vestibular nuclei and flocculus activity alone. (From Büttner, Boyle and Markert, 1986).

completely (Zee *et al.*, 1981) but total cerebellectomy does (Westheimer and Blair, 1974). It is therefore likely that other cerebellar structures besides the flocculus are involved in smooth pursuit generation. One likely candidate is the posterior vermis (lobule VI and VII). Here Purkinje cells have been found in the alert monkey, which are modulated during SPEM (Suzuki, Noda and Kase, 1981). In contrast to Purkinje cells in the flocculus, those in the vermis are also activated by moving visual stimuli.

16.4 Comments and unsolved problems

For all clinical purposes the results of SPEM and optokinetic nystagmus investigations are comparable, since optokinetic nystagmus in man is mainly determined by the 'direct' (smooth pursuit) component. The 'velocity storage' component of optokinetic nystagmus is weak and very variable; and furthermore it requires optokinetic stimulation which must last 10–20 s, and must be of high and constant-velocity before a definite contribution of the 'velocity storage' optokinetic nystagmus component can be demonstrated (Simons and Büttner, 1985). Even in the monkey with a much stronger 'velocity storage' component, sinusoidal optokinetic stimulation at a frequency as low as 0.05 Hz is insufficient to drive the 'velocity storage' component (Boyle, Büttner and Markert, 1985). These are parameters generally not applied during bedside examination with a hand-held optokinetic cylinder.

On the other hand, in an evaluation of the experimental literature, smooth pursuit mechanisms and optokinetic nystagmus have to be clearly distinguished. Most work on optokinetic nystagmus has been done on species which have no smooth pursuit mechanism. Thus an optokinetic nystagmus study in the rabbit cannot be compared with studies in man.

An isolated disturbance of smooth pursuit has clinically very little localizing value since, as pointed out, the cerebral cortex as well as the brainstem and the cerebellum are involved in its generation. Therefore additional oculomotor signs like spontaneous nystagmus, gaze-holding nystagmus, vestibular responses and other neurological symptoms are required to provide a definitive topographical diagnosis.

Since a disturbance in smooth pursuit can be the result of a lesion in either the visual motion processing system or the immediate premotor structures, investigations in which visual motion sensitivity is tested in conjunction with SPEM might be helpful in distinguishing between cortical and infratentorial lesions. Another problem could be the relation of target and background motion in patients. Smooth pursuit performance is normally little affected by the background (i.e. SPEM in dark, background moving in the same or opposite direction) (Collewijn *et al.*, 1982), but extended studies in patients have not so far been performed.

Acknowledgements

The author wishes to thank Ms B. Liebold and B. Pfreunder for typing the manuscript.

References

Baloh, R.W., Yee, R.D. and Honrubia, V. (1980) Optokinetic nystagmus and parietal lobe lesions. *Ann. Neurol.*, **7**, 269–76.

Barnes, G.R., Benson, A.J. and Prior, A.R.J. (1978) Visual-vestibular interaction in the control of eye movement. *Aviat. Space Environ. Med.*, **49**, 557–64.

Boyle, R. Büttner, U. and Markert, G. (1985) Vestibular nuclei activity and eye movements in the alert monkey during sinusoidal optokinetic stimulation. *Exp. Brain Res.*, **57**, 362–9.

Brodal, P. (1979) The pontocerebellar projection in the rhesus monkey: an experimental study with retrograde axonal transport of horseradish peroxidase. *Neuroscience*, **4**, 193–208.

Buettner, U.W. and Büttner, U. (1979) Vestibular nuclei activity in the alert monkey during suppression of vestibular and optokinetic nystagmus. *Exp. Brain Res.*, **37**, 581–93.

Büttner, U. and Waespe, W. (1984) Purkinje cell activity in the primate flocculus during optokinetic stimulation, smooth pursuit eye movements and VOR-suppression. *Exp. Brain Res.*, **55**, 97–104.

Büttner, U., Boyle, R. and Markert, G. (1986) Cerebellar control of eye movements, in *The Oculomotor and Skeletalmotor Systems: Differences and Similarities* (eds H.-J. Freund, U. Büttner, B. Cohen and J. Noth). Elsevier, Amsterdam, pp. 225–33.

Büttner, U., Meienberg, O. and Schimmelpfennig, B. (1983) The effect of central retinal lesions on optokinetic nystagmus in the monkey. *Exp. Brain Res.*, **52**, 248–56.

Chambers, B.R. and Gresty, M.A. (1983) The relationship between disordered pursuit and vestibulo-ocular reflex suppression. *J. Neurol. Neurosurg. Psychiat.*, **46**, 61–6.

Cohen, B., Matsuo, V. and Raphan, T. (1977) Quantitative analysis of the velocity characteristics of optokinetic nystagmus and optokinetic after-nystagmus. *J. Physiol.*, **270**, 321–44.

Collewijn, H., Conijn, P., Martins, A.J., Tamminga, E.P. and Van Die, G.C. (1982) Control of gaze in man: synthesis of pursuit, optokinetic and vestibulo-ocular systems, in *Physiological and Pathological Aspects of Eye Movements* (eds A. Roucoux and M. Crommelinck). Junk Publishers, The Hague, pp. 3–22.

Crandall, W.F. and Keller, E.L. (1985) Visual and oculomotor signals in nucleus reticularis tegmenti pontis in alert monkey. *J. Neurophysiol.*, **54**, 1326–45.

Daroff, R.B. and Hoyt, W.F. (1971) Supranuclear disorders of ocular control systems in man: clinical, anatomical, and physiological correlations, in *The*

Control of Eye Movements (eds P. Bach-y-Rita, C.C. Collins and J.E. Hyde). Academic Press, New York, pp. 175–236.

Davidoff, R.A., Atkin, A., Anderson, P.J. and Bender, M.B. (1966) Optokinetic nystagmus and cerebral disease. *Arch. Neurol.* (*Chicago*), **14**, 73–81.

Dichgans, J. and Jung, R. (1975) Oculomotor abnormalities due to cerebellar lesions, in *Basic Mechanisms of Ocular Motility and their Clinical Implications* (eds G. Lennerstrand and P. Bach-y-Rita). Pergamon, Oxford, pp. 281–98.

Dichgans, J., Kolb., B. and Wolpert, E. (1974) Provokation optokinetischer Seitendifferenzen durch Einschränkung der Reizfeldbreite und ihre Bedeutung für die Klinik. *Arch. Psychiat. Nervenkr.*, **219**, 117–31.

Dichgans, J., von Reutern, G.M. and Römmelt, U. (1978) Impaired suppression of vestibular nystagmus by fixation in cerebellar and non-cerebellar patients. *Arch. Psychiat. Nervenkr.*, **226**, 183–99.

Evinger, C. and Fuchs, A.F. (1978) Saccadic, smooth pursuit and optokinetic eye movements of the trained cat. *J. Psysiol.* (*Lond.*), **285**, 209–29.

Fuchs, A.F. (1967) Periodic eye tracking in the monkey. *J. Physiol.* (*Lond.*), **193**, 161–71.

Glickstein, M., Cohen, J.L., Dixon, B., Gibson, A., Hollins, M., Labossiere, E. and Robinson, F. (1980) Corticopontine visual projections in macaque monkeys. *J. Comp. Neurol.*, **190**, 209–29.

Henn, V. and Büttner, U. (1982) Disorders of horizontal gaze, in *Functional Basis of Oculomotor Motility Disorders* (eds G. Lennerstrand, E. Zee and E. Keller), Pergamon, Oxford, pp. 431–9.

Keller, E.L. and Daniels, P.D. (1975) Oculomotor related interaction of vestibular and visual stimulation in vestibular nucleus cells in alert monkey. *Exp. Neurol.*, **46**, 187–98.

Keller, E.L. and Precht, W. (1978) Persistence of visual response in vestibular nucleus neurons in cerebellectomized cat. *Exp. Brain Res.*, **32**, 591–4.

Kömpf, D. (1985) The significance of optokinetic nystagmus asymmetry in hemispheric lesions. *Neuro-Ophthalmology*, **6**, 61–4.

Kommerell, G. and Täumer, R. (1972) Investigations of the eye tracking system through stabilized retinal images, in *Cerebral Control of Eye Movements and Motion Perception* (eds J. Dichgans and E. Bizzi). Karger, Basel, *Bibliothec Ophthalmol.*, **82**, 288–97.

Langer, T., Fuchs, A.F., Scudder, C.A. and Chubb, M.C. (1985) Afferents to the flocculus of the cerebellum in the rhesus macaque as revealed by retrograde transport of horseradish peroxidase. *J. Comp. Neurol.*, **235**, 1–25.

Lisberger, S.G., Evinger, C., Johanson, G.W. and Fuchs, A.F. (1981) Relationship between eye acceleration and retinal image velocity during foveal smooth pursuit in man and monkey. *J. Neurophysiol.*, **46**, 229–49.

Lisberger, S.G. and Fuchs, A.F. (1978) Role of primate flocculus during rapid behavioral modification of vestibuloocular reflex. I. Purkinje cell activity during visually guided horizontal smooth-pursuit eye movements and passive head rotation. *J. Neurophysiol.*, **41**, 733–63.

Lisberger, S.G. and Pavelko, T.A. (1984) Functional properties of brainstem cells inhibited from the cerebellar flocculus in monkey. *Soc. Neurosci., Abstr.*, **10**, 988.

Maunsell, J.H.R. and van Essen, D.C. (1983) The connections of the middle temporal visual area (MT) and their relationship to a cortical hierarchy in the macaque monkey. *J. Neurosci.*, **3**, 2563–86.

May, J.G., Keller, E.L. and Crandall, W.F. (1985) Changes in eye velocity during smooth pursuit tracking induced by microstimulation in the dorsolateral pontine nucleus of the macaque. *Soc. Neurosci., Abstr.*, **11**, 79.

Michalski, A., Kossut, M. and Zernecki, B. (1977) The ocular following reflex elicited from the retinal periphery in the cat. *Vision Res.*, **17**, 731–6.

Paige, G.D. (1983) Vestibuloocular reflex and its interactions with visual following mechanisms in the squirrel monkey. I. Response characteristics in normal animals. *J. Neurophysiol.*, **49**, 134–51.

Precht, W. (1982) Anatomical and functional organisation of optokinetic pathways, in *Functional Basis of Ocular Motility Disorders* (eds G. Lennerstrand, D.S. Zee and E.L. Keller). Pergamon, Oxford, pp. 291–302.

Robinson, D.A. (1965) The mechanics of human smooth pursuit eye movement. *J. Physiol. (Lond.)*, **180**, 569–91.

Robinson, D.A. (1981) Control of eye movements, in *Handbook of Physiology. Section 1: The Nervous System* (ed. V.B. Brooks), vol. II, part 2. American Physiology Society, Bethesda, MD, pp. 1275–320.

Sharpe, J.A. and Sylvester, T.O. (1978) Effect of aging on horizontal smooth pursuit. *Invest. Ophthalmol.*, **17**, 465–8.

Simons, B. and Büttner, U. (1985) The influence of age on optokinetic nystagmus. *Eur. Arch. Psychiat. Neurol. Sci.*, **234**, 369–73.

Suzuki, D.A. and Keller, E.L. (1984) Visual signals in the dorsolateral pontine nucleus of the alert monkey: their relationship to smooth pursuit eye movements. *Exp. Brain Res.*, **53**, 473–8.

Suzuki, D.A., Noda, H. and Kase, M. (1981) Visual and pursuit eye movement-related activity in posterior vermis of monkey cerebellum. *J. Neurophysiol.*, **46**, 1120–39.

Trincker, D., Sieber, J. and Bartual, J. (1961) Schwingungsanalyse der vestibulär, optokinetisch und durch elektrische Reizung ausgelösten Augenbewegungen beim Menschen. I. Mitteilung. Stetige Augenbewegungen: Frequenzgänge und Ortskurven. *Kybernetik*, **1**, 21–8.

Waespe, W. and Henn, V. (1977) Vestibular nuclei activity during optokinetic after-nystagmus (OKAN) in the alert monkey. *Exp. Brain Res.*, **30**, 323–30.

Waespe, W. and Henn, V. (1981) Visual-vestibular interaction in the flocculus of the alert monkey. II Purkinje cell activity. *Exp. Brain Res.*, **43**, 349–60.

Westheimer, G. and Blair, S.M. (1974) Functional organization of primate oculomotor system revealed by cerebellectomy. *Exp. Brain Res.*, **21**, 463–72.

Winterson, B.J. and Steinman, R.M. (1978) The effect of luminance on human smooth pursuit of perifoveal and foveal targets. *Vision Res.*, **18**, 1165–72.

Wurtz, R.H. and Newsome, W.T. (1985) Divergent signals encoded by neurons in extrastriate areas MT and MST during smooth pursuit eye movements. *Soc. Neurosci., Abstr.*, **11**, 1246.

Yee, R.D., Baloh, R.W., Honrubia, V., Lau, C.G.Y. and Jenkins, H.A. (1979) Slow build-up of optokinetic nystagmus associated with downbeat nystagmus. *Invest. Ophthalmol. Vis. Sci.*, **18**, 622–9.

Zackon, D.H. and Sharpe, J.A. (1984) Midbrain paresis of horizontal gaze. *Ann. Neurol.*, **16**, 495–504.

Zee, D.S., Yamazaki, A., Butler, P.H. and Gücer, G. (1981) Effects of ablation of flocculus and paraflocculus on eye movements in primates. *J. Neurophysiol.*, **46**, 878–99.

CHAPTER 17

The vestibulo-ocular reflex

H. COLLEWIJN AND L. FERMAN

The vestibulo-ocular reflex (VOR) is one of the earliest recognized and most extensively studied neuronal systems so that any attempt to review the vast literature dealing with its many aspects would far exceed the scope of this chapter. General reviews covering the work up to the early seventies have been compiled by Cohen (1971, 1974), and more recent comprehensive sources are Wilson and Melvill Jones (1979), Granit and Pompeiano (1979), Cohen (1981) and Berthoz and Melvill Jones (1985).

Clinical interest in the VOR has been intense ever since Bárány's work early in this century, mainly because the VOR can be used as a tool for assessing function of the otherwise inaccessible vestibular organ. Malfunction of the VOR can express itself in oculomotor problems such as nystagmus or oscillopsia (for reviews of the clinical aspects of VOR, see Baloh and Honrubia, 1979, and Leigh and Zee, 1983). In this chapter we shall concentrate first on the intricacy of the VOR as a highly sophisticated control system, which makes it much more elaborate than a simple reflex. Subsequently, we shall summarize our recent work on the performance of the VOR – in the widest sense – under physiological conditions.

The functional significance of the VOR is the generation of compensatory eye movements which stabilize the direction of gaze. Whenever the head moves in space, similar but opposite movements of the eye in the head should be generated to prevent intolerable motion of the retinal image. In a simple view of the VOR, head motions will be sensed by the accelerometers of the vestibular organ; the relevant signals may be transmitted within milliseconds to the extra-ocular muscles through reflex arcs which may be as short as three neurones. Pioneers exploring this three-neurons reflex arc (Lorente de Nó, 1933; Szentágothai, 1950) were well aware that it represented the mere skeleton of the VOR. Nevertheless, in subsequent years, there has been a tendency to neglect the complexities of neuronal processing and to account for induced eye movements mainly in terms of vestibular mechanics. The mechanical properties of sensory and effector organs undoubtedly have functional consequences for the VOR, but in recent years we have become much more aware of the complexity and flexibility of central data processing required to optimize the performance of the VOR.

The VOR in the narrow sense uses only the labyrinth as its sensory input; therefore it is measured in total darkness. Paradoxically, by thus isolating the VOR as a system we also deprive it of its only function, the stabilization of gaze. The testing of any system under non-functional circumstances is problematic, and we shall see that the VOR is no exception. The elimination of vision deprives the VOR not only of its goal, but also of a considerable part of its specifications and instructions. As a consequence, the significance of data obtained in darkness is doubtful.

17.1 Maculo-ocular and canal-ocular reflexes

The labyrinth provides two kinds of signals (for detailed description, see Wilson and Melvill Jones, 1979). The otolith organs, utriculus and sacculus, contain hair cells organized in maculae that respond to linear accelerations. There are various sectors in which the hair cells are oriented systematically in different directions. Therefore, in the assembly of macular afferents both the magnitude and the direction of the linear acceleration vector can be properly encoded in three dimensions. The main, continuously present stimulus for the otolith organs is the gravity vector, representing the objective vertical. This parameter is of primary importance in the regulation of posture, and the principal function of the otolith organs is to signal the orientation of the head with respect to the vertical. In addition to functioning in postural control, these signals can be used in maculo-ocular reflexes to maintain an upright position of the eye. The relevant directions of control are obviously vertical and torsional, not horizontal. The ocular displacements should offset head tilt in a sideways or antero-posterior direction. Such responses are usually well developed in animals with a relatively primitive visual system; among mammals the rabbit is a good example (Van der Hoeve and De Kleijn, 1917; Baarsma and Collewijn, 1975; Van der Steen and Collewijn, 1984). In humans the maculo-ocular reflexes are vestigial; they can, however, be observed as a consistent but very small sustained counter-roll of the eye when the head is tilted around the sagittal axis (see Collewijn *et al.*, 1985a; Simonsz, 1985).

The three pairs of semicircular canals, oriented in three almost orthogonal planes, are normally only sensitive to rotatory accelerations. The mechanical properties of the canal–endolymph–cupula system result essentially in an integration of the forces exerted by the rotatory acceleration over time, at least in the physiological frequency range of head movements. As a result, the modulation of the discharge rate in the primary canal afferent corresponds closely to the changes in the head's angular velocity. The processing of such signals in the canal-ocular reflexes should generate eye velocities exactly opposite in direction and magnitude to the head velocity. Velocity, not position, is the relevant parameter in this reflex. Although velocity compensation implies positional stabilization, the latter is not absolute. Especially during rotations through larger angles the smooth, compensatory eye movement is frequently interrupted by saccadic resets. The alternating saccadic and smooth components, which have opposite directions with respect to the head, constitute the characteristic waveform of vestibular nystagmus. In relation to stationary surroundings, gaze is stabilized in the intersaccadic intervals and rapidly displaced during the saccades.

The canal-ocular reflexes are highly active in most vertebrates, including man, which suggests that velocity compensation is a highly effective way to fulfil the visual system's needs for a restricted range of retinal image slip. In contrast to maculo-ocular reflexes, canal-ocular reflexes can stabilize the retinal image in any plane, including the horizontal one, without enforcing any particular position of the eye.

17.2 First requirements of neuronal processing

The task of the nervous system is to relay the vestibular signals to the extra-ocular muscles in such a way that eye movements are commensurate with head movements at all times. The eye movements should have the appropriate dimension, direction and magnitude.

Correct dimensionality means that a change in head tilt position should result in a similar change in eye position, but a head velocity should be expressed in a similar eye velocity, not an eye position. This requires neuronal operations which are by no means trivial. The vestibular organs as well as the eye in the orbit (often called 'the plant') have complex, dissimilar transfer functions (frequency responses). The canals produce a velocity signal which lags head acceleration by about 90° in the usual range of head movements, but phase is progressively advanced at low frequencies. This is caused by the 'leakiness' of the mechanical process of integration in the canals, which has a time constant of 3–5 s in most animals (Fernandez and Goldberg, 1971; Blanks, Estes and Markham, 1975). The transfer function between oculomotor neurone discharge rate and eye position is entirely different. At lower frequencies, motoneurones code primarily position, but at higher frequencies of modulation the eye position shows an increasing lag due to the visco-elastic properties of the eye in the orbit, which has low pass characteristics with a time constant of about 1 s. Since the vestibular and oculomotor frequency responses do not match, the neuronal circuits will have to make up for the difference (Skavenski and Robinson, 1973; Robinson, 1975; Miles, Optican and Lisberger, 1985). These processes have to be totally different for the maculo-ocular and canal-ocular reflexes; in the latter case a process of mathematical integration (velocity to position) is absolutely necessary. Several circuits which could accomplish such an integration have been proposed (Cannon and Robinson, 1985) but the tracing of this operation in neurophysiological experiments is very difficult.

Correct directionality is another major problem. To be appropriate, compensatory eye movements have to be made in the same plane as the head movements. In the case of the canal-ocular reflexes there is a certain congruence between the orientation of the canals and the several pairs of ocular muscles. This relation is quite close in the rabbit (Simpson and Graf, 1981, 1985) but even in humans it has been conserved to a certain degree. However, it has long been known that all canals can influence the activity in all eye muscles. To achieve the right amount of coupling between the several input and output components for an appropriate co-ordinate transformation, mutli-dimensional matrix operations have to be executed (Robinson, 1982b, 1985). Some investigators prefer to model such operations in terms of tensor networks (Pellionisz and Llinás, 1982), although this approach has been under some attack (Arbib and Amari, 1985). The details of the neuronal operations affecting the proper corrections of co-ordinate systems and transfer functions are virtually unknown, although it is most likely that vestibular nuclei, parts of the cerebellum and the reticular formation, and the prepositus hypoglossi nucleus are involved.

The operation of a corrective network with the properties just described would enable the functioning of a primitive, unsophisticated type of VOR, if at least a system for the appropriate insertion of saccades is also added. What is still lacking is the correct magnitude of the responses.

17.3 Gain regulation of the VOR

Proper scaling is, of course, essential to a meaningful function of the VOR, especially in primates with foveal vision. An incorrect ratio between eye and head movements (gain) would result in the inability of a subject to keep a visual target within the fovea in the presence of any substantial head motion. However, the specification of an optimal gain for the VOR is neither simple nor constant. Although at first glance a unity gain would seem ideal to maintain retinal image stability, this is not the case, since it would be true only if the head and the eyes would rotate around coinciding axes. Such a situation does not occur physiologically. The two eyes have centres of rotation separated by about 65 mm; each of them is separated from the rotatory axes of the head by distances of the order of 10 cm. Thus, the rotatory axes of head and eye have different distances to a fixed target and, in addition, any head rotation will cause a translation (linear displacement) of the eyes in space. As a result, a one-to-one relation between the angular rotations of eye and head will be inappropriate to maintain fixation, except for targets at optical infinity. For closer targets ocular rotations should be larger than head rotations; the difference is already about 10% for targets at a distance of 1 m. These elementary geometrical relations alone necessitate great flexibility of VOR gain (Blakemore and Donaghy, 1980; Collewijn, Conijn and Tamminga, 1982).

There is no doubt that humans have the ability to control the effective gain of the VOR over a wide range. For instance, during head movements we can easily fixate a target which moves through the same angle as the head. Effectively, we suppress the VOR under such circumstances, and this paradigm has been studied fairly extensively in recent years (see Robinson, 1982a).

We can ensivage two possible mechanisms to accomplish the adjustment of the eye movements to the appropriate size. First, the VOR might generate a rough correction, which compensates a lot of the head motion but leaves errors, to be acted upon secondarily by other systems, such as the optokinetic and smooth pursuit system. In this view, the VOR and visual pursuit would interact in an essentially *additive* way, with each system retaining its own characteristics of operation. Secondly, non-vestibular (e.g. visual) information could actually *change* the operational parameters of the VOR, setting the gain and possibly other parameters to a different level (see, e.g., Schmid, Zambarbieri and Magenes, 1981). This type of interaction would be essentially non-linear.

The first type of interaction undoubtedly occurs. Whenever VOR gain is inappropriate the retinal displacement of a fixated target will activate the smooth pursuit system. A simple analysis of this interaction shows that it is self-corrective and safe to use. The VOR is a feed-forward system; vestibular input drives the eyes but there is no direct feedback from the eye muscles to the labyrinth. In contrast, visual pursuit is initiated by retinal image motion and acts also on retinal position. Thus, it is a negative feedback system, which will in principle always reduce errors and adjust the eye movements towards an appropriate velocity. Although feedback systems are ideal in this respect, they are often relatively slow and when they contain a delay their response to high frequencies must be restricted to prevent unstable, oscillatory behaviour.

Feed-forward systems are fast and stable, but they have one large problem. Whereas in feedback systems the gain is not very critical, and should be essentially as high as compatible with stability, the output of a feed-forward system is directly proportional to its gain. If the VOR would really operate as a feed-forward system, how could it ever have an even approximately correct gain? Genetic design usually needs environmental correction; moreover, in the span of time of a human life many changes occur such as growth, illness, trauma and ageing, involving substantial changes of tissues and neurones.

Once more it is clear that a rigid layout of vestibulo-oculomotor coupling would be functionally disastrous. This line of thinking has led in the past decade to numerous experiments on adaptation and plasticity which strongly support the second, non-linear kind of interaction between the visual and vestibular system. These experiments have clearly shown that on a medium (minutes–hours) and long-term (days–weeks) basis the properties of the VOR can be altered such that retinal image stability is improved (for review, see Berthoz and Melvill Jones, 1985).

17.4 Adaptation of the VOR

The general design of adaptation experiments is as follows. First, the VOR is measured in isolation, in darkness. Then head movements are made for some time (minutes–days) with a modified visual input. From time to time the VOR is tested again in darkness, and systematic changes related to the visual modification are evaluated. The visual modifications consist of a change in the magnitude or direction of the visual motion signals associated with the head movement. Changes in magnification are usually induced by the wearing of magnifying or minifying spectacles, which are a common reason for the adjustment of VOR gain in man. Changes in the expected direction have indeed been found in a variety of experiments of this kind on animals and humans (Miles and Fuller, 1974; Gauthier and Robinson, 1975; Miles and Eighmy, 1980; Collewijn, Martins and Steinman, 1983; Cannon *et al.*, 1985).

A change in the direction of the VOR, e.g. the induction of a vertical oculomotor component in response to horizontal head motion, is also readily achieved (Schultheis and Robinson, 1981; Callan and Ebenholtz, 1982; Baker *et al.*, 1986; Harrison *et al.*, 1986). Even complete reversal of VOR direction (180° phase shift) by adaptation to inverting prisms (actually one of the first paradigms tested) is attainable, though with considerable difficulty (Melvill Jones, 1985).

In other types of experiment, continuous unidirectional drifting of the visual surroundings induced a sustained drift of the eyes and a directional bias of the VOR, probably due to an unbalancing of the VOR (Clément *et al.*, 1981; Harris and Cynader, 1981). Thus, it is evident that the neuronal matrix controlling the VOR can be reprogrammed to a large, although probably limited, extent. The induced changes are sustained for a relatively long time in the absence of visual information conflicting with the new condition.

The time course of these adaptations is of great interest. We can distinguish the changes in the light, with the modified visual conditions present, from those in the dark. The changes in the light reflect the adaptation to the new situation where it really matters, i.e. when vision is used. Performance in the dark reflects the level to which the new conditions have changed the system more permanently. One might consider these as situations with new instructions being actually presented (light) or being memorized (dark). The adaptation while the light is on is much faster – though not necessarily instantaneous – than the more permanent changes recorded in darkness. Examples are shown in Fig. 17.1 for two myopic subjects who changed their normal, negative glasses for +5 diopter spectacles (Collewijn, Martins and Steinman, 1983).

In the light, a large part (subject AM) or even all (subject HC) of the required increase in gain was reached immediately, with some further, slower adaptation over the next 10–30 min (subject AM). The adaptive changes measured for the VOR in darkness were slower in the beginning, but for this modest change (magnification by about 35%) they were fairly complete after 40 min. Although it is possible that the quick adaptation in the light is simply due to the additive activity of separate VOR and smooth pursuit circuits, it may be more fruitful to hypothesize that the fast adaptation in the light and the slow adaptation in the dark actually use the same circuits. The only difference would be in the permanence of the changes.

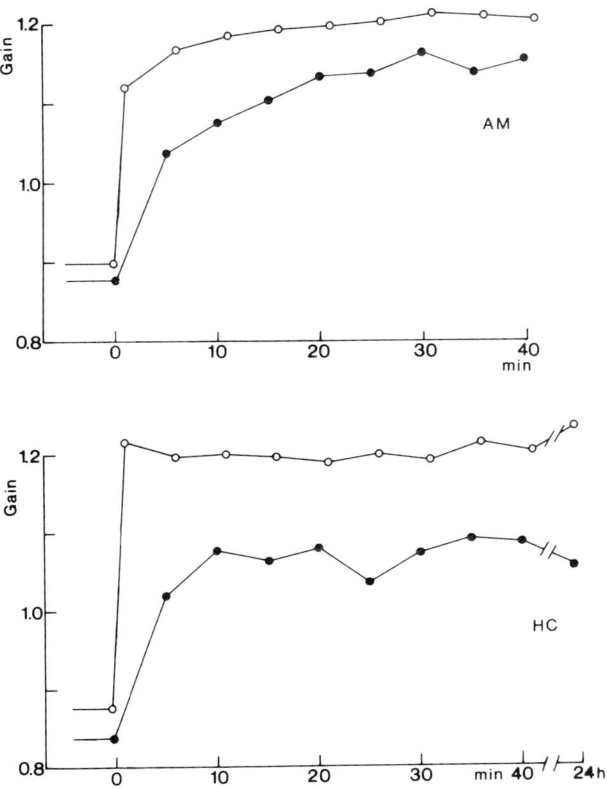

Fig. 17.1 Adaptation of VOR gain in the light (open circles) and dark (dots) after switching from normal, negative to + 5 D spectacles by two myopic subjects. By this procedure magnification was changed by a factor 1.35. In subject HC the VOR was also evaluated after 24 h continuous wearing of the + 5 D glasses. (After Collewijn, Martins and Steinman, 1983.)

17.5 The VOR as a more general system

It is clear that visual information is used to assist and/or adjust the VOR in all its aspects on a short- and long-term basis. Other types of information can also be used to assist or modify the VOR. One source is neck proprioception. Although most authors have found cervico-ocular reflexes to be insignificant under normal circumstances (Barnes and Forbat, 1979; Barlow and Freedman, 1980), their contribution seems to improve dramatically in the absence of functioning labyrinths (Dichgans *et al.*, 1973; Kasai and Zee, 1978; Bronstein and Hood, 1986). Also the fact that a subject produces active head movements rather than being passively oscillated may improve compensatory eye movements.

It may be appropriate to hypothesize that the VOR in the narrow sense is just a part of a larger, comprehensive system which generates compensatory eye movements in order to stabilize gaze. We may call this the 'generalized VOR'. This system uses various kinds of information, of which vestibular signals are normally the most relevant. In addition retinal slip, neck proprioception, motor commands, and even auditory (Schmid, Zambarbieri and Magenes, 1981) and somatosensory (Bles *et al.*, 1983) information could be used. The magnitude and directions of the outputs, and the strength of coupling of the different inputs are controlled by visual feedback using short- and long-term adjustments. The successful orchestration of all these parameter settings requires in addition cognitive decisions, as soon as selective use of vision is made. The retina does not know whether we want to look at a distant target, a close target or something moving with us, while we move our head. We have to make this decision at a cognitive level and instruct the system.

It has been established that such cognitive decisions can markedly change the parameters of the VOR, even in the absence of actual visual information. Barr, Schultheis and Robinson (1976) showed that the gain of the human VOR, measured in darkness, could be set at low or high levels by purely mental factors. When subjects were instructed to fixate an imagined target which was stationary in space, VOR gain reached high values (although below unity). When, on the contrary, subjects were instructed to fixate an imagined target attached to the chair and moving with them, VOR gain was very low (although not zero). Such observations have been confirmed and extended (Baloh *et al.*, 1984; McKinley and Peterson, 1985). When subjects received no instruction at all, VOR gain was unpredictable and variable. Melvill Jones, Berthoz and Segal (1984) have even shown that such an entirely cognitive manipulation can lead to a plastic change in VOR gain.

17.6 The VOR in the dark: a system with unspecified parameters

Where does this leave us with regard to the measurement of the VOR as an isolated system? We have to conclude that by recording the VOR in the absence of vision, we literally leave the system in the dark as to what to do. If the system receives neither visual input nor specific instructions, its output will be variable and unpredictable. This is entirely borne out by the literature. In Fig. 17.2, a number of data from the literature have been compiled, all showing the frequency response of the VOR in the dark in

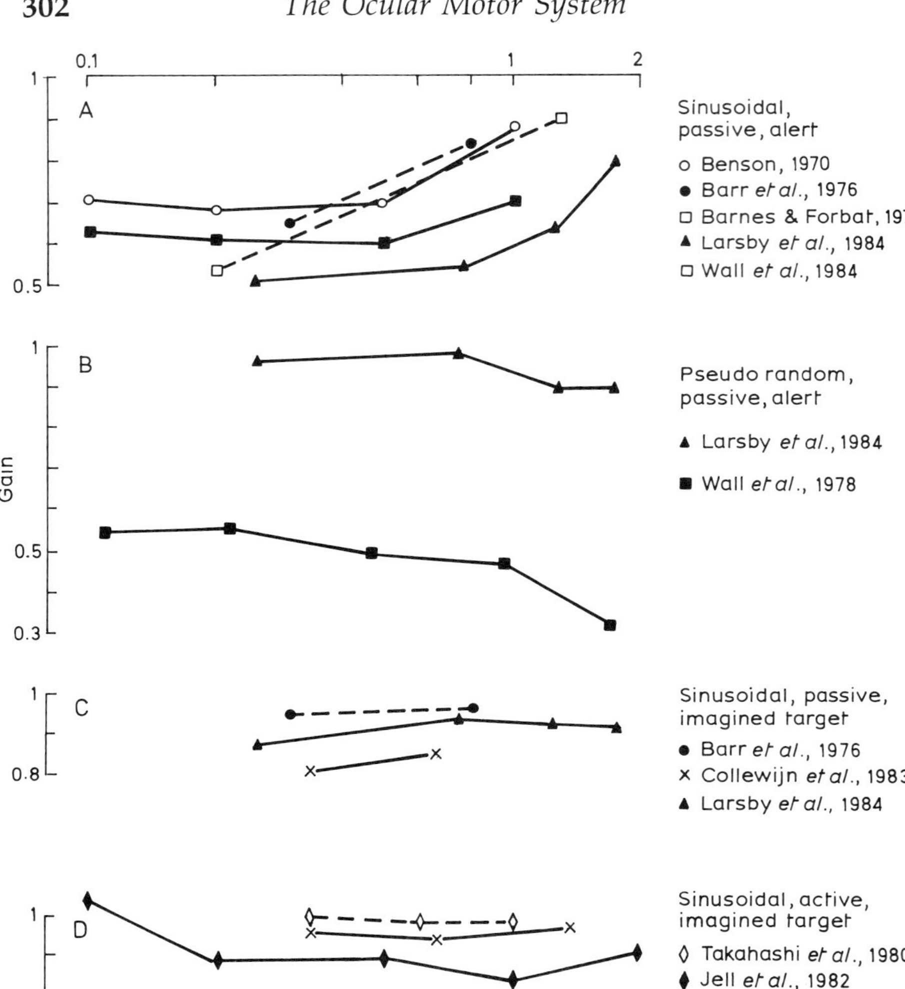

Fig. 17.2 Some data from the literature on VOR gain in the dark, as a function of frequency, for different instructions and ways of moving.

subjects that were kept alert by the performance of mental arithmetic or similar methods. In the absence of any more specific instructions, sinusoidal, passive oscillation in the dark (Fig. 17.2A) produces a VOR with a low gain (0.5–0.7) for frequencies up to about 0.5 Hz, with a progressive increase for higher frequencies, differences between authors being minor in this respect (Benson, 1970; Barr, Schultheis and Robinson, 1976; Barnes and Forbat, 1979; Larsby, Hydén and Ödkvist, 1984; Wall, Black and Hunt, 1984). In recent years the use of pseudo-random movement programmes has been advocated as a more efficient and shorter test, but there is a discrepancy (Fig. 17.2B) in the gains obtained with such movement by different groups: Wall, Black and O'Leary (1978) reported data corresponding to velocity gains of 0.3–0.55, whereas Larsby, Hydén and Ödkvist (1984) found gains of 0.9 and higher in a similar frequency range. These variations suggest that there were differences in the mental set of the subjects, and that the use of pseudo-random motion alone does not guarantee a high VOR gain. In contrast, passive, sinusoidal oscillation combined with the instruction to fixate an imagined, stationary target (Fig. 17.2C) has consistently yielded high gains (Barr, Schultheis and Robinson, 1976; Collewijn, Martins and Steinman, 1983; Larsby, Hydén and Ödkvist, 1984), the highest being reached probably by the combination (Fig. 17.2D) of voluntary (instead of passive) head oscillation with attempted fixation (Takahashi, Uemura and Fujishiro, 1980; Jell, Guedry and Hixson, 1982; Collewijn, Martins and Steinman, 1983). All the measurements cited were obtained with the relatively inaccurate electro-oculographic (EOG) method, except those by Collewijn, Martins and Steinman (1983), who used a scleral coil method and found a clearly higher gain of the VOR in the dark with active than with passive head movement. In addition, the data obtained with passive motion showed a much larger variance. Variability is one of the striking features encountered during examination of the literature on the human VOR and, although some of it may be attributed to unreliability of the EOG, a substantial part is real.

Even when the very best conditions were applied, i.e. use of voluntary head motion, attempted fixation and completely reliable recording with scleral coil techniques, we find that variability of the VOR in darkness remains a problem. In Fig. 17.3 a number of long-term (30-min) recordings are shown in which four highly motivated and informed subjects continuously oscillated their heads at 0.66 Hz, while fixating a point target at infinity. Every 2 min VOR gain was assessed in the light, as well as during a brief dark interval in which subjects continued to oscillate their heads in the horizontal plane. Compensatory eye movement gain was calculated by the computer after elimination of saccades. In the light, gain was reasonably constant and close to unity in all four subjects. The lower value (about 0.9) in subject HC was due to his negative, minifying glasses. In the dark, gain was always lower than in the light. It appeared to be rather constant only in subject HC, rather variable (over a range of 0.2) in subjects DP and HS, and extremely variable with a downward

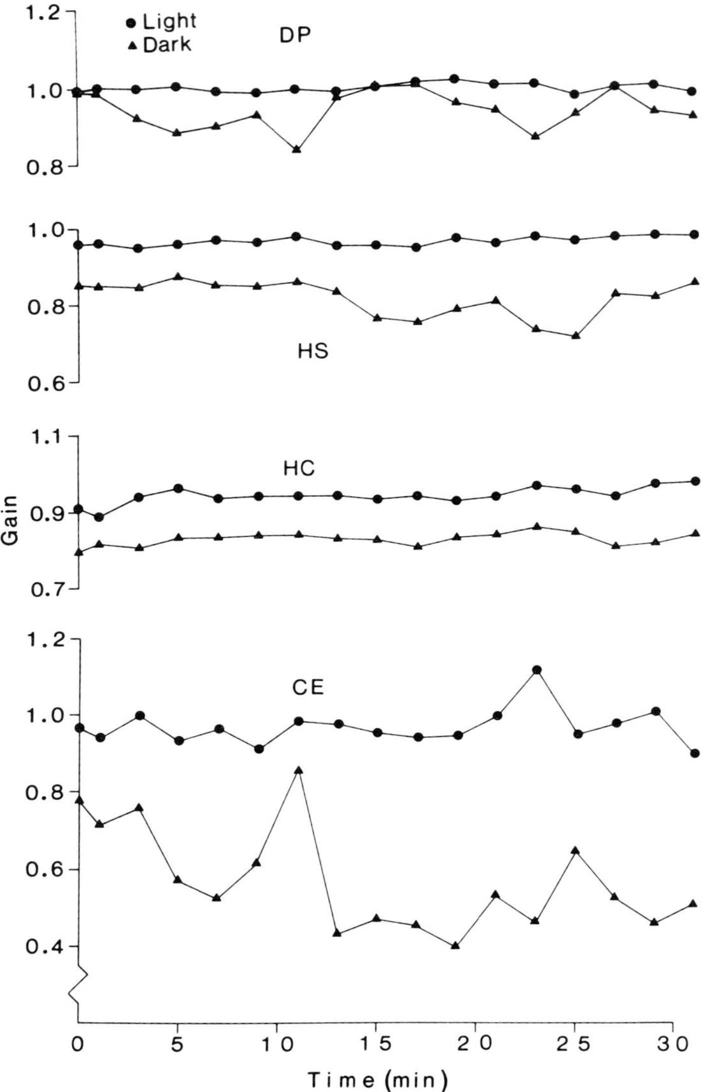

Fig. 17.3 Variability of VOR gain in light (circles) and dark (triangles) in the course of a 30 min session during which subjects continuously oscillated their head horizontally at 0.66 Hz, while fixating a point target at optical infinity. Subjects DP and HS were emmetropic, HC was myopic and wore his normal, negative glasses; CE was myopic and wore contact lenses.

trend in subject CE, who showed a similar result in a replication of the experiment. This happened even though CE was a very motivated, informed subject who was repeatedly reminded of his task during the session. Such results severely undermined our confidence in a consistent determination of VOR in darkness. Three of the four tracings in Fig. 17.3 were too erratic to form a firm baseline against which adaptive changes could be reliably assessed. If random fluctuations in VOR gain in darkness by 10–20% and more cannot be avoided, then the search for subtle adaptations becomes very questionable and clinical application especially would seem unpromising.

17.7 The VOR in the light

A much more promising approach is the functional assessment of the generalized VOR, i.e. gaze stability with vision in the light. This parameter can be measured reliably and is functionally relevant, both for normal physiology and clinical problems, but requires great precision and accuracy of the methods. The fact that compensatory eye movements have a consistent and high gain in the light has been reported by all investigators, and a unity gain has often been mentioned or implicitly assumed. However, we should consider this as 'unity gain' only in a loose manner of speaking, since neither the recording methods nor the visual stimulus conditions would allow very precise statements in this respect. Any method which records the eye position with respect to the head, and in addition the head position, has to rely on the difference of these data in assessing gaze stability. As a small difference between two fairly large numbers is very sensitive to errors and inconstancies of calibration, gaze instability cannot be reliably measured in this way. This is particularly true for the EOG, but not much better for infrared reflection methods. The only reliable, existing method for measuring gaze direction (eye in space) directly is by using a scleral search coil in a large, homogeneous magnetic field (see Collewijn, Martins and Steinman, 1981; Steinman, Cushman and Martins, 1982). With this method, the groups of Steinman in College Park, Maryland, and Collewijn in Rotterdam have in collaboration measured gaze stability with increasing accuracy in the past several years.

The traditional measurements of precision of fixation with the head immobilized on a biteboard show typically standard deviations of eye position smaller than 5 minarc and retinal image velocities smaller than 0.25°/s (for reviews, see Steinman *et al.*, 1973; and Steinman, Cushman and Martins, 1982). As shown first by Skavenski *et al.* (1979), getting off the biteboard and keeping the head as still as possible was sufficient to double the speeds of retinal image slip. Measurements of gaze stability with the scleral coil system while the head was oscillated passively or actively were initiated by Steinman and Collewijn (1980) and further refined later on (Collewijn, Martins and Steinman, 1981, 1983; Steinman, Cushman and Martins, 1982). These investigations led to estimates of the standard deviation of gaze and of retinal image speed of the order of 30 minarc and 1–2°/s, respectively.

17.8 Recent measurements of gaze stability in the light

In recent investigations in our laboratory (Collewijn *et al.*, 1985a; Ferman *et al.*, 1987) we have extended and refined this type of measurement. The extension consisted of the addition of the two other dimensions: modification of the search coil (Collewijn, Van der Mark and Jansen, 1975) according to principles described by Robinson (1963) enabled us to measure horizontal, vertical and torsional eye movements simultaneously. The main refinements were: (1) the target (a red spot, formed by a laser beam) was placed in the focal point of a large lens, and thus viewed at optical infinity, which eliminates problems due to non-coincidence of rotational centres and places the ideal value of VOR gain unambiguously at unity. (2) The raw data were completely corrected (off-line) for goniometric non-linearities and cross-coupling effects between dimensions due to misalignments of the coil on the eye. As a result, veridical co-ordinates in Fick's axial system were obtained. (3) The homogeneity of the magnetic field, resulting in complete insensitivity to translation of the head, was confirmed. (4) Only emmetropic subjects ($n = 8$) with 20/20 visual acuity were tested, to avoid the extra complications of a non-unity magnification factor between head rotation and the associated relative rotation of the surroundings.

For full details of methodology and results, see Ferman *et al.* (1987); Table 17.1 summarizes our results and examples of recordings are shown in Figs 17.4–17.7. Three-dimensional recordings of eye and head position were obtained with search coil techniques. Recordings were made with the head held stationary (frequency zero) or actively moved by the subject in a sinusoidal way (frequency 0.16, 0.33 or 0.66 Hz, paced by a metronome; amplitude about 10°). To compare dynamic with static accuracy of fixation, and as an internal control on the reliability of the data, we recorded gaze positions also during static head deviations of 10–15°, and calculated a 'VOR gain' for the static case. Obviously this value should be very close to unity. For all frequencies we determined the mean speeds of head motion and of retinal image (= gaze) motion in the time domain, using a sliding window technique to calculate velocities, which were

Table 17.1 Retinal image motion and VOR gain in the light found for voluntary head oscillation (amplitude about 10°) in horizontal, vertical or torsional direction during fixation of a point target at optical infinity. Means (±SD) of eight subjects. (Data from Ferman *et al*. (1987)).

Head motion			*Retinal image motion in plane of head motion*		*VOR gain*
Main direction	*Frequency (Hz)*	*Mean speed (°/s)*	*SD of position (minarc)*	*Mean speed (minarc/s)*	
Horizontal	0	0.54±0.20	6.86± 3.79	23.17± 5.18	0.991±0.011*
	0.16	7.08±1.98	16.53± 8.39	33.62± 7.87	0.983±0.021
	0.33	13.04±3.10	15.49± 5.02	42.32± 11.63	0.981±0.020
	0.66	22.42±7.61	16.12± 5.49	55.60± 21.50	0.979±0.018
Vertical	0	0.69±0.19	8.05± 3.17	29.81± 12.46	0.993±0.01*
	0.16	6.21±2.21	12.36± 3.54	42.36± 14.81	0.989±0.012
	0.33	9.64±2.51	16.89± 10.02	46.71± 20.53	0.982±0.016
	0.66	22.64±7.09	19.93± 10.28	72.88± 23.57	0.983±0.013
Torsional	0	0.55±0.13	16.67± 7.09	45.60± 9.00	0.26±0.24*
	0.16	8.09±3.37	360.13±202.40	297.60±166.20	0.418±0.110
	0.33	13.54±4.65	282.04±121.90	397.80±175.20	0.520±0.134
	0.66	21.87±6.59	196.46± 93.28	514.20±208.20	0.638±0.076

* VOR gain values determined for static head deviations.

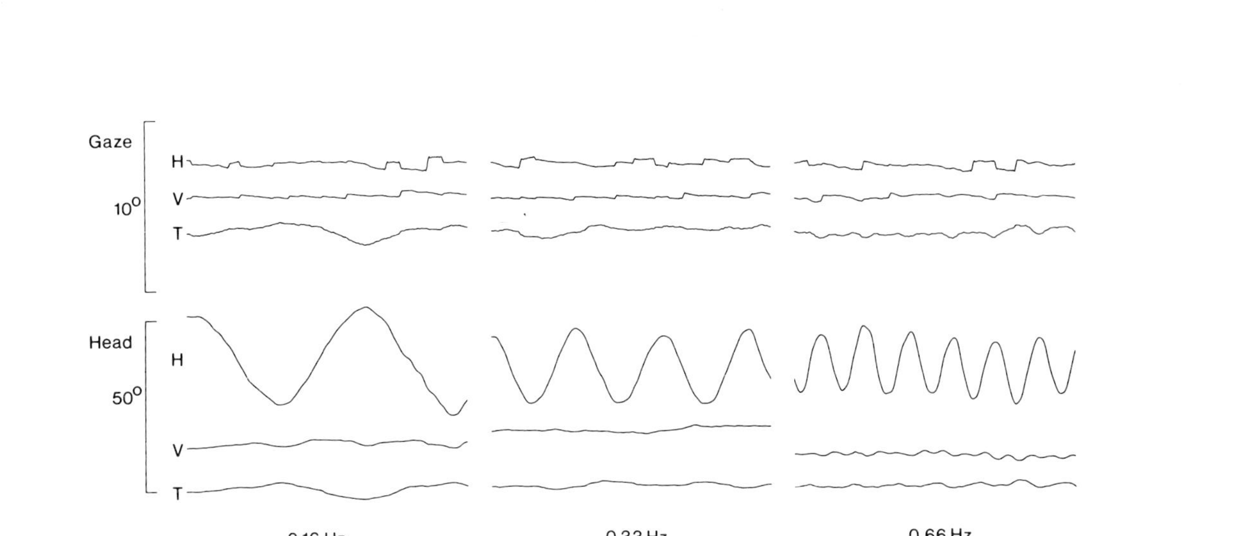

Fig. 17.4 Gaze and head movements (after full correction of coordinates) of subject EF (one of our most stable subjects) during voluntary oscillation of the head in the horizontal plane, at 0.16, 0.33 or 0.66 Hz. H = horizontal; V = vertical; T = torsion.

converted into absolute values (speed). All saccades were eliminated before this calculation; the speeds refer to the non-saccadic gaze movements. Furthermore, the standard deviations of gaze position were calculated, inclusive of saccades; these values represent the overall precision of fixation. Finally, VOR gains were calculated as the ratio smooth eye-in-head movement/head movement (eye-in-head being equal to gaze minus head). These gains were calculated in the frequency domain; cumulative smooth eye positions were obtained by removal of saccades; bias and trend were corrected and the data for head and eye were fast-fourier transformed. Gain and phase were determined for the fundamental component of head oscillation. Phase errors were not larger than 2° for the horizontal and vertical VOR and not larger than 13° for the torsional VOR. These values are so small that they can be safely neglected in the further discussion of precision of gaze.

17.8.1 THE PRECISION OF HORIZONTAL GAZE

For static head deviations, mean counter-rotation had a gain of 0.991 ± 0.011 (SD) for all eight subjects. Actually, these values were affected adversely by a few subjects who fixated less precisely in eccentric positions. For the best four subjects, average static horizontal gain was better than 0.999. In all subjects, dynamic head oscillation reduced retinal image stability. Examples of (fully corrected) recordings for our most stable subject (EF) are shown in Fig. 17.4, for voluntary horizontal head oscillations at 0.16, 0.33 and 0.66 Hz. The head position recordings reveal some cross-coupling to vertical and torsional motion (mean values 4.6 and 11.1% for all subjects). The horizontal gaze position shows very good compensation for the head oscillation; the mean horizontal VOR gain for all subjects was in the order of 0.98 (see Table 17.1). Thus, for the average subject, a part in the order of 2% of horizontal head oscillation remains uncompensated by the VOR, but this finding cannot be directly translated into retinal image motion, because position is corrected by saccades as well as the smooth component, and retinal image speed contains components unrelated to head motion. The standard deviation of gaze position (inclusive of saccades) increased from about 7 minarc with the head stationary to about 16 minarc during horizontal oscillation, independently of frequency, and was thus roughly doubled. Mean retinal image speeds increased from about 23 minarc/s with the head stationary to 34–56 minarc/s, speed being clearly correlated with frequency.

Our present findings are basically in agreement with our previous work (Collewijn, Martins and Steinman, 1981; Steinman, Cushman and Martins, 1982). Smaller values of the SD of gaze during active head oscillation were found by Duwaer (1982), using an after-image method. It

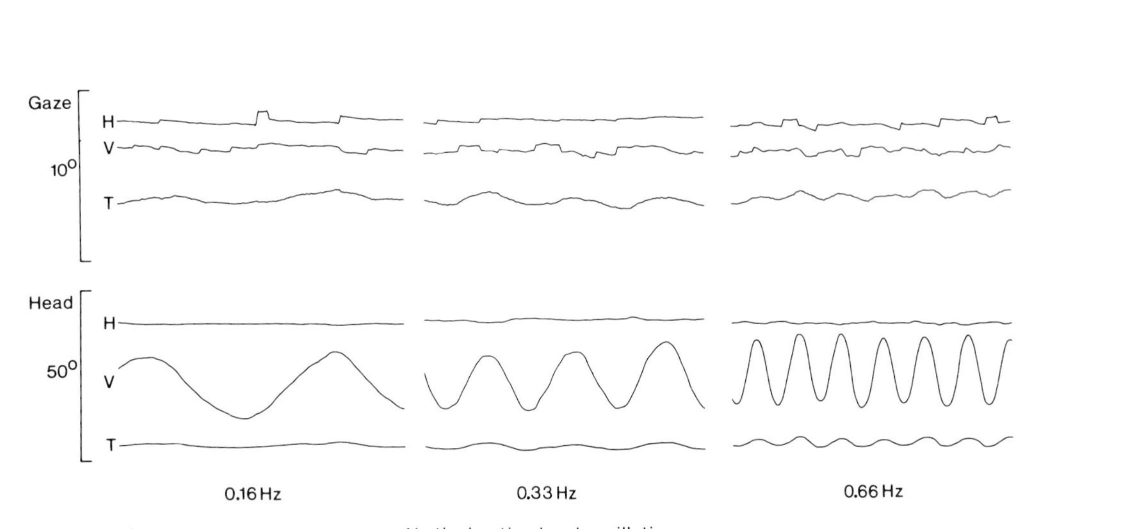

Fig. 17.5 As Fig. 17.4 (same subject) for vertical head oscillation.

is interesting to speculate that this discrepancy could be due to central processes controlling constancy of subjective localization of a fixed target.

17.8.2 THE PRECISION OF VERTICAL GAZE

The findings for vertical gaze stability during vertical head movements were virtually identical to the ones described above for the horizontal plane. Both the absolute levels and the dynamic effects were entirely similar. Vertical head motion was relatively pure; cross-coupling to horizontal and torsional planes amounted to 3.4 and 5.4% (mean values). Recordings for one of the most stable subjects (same as in Fig. 17.4) are shown in Fig. 17.5. In all subjects, dynamic instability was larger than static gaze errors.

Data in the literature on the human vertical VOR are scarce and not very reliable due to the use of EOG, which is strongly affected by lid artefacts (Barry and Melvill Jones, 1965; Collewijn, Van der Steen and Steinman, 1985b) in the vertical direction. Asymmetries of various kinds have been described (see Baloh *et al.*, 1983, also for review). No such asymmetries were obvious in our gaze tracings but our data have not been rigorously analysed in this respect.

17.8.3 STABILITY OF TORSIONAL GAZE POSITION

Stability of the retinal image for rotation around the visual axis is much inferior to stability in the horizontal and vertical direction. Even when the head is held still and upright, the SD of position and retinal image speed in torsion are about twice as high as for the horizontal and vertical direction (Table 17.1). For static tilt (roll) of the head, only a small percentage is compensated by counter-roll. This is well known from the literature, where values around 10% are usually mentioned (see Collewijn *et al.*, 1985a, for a survey and some earlier measurements in our laboratory). In the present experiments static counter-roll had a mean gain of 0.26 ± 0.24 (SD), which is rather high.

A possible reason for these relatively favourable values may be seen in Fig. 17.6, which shows static gaze positions (top traces) in steps of about 10° (subject CE). Due to the small counter-roll, gaze rolls in the same direction as the head, although over a smaller angle. However, a dynamic aspect can be seen. Whereas head torsion positions remained virtually constant after the displacement, Fig. 17.6 shows that gaze positions tended to drift slowly back towards the mid-position. Therefore, smaller values for static counter-roll would have been found if the measurements had been made somewhat later after reaching a new head position in roll. Static counter-roll depends entirely on maculo-ocular reflexes, especially

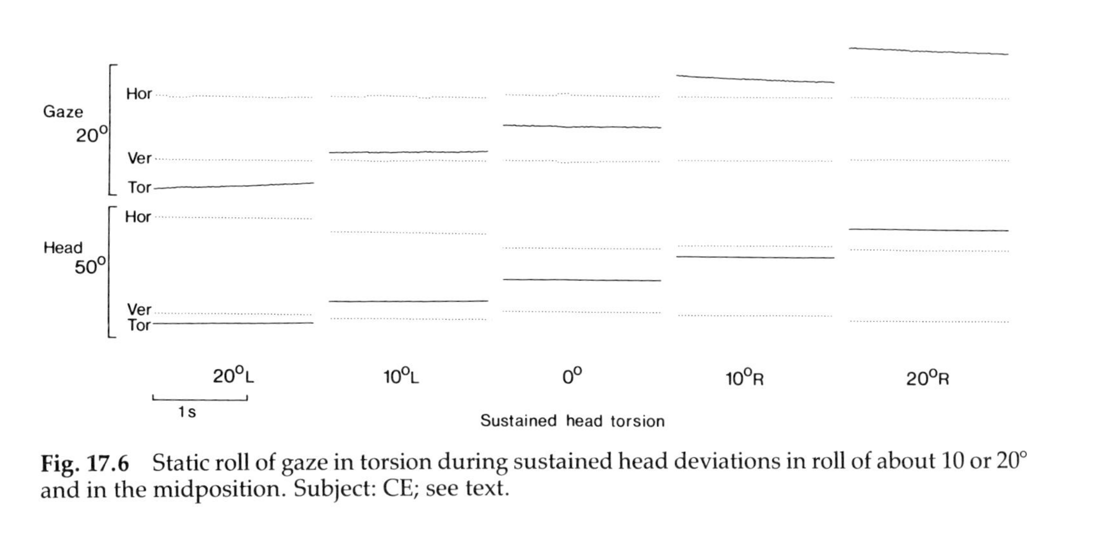

Fig. 17.6 Static roll of gaze in torsion during sustained head deviations in roll of about 10 or 20° and in the midposition. Subject: CE; see text.

when the visual target is a single point. It is hardly improved by a structured visual background (see Collewijn *et al.*, 1985a); the visual drive of torsional eye position (e.g. to keep vertical contours vertically on the retina) is apparently negligible. This is confirmed by the very low gain of optokinetic nystagmus in torsion (Collewijn *et al.*, 1985a).

However, a considerably better compensation occurs during dynamic head motion in roll. This was found by Collewijn *et al.* (1985a) and is confirmed in the present experiments for a larger number of subjects. Figure 17.7 illustrates these effects for voluntary head oscillation in the torsional plane. It is very difficult to make such a movement with any purity, and a large amount of cross-coupling to the horizontal and vertical planes was found (mean percentages 49.1 and 6.6%). Whereas these horizontal and vertical components were largely compensated (Fig. 17.7), as discussed previously, a large residual motion of gaze in torsion was seen. Torsional gaze motion showed many saccades, running in the same direction as the smooth movement. This is because the partial smooth compensatory movements of the eye in the head are reset by opposite saccades (see Collewijn *et al.*, 1985a, for clear illustrations of this effect). The gain of the smooth, dynamic counter-roll increased markedly with the frequency of the head movement. It rose from about 0.42 at 0.16 Hz to about 0.64 at 0.66 Hz, in agreement with our previous findings. SD of torsional gaze during oscillation was inversely proportional with frequency and at least an order of magnitude higher than in horizontal and vertical direction. Mean torsional slip speeds are also an order of magnitude larger than in the other dimensions, and increase with frequency (Table 17.1). The considerable improvement of torsional gain with dynamic rather than static stimuli is probably due to a significant canal-ocular reflex in torsion, compared to a vestigial maculo-ocular component. The relatively high initial values of counter-roll after a step input, followed by drift back to the mid-position when the head deviation is sustained (Fig. 17.6) is undoubtedly due to the canal-ocular component, which dies out rapidly. The relatively poor stabilization of gaze in torsion is also evident in Figs 17.4 and 17.5, where the small accidental head movements in torsion are clearly reflected in torsional gaze movements.

17.9 Conclusions

Although the performance of the VOR in the dark can be improved by attempted fixation and active generation of head movements as a means of providing the system with a specified frame of reference, there is no real substitute for vision. Only in the light is the true potential of the VOR

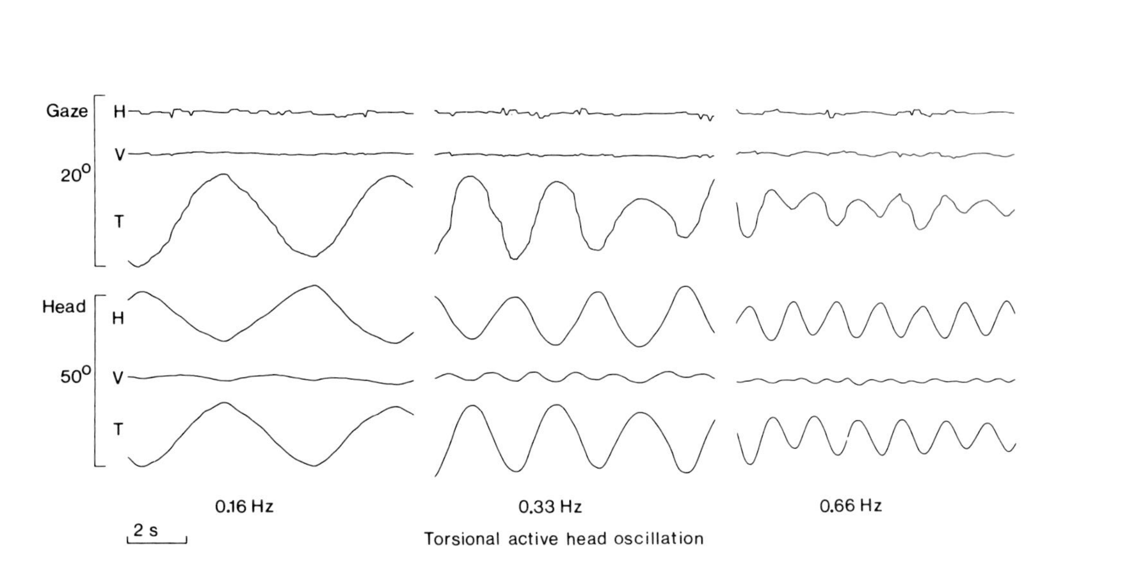

Fig. 17.7 Gaze and head movements (after full correction of coordinates) of subject CE during voluntary oscillation of the head in the torsional plane.

revealed. Its performance is not perfect, but clearly good enough to maintain visual acuity during head motion. A minimum amount of retinal image instability is necessary to achieve maximum contrast sensitivity, and this minimum is probably about 10–15 minarc/s (King-Smith and Riggs, 1978). Our recordings show just this amount of retinal image speed when the head is stationary. On the other hand, retinal image slip speeds up to 100–150 minarc/s do not impair visual acuity (Westheimer and McKee, 1975; King-Smith and Riggs, 1978; Murphy, 1978). In our conditions, horizontal and vertical retinal image speeds did not exceed 60 minarc/s, but they will become higher when the frequency of the head movement is raised further. It seems safe to conclude that most of the time the VOR in the light is good enough to keep retinal image slip velocities within the range optimal for vision, although VOR gain is not unity.

For a better understanding of pathophysiology of the VOR, it seems necessary to measure the performance of the VOR with vision, to reveal true functional deficits that are not simply due to non-specific programming of the system. It is clear that to discover subtle defects, very precise methods have to be used. A second important goal would be to explore the adaptivity of human compensatory eye movements in greater depth. Although we know that modifications of magnitude and direction are possible, we have insufficient knowledge of the time course and the limits of adaptation. Assessment of the range over which the VOR can be adapted could be informative, because for a long time pathology could be compensated by adaptive processes without the manifestation of overt functional loss.

Especially in slowly progressive disease, the onset of deficient function might signal the exhaustion of the available range of adaptation. Measurement of the available range of adaptation might therefore give a clue to hidden damage that is being repaired and give an indication of the functional reserves of the system.

Acknowledgement

These investigations were supported by the Foundation for Medical Research MEDIGON (grant nr.900-550-092).

References

Arbib, M.A. and Amari, S.I. (1985) Sensori-motor transformations in the brain (with a critique of the tensor theory of cerebellum). *J. Theor. Biol.*, **112**, 123–55.

Baarsma, E.A. and Collewijn, H. (1975) Eye movements due to linear accelerations in the rabbit. *J. Physiol. (Lond.)*, **245**, 227–47.

Baker, J., Harrison, R.E.W., Isu, N., Wickland, C. and Peterson, B. (1986) Dynamics of adaptive change in vestibulo-ocular reflex direction. II. Sagittal plane rotations. *Brain Res.*, **371**, 166–70.

Baloh, R.W. and Honrubia, V. (1979) *Clinical Neurophysiology of the Vestibular System*. Davis, Philadelphia.

Baloh, R.W., Lyerly, K., Yee, R.D. and Honrubia, V. (1984) Voluntary control of the human vestibulo-ocular reflex. *Acta Otolaryngol.*, **97**, 1–6.

Baloh, R.W., Richman, L., Yee, R.D. and Honrubia, V. (1983) The dynamics of vertical eye movements in normal human subjects. *Aviat. Space Environ. Med.*, **54**, 32–8.

Barlow, D. and Freedman, W. (1980) Cervico-ocular reflex in the normal adult. *Acta Otolaryngol.*, **89**, 487–96.

Barnes, G.R. and Forbat, L.N. (1979) Cervical and vestibular afferent control of oculomotor response in man. *Acta Otolaryngol.*, **88**, 79–87.

Barr, C.C., Schultheis, L.W. and Robinson, D.A. (1976) Voluntary, non-visual control of the human vestibulo-ocular reflex. *Acta Otolaryngol.*, **81**, 365–75.

Barry, W. and Melvill Jones, G. (1965) Influence of eye lid movement upon electro-oculographic recording of vertical eye movements. *Aerospace Med.*, **36**, 855–8.

Benson, A.J. (1970) Interactions between semicircular canals and graviceptors, in *Recent Advances in Aerospace Medicine* (ed. D.E. Busby). Reidel, Dordrecht, pp. 249–61.

Berthoz, A. and Melvill Jones, G. (1985) *Adaptive Mechanisms in Gaze Control*. Elsevier, Amsterdam.

Blakemore, C. and Donaghy, M. (1980) Coordination of head and eyes in the gaze changing behaviour of cats. *J. Physiol. (Lond.)*, **300**, 317–35.

Blanks, R.H., Estes, M.S. and Markham, C.H. (1975) Physiologic characteristics of vestibular first-order canal neurons in the cat. II. Response to constant angular acceleration. *J. Neurophysiol.*, **38**, 1250–68.

Bles, W., Klören, T., Büchele, W. and Brandt, T. (1983) Somatosensory nystagmus: physiological and clinical aspects. *Adv. Oto.-Rhino.-Laryngol.*, **30**, 30–3.

Bronstein, A.M. and Hood, J.D. (1986) The cervico-ocular reflex in normal subjects and patients with absent vestibular function. *Brain Res.*, **373**, 399–408.

Callan, J.W. and Ebenholtz, S.M. (1982) Directional changes in the vestibular ocular response as a result of adaptation to optical tilt. *Vision Res.*, **22**, 37–42.

Cannon, S.C. and Robinson, D.A. (1985) An improved neural-network model for the neural integrator of the oculomotor system: more realistic neuron behavior. *Biol. Cybern.*, **53**, 93–108.

Cannon, S.C., Leigh, R.J., Zee, D.S. and Abel, L.A. (1985) The effect of the rotational magnification of corrective spectacles on the quantitative evaluation of the VOR. *Acta Otolaryngol.*, **100**, 81–8.

Clément, G., Courjon, J.H., Jeannerod, M. and Schmid, R. (1981) Unidirectional habituation of vestibulo-ocular responses by repeated rotational or optokinetic stimulations in the cat. *Exp. Brain Res.*, **42**, 34–42.

Cohen, B. (1971) Vestibulo-ocular relations, in *The Control of Eye Movements* (eds P. Bach-y-Rita, C.C. Collins and E. Hyde). Academic Press, New York, pp. 105–48.

Cohen, B. (1974) The vestibulo-ocular reflex arc, in *Handbook of Sensory Physiology* (ed. H. Autrum), vol. VI/1. Springer, Berlin, pp. 477–540.

Cohen, B. (1981) Vestibular and oculomotor physiology. *Int. Meet. Barony. Soc., Ann. NY Acad. Sci.*, **374**, 892.

Collewijn, H., Conijn, P. and Tamminga, E.P. (1982) Eye–head coordination in man during the pursuit of moving targets, in *Functional Basis of Ocular Motility Disorders* (eds G. Lennerstrand, D.S. Zee and E.L. Keller). Pergamon, Oxford, pp. 369–78.

Collewijn, H., Martins, A.J. and Steinman, R.M. (1981) Natural retinal image motion: origin and change. *Ann. NY Acad Sci.*, **374**, 312–29.

Collewijn, H., Martins, A.J. and Steinman, R.M. (1983) Compensatory eye movements during active and passive head movements: fast adaptation to changes in visual magnification. *J. Physiol.*, **340**, 259–86.

Collewijn, H., Van der Mark, F. and Jansen, T.C. (1975) Precise recording of human eye movements. *Vision Res.*, **15**, 447–50.

Collewijn, H., Van der Steen, J., Ferman, L. and Jansen, T.C. (1985a) Human ocular counterroll: assessment of static and dynamic properties from electromagnetic scleral coil recordings. *Exp. Brain Res.*, **59**, 185–96.

Collewijn, H., Van der Steen, J. and Steinman, R.M. (1985b) Human eye movements associated with blinks and prolonged eyelid closure. *J. Neurophysiol.*, **54**, 11–27.

Dichgans, J., Bizzi, E., Morasso, P. and Tagliasco, V. (1973) Mechanisms underlying recovery of eye–head coordination following bilateral labyrinthectomy in monkeys. *Exp. Brain Res.*, **18**, 548–62.

Duwaer, A.L. (1982) Assessment of retinal image displacement during head movement using an afterimage method. *Vision Res.*, **22**, 1379–88.

Ferman, L., Collewijn, H., Jansen, T.C. and Van den Berg, A.V. (1987) Human gaze stability in horizontal, vertical and torsional direction during voluntary head movements, evaluated with a three-dimensional scleral induction coil technique. *Vision Res.*, **27**, 811–28.

Fernandez, C. and Goldberg, J.M. (1971) Physiology of peripheral neurons innervating semicircular canals of the squirrel monkey. II. Response to sinusoidal stimulation and dynamics of peripheral vestibular system. *J. Neurophysiol.*, **34**, 661–75.

Gauthier, G.M. and Robinson, D.A. (1975) Adaptation of the human vestibulo-ocular reflex to magnifying lenses. *Brain Res.*, **92**, 331–5.

Granit, R. and Pompeiano, O. (1979) *Reflex Control of Posture and Movement*. Elsevier/North-Holland, Amsterdam.

Harris, L.R. and Cynader, M. (1981) Modification of the balance and gain of the vestibulo-ocular reflex in the cat. *Exp. Brain Res.*, **44**, 57–70.

Harrison, R.E.W., Baker, J.F., Isu, N., Wickland, C.R. and Peterson, B. (1986) Dynamics of adaptive change in vestibulo-ocular reflex direction. I. Rotations in the horizontal plane. *Brain Res.*, **371**, 162–5.

Jell, R.M., Guedry, F.E. and Hixson, W.C. (1982) The vestibulo-ocular reflex in man during voluntary head oscillation under three visual conditions. *Aviat. Space Environ. Med.*, **53**, 541–8.

Kasai, T. and Zee, D.S. (1978) Eye–head coordination in labyrinthine-defective human beings. *Brain Res.*, **144**, 123–41.

King-Smith, P.E. and Riggs, L.A. (1978) Visual sensitivity to controlled motion of a line or edge. *Vision Res.*, **18**, 1509–20.

Larsby, B., Hydén, D. and Ödkvist, L.M. (1984) Gain and phase characteristics of compensatory eye movements in light and darkness. *Acta Otolaryngol.*, **97**, 223–32.

Leigh, R.J. and Zee, D.S. (1983) *The Neurology of Eye Movements*. Davis, Philadelphia.

Lorente de Nó, R. (1933) Vestibulo-ocular reflex arc. *Arch. Neurol. Psychiat.*, **30**, 245–91.

McKinley, P.A. and Peterson, B.W. (1985) Voluntary modulation of the vestibuloocular reflex in humans and its relation to smooth pursuit. *Exp. Brain Res.*, **60**, 454–64.

Melvill Jones, G. (1985) Adaptive modulation of VOR parameters by vision, in *Adaptive Mechanisms in Gaze Control* (eds A. Berthoz and G. Melvill Jones). Elsevier, Amsterdam, pp. 21–50.

Melvill Jones, G., Berthoz, A. and Segal, B. (1984) Adaptive modification of the vestibulo-ocular reflex by mental effort in darkness. *Exp. Brain Res.*, **56**, 149–53.

Miles, F.A. and Eighmy, B.B. (1980) Long-term adaptive changes in primate vestibuloocular reflex. I. Behavioral observations. *J. Neurophysiol.*, **43**, 1406–25.

Miles, F.A. and Fuller, J.H. (1974) Adaptive plasticity in the vestibulo-ocular responses of the rhesus monkey. *Brain Res.*, **80**, 512–16.

Miles, F.A., Optican, L.M. and Lisberger, S.G. (1985) An adaptive equalizer model of the primate vestibulo-ocular reflex, in *Adaptive Mechanisms in Gaze Control* (eds A. Berthoz and G. Melvill Jones). Elsevier, Amsterdam, pp. 313–26.

Murphy, B.J. (1978) Pattern thresholds for moving and stationary gratings during smooth eye movements. *Vision Res.*, **18**, 521–30.

Pellionisz, A. and Llinás, R. (1982) Space–time representation in the brain. The cerebellum as a predictive space–time metric tensor. *Neuroscience*, **7**, 2949–70.

Robinson, D.A. (1963) A method of measuring eye movement using a scleral search coil in a magnetic field. *IEEE Trans. Biomed. Electron*, BME-10, 137–45.

Robinson, D.A. (1975) Oculomotor control signals, in *Basic Mechanisms of Ocular Motility and their Clinical Implications* (eds G. Lennerstrand and P. Bach-y-Rita). Pergamon, Oxford, pp. 337–74.

Robinson, D.A. (1982a) A model of cancellation of the vestibulo-ocular reflex, in *Functional Basis of Ocular Motility Disorders* (eds G. Lennerstrand, D.S. Zee and E.L. Keller). Pergamon, Oxford, pp. 5–13.

Robinson, D.A. (1982b) The use of matrices in analyzing the three-dimensional behavior of the vestibulo-ocular reflex. *Biol. Cybern.*, **46**, 53–66.

Robinson, D.A. (1985) The coordinates of neurons in the vestibulo-ocular reflex, in *Adaptive Mechanisms in Gaze Control* (eds A. Berthoz and G. Melvill Jones). Elsevier, Amsterdam, pp. 297–311.

Schmid, R., Zambarbieri, D. and Magenes, G. (1981) Modifications of vestibular

nystagmus produced by fixation of visual and nonvisual targets. *Ann. NY Acad. Sci.*, **374**, 689–705.
Schultheis, L.W. and Robinson, D.A. (1981) Directional plasticity of the vestibulo-ocular reflex in the cat. *Ann. NY Acad. Sci.*, **374**, 504–12.
Simonsz, H.J. (1985) The history of the scientific elucidation of ocular counter-rolling. *Doc. Ophthalmol.*, **61**, 183–9.
Simpson, J.I. and Graf, W. (1981) Eye-muscle geometry and compensatory eye movements in lateral-eyed and frontal-eyed animals. *Ann. NY Acad. Sci.*, **374**, 20–30.
Simpson, J.I. and Graf, W. (1985) The selection of reference frames by nature and its investigators, in *Adaptive Mechanisms in Gaze Control* (eds A. Berthoz and G. Melvill Jones). Elsevier, Amsterdam, pp. 3–16.
Skavenski, A. and Robinson, D.A. (1973) Role of abducens neurons in vestibulo-ocular reflex. *J. Neurophysiol.*, **36**, 724–38.
Skavenski, A.A., Hansen, R.M., Steinman, R.M. and Winterson, B.J. (1979) Quality of retinal image stabilization during small natural and artificial body rotations in man. *Vision Res.*, **19**, 675–83.
Steinman, R.M. and Collewijn, H. (1980) Binocular retinal image motion during active head rotation. *Vision Res.*, **20**, 415–29.
Steinman, R.M., Cushman, W.B. and Martins, A.J. (1982) The precision of gaze. *Human Neurobiol.*, **1**, 97–109.
Steinman, R.M., Haddad, G.M., Skavenski, A.A. and Wyman, D. (1973) Miniature eye movements. *Science*, **181**, 810–19.
Szentágothai, J. (1950) The elementary vestibulo-ocular reflex arc. *J. Neurophysiol.*, **13**, 395–407.
Takahashi, M., Uemura, T. and Fujishiro, T. (1980) Studies of the vestibulo-ocular reflex and visual-vestibular interactions during active head movements. *Acta Otolaryngol.*, **90**, 115–24.
Van der Hoeve, J. and De Kleijn, A. (1917) Tonische Labyrinthreflexe auf die Augen. *Pflügers Arch.*, **169**, 241–62.
Van der Steen, J. and Collewijn, H. (1984) Ocular stability in the horizontal, frontal and sagittal planes in the rabbit. *Exp. Brain Res.*, **56**, 263–74.
Wall, C., Black, F.O. and Hunt, A.E. (1984) Effects of age, sex and stimulus parameters upon vestibulo-ocular responses to sinusoidal rotation. *Acta Otolaryngol.*, **98**, 270–8.
Wall, C., Black, F.O. and O'Leary, D.P. (1978) Clinical use of pseudorandom binary sequence white noise in assessment of the human vestibulo-ocular system. *Ann. Otol.*, **87**, 845–52.
Westheimer, G. and McKee, S.P. (1975) Visual acuity in the presence of retinal-image motion. *J. Opt. Soc. Am.*, **65**, 847–50.
Wilson, V.J. and Melvill Jones, G. (1979) *Mammalian Vestibular Physiology*. Plenum Press, New York, London.

CHAPTER 18

Oscillopsia and motion perception

THOMAS BRANDT AND MARIANNE DIETERICH

Patients with external ophthalmoplegia are often unable to recognize faces or read while walking, and report motion of stationary visual scenes during head motion or locomotion, a phenomenon termed oscillopsia (Brickner, 1936). Oscillopsia also occurs in diseases causing involuntary ocular oscillations, e.g. acquired pendular nystagmus, downbeat nystagmus and superior oblique myokymia (Bender, 1965). It is either the deficiency of compensatory eye movements (due to an inappropriate vestibulo-ocular reflex) or the deficiency of visual fixation (due to ocular oscillation) which cause undesired retinal image motion with disturbing oscillopsia.

Angular displacement of the apparent motion perceived by the subject does not quantitatively match the net retinal slip (Brandt, 1982; Wist, Brandt and Krafczyk, 1983; Büchele, Brandt and Degner, 1983), and it will be demonstrated that the dissociation between the two can be explained by the combination of two separate mechanisms which involve motion perception:

1. A physiological elevation of thresholds to detect object motion with moving eyes.
2. A pathological elevation of thresholds to detect object motion with either infranuclear ocular motor palsy or supranuclear ocular oscillations.

In a teleological sense, this 'adaptive suppression' of the detection of retinal image motion is beneficial to the organism to the extent that it alleviates the distressing oscillopsia with the disadvantageous side-effect of impaired motion perception in general.

18.1 Oscillopsia is smaller than retinal image slip

18.1.1 DEFICIENT VESTIBULO-OCULAR REFLEX

The cause for apparent motion due to retinal image motion in cases of infranuclear eye movement defects is an inappropriate gain of the vestibulo-ocular reflex (VOR). The VOR normally serves to hold the direction of gaze in space constant during head movements by driving the eyes to move in their orbits in the direction opposite to that of head motion, with a velocity and amplitude which 'compensates' for the head motion. If the amplitude and/or velocity of eye movements are inappropriate, the result is a shift in the direction of gaze causing a displacement or slip of the retinal image which may be perceived as an apparent motion of the fixated object. As appealing and simple as this model is, it is not fully supported by recent studies. It has been shown that for healthy subjects even under optimal fixation conditions, either with a biteboard or with subjects sitting or standing as still as possible (Stavenski *et al.*, 1979), or with head oscillations (Steinman and Collewijn, 1980), appreciable displacements of retinal images result. Velocities of retinal slip ranged between 20 minarc/s with the head fixed by a biteboard to an average of 4°/s with head oscillations. Moreover, retinal image slip was found to be different in each eye with considerable relative binocular motion of the fixated (objectively) stationary visual scene. In spite of such retinal image velocities, oscillopsia is not reported. Thus, a stable world may be perceived even if the 'compensatory' eye movements initiated by the VOR are insufficient to cancel the retinal image motion.

Bender and his co-workers described clinical cases of patients in which oscillopsia was presumably due to a deficient VOR as well as cases without any measurable oculomotor disturbances (Bender, 1965; Bender and Feldman, 1967; Atkin and Bender, 1968; Gresty, Hess and Leech, 1977). Functional tests of inappropriate compensatory eye movements have been reported by Benson and Barnes (1978) using visual acuity, by Wist, Brandt and Krafczyk (1983) using a bedside test of oscillopsia and by Zee (1978) who observed relative movements of the optic disc by means of ophthalmoscopy during active head movements.

In order to compare the relationship between oscillopsia and retinal slip quantitatively, we recorded head and eye movements simultaneously during sinusoidal oscillations about the vertical z-axis (±20°; 1 Hz) with subjects fixating on a stationary target at a distance of 120 cm (Figs 18.1 and 18.2). For the VOR to be completely compensatory (maintaining a constant gaze direction in space), the eye must rotate with an angle exceeding that of the head since the eye and head have different axes (Fig. 18.1). The additional angle of eye motion (β) depends on the

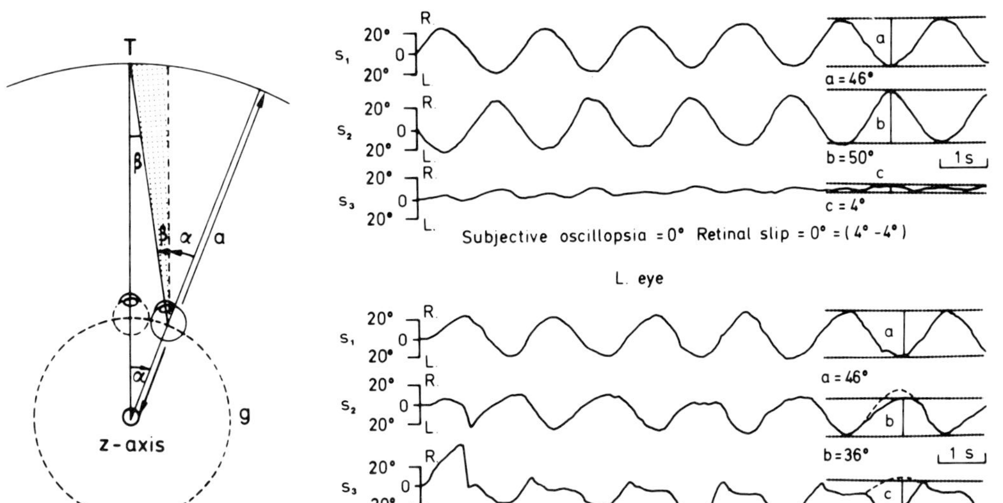

Fig. 18.1 Schematic representation of the experimental procedure for the measurement of eye–head coordination and retinal slip during sinusoidal oscillatory head movements about the vertical z-axis with fixation of a stationary target. In order to maintain fixation on the target during head oscillation additional rotation of the eye is required (β) which results from the different axis of rotation of eye and head. α = Angle of head rotation. $\alpha + \beta$ = Angle of eye rotation. β = Additional angle of eye rotation. g = Head circumference ($g_1 = 0.51\,\text{m}$, $g_2 = 0.61\,\text{m}$). a = Target-z-axis distance (a = 1.2 m).

$$\beta = \text{arc cos}\,\frac{2\pi a - g\cos\alpha}{\sqrt{(2\pi a)^2 + g^2 - 4\pi a g\cos\alpha}}$$

Original recording obtained from a patient with a partial left third nerve palsy (Tolosa-Hunt syndrome). Records for the normal right eye are shown above. In the third line, β was equal to 4° and retinal slip was 0. No oscillopsia was reported. For the left eye a retinal slip of 10° was demonstrated with a maximal retinal velocity of 20° L/S. In spite of this, no oscillopsia was reported. Subjective oscillopsia = 0°. Retinal slip = 10° (14° − 4°). S_1 = head oscillation, S_2 = eye oscillation, $S_3 = S_1 + S_2$. (Modified after Wist, Brandt and Krafczyk, 1983.)

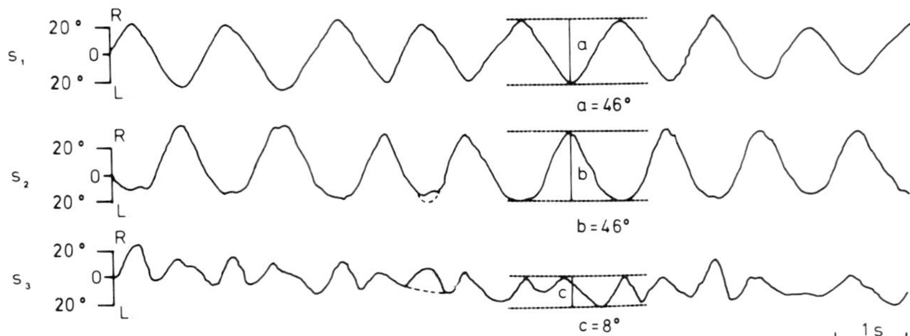

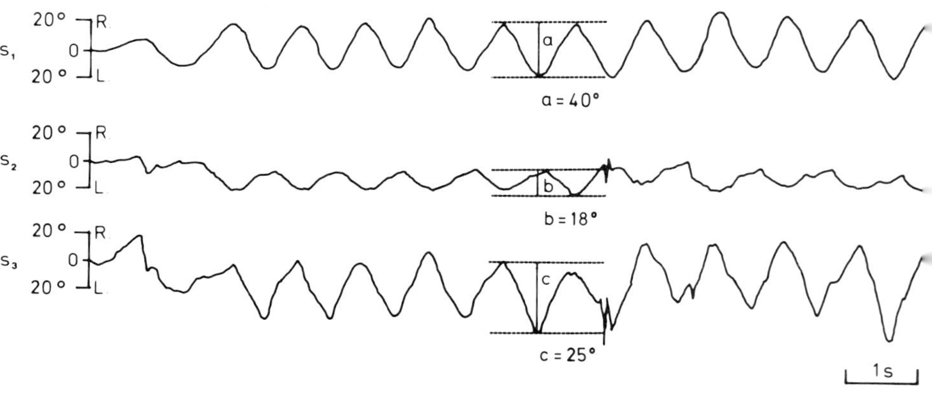

Fig. 18.2 Top: Original recording obtained from a patient with a subacute left abducens palsy. As shown in the second line the displacement of the eye to the left was too small. The amplitude of head displacement was ±23° at a frequency of 0.8 Hz. For this head movement, β was 4°, while the mean excess eye displacement was in fact 8°. Thus this patient showed a retinal slip of 4° but reported no oscillopsia. Subjective oscillopsia = 0°. Retinal slip = 4° = (8° − 4°).
Bottom: Original recording obtained from a patient (aged 53 yrs) with chronic ocular myasthenia of varying severity. Because of weakness of all eye muscles, the amplitude of lateral eye deviation was only ±9° (second tracing). The result of this was a calculated retinal slip of ±11° corresponding to a maximal retinal velocity of 66° L/S. This patient reported oscillopsia which was indicated subjectively as ±10° in amplitude. Subjective oscillopsia = 10°. Retinal slip = 22° (25° − 3°). S_1 = head oscillation, S_2 = eye oscillation, $S_3 = S_1 + S_2$. (Modified after Wist, Brandt and Krafczyk, 1983.)

circumference of the head (*g*) as well as the distance between the head and the fixated target (*a*). In patients with subacute peripheral ocular muscle paresis, the psychophysically determined angle of subjective oscillopsia was considerably smaller or even absent (Figs 18.1 and 18.2) when compared to the calculated net retinal slip (Brandt, 1982; Wist, Brandt and Krafczyk, 1983). The patients were not able to detect the amount of actual displacement of the visual scene on the retina.

18.1.2 ACQUIRED OCULAR OSCILLATIONS

Oscillopsia may also occur in disorders involving involuntary ocular movements which override fixation in the absence of concomitant head motion, and therefore without the involvement of the VOR. Here it is excessive rather than deficient eye movements which lead to the retinal motion of objectively stationary objects. The retinal slip in downbeat nystagmus is misinterpreted as motion of the visual scene, because the involuntary ocular movements are not associated with an appropriate efference-copy signal.

Simultaneous psychophysical and electronystagmographic measurements have been performed in patients with downbeat nystagmus in order to elucidate the relationship between retinal image slip and oscillopsia (Büchele, Brandt and Degner, 1983). Oscillopsia is a permanent symptom but the illusory motion is smaller than that which would be expected from the amplitude of the nystagmus; oscillopsia is dependent on the direction of gaze as is nystagmus amplitude; it increases with increasing nystagmus amplitude (Fig. 18.3) with a mean ratio between the two of 0.37; the individual ratio is relatively consistent for each patient with an interindividual range from 0.13 to 0.61.

Thresholds for egocentric detection of object motion are significantly raised in patients with downbeat nystagmus as compared to healthy subjects; thresholds increase with increasing nystagmus amplitude (Figs 18.3 and 18.8). Thus, there is a partial suppression of visual motion perception for both the retinal slip due to the involuntary eye movements as well as for single objects moving within the visual scene.

18.2 Physiological impairment of motion perception with moving eyes

When Steinman and Collewijn (1980) considered how perceptually a stable world is deduced in the presence of considerable retinal image motion during head oscillation they were particularly intrigued 'by the possibility that vestibular signals are monitored by the visual system and

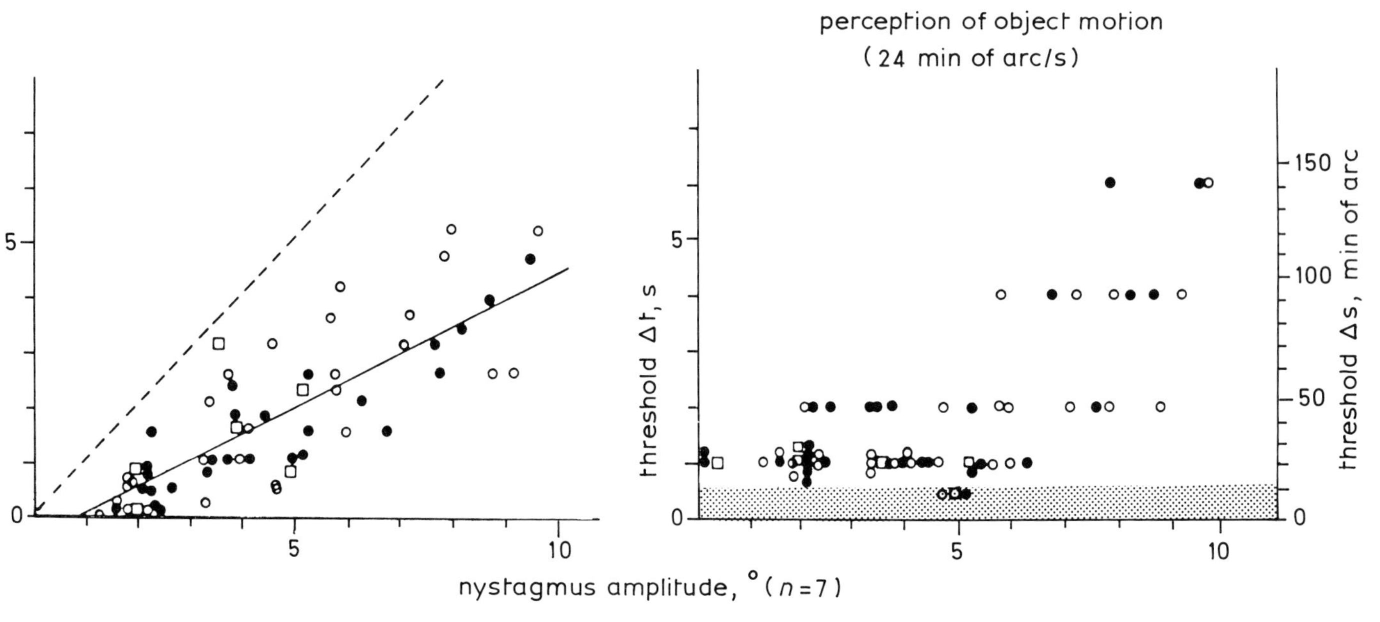

Fig. 18.3 Downbeat nystagmus and concurrent subjective oscillopsia as a function of lateral gaze in seven patients (0 = gaze right; ● = gaze left, □ = gaze straight ahead). Oscillopsia is depicted as a function of nystagmus amplitude (left). Thresholds for the perception of object motion (24 min of arc/s) as a function of nystagmus amplitude (right). Shaded area represents mean thresholds of normals. cillopsia, always smaller than the net retinal slip, increases with increasing nystagmus amplitude with a mean ratio of 0.37. resholds to detect object motion are significantly raised and increase according to nystagmus amplitude.

used to compensate for retinal image motion that accompanies bodily movement'. We do not believe in such a mechanism but have experimental evidence (Fig. 18.4) for a differing mechanism they considered as a seemingly less interesting explanation: 'we may simply find that vision under the conditions of retinal image motion described in the present paper is actually much less keen than our phenomenological observations suggest'.

There is a phenomenon of a physiological impairment of retinal image motion detection during eye movements. This contributes to the partial suppression of oscillopsia under perceptual conditions with inappropriate compensatory eye movements (deficient VOR) or acquired ocular oscillation such as downbeat nystagmus. We have shown that the thresholds for egocentric perception of object motion are significantly raised during concurrent head oscillations of ±20° about the vertical *z*-axis and fixation of the target (Degner and Brandt, 1981; Brandt, 1982). Subjects were exposed to the target which randomly moved either to the right or to the left at a constant angular velocity of 24 minarc/s with a stepwise increase in exposure times from 0.25 to 10 s (20 repetitions of each stimulus condition). Conservative determination of threshold was based on 18 out of 20 possible correct perceptions of movement as well as direction. Sinusoidal active head oscillations raised the detection threshold for object motion by a factor of 2.9 at 1 Hz and 6.4 at 2 Hz oscillations (Fig. 18.4) despite intended stabilization of the target on the retina (VOR). This effect increases disproportionately with increasing eccentricity of the image of the moving stimulus on the retina (Fig. 18.5). Independently, Wertheim (1981) was able to demonstrate that, during smooth pursuit of a target (head stationary), the threshold to detect motion of a visual background increases proportionally to ocular velocity, irrespective of whether the stimulus and the eyes move in the same or opposite directions.

The 'new' phenomenon of visual motion perception suppression during eye movements may reflect a basic sensory-motor mechanism because it has a somatosensory analogue. Elevated thresholds are reported for the perception of electrical stimuli applied to a fingertip as well as partially suppressed somatosensory evoked potentials with simultaneous movement of the stimulated finger in man (Coquery, 1978). The suppression of response activity in the medial lemniscus to contralateral electrical stimulation 100 ms before the onset of active movement in the cat (Ghez and Pisa, 1972; Coulter, 1973) seems to support the view of an efferent inhibition of sensory inflow. Since suppression also occurs with passive movements of the limbs, 'afferent inhibition' must also be possible (Angel and Malenka, 1982). Furthermore, analysis of EMG responses evoked in the leg in man by perturbations revealed that

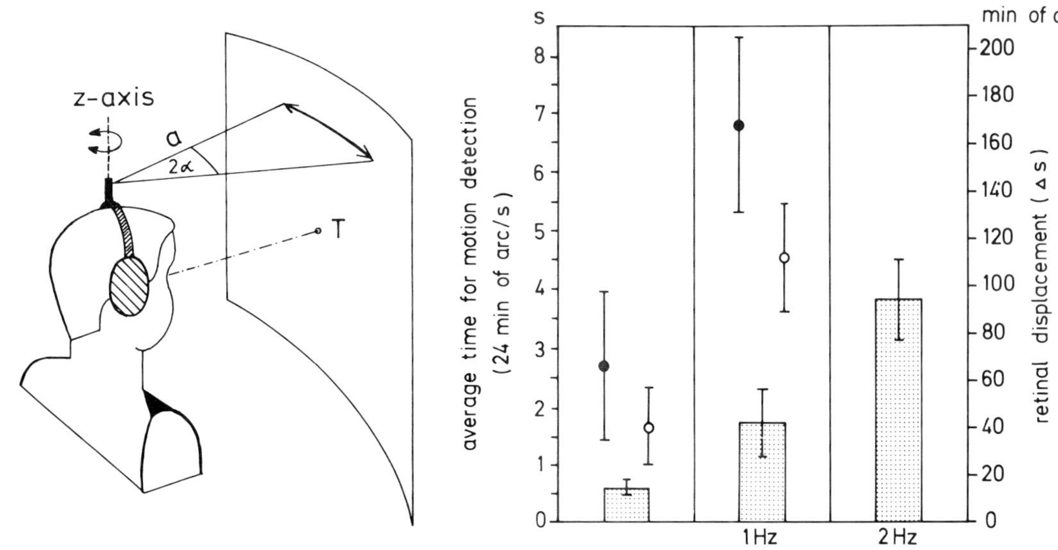

Fig. 18.4 Thresholds for detection of object-motion (means ±SD) in 12 normal subjects (columns) as compared to 8 patients suffering from acquired peripheral ocular motor palsies (●: paretic eye; ○: unaffected eye). During the measurements the moving target (24 min of arc/s; left or right) was fixated by the subject and the head was either fixed by a biteboard or voluntarily oscillated about the vertical *z*-axis at 1 or 2 Hz with an amplitude of ±20° (motion perception during vestibulo-ocular reflex). Physiologically thresholds for object motion detection significantly increase in normal subject with increasing frequency of head oscillation (columns). With peripheral ocular-motor palsies a further pathological elevation of thresholds can be obtained for both the head-fixed condition and head oscillation in both eyes, and is obviously more pronounced in the affected eye. (Modified after Brandt and Dieterich, 1986.)

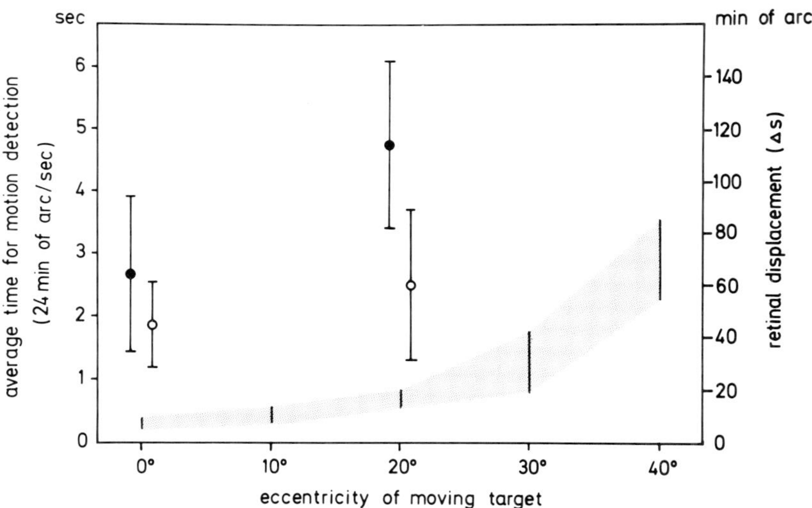

Fig. 18.5 Thresholds for detection of object motion (means ±SD) as a function of the horizontal eccentricity of the moving target on the retina (0°–40°) in 12 normal subjects (shaded area) and 8 patients with acquired peripheral ocular motor palsies (●: paretic eye; ○: unaffected eye). Average time to detect motion increases with increasing eccentricity of the retinal area stimulated in healthy subjects. Thresholds of patients are significantly higher for both eyes with foveal as well as with parafoveal motion stimulation as compared to normal subjects. Thus acquired extraocular muscle paresis seems to impair object motion perception within the entire visual field.

monosynaptic stretch reflex responses as well as supraspinal pathways of group I afferents are suppressed during gait (Dietz, 1986). Chapin and Woodward (1981) have speculated about an inhibitory interaction within the cortex itself (between motor area 4 and somatosensory area 3) since the reduction of afferent signals was more pronounced in cortex neurones as compared to corresponding nuclei within the spinal cord.

18.3 Physiological inhibitory interaction between self-motion and object-motion perception

The incidental observation that one has considerable difficulty in seeing the treetops moving in the wind while driving a vehicle led us to a systematic study of egocentric object-motion perception during concurrent self-motion. In a series of laboratory experiments we found significantly increased thresholds of object-motion perception during simultaneous self-motion under various stimulus conditions. These were vestibular, optokinetic or cervico-proprioceptive stimulation (Brandt, 1982; Probst *et al.*, 1984) and the results resemble the phenomenon described in the previous section.

That real motion of the eyes or the head is not the essential stimulus to suppress object-motion perception was demonstrated by slow trunk oscillations (cervical stimulation) relative to the head fixed by a biteboard (Probst, Brandt and Degner, 1986), and by circularvection studies (Brandt, 1982) with objectively stationary subjects for whom apparent self-motion was visually induced by full-field optokinetic stimulation with the head fixed, the subjects experiencing horizontal optokinetically induced circularvection. The thresholds for perceiving vertical target motion were raised by a factor of 5.5; here the target motion was perpendicular to the direction of the horizontal pattern motion. However, with concurrent horizontal target motion during horizontal pattern motion, the thresholds were raised by a factor of 17.8.

The physiological inhibitory interaction between object-motion and self-motion perception may reflect lack of specificity (or a side-effect) of a space constancy mechanism (efference-copy?) which provides us with a stable picture of the world during locomotion. It has practical implications when one is riding a vehicle with the twofold perceptual task of controlling self-motion (preferably by linearvection) and perceiving object-motion simultaneously. Authorities on road traffic accidents should consider an additional perceptual time of at least 300 ms for detecting critical changes in intercar distances beyond the usual reaction time as expected from laboratory data with the subject's head fixed by a biteboard (Probst *et al.*, 1984). This hypothesis was proven with a field study (vehicle guidance under natural conditions) and a corresponding simulation in the laboratory, in which a stationary surround eliminated the perception of self-motion. Detection times thus corrected consequently lead to an alteration of our concept of safe intervehicle distance in a convoy.

18.4 Pathological (adaptive?) binocular impairment of motion perception caused by monocular external eye muscle paresis

It was the amount of net retinal slip tolerated by the patients (Figs 18.1 and 18.2) without causing oscillopsia, as well as the interindividual differences with respect to the degree and acuteness of paresis which led us to suspect an additional pathological impairment of motion perception. The latter is dependent on the particular disease distinct from the physiological phenomena described above (Brandt and Dieterich, 1986).

Motion perception was investigated separately for the affected and unaffected eye while fixating a horizontally moving target 1° in diameter, with a constant velocity of 24 minarc/s in a total of 24 patients suffering from abducens ($n = 14$), oculomotor ($n = 6$), trochlear palsy ($n = 2$) or monocular myasthenic weakness ($n = 2$).

Thresholds for the detection of object motion (eight patients) with the head fixed were significantly raised up to a factor of 5 for the paretic eye and a factor of 3.3 for the normal eye (Fig. 18.4). With sinusoidal head oscillations at 1 Hz (which physiologically elevates thresholds) the ratio between thresholds in patients and normals is about 4 for the paretic eye and 2.7 for the unaffected eye (Fig. 18.4). This clearly suggests that in patients with acquired peripheral ocular motor palsies both the physiological and the pathological impairment of motion perception summate when the moving target is fixated during voluntary head motion. These effects are not restricted to the fovea but also apply to perception of motion within the peripheral retina (Fig. 18.5). In normal subjects thresholds increase with increasing eccentric location of the target on the retina (factor of 1.23 for 20° eccentricity); accordingly pathological thresholds in patients are further elevated when a moving stimulus is viewed from the peripheral retina (factor of 1.7 for 20° eccentricity in paretic eye). A central mechanism must be assumed which affects motion perception since perception of both eyes is involved even though the paretic eye tends to perform more poorly.

In a second series of experiments (19 patients) mean response times (20 repetitions for each direction) to the detection of motion of a projected target were determined instead of conventional threshold measurements which require bothersome attention of the patient for hours. Response times were determined as a function of age ($n = 10$ for each decade from 10 to 70 years) in a control group of 60 neurological patients without ocular motor disturbances. Again, response times of most patients with acquired ocular muscle paresis were longer and exhibited larger standard deviations compared with the range of patients of the same age without ocular motor dysfunction (Fig. 18.6). Three patients, however, did not show abnormal prolongation of response times; one of them (●) was the only patient with a congenital abducens palsy. Prolongation of response times to motion stimuli in patients was not simply due to a 'retarded reaction' since mean net reaction times to suprathreshold stimuli were the same for the ocular motor and the control group (266 ± 79 ms and 265 ± 58 ms, respectively). Differences between affected and unaffected eyes were significant but there was no direction-specific suppression of motion perception (right vs left) with respect to the direction of eye movement dysfunction in right or left abducens palsies (Fig. 18.7).

Thus, there is a central binocular impairment of motion perception in

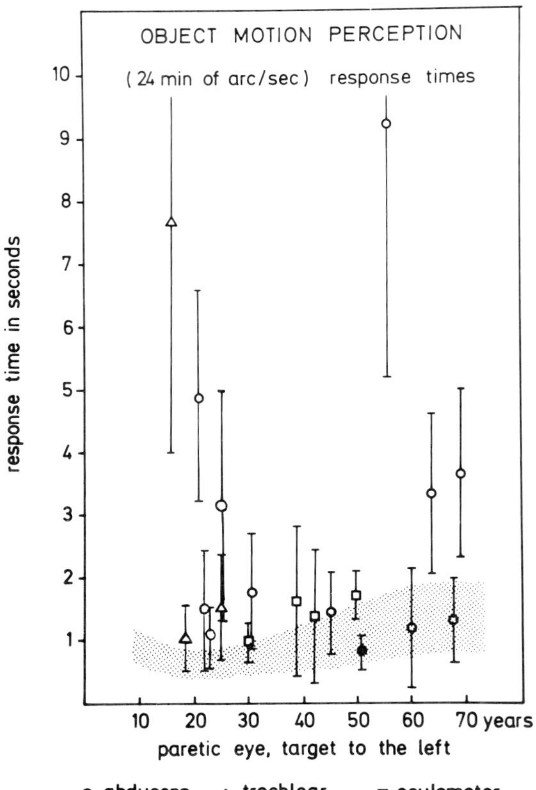

Fig. 18.6 Response times (means ±SD) to detect horizontal object motion at constant angular velocity of 24 min of arc/s. The shaded area represents a control group of 60 neurological patients without ocular motor disturbances (n = 10 for each decade from 10 to 70 years). Response times are shortest at about 20 years of age with increasing mean values and standard deviations in the elderly. Most of the 19 patients with acquired peripheral ocular motor disorders have higher response times for monocular vision of the affected eye. Three patients (one with a congenital abducens palsy, ●) between 52 to 70 years appeared normal with respect to motion perception. (Modified after Brandt and Dieterich, 1986.)

patients with acquired peripheral ocular motor palsies which lasts as long as the palsy lasts, the underlying mechanism of which is unknown. The amount of suppression of motion perception seems for the most part to be independent of the degree of the individual palsy, but the time course, in particular the improvement of motion perception during the recovery of the palsy, has yet to be systematically studied.

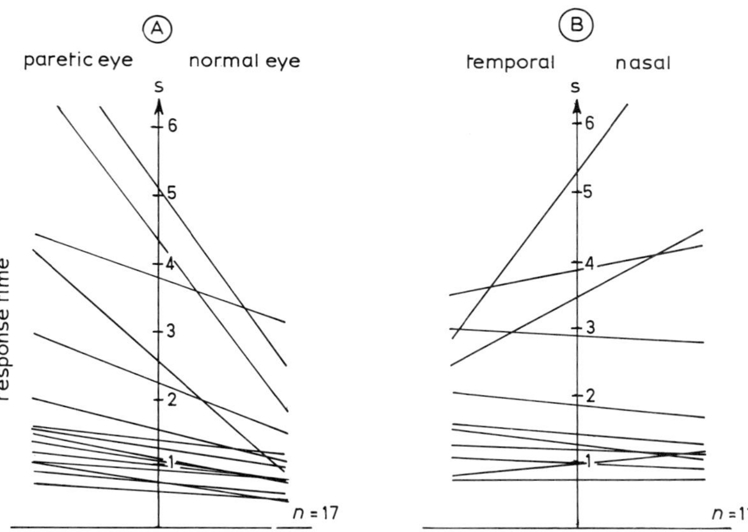

Fig. 18.7 A, Response times (means) to detect horizontal motion of a target at a constant angular velocity (24 min of arc/s) in 17 patients suffering from acquired external eye muscle paresis (abducens 11; trochlear 3; oculomotor 3). Comparison between the paretic and the normal eye shows that impairment of motion perception is always greater in the paretic eye. B, Response times of 11 patients with acquired abducens palsies exhibit no significant differences for the direction of target motion (temporal versus nasal) with respect to the functional deficit of eye movement.

18.5 Oscillopsia and motion perception in congenital nystagmus

Oscillopsia is widely suppressed in congenital nystagmus being usually absent in the primary position of gaze and the null-zone of nystagmus, but still detectable by most sufferers as a subtle oscillation of fixated objects when eccentric gaze precipitates maximal amplitudes of the nystagmus.

This raises the question of the capability of motion perception in congenital nystagmus, since in all instances of ocular motor disturbances so far discussed partial suppression of oscillopsia amplitudes was linked to impaired motion perception in general. It was the typical defect of optokinetic nystagmus in congenital nystagmus which stimulated Kommerell and Mehdorn (1982) to speculate that a dysfunction of the feedback system that controls shifts of the images across the retina might be the basic abnormality underlying the development of congenital nystagmus.

From their experiments with magnitude estimation of perceived motion – in which the patients managed to differentiate velocities within the range between 15 and 100°/s almost as precisely as normal controls – they infer that dysfunction of the feedback system is not caused simply by a sensory defect (Kommerell, Horn and Bach, 1986). The differentiation between gross image shifts as caused by the congenital nystagmus and the velocities of viewed pattern motion were surprisingly good even with the exposure time (0.2 s) kept shorter than one cycle of nystagmus (0.5 s).

The data by Kommerell, Horn and Bach (1986), however, do not allow the conclusion that motion perception is normal in these individuals because of the method used. In psychophysical magnitude estimation experiments, a standard stimulus (here 40°/s) serves as a modulus with an arbitrary value and subjects are asked to indicate all subsequent stimulus velocities presented as a multiple or a fraction of this modulus. This method implies that, if the standard stimuli were perceived slower by the congenital nystagmus patients as compared to normals, it is still possible that the differentiation within the velocity range of stimulation is preserved. Thus, the power function of velocity perception (magnitude estimation after Stevens, 1957) would then appear normal despite the pathology that with respect to absolute velocity all single pattern motions were underestimated by congenital nystagmus patients.

On the basis of our own preliminary data on congenital nystagmus we have reason to believe that there is in fact an impairment of motion perception in these individuals (Dieterich and Brandt, 1987). Thresholds to detect object motion of a fixated target straight ahead (24 minarc/s) were raised by a factor of 2–3 as compared to normals and were even higher than those of patients with acquired downbeat nystagmus (factor 1.46). With increasing horizontal eccentricity of gaze thresholds became increasingly higher in congenital as well as acquired downbeat nystagmus due to the progressive increase of nystagmus amplitude in both 'disorders' (Fig. 18.8). There are considerable differences in the accuracy to perceive object motion either to the right or to the left with either the right or the left eye (Fig. 18.9). The correspondence with characteristics of the individual nystagmus (such as wave-form) is still a matter for speculation and the object of current investigations.

Oscillopsia, and consequently the sensitivity to detect retinal image slip due to the nystagmus, is obviously lower in congenital nystagmus than in downbeat nystagmus, which suggests more powerful adaptation in the congenital abnormality. If the congenital nystagmus patients were able to subtract their current eye motion from the change in position of a viewed target on the retina (by efference-copy mechanism) one would expect them to see an after-image oscillate in darkness according to their

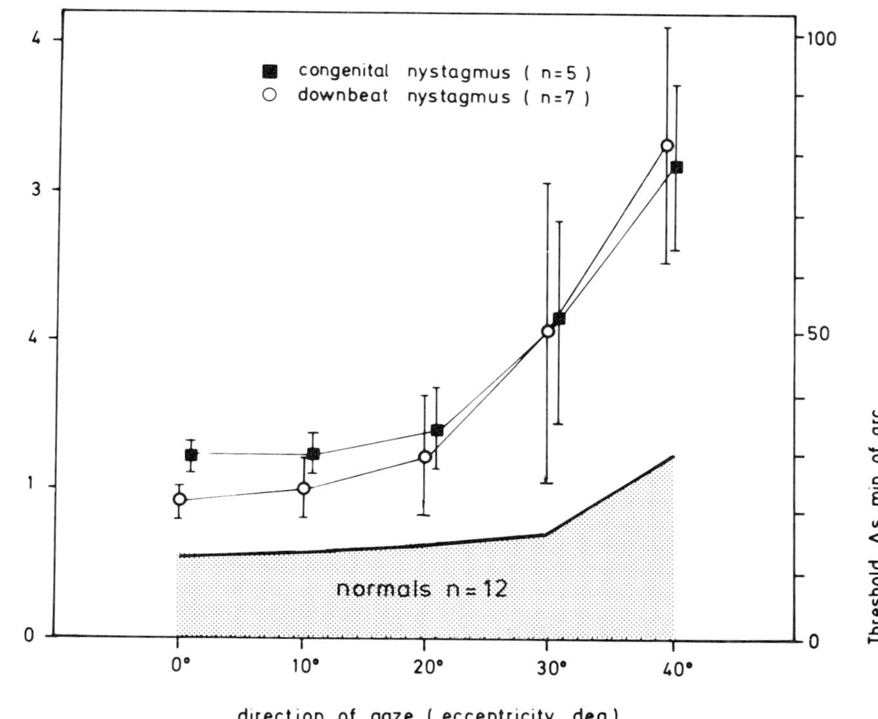

Fig. 18.8 Thresholds for detection of object motion (24 min of arc/s; means ±SD) as a function of the eccentricity of horizontal gaze (0–40°) in patients suffering from congenital nystagmus (n = 5) and acquired downbeat nystagmus (n = 7) as compared to normals (n = 12). Normals show only a slight increase in thresholds with eccentric gaze which becomes more pronounced on lateral gaze of 40°. The thresholds for the patients are significantly raised irrespective of whether the ocular oscillation is congenital or acquired. There is a disproportionate increase on lateral gaze beyond 20° which simultaneously activates nystagmus amplitude in both disorders.

nystagmus. Surprisingly enough this was not observed by vom Hofe (1941) and particularly by Goddé-Jolly and Larmande (1973) who reported on patients with congenital nystagmus who were able to fixate a stationary object with a foveal after-image without seeing either one oscillate. In contrast Kommerell, Horn and Bach (1986) found some patients with congenital nystagmus who did observe oscillation of an after-image in darkness with an amplitude about half of the nystagmus amplitude. The latter fits recent observations by Leigh and Dell'Osso

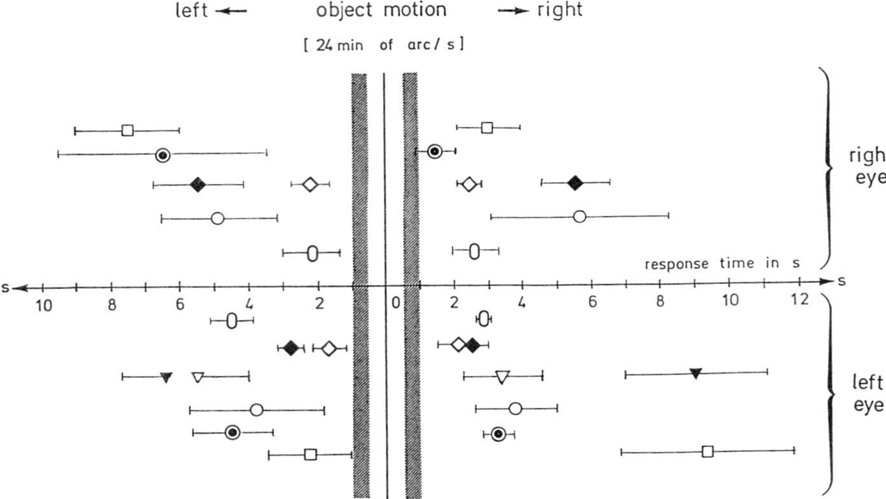

Fig. 18.9 Response times (means ±SD) to detect horizontal object motion (24 min of arc/s) with right or left eye separately for motion stimulation to the right or to the left in six patients (○, □, ▽, 0, ◇, ◉) with congenital nystagmus (patients are not identical with those in Fig. 18.8). There are considerable differences for each eye and stimulus directions (○, □, ◉, 0 = primary position of gaze; ▽, ◇ = nullzone; ▼, ◆ = maximal-'zone'). Shaded area represents means ±SD of normal controls (n = 10).

(personal communication) in which oscillopsia (completely suppressed under natural conditions) was elicited in congenital nystagmus by use of a combined lens device which enables an approximate stabilization of vision of the real world despite moving eyes. This device is being currently tested for the optical treatment of oscillopsia due to acquired ocular oscillation in order to regain reading ability and to watch television more comfortably (Leigh *et al.*, 1986). It consists of two parts, a field lens and a strongly divergent contact lens. The field lens is so placed that its own principal focus would be at the centre of rotation of the eye ball such that a ray from the fixation point traverses the optical axis of the eye regardless of the direction in which the eye is pointing (Rushton and Rushton, 1984).

The powerful suppression of oscillopsia in chronic ocular oscillations as well as the re-occurrence of oscillopsia when stabilizing retinal images (which interrupts continuous motion stimulation) is reminiscent of the well-known velocity habituation and motion after-effects following prolonged motion stimulation.

18.6 Conclusions

Undesired retinal image slips of the fixated visual scene are caused by a deficient VOR during head movements as well as involuntary ocular oscillations which override fixation with the head stationary (Fig. 18.10). In all instances of ocular motor disorders investigated so far (whether supranuclear or infranuclear, congenital or acquired) the amplitude of perceived motion of the visual scene was considerably smaller than the calculated net retinal slip. This partial suppression of distressing oscillopsia was inevitably linked to impaired motion perception in general. There is a physiological mechanism of impaired motion perception with moving eyes which contributes to the suppression of oscillopsia but does not completely account for it. An additional adaptive binocular impairment of motion perception must be involved which is separate from the physiological phenomenon and initiated by the particular ocular motor disorder. The characteristics of the latter have yet to be studied more thoroughly.

Patients with chronic ocular oscillations and largely suppressed oscillopsia may (paradoxically) experience oscillopsia of stabilized retinal images. Both findings, impaired motion perception with continuous oscillation of retinal images as well as apparent motion perception with artificial stabilization of retinal images, reflect the well-known

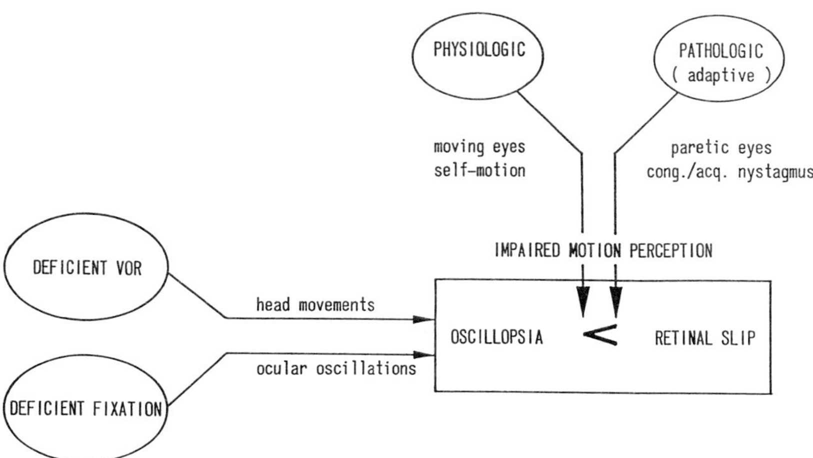

Fig. 18.10 Oscillopsia is caused either by inappropriate compensatory eye movements (VOR) during head motion or by oscillations which override fixation. Oscillopsia amplitudes are always smaller than net retinal slip because of partial suppression of motion perception under these conditions. Suppression of motion perception is due to the summation of physiological and pathological (adaptive) elevation of thresholds to detect retinal image shifts of the viewed visual scene.

mechanisms of motion habituation and motion after-effects as dependent on the duration of stimulation.

References

Angel, R.W. and Malenka, R.C. (1982) Velocity dependent suppression of cutaneous sensitivity during movement. *Exp. Neurol.*, **77**, 266–74.

Atkin, A. and Bender, M.B. (1968) Ocular stabilization during oscillatory head movements. *Arch. Neurol. (Chicago)*, **19**, 559–66.

Bender, M.B. (1965) Oscillopsia. *Arch. Neurol. (Chicago)*, **13**, 204–13.

Bender, M.B. and Feldman, M. (1967) Visual illusions during head movement in lesions of the brain stem. *Arch. Neurol. (Chicago)*, **17**, 354–64.

Benson, A.J. and Barnes, G.R. (1978) Vision during angular oscillation: the dynamic interaction of visual and vestibular mechanism. *Aviat. Space Environ. Med.*, **49**, 340–5.

Brandt, Th. (1982) The relationship between retinal image slip, oscillopsia and postural imbalance, in *Functional Bases of Ocular Motility Disorders* (eds G. Lennerstrand, D.S. Zee and E.L. Keller), Pergamon, Oxford, New York, pp. 379–85.

Brandt, Th. and Dieterich, M. (1986) Peripheral ocular motor palsy impairs motion perception, in *Adaptive Processes in Visual and Oculomotor Systems* (eds E.L. Keller and D.S. Zee). Pergamon, Oxford, New York, pp. 457–64.

Brickner, R. (1936) Oscillopsia: a new symptom commonly occurring in multiple sclerosis. *Arch. Neurol. Psychiat. (Chicago)*, **36**, 586–9.

Büchele, W., Brandt, Th. and Degner, D. (1983) Ataxia and oscillopsia in downbeat-nystagmus vertigo syndrome. *Adv. Oto.-Rhino.-Laryngol.*, **30**, 291–7.

Chapin, J.K. and Woodward, D.J. (1981) Modulation of sensory responsiveness of single somatosensory cortical cells during movement and arousal behaviours. *Exp. Neurol.*, **72**, 164–78.

Coquery, J.-M. (1978) Role of active movement in control of afferent input from skin in cat and man, in *Active Touch – The Mechanism of Recognition of Objects by Manipulation* (ed. G. Gordon), Elmsford, New York, pp. 161–9.

Coulter, J.D. (1973) Sensory transmission through lemniscal pathway during voluntary movement in the cat. *J. Neurophysiol.*, **37**, 831–45.

Degner, D and Brandt, Th. (1981) Interaction between self- and object-motion perception. *Pflügers Arch.* Suppl. **389**, R 30, 118.

Dieterich, M. and Brandt, Th. (1987) Impaired motion perception in congenital nystagmns and acquired ocular motor palsy. *Clin. Vision Sci.*, **1**, 337–45.

Dietz, V. (1986) Afferent and efferent control of posture and gait, in *Disorders of Posture and Gait* (eds W. Bles and Th. Brandt), Elsevier, Amsterdam, pp. 69–81.

Ghez, G. and Pisa, M. (1972) Inhibition of afferent transmission in cuneate nucleus during voluntary movement in the cat. *Brain Res.*, **40**, 145–51.

Goddé-Jolly, D. and Larmande, A. (1973) *Les Nystagmus*, Masson, Paris.

Gresty, M.A., Hess, K. and Leech, J. (1977) Disorders of the vestibulo-ocular reflex producing oscillopsia and mechanisms compensating for loss of labyrinthine function. *Brain*, **100**, 693–716.

vom Hofe, K. (1941) Untersuchungen über das Verhalten eines zentralen optischen Nachbildes bei und nach unwillkürlichen Bewegungen sowie mechanischen Verlagerungen des Auges. *Graefe's Arch. Ophthalmol.*, **144**, 164–9.

Kommerell, G., Horn, R. and Bach, M. (1986) Motion perception in congenital nystagmus, in *Adaptive Processes in Visual and Oculomotor Systems* (eds E.L. Keller and D.S. Zee), Pergamon, Oxford, New York, pp. 485–92.

Kommerell, G. and Mehdorn, E. (1982) Is an optokinetic defect cause of congenital nystagmus? in *Functional Basis of Ocular Motility Disorders* (eds G. Lennerstrand, D.S. Zee and E.L. Keller), Pergamon, Oxford, New York, pp. 159–67.

Leigh, R.J., Rushton, D.N., Thurston, S.E. and Hertle, R.W. (1986) Optical treatment of oscillopsia due to acquired nystagmus. *Neurology*, **36** (Suppl. 1), 252.

Probst, Th., Brandt, Th. and Degner, D. (1986) Object-motion detection affected by concurrent self-motion perception: Psychophysics of a new phenomenon. *Behav. Brain Res.* (in press).

Probst, Th., Krafczyk, S., Brandt, Th. and Wist, E.R. (1984) Interaction between perceived self-motion and object-motion impairs vehicle guidance. *Science*, **225**, 536–8.

Rushton, D.N. and Rushton, R.H. (1984) An optical method for approximate stabilization of vision of the real world. *J. Physiol. (Lond.)*, **357**, 3 RP.

Stavenski, A.A., Hansen, R.N., Steinman, R.M. and Winterson, B.J. (1979) Quality of retinal image stabilization during small natural and artificial body rotations in man. *Vision Res.*, **19**, 675–83.

Steinman, R.M. and Collewijn, H. (1980) Binocular retinal image motion during active head rotation. *Vision Res.*, **20**, 415–29.

Stevens, S.S. (1957) On the psychophysical law. *Psychol. Rev.*, **64**, 153–81.

Wertheim, A.H. (1981) On the relativity of perceived motion. *Acta Psychol.*, **48**, 97–110.

Wist, E.R., Brandt, Th. and Krafczyk, S. (1983) Oscillopsia and retinal slip: Evidence supporting a clinical test. *Brain*, **106**, 153–68.

Zee, D.S. (1978) Ophthalmoscopy in examination of patients with vestibular disorders. *Ann. Neurol.*, **3**, 373–4.

CHAPTER 19

Cerebellar involvement in smooth pursuit eye movement generation: flocculus and vermis

EDWARD L. KELLER

19.1 Introduction

The more frequent application of sensitive and accurate eye movement recording systems and other technical advances in the clinic has led to a steady increase in the number of types of oculomotor disturbances reported in patients with cerebellar lesions. Thus, a recent review (Daroff, 1982) lists 32 types of clinical eye signs of cerebellar dysfunction. Daroff's review also points out the problem of distinguishing those types of oculomotor disturbance which are due to isolated cerebellar lesions from those that also include co-existing brainstem involvement, since pure cerebellar lesions are a relatively rare occurrence in clinical cases. This problem has been clarified, and the size of the list has been pruned considerably by quantitative oculomotor studies in several groups of patients affected with selective cerebellar cortical atrophy (Baloh, Konrad and Honrubia, 1975; Baloh, Yee and Honrubia, 1986; Zee *et al.*, 1976). This approach has been also aided by careful comparative experimental lesion studies in monkeys that have oculomotor systems similar to those in man. Recent reviews have taken the position that only those oculomotor disturbances seen in the human cerebellar atrophy cases, and those also found in the experimental monkey cerebellar lesion studies, are true signs of cerebellar dysfunction (Zee, 1982; Zee, 1984; Keller, in press).

The most revealing result that has emerged from the experimental cerebellar lesions is that the cerebellum plays a vital role in the control of long-term, plastic, adaptive oculomotor changes that allow the nervous system to adjust performance in the face of internal lesions or external physical changes (Robinson, 1976; Optican and Robinson, 1980; Optican *et al.*, 1980). These findings raise the problem for interpretation of the clinical material that the onset of a selective cerebellar lesion can unmask a previously incurred brainstem lesion which is being compensated by that piece of cerebellar tissue. The later cerebellar lesion might then produce an oculomotor deficit that would not have been present with either lesion alone.

The experimental cerebellar lesion studies and the selective cerebellar atrophy cases have also produced evidence that the cerebellum is involved in a number of specific on-line oculomotor functions. The term on-line is used here to refer to a direct neurological control function on a movement-to-movement basis. Zee (1982) has summarized these cerebellar oculomotor functions in a particularly effective manner. They include aiding retinal-image stabilization (smooth pursuit tracking, suppression of inappropriate vestibular nystagmus, gaze holding) and control of saccadic amplitude.

One further advance has been facilitated by the experimental lesion studies. Selective localized lesions of just certain portions of the cerebellum have produced differential oculomotor deficits which suggest that different oculomotor control functions may be localized in certain regions of the cerebellum. The greater resolving power inherent in the newer tissue-imaging techniques have also begun to present clinical researchers with the ability to localize the exact region of cerebellar lesions in humans and then to associate each type of oculomotor deficit with specific cerebellar regions (Baloh, Yee and Honrubia, 1986). Zee (1982) has summarized the earlier work and suggests that the control of image stabilization and the long-term adaptation of the vestibulo-ocular reflex and the adjustment of post-saccadic gaze holding are the function of the flocculo-nodular lobe. The immediate control and long-term adjustment of saccadic movement amplitude is mediated by the posterior vermis (lobules VI and VII) and this region's connections with the midline deep cerebellar nuclei (fastigial nuclei).

The main purpose of this chapter is to examine critically the hypothesis that smooth pursuit eye movement control is localized exclusively in flocculus in contradistinction to the notion that this function is more widely distributed across the cerebellar cortex including in particular the posterior vermis. However, in order to make the chapter more complete as a reference source, a brief discussion of the cerebellar control of saccadic eye movements will be included.

A marked deficit in the performance of smooth pursuit tracking occurs without exception as a concomitant of all the experimental primate, total cerebellar lesion studies and in all the human selective cerebellar atrophy cases (Westheimer and Blair, 1973; 1974; Baloh, Konrad and Honrubia, 1975; Burde *et al.*, 1975; Zee *et al.*, 1976; Baloh, Yee and Honrubia, 1986). The degree of saccadic dysmetria observed following cerebellar lesions is more variable, particularly in the human studies (Baloh, Yee and Honrubia, 1986).

According to Zee's (1982) hypothesis, the control of pursuit eye movements – a neural mechanism that stabilizes the image of a moving selective point on the fovea even in the presence of a stationary background texture – is localized in the flocculo-nodular lobe of the cerebellum. While a great deal of evidence supports this view, this chapter presents additional evidence, based on single-unit recordings and experimental lesions in primates, that the vermis, lobules VI and VII, may also be important in the control of pursuit eye movements. These findings suggest a more widespread distribution of pursuit control over the cerebellar cortex.

19.2 Evidence for floccular involvement in pursuit eye movements

Single-unit recording studies in the alert monkey have shown that many floccular Purkinje cells discharge during pursuit eye movements (Lisberger and Fuchs, 1978; Miles *et al.*, 1980). When the temporal characteristics of this discharge were quantified, it was shown to be closely in phase with eye velocity signals and its modulation increased monotonically and often linearly with the magnitude of eye velocity. Since the modulation in these cells' discharge remains the same during smooth tracking of small moving targets whether the head is still (oculomotor pursuit) or moving (cancellation of the VOR), they have been called gaze velocity cells.

These floccular Purkinje cells project directly to various regions of the vestibular nuclei including the y-group, the superior and the medial vestibular nuclei (Balaban, Ito and Watanabe, 1981; Langer *et al.*, 1985a). Since these same regions of the vestibular nucleus complex are well known to contain neurones with direct and polysynaptic oculomotor neurone projections, it is clear that the flocculus is anatomically closely linked to oculomotor control.

Surgical ablations (bilateral) of the flocculus (and portions of the paraflocculus) in monkeys lead to major deficits in smooth pursuit control (Zee *et al.*, 1981). When this deficit was quantified by calculating gain (eye velocity/target velocity) an average value of 0.64 was found in four lesioned animals. This compares to a normal value of very close to one in the intact monkey. This deficit showed only partial recovery to a value of 0.78 after a post-operative period of 6 to 12 weeks.

Electrical stimulation of the monkey flocculus leads to slow, smooth eye movements that were interpreted to be pursuit (Ron and Robinson, 1973) although it would be difficult to distinguish between slow ocular drifts set up by vestibular system imbalance and visual smooth pursuit on the basis of these results. More convincing evidence of the floccular link to pursuit control resulted from a focal microstimulation study of the flocculus during ongoing pursuit (Belknap, Noda and Ohno, 1983).

The flocculus is also a terminal target of the mossy fibre input from the visual portions of the pontine nuclei (Brodal, 1982; Langer *et al.*, 1985b). In particular the dorsolateral and lateral pontine nuclei project, primarily in a contralateral fashion, to the flocculus in monkey. These regions of the pons contain neurones carrying retinal slip signals with foveal receptive fields (Suzuki and Keller, 1984), and are the primary regions of the pons receiving input from the extrastriate cortex visual motion processing areas (Glickstein *et al.*, 1980; Van Essen, Maunsell and Bixley, 1981). These afferent links complete the anatomical picture that further suggests the central role of the flocculus in smooth pursuit generation.

When all these experimental results are taken together the evidence is rather strong that the major locus of pursuit control within the cerebellum is in the flocculus. However, the fact that complete cerebellectomies in the monkey create a total pursuit deficit (Westheimer and Blair, 1973) or almost total deficit (Optican and Robinson, 1980), while the flocculectomies produced only a 36% decrement in pursuit gain is evidence that other regions of the cerebellum may be contributing to normal pursuit behaviour.

19.3 Evidence for vermal involvement in pursuit eye movements

19.3.1 SINGLE-UNIT RECORDING STUDIES

The discharge pattern of a subset of Purkinje cells in the cerebellar vermis, lobules VI and VII (hereafter called just vermis), have recently been shown to resemble that of floccular gaze velocity cells during pursuit (Suzuki and Keller, in press). The discharge modulation in these cells is approximately in phase, and increased, with eye velocity. On average their sensitivity to eye velocity (0.64 spikes/s per deg/s) was somewhat lower than that reported in the average floccular gaze velocity cell

(0.92 spikes/s per deg/s) (Lisberger and Fuchs, 1978; Miles *et al.*, 1980). In addition, the fidelity of the modulation was not as clear in the vermis as that observed in the flocculus, a fact reflected in the relatively high harmonic distortions present in vermal Purkinje cells (typically 30–40%) during sinusoidal smooth pursuit.

Most posterior vermis Purkinje cells that carried an eye velocity signal also were modulated by head velocity paradigms (VOR suppression) in a similar manner to floccular gaze velocity cells. In these cells the direction of eye and head velocity associated with increased cellular discharge was the same. Sensitivities to the two signals were usually similar but, on average, the sensitivity to eye velocity was 1.4 times that to head velocity. In floccular gaze velocity cells the sensitivities to these two signals were more closely matched.

This group of vermal Purkinje cells showed one very pronounced difference in their behaviour from that reported for floccular gaze velocity cells. Most vermal Purkinje cells showed a clear modulation of discharge correlated with retinal slip velocity (Suzuki, Noda and Kase, 1981), while such signals have never been unambiguously demonstrated in the flocculus. In general, this visual slip signal had the same directional preference as the eye and head velocity directional preference in any given unit. In 65 vermal cells tested with all three paradigms, 39 cells (60%) contained all three signals. The sensitivities to retinal slip velocity were, on average, about 80% of the sensitivities to eye velocity.

If the small differences in sensitivity to head and eye velocity are ignored, then during pursuit eye movements and combined eye/head tracking when the tracking closely matches target velocity (i.e. retinal slip is negligible), vermal Purkinje cells function as gaze velocity cells in a similar fashion to floccular neurones. Only during episodes of poor tracking or when the target suddenly changes speed or direction, do vermal cells manifest their basic difference in behaviour. At these particular times retinal slip increases as eye and/or head velocity falls. In vermal Purkinje cells the discharge remains proportional to target velocity (Suzuki and Keller, in press) while floccular discharge decreases in parallel with eye and/or head velocity (Lisberger and Fuchs, 1978; Miles *et al.*, 1980). In mathematical terms the vermal signal can be viewed as coding actual target velocity in space, a signal not directly accessible from any of the nervous system's afferent or efferent signals. Target velocity can be computed from the summation of eye velocity, head velocity and retinal slip, exactly the combination of signals found to be present on many vermal Purkinje cells.

Most current models of the pursuit system use positive feedback of an efferent copy of eye velocity and feed-forward of a vestibular signal proportional to head velocity to sustain steady gaze velocity during pursuit movements (Miles *et al.*, 1980). Neurones involved in this circuitry, which seems to include the flocculus, closely reflect the ongoing gaze velocity. On the other hand, a reconstructed target velocity signal is clearly a higher level of abstraction than a motor-related gaze velocity signal. It is the signal required to guide combined limb/eye or eye/head movements in target space. The existence of an internal circuit to 'regenerate' target velocity has been proposed on theoretical grounds by Young (1977). The demonstration of the required composite signals on vermal Purkinje cells is the first experimental evidence that such a combination exists on single central neurones.

Based on the foregoing evidence it is logical to hypothesize that the flocculus acts to maintain pursuit eye movements particularly in the steady state, while the vermis is particularly important during certain conditions of pursuit when the target velocity is changed or pursuit is initiated in response to auditory or other non-visual inputs. Since the types of signals present in the vermis and flocculus are so similar, it also seems logical that the vermis could partially compensate for the deficit produced in pursuit eye movements by floccular lesions. This line of reasoning would also suggest that eye movement studies of patients with vermal lesions as opposed to floccular lesions would show greater deficits in initiating pursuit to non-visual targets.

19.3.2 EXPERIMENTAL LESIONS IN THE VERMIS OF MONKEYS

Some experimental evidence exists on the effect of selective vermal lesions in monkeys on smooth pursuit behaviour. Both Ritchie (1976) and Optican and Robinson (1980) reported anecdotally that smooth pursuit appeared normal in their monkeys with large vermal lesions that included lobules VI and VII. However, since the focus of both of these studies was on saccadic eye movements, neither set of authors gave any details about how pursuit was measured, the velocity range examined or the visual targets used. More recently in our laboratory (Suzuki and Keller, 1983), the effect of vermal lesions on smooth pursuit eye movements has been reinvestigated. Animals were trained to track a small moving visual spot presented on a dim homogeneous background. After the animals' tracking behaviour had stabilized the gain of their smooth pursuit systems was measured over a frequency range of 0.1 to 2.0 Hz (target amplitude $\pm 10°$). Surgical lesions were made in two monkeys and similar post-surgical effects on smooth pursuit were noted in both animals. Saccades made to stationary visual targets were frequently dysmetric as has previously been reported in the earlier vermis lesion papers. In addition substantial deficits in each animal's smooth pursuit ability appeared following the vermal lesion. This effect for one animal is illustrated in Fig. 19.1. Following the surgical ablation of the posterior vermis this animal's smooth pursuit gain was only about 60–70% of the control values. This behaviour recovered somewhat by 22 days following the lesion at which time the animal was killed to obtained histological verification of the extent of the lesion. The lesion was found to include the

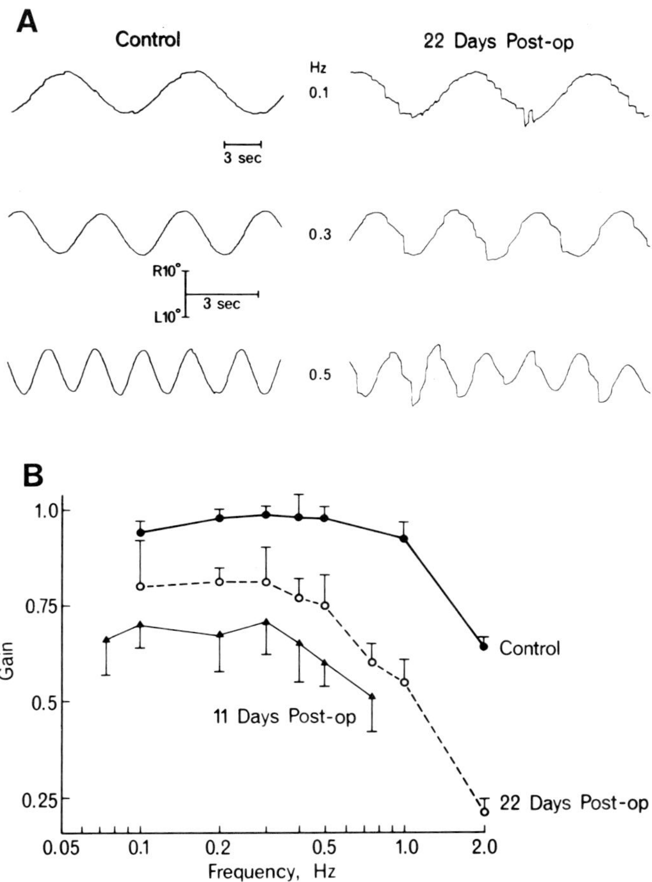

Fig. 19.1 The effect of vermisectomy on smooth pursuit eye movements in one monkey. A: specimen eye movement records during sinusoidal tracking of a small, one-half degree, target spot at three different sinusoidal frequencies. Behaviour prior to the lesion is shown on the left and that following the lesion on the right. Traces shown are horizontal eye position. B: Frequency response of gain defined as peak smooth eye velocity divided by peak target velocity for the same animal shown in A. Separate curves show the gain values for the monkey prior to the lesion, at 11 days following the lesion, and at 22 days following the lesion.

vermis and paravermis of lobules IV to VI (complete) and major portions of the vermis and paravermis of lobules VII and VIII. The deep cerebellar nuclei were all spared. Similar results were obtained in the other animal.

19.3.3 ANATOMICAL CONNECTIONS OF THE VERMIS

The source of a number of the important afferent inputs to the vermis, lobules VI and VII, supports the view that this region also plays a role in controlling smooth pursuit behaviour. In similarity to the flocculus, this region of vermis receives extensive inputs from the dorsolateral pontine nuclei (Brodal, 1978). This latter region has been implicated as the major pontine region involved in relaying visual motion and visuo-oculomotor signals to the cerebellum (Mustari, Fuchs and Wallman, 1984; Suzuki and Keller, 1984; Suzuki, May and Keller, 1984; May, Keller and Crandall, 1985). It is not clear at this time whether the same types of signals are projected to both the vermis and flocculus or whether each region receives a selective subset of the many types of discrete spot, moving background and oculomotor signals shown to exist in the dorsolateral pons.

In terms of efferent projections the vermal Purkinje cells all project exclusively to the midline deep cerebellar nuclei (fastigial nuclei). Therefore actions of the vermis on pursuit behaviour have to take place through projections of the fastigial nuclei. Projections of the monkey fastigial nuclei have been studied by Batton *et al.* (1977) using the autoradiographic technique. The projections of this nucleus do not seem to include brainstem regions closely associated with pursuit, as was the case for the floccular projections. There are heavy projections to the vestibular nuclei, but only to the inferior and lateral parts, areas not involved directly with oculomotor neurones. There are some projections to the reticular formation near the abducens nuclei that might include a region in which smooth pursuit neurones have been recorded (Eckmiller, 1982). Finally, there is an interesting projection to the dorsolateral pontine nuclei. These connections provide a possible pathway for the feedback of eye movement signals onto neurones that are the recipient of cortical visual motion detector inputs.

19.4 Evidence for cerebellar involvement in saccadic eye movements

Both animal and human studies indicate that, in contrast to its role in the generation of pursuit eye movements, the cerebellum is not essential for the production of saccades. Both memory and visually guided saccades can be produced with normal latencies and dynamics (i.e. normal durations and velocities for the size of the movement) following cerebellar lesions (Optican and Robinson, 1980; Zee, 1982). The specialized role of the cerebellum for this particular system is a modulatory influence in assuring the amplitude accuracy of saccadic eye movements. This auxiliary role ensures that saccades are consistently made to the precise location of selected visual targets. It carries out this function within two separate time frames. The first is an on-line or movement coincident correction which affects individual saccades. The presence of modulatory cerebellar signals is particularly important for large saccades and to ensure the equal accuracy of movements from different initial eye positions (perhaps to compensate for orbital non-linearities (Vilis and Hore, 1981)). The second time frame for cerebellar influence is a longer-term adaptive modulation that compensates for saccadic dysmetrias due to orbital or central lesions or other changes in system characteristics such as growth or metabolism (Optican and Robinson, 1980).

When attempts are made to localize further this cerebellar function into the various anatomic divisions of this organ, the evidence strongly supports the notion that the vermis (lobules VI and VII and perhaps parts of V), and its associated fastigial nuclei are the parts of the cerebellum involved in saccadic regulation (Keller, in press).

This influence on the saccadic system is mediated primarily through fastigial nucleus outflow that decussates to the contralateral saccadic, brainstem pulse generator. This influence does not directly change the discharge characteristics of brainstem short-lead burst cells, but more likely affects the generation of a veridical internal estimate of current eye position, a signal necessary for the control of saccadic amplitude (Keller, Slakey and Crandall, 1983). Thus, clinical observations of eye movement pathology that include slow saccades most likely indicate that brainstem structures in addition to the cerebellum are affected.

Single-unit recordings from Purkinje cells in the vermis show cellular activity during saccades that is very dependent on initial eye position before the saccade, an observation consistent with the on-line corrections. Other cells show late responses after the saccade that could play a role in longer-term calibration (McElligott and Keller, 1982).

Focal electrical stimulation of both the posterior vermis and the floccular lobes in alert monkey leads to short-latency evoked saccades (Ron and Robinson, 1973; McElligott and Keller, 1984). The size and direction of these evoked saccades depended dramatically on initial eye position, an observation which again emphasizes the cerebellum's involvement with compensation for the effects of initial position. These electrical stimulation studies showed that a crude map for direction of the evoked saccades existed over the vermal cortex such that oblique movements with an upward component were represented more rostrally in the vermis and downward components most caudally. Horizontal components were always towards the side ipsilateral to the stimulation site. Evoked saccades were conjugate.

Most importantly, the amplitude of the saccade evoked at a given vermal site was proportional to stimulating current strength. This effect is quite different from that observed with increased current strengths in other saccadic control areas (superior colliculus and frontal eye fields), where saccade size depends primarily on the neural location of the stimulation and not its temporal or magnitude characteristics. The inference that may be made from this result is that the cerebellum influences the saccadic system closer to its final output where the system's neural interactions are coded in the temporal and not the spatial domain, whereas the collicular and frontal eye field effects are clearly spatial in nature.

In terms of human studies, Selhorst *et al.* (1976a,b) provided the first exceptionally clear eye movement recordings employing a registration technique of sufficient time resolution, lack of drift and sensitivity to define quantitatively the characteristics of overshoot dysmetria and saccadic oscillations in a group of cerebellar patients. From this study one may conclude that patients with these disorders produce saccades with normal latencies and velocities, that when oscillations occur they consist of saccades separated by short intersaccadic intervals, that intersaccadic slow drifts can occur in some records and that some degree of disconjugacy between the two eyes can result. The majority of these patients had been operated on for cerebellar tumours, and at least some showed recovery from the saccadic disorder after a period of several months.

Related studies by Baloh, Konrad and Honrubia (1975) and Zee *et al.* (1976) show somewhat similar results in a different class of cerebellar patients. In these studies the patients suffered from hereditary cerebellar ataxia, a highly selective atrophy of the cerebellar cortex. A variety of oculomotor abnormalities were present, with saccadic deficits being dysmetria and square-wave jerks. The metrics of the dysmetria (hypo or hyper) varied from individual to individual, but velocities and latencies were normal. Another important observation in the latter study was that the degree and metrics of the dysmetria were often initial eye position dependent.

More recent studies (Avanzini *et al.*, 1979; Hotson, 1982; Ranalli and Sharpe, 1986) reported similar results of dysmetria, saccadic oscillations and intrusions. The last study is interesting because the site of damage of the distal left superior cerebellar artery (as demonstrated by CT and MRI imaging) was limited to the ipsilateral cerebellum. The effect was to produce hypermetric saccades to the contralateral side and hypometric saccades to the ipsilateral side. In addition, attempted vertical saccades contained contralateral, horizontal saccadic intrusions.

In summary, the literature on human cerebellar patients suggests that the exact pattern of saccadic dysmetria (the direction, metrics and dependency on initial eye position) cannot be precisely predicted from the site of the cerebellar lesion. Furthermore, a patient reported by Estanol, Romero and Covero (1979), who had undergone hemicerebellectomy for a tumour which then recurred in the opposite cerebellar hemisphere, surprisingly showed no saccadic dysmetria. These seemingly inconsistent effects of cerebellar lesions on the patterns of saccadic dysmetria, while possibly due to variations in the location of lesions, may in fact be related to a more basic role of the cerebellum in the control of adaptive recovery processes (Optican and Robinson, 1980).

19.5 Summary

In this chapter the experimental evidence concerning the possible localization of smooth pursuit function to specific portions of the primate cerebellar cortex has been summarized. The goal of this line of inquiry is to determine whether clinical measurements of smooth pursuit deficits in humans are diagnostic for a specific location of a suspected cerebellar lesion. Overall the evidence, gathered from neural recording studies, experimental lesions and anatomical tracing studies, consistently indicates that the flocculus is the primary locus of pursuit-related neural circuits within the cerebellum. The evidence with regard to the posterior vermis, lobules VI and VII, is more preliminary and inconsistent. Zee (1982) has suggested that the presence of eye velocity and target velocity neurones in the vermis might be a reflection of the use of these signals in planning accurate foveating saccades to moving targets during pursuit movements. This argument would preserve the hypothesized division of labour in the cerebellum, with slow and holding-type eye movements under floccular control and saccades under vermal control. While this argument would explain the necessity for eye velocity and target velocity signals in the vermis, it would not explain why steady-state, sinusoidal pursuit eye velocity is so affected by vermal lesions.

It would be nice to find cases in the clinic with selective lesions of one or the other of these areas. Unfortunately, familial cerebellar atrophy, which is highly selective for the cerebellar, seems to affect indiscriminately large regions of the cerebellar cortex (Zee *et al.*, 1976) including both flocculus and vermis. Likewise the late onset, adult type of cerebellar atrophy produces severe cell loss in both the flocculo-nodular lobe and the vermis (Marie, Foix and Alajouanine, 1922). These authors found relatively greater loss of cells in the anterior vermis, a region not presently associated with eye movements, than in the posterior vermis. However, more recent magnetic resonance images in patients with this disorder show remarkably clear lesions in the vermis, lobules VI and VII, as well as anterior vermis lesions (Baloh, Yee and Honrubia, 1986).

The conclusion of this summary is that the posterior vermis may very well play an important role in smooth pursuit control in the primate. This role may run in parallel with that provided by the flocculus or it may be involved only in special aspects of pursuit which particularly require the target velocity signal seen selectively in vermal Purkinje cells.

Acknowledgements

Work described in this chapter was partially supported by NIH Research Grant EY-06860 and Core Grant for Vision Research EY-01186 and by The Smith-Kettlewell Eye Research Foundation.

References

Avanzini, G., Girotti, F., Crenna, P. and Negri, S. (1979) Alterations of ocular motility in cerebellar pathology. *Arch. Neurol.*, **36**, 274–80.

Balaban, D.C., Ito, M. and Watanabe, E. (1981) Demonstration of zonal projections from the cerebellar flocculus to vestibular nuclei in monkeys (*Macaca fuscata*). *Neurosci. Lett.*, **27**, 101–5.

Baloh, R.W., Konrad, H.R. and Honrubia, V. (1975) Vestibulo-ocular function in patients with cerebellar atrophy. *Neurology*, **25**, 160–8.

Baloh, R.W., Yee, R.D. and Honrubia, V. (1986) Late cortical cerebellar atrophy. Clinical and oculographic features. *Brain*, **109**, 159–80.

Batton, R.R., Jayaraman, A., Ruggiero, D. and Carpenter, M.B. (1977) Fastigial efferent projections in the monkey: an autoradiographic study. *J. Comp. Neurol.*, **174**, 281–306.

Belknap. D., Noda, H. and Ohno, M. (1983) Unit activity and responses to microstimulation in the macaque flocculus during smooth pursuit eye movements. *Soc. Neurosci., Abst.*, **9**, 609.

Brodal, P. (1978) The corticopontine projection in the rhesus monkey. Origin and principles of organization. *Brain*, **101**, 251–83.

Brodal, P. (1982) Further observations on the cerebellar projections from the pontine nuclei and the nucleus reticularis tegmenti pontis in the rhesus monkey. *J. Comp. Neurol.*, **204**, 44–55.

Burde, R.M., Stroud, M.H., Roper-Hall, G., Wirth, F.P. and O'Leary, J.L. (1975) Ocular motor dysfunction in total and hemicerebellectomized monkeys. *Br. J. Ophthalmol.*, **59**, 560–5.

Daroff, R.B. (1982) Eye signs in humans with cerebellar dysfunction, in *Functional Basis of Ocular Motility Disorders* (eds G. Lennerstrand, D.S. Zee and E.L. Keller). Pergamon, Oxford, pp. 463–6.

Eckmiller, R. (1982) The transition between pre-motor eye velocity signals and oculomotor eye position signals in primate brain stem neurons during pursuit, in *Adaptive Processes in Visual and Oculomotor Systems* (eds E.L. Keller and D.S. Zee). Pergamon, Oxford, pp. 301–6.

Estanol, B., Romero, R. and Covero, J. (1979) Effects of cerebellectomy on eye movements in man. *Arch. Neurol.*, **36**, 281–4.

Glickstein, M., Cohen, J.L., Dixon, B., Gibson, A., Hollins, M., Labossiere, E. and Robinson, A. (1980) Corticopontine visual projections in macaque monkeys. *J. Comp. Neurol.*, **190**, 209–29.

Hotson, J.R. (1982) Visual suppression and activation of fixation eye movements in cerebellar disorders, in *Functional Basis of Ocular Motility Disorders* (eds G. Lennerstrand, D.S. Zee and E.L. Keller). Pergamon, Oxford, pp. 471–3.

Keller, E.L. (in press) Role of the cerebellum in the control of saccadic eye movements, in *The Neurobiology of Saccadic Eye Movements* (eds R. Wurtz and M.E. Goldberg). Elsevier, Amsterdam.

Keller, E.L., Slakey, D.P. and Crandall, W.F. (1983) Microstimulation of the primate cerebellar vermis during saccadic eye movements. *Brain Res.*, **288**, 131–43.

Langer, T., Fuchs, A.F., Chubb, M.C., Scudder, C.A. and Lisberger, S.G. (1985a) Floccular efferents in the rhesus macaque as revealed by autoradiography and horseradish peroxidase. *J. Comp. Neurol.*, **235**, 26–37.

Langer, T., Fuchs, A.F., Scudder, C.A. and Chubb, M.C. (1985b) Afferents to the flocculus of the cerebellum in the rhesus macaque as revealed by retrograde transport of horseradish peroxidase. *J. Comp. Neurol.*, **235**, 1–25.

Lisberger, S.G. and Fuchs, F.A. (1978) Role of primate flocculus during rapid behavioral modification of vestibuloocular reflex. I. Purkinje cell activity during visually guided horizontal smooth-pursuit eye movements and passive head rotation. *J. Neurophysiol.*, **41**, 733–63.

Marie, P., Foix, C. and Alajouanine, T. (1922) De l'atrophie cérébelleuse tardive a prédominance corticale. *Rev. Neurol.*, **38**, 849–85.

May, J.G., Keller, E.L. and Crandall, W.F. (1985) Changes in eye velocity during smooth pursuit tracking induced by microstimulation in the dorsolateral pontine nucleus of the macaque. *Soc. Neurosci., Abst.*, **11**, 79.

McElligott, J.G. and Keller, E.L. (1982) Neuronal discharge in the posterior cerebellum: its relationship to saccadic eye movement generation, in *Functional Basis of Ocular Motility Disorders* (eds G. Lennerstrand, D.S. Zee and E.L. Keller). Pergamon, Oxford, pp. 453–61.

McElligott, J.G. and Keller, E.L. (1984) Cerebellar vermis involvement in monkey saccadic eye movements: microstimulation. *Exp. Neurol.*, **86**, 543–58.

Miles, F.A., Fuller, J.H., Braitman, D.J. and Dow, B.M. (1980) Long-term adaptive changes in primate vestibuloocular reflex. III. Electrophysiological observation in flocculus of normal monkeys. *J. Neurophysiol.*, **43**, 1437–76.

Mustari, M.J., Fuchs, A.F. and Wallman, J. (1984) Smooth-pursuit related units in the dorsolateral pons of the rhesus macaque. *Soc. Neurosci., Abst.*, **10**, 987.

Optican, L.M. and Robinson, D.A. (1980) Cerebellar-dependent adaptive control of primate saccadic system. *J. Neurophysiol.*, **44**, 1058–76.

Optican, L.M., Zee, D.S., Miles, F.A. and Lisberger, S.G. (1980) Oculomotor deficits in monkeys with floccular lesions. *Soc. Neurosci., Abst.*, **6**, 474.

Ranalli, P.J. and Sharpe, J.A. (1986) Contrapulsion of saccades and ipsilateral ataxia. *Ann. Neurol.*, **20**, 311–16.

Ritchie, L. (1976) Effects of cerebellar lesions on saccadic eye movements. *J. Neurophysiol.*, **39**, 1246–56.

Robinson, D.A. (1976) Adaptive gain control of vestibuloocular reflex by the cerebellum. *J. Neurophysiol.*, **39**, 954–69.

Ron, S. and Robinson, D.A. (1973) Eye movements by cerebellar stimulation in the alert monkey. *J. Neurophysiol.*, **36**, 1004–22.

Selhorst, J.B., Stark, L., Ochs, A.L. and Hoyt, W.F. (1976a) Disorders in cerebellar ocular motor control. I. Saccadic overshoot dysmetria: an oculographic, control system and clinico-anatomical analysis. *Brain*, **99**, 497–508.

Selhorst, J.B., Stark, L., Ochs, A.L. and Hoyt, W.F. (1976b) Disorders in cerebellar ocular motor control. II. Macrosaccadic oscillation: an oculographic, control system and clinico-anatomical analysis. *Brain*, **99**, 509–22.

Suzuki, D., Noda, H. and Kase, M. (1981) Visual and pursuit eye movement-related activity in posterior vermis of monkey cerebellum. *J. Neurophysiol.*, **46**, 1120–39.

Suzuki, D.A. and Keller, E.L. (1983) Sensory-oculomotor interactions in primate cerebellar vermis: a role in smooth pursuit control. *Soc. Neurosci., Abst.*, **9**, 606.

Suzuki, D.A. and Keller, E.L. (1984) Visual signals in the dorsolateral pontine nucleus of the alert monkey: their relationship to smooth-pursuit eye movements. *Exp. Brain Res.*, **53**, 473–8.

Suzuki, D. and Keller, E.L. (in press) The role of the posterior vermis of monkey cerebellum in smooth-pursuit eye movement control. II. Target velocity-related Purkinje cell activity. *J. Neurophysiol.*

Suzuki, D.A., May, J. and Keller, E.L. (1984) Smooth-pursuit eye movement deficits with pharmacological lesions in monkey dorsolateral pontine nucleus. *Soc. Neurosci., Abst.*, **10**, 58.

Van Essen, D.C., Maunsell, J.H.R. and Bixley, J.L. (1981) The middle temporal visual area in the macaque: myeloarchitecture, connections, functional properties and topographic organization. *J. Comp. Neurol.*, **199**, 293–326.

Vilis, T. and Hore, J. (1981) Characteristics of saccadic dysmetria in monkeys during reversible lesions of medial cerebellar nuclei. *J. Neurophysiol.*, **46**, 828–38.

Westheimer, G. and Blair, S.M. (1973) Oculomotor defects in cerebellectomized monkeys. *Invest. Ophthalmol.*, **12**, 618–21.

Westheimer, G. and Blair, S.M. (1974) Functional organization of primate oculomotor system revealed by cerebellectomy. *Exp. Brain Res.*, **21**, 463–72.

Young, L.R. (1977) Pursuit eye movement – what is being pursued?, in *Control of Gaze by Brain Stem Neurons* (eds R. Baker and A. Berthoz). Elsevier, Amsterdam, pp. 29–36.

Zee, D.S. (1982) Ocular motor control: the cerebellum, in *Neuro-ophthalmology* (eds S. Lessell and J.T.W. van Dalen), vol. 2. Excerpta Medica, Amsterdam, pp. 136–47.

Zee, D.S. (1984) New concepts of cerebellar control of eye movements. *Otolaryngol.-Head Neck Surg.*, **92**, 59–62.
Zee, D.S., Yamazaki, A., Butler, P.H. and Gucer, G. (1981) Effect of ablation of flocculus and paraflocculus on eye movement in primate. *J. Neurophysiol.*, **46**, 878–99.
Zee, D.S., Yee, R.D., Cogan, D.G., Robinson, D.A. and Engel, K. (1976) Ocular motor abnormalities in hereditary cerebellar ataxia. *Brain*, **99**, 207–34.

CHAPTER 20

Ocular motor phenomena in infantile strabismus

G. KOMMERELL

20.1 Introduction

The occurrence of early onset strabismus, asymmetry of pursuit and optokinetic nystagmus, latent nystagmus and dissociated vertical divergence is highly correlated (Roelofs, 1928; Keiner and Roelofs, 1955; Nicolai, 1959; Kornhuber, 1960; Doden, 1961; Loewer-Sieger, 1962; Mein, 1983; Schor, 1983). The combination of these signs has therefore been defined as a syndrome, the so-called 'congenital squint syndrome' (Lang, 1968). Because strabismus is rarely present at birth and usually becomes manifest during the first three months of life, the term 'infantile strabismus syndrome' may be more appropriate.

Although a cause common to all four signs has to be considered, a causal interdependence between them appears to be more likely. Indeed, a wealth of evidence indicates that strabismus is the primary abnormality which secondarily leads to an asymmetry of the pursuit and optokinetic systems, and it is a plausible hypothesis that the asymmetry of these smooth tracking systems ultimately leads to latent nystagmus. Less clear is the causal relationship between dissociated vertical divergence and strabismus, but it also seems to occur secondarily to the strabismus.

20.2 Asymmetry of pursuit and optokinetic nystagmus

The asymmetry of pursuit and optokinetic nystagmus is defined as a reduction of gain for uniocular stimuli directed to the temporal side, while the gain for nasally directed stimuli is normal or only moderately reduced. Healthy infants show such an asymmetry of the smooth tracking systems (Atkinson, 1979; Atkinson and Braddick, 1981; Naegele and Held, 1982; Hainline *et al.*, 1984), but the asymmetry disappears by about six months of age if signs of normal binocularity appear (Atkinson, 1979; Naegele and Held, 1982). In the adult human, a slight nasally directed preponderance can be shown only if the optokinetic stimulation is confined to the temporal half-field; this asymmetry is counterbalanced by a temporally directed preponderance of the nasal hemifield (Ohmi, Howard and Eveleigh, 1986).

The reduced, not necessarily absent (Sorsby, 1931; Flynn, Pritchard and Lasley, 1984), binocularity brought about by strabismus could prevent maturation of the smooth tracking systems (van Hof-van Duin, 1978), an hypothesis supported by the persistence of the nasal-temporal asymmetry in each eye of cats which were deprived of binocular vision by unilateral lid suture early in life (van Hof-van Duin, 1976; Hoffman, 1979).

The critical factor in producing asymmetry of pursuit and optokinetic nystagmus appears to be the reduced binocularity rather than monocular or binocular deprivation. At least in strabismic humans, amblyopia is not a prerequisite for the asymmetry of the smooth tracking systems (Tychsen, Hurtig and Scott, 1985; Mohn, Sireteanu and van Hof-van Duin, 1986; Tychsen and Lisberger, 1986; van Hof-van Duin and Mohn, 1986). In monkeys an adequate model still seems to be lacking. However, cats rendered exotropic, but not amblyopic, by early surgery, show a reduction of the optokinetic nystagmus, predominately of the temporally directed slow phases (Cynader and Harris, 1980). In the monocularly deprived (i.e. amblyopic) monkey nasal-temporal asymmetry of the optokinetic nystagmus is present when the deprived eye is stimulated with a rotating drum, but stimulation of the non-deprived eye results in normal optokinetic nystagmus (Sparks *et al.*, 1986).

The neural mechanism by which the loss of binocularity leads to the asymmetry of the smooth tracking systems could be 'functional suppression' (Schor, 1983) of the cortical projection to the nucleus of the optic tract (NOT) which is located in the pretectum. The NOT is an important relay station of the optokinetic system that receives direct input from the contralateral eye and indirect input from both eyes via both occipital lobes (Hoffmann, 1982). Lesions of the visual cortex drastically reduce the optokinetic response to temporally directed motion under conditions of monocular viewing in the cat (Hoffman, 1982; Strong *et al.*, 1984) and in the monkey (Zee *et al.*, 1986). Dark rearing of cats also results in asymmetry of the smooth tracking systems and may be equivalent to a surgical lesion of the visual cortex (van Hof-van Duin, 1978; Harris and Cynader, 1981). The relative preservation of responses to nasally directed motion appears to be due to direct connections from the retina to the contralateral NOT both in the cat (Hoffmann, 1982) and in the monkey (Hoffmann and Distler, 1986). In the normal adult human, the subcortical projection alone seems to be insufficient to drive the NOT, as most cortically blind patients do not show any optokinetic response (Jung and Kornhuber, 1964). But the relative preservation of responses to nasally directed stimuli in patients with incomplete bilateral occipital lobe destruction (Mehdorn, 1982) could be due to remnants of the subcortical projection to the NOT which might have been released from cortical control.

Although a cortical defect of binocularity induced by infantile strabismus may be responsible for the impairment of temporally directed tracking, this defect does not imply major difficulties in motion perception. Indeed, patients are able to differentiate between various stimulus velocities. We ascertained this in a patient with infantile esotropia who had a marked asymmetry of the smooth tracking systems (Fig. 20.1). Using optokinetic stimuli and Stevens' (1957) magnitude estimation, the

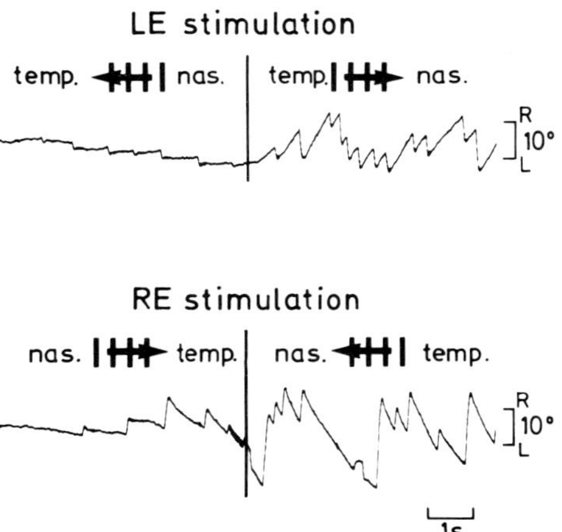

Fig. 20.1 Full-field temporally directed optokinetic stimulation of either eye at 60°/s does not overcome the nasally directed slow phases of the latent nystagmus in patient CW 130360. Nasally directed stimulation evokes a strong optokinetic nystagmus. DC-Electro-oculogram.

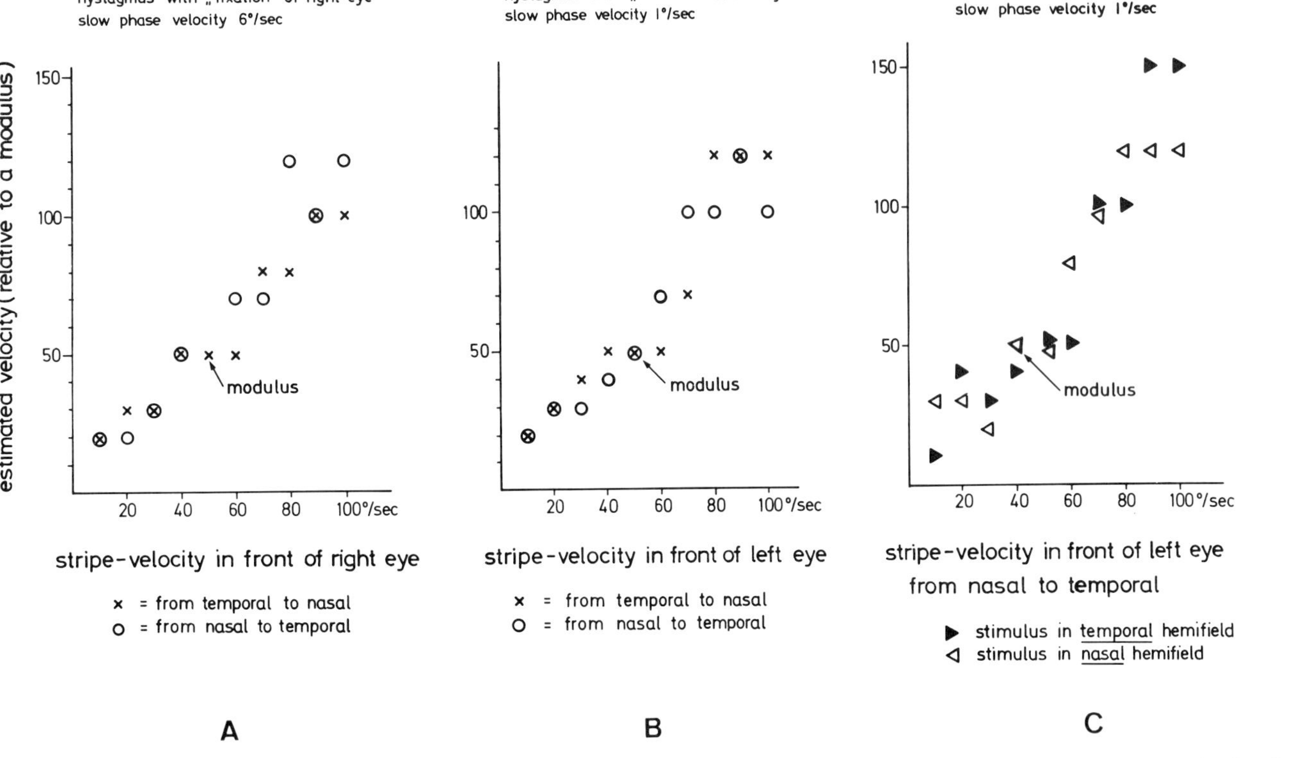

Fig. 20.2 Unimpaired velocity perception of an image slipping across the retina. The same patient as in Fig. 20.1 was asked to look monocularly at a fixation point in the middle of a full-field optokinetic stimulus. Under this condition, his eyes were nearly stationary, except for a persisting latent nystagmus, as indicated on the top of each panel. The stripes were moved either nasally or temporally at various velocities in random order. Exposure time was 10 s. The patient had to estimate the velocity relative to a 'modulus' which was presented three times at the beginning of the test series for each eye (A and B). In C, only one half field of the left eye was stimulated. Velocity estimation was equally good independent of whether the stimulus was presented in the temporal or nasal hemifield. The method is similar to the one employed by Körner and Dichgans (1967) in normal subjects.

patient could clearly distinguish between fast and slow slip velocities of the retinal image. The performance was equal regardless of whether the stimuli were nasally or temporally directed (Fig. 20.2A and B). There was also equally good velocity discrimination independent of whether the optokinetic stimulus was applied in the nasal or temporal hemifield (Fig. 20.2C).

This result is compatible with recent work of Tychsen and Lisberger (1986) who presented to patients with infantile strabismus a nasally or temporally moving single target whilst fixating a central stationary target (technique of McKee and Welch, 1985). The ability to discriminate differences in velocity was normal when nasally and temporally directed motion were considered separately. Only when the patients compared target speed in the two directions did they judge temporally directed stimuli to be slightly slower than nasally directed stimuli. The authors regard this perceptual asymmetry as an indication of a defect in the cerebral pathways responsible for velocity perception, but an alternative interpretation is tenable. Patients may have underestimated temporally directed stimuli secondarily because of adaptation to their 'latent' nystagmus which may have been partly manifest under natural viewing conditions, i.e. the patients may have had so-called manifest latent nystagmus.

The patients' unimpaired ability to distinguish between fast and slow slip velocities of full-field (Fig. 20.2) and small (Tychsen and Lisberger, 1986) retinal images in both horizontal directions argues against a defect in the retinocortical pathway which could be responsible for the asymmetry of the smooth tracking systems. Rather, the visual cortex seems to lose the ability to transmit temporally directed object motion to the premotor structures of the brainstem if binocularity fails to develop in the first months of life.

20.3 Latent nystagmus

Latent nystagmus is defined as a jerk nystagmus whose rapid phases are directed to the side of the visually dominant eye. With the left eye occluded the slow phases are directed to the left, and with the right eye occluded the slow phases are directed to the right (Fig. 20.3). We suggested the hypothesis that asymmetry of the smooth tracking systems

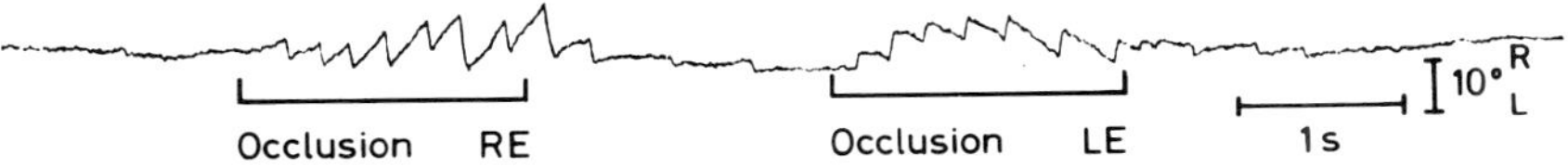

Fig. 20.3 Latent nystagmus in patient FU180771. Infrared reflection recording.

might be the cause of latent nystagmus (Kommerell, 1978; Kommerell and Mehdorn, 1982). According to this concept, the nasally directed vector of the smooth tracking systems would be preponderant, even in the presence of stationary patterns. This directional preponderance could drive the slow phases of the latent nystagmus as soon as only one eye has a visual input. Total occlusion of one eye is the strongest means to skew the smooth tracking systems but, as most patients with latent nystagmus also have strabismus, part of the directional preponderance becomes manifest with spontaneous suppression of the squinting eye. This results in the above-mentioned 'manifest latent nystagmus' (Roelofs, 1928; Kestenbaum, 1961; Dell'Osso, Schmidt and Daroff 1979) but, with binocular viewing, the normal-functioning nasally directed smooth tracking systems of both eyes complement each other and largely prevent drifting of the eyes.

The neural basis of latent nystagmus may be a drift bias introduced by functional suppression of the cortical projection to the NOT. The term functional suppression is used because axonal connections can still be demonstrated by spike potentials in the NOT during electrical stimulation of the ipsilateral cortex in the monocularly deprived cat (Hoffmann, 1983).

There are two analogues of latent nystagmus in which a directional preponderance of the smooth tracking systems may also cause spontaneous nystagmus in humans. The first is downbeat nystagmus (Zee, Friendlich and Robinson, 1974), and the second is a lesion of the cerebral hemispheres which leads to slow phases directed to the contralateral side (Sharpe, Lo and Rabinovitch, 1979). Lesions of one cerebral hemisphere in the monkey also produce nystagmus (see Chapter 14) which may be due to directional preponderance of the smooth tracking systems.

The hypothesis that the asymmetry of the smooth tracking systems might be the cause of latent nystagmus is supported by a high correlation between the intensity of latent nystagmus and the magnitude of pursuit asymmetry. Tychsen and Lisberger (1986) found this in seven patients by comparing the velocity of the slow phases of the latent nystagmus with the eye acceleration in response to a ramp stimulus, and with sinusoidal tracking.

Comparing latent nystagmus with the asymmetry of full-field optokinetic nystagmus, we were unable to find a clear correlation (Mehdorn and Kommerell, 1983; Fig. 20.4). It may well be that the asymmetry of pursuit or small-field optokinetic nystagmus (Schor and Levi, 1980; Schor, 1981) is more relevant to the latent nystagmus than large-field optokinetic nystagmus.

It is questionable, however, whether a very high correlation between the intensity of latent nystagmus and the magnitude of the asymmetry of the smooth tracking systems should be expected, because the intensity of latent nystagmus can be very variable (Sorsby, 1931). Particularly during occlusion therapy for strabismic amblyopia, the nystagmus in the viewing amblyopic eye can decrease considerably in a few days (unpublished observation).

Cognitive factors also modify latent nystagmus; for instance, the slow phases can be reversed if the patient alternately occludes his right and left eyes in total darkness (Jung and Kornhuber, 1964; van Vliet, 1973; Schor, 1981; Kommerell and Mehdorn, 1982; Hain, Kelman and Zee, 1985).

The cognitive influence is further exemplified by an unusual patient who was able to manifest his latent nystagmus volitionally. When asked to 'wiggle' his eyes he evoked a strong nystagmus with the fast phases directed to his leading left eye (Fig. 20.5). Binocular vision was tested with Bagolini's striated glasses. In the everyday condition when the nystagmus was not obvious (only occasionally was there a slight 'manifest latent' nystagmus), the patient reported the streak of the squinting right eye to be faintly visible. When he volitionally aroused the left-beating nystagmus, he completely suppressed the streak of the squinting right eye. This result suggests that some residual binocularity was available to the patient under normal circumstances, but that he was able to concentrate fully on his leading left eye. The concentration on the left eye may have skewed his pursuit balance so much that a strong nystagmus appeared. Our patient required visual contours volitionally to arouse the nystagmus. He could not produce it in darkness or when he was looking at a contourless light screen.

A remarkable cognitive influence on latent nystagmus in the dark was demonstrated by Abel *et al.* (1986) in a patient who had been blind in the right eye from birth because of a malformation of the eye. The right eye had been enucleated. In darkness, the patient's 'latent nystagmus' beat as though his right prosthesis were viewing (similar to the case described by Ohm, 1928); he could, however, volitionally intend to 'view' with either eye, producing the appropriate reversals of direction.

We do not believe that cognitive, i.e. non-visual, influences are at variance with our hypothesis that latent nystagmus is related to the asymmetry of the smooth tracking systems, because the smooth tracking systems of normal observers can also be influenced by cognitive effort. For instance, Zikmund (1966) has shown that trained subjects, studied in total darkness, can elicit optokinetic nystagmus by visual imagery of a moving stimulus pattern.

Summing up the arguments presented so far, we have suggested the following causal relationship. Infantile strabismus impairs the development of binocularity in the visual cortex. The reduced binocularity prevents oculomotor maturation in that the nasal-temporal asymmetry of

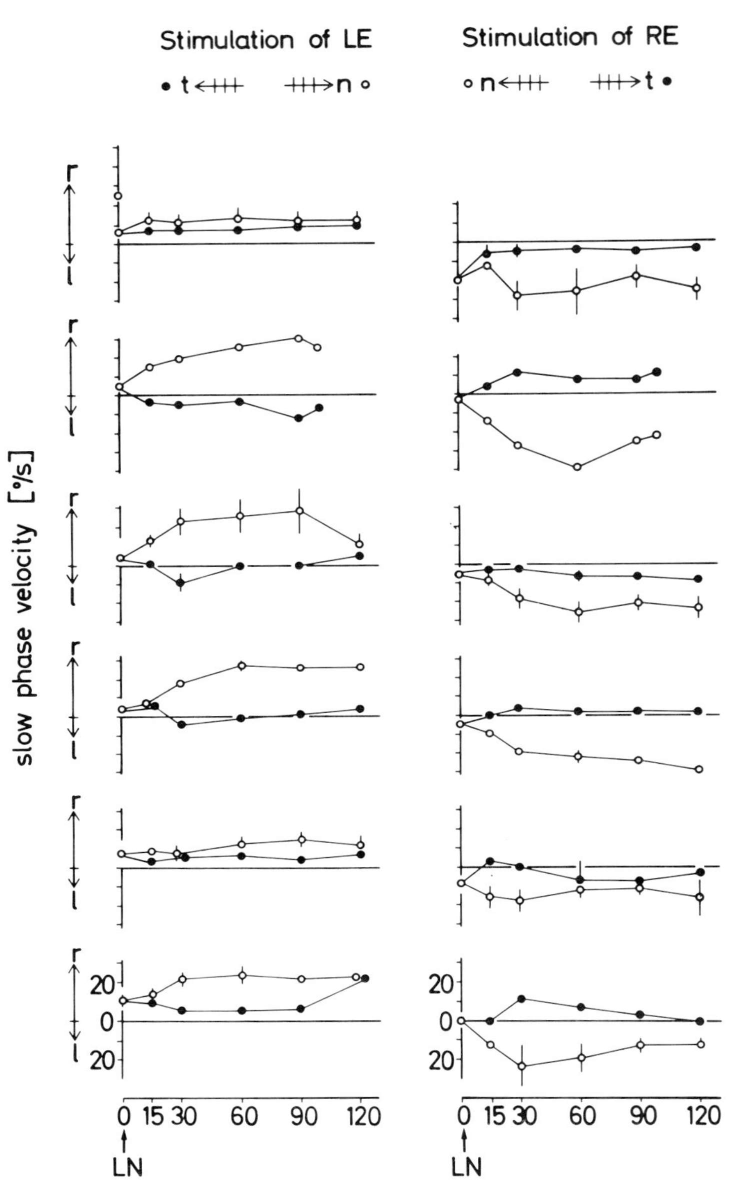

Stimulation of LE
• t ←+++
+++→ n ○
Stimulation of RE
○ n ←+++
+++→ t •
slow phase velocity [°/s]
r
l
20
0
20
0 15 30 60 90 120
LN
Stimulus velocity [°/s]

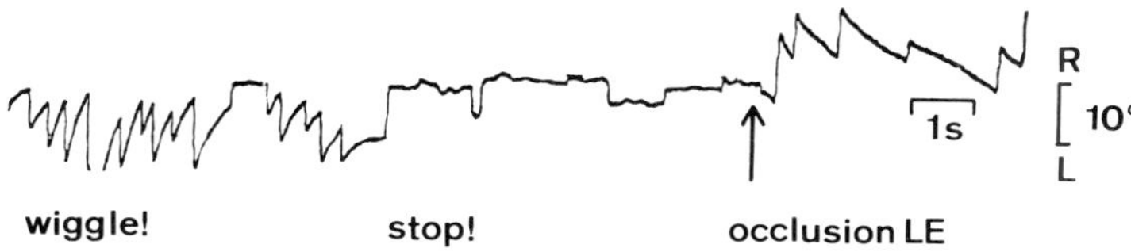

Fig. 20.5 Volitionally elicited 'manifest latent' nystagmus. The patient had an infantile convergent strabismus with a slight amblyopia in the right eye. When he was asked to 'wiggle' his eyes, a marked left-beating nystagmus appeared. It is remarkable that the rapid phases overshot the target. With both eyes open, the patient was unable to produce a nystagmus corresponding to a dominance of his squinting right eye, i.e., he could not volitionally reverse the slow phases. Right-beating nystagmus only appeared when the leading left eye was occluded. Infrared reflection recording. The same patient is represented also in the first panel of Fig. 20.4. The volitionally elicited 'manifest latent' nystagmus of this patient should not be confused with the well-known 'voluntary nystagmus' that occurs in otherwise normal subjects. Voluntary nystagmus shows a high frequency (often above 10 Hz) of to and fro saccades without intersaccadic intervals, and convergence is often superimposed. In the patient depicted here, there was no change of vergence or pupil size when he 'wiggled' his eyes.

the smooth tracking systems which is a normal feature in the first few months of life remains as a permanent defect. Finally, the asymmetry of the smooth tracking systems produces latent nystagmus.

The reverse relationship suggested by Tychsen and Lisberger (1986), that latent nystagmus might constitute a tonic drive which leads to convergent strabismus appears unlikely to us. It has to be borne in mind that the drift directed to the nose refers only to the viewing eye. The drift is always conjugate, i.e. at the same time, the non-viewing eye drifts temporally. It is hard to see how such a conjugate drift could lead to convergent strabismus. Moreover, asymmetry of the smooth tracking systems and latent nystagmus also occur in patients who have had

---

Fig. 20.4 Asymmetry of the optokinetic nystagmus in six patients with latent nystagmus. A full-field stimulus with 7° wide stripes was presented monocularly for 15 s. The average velocity of the ten fastest slow phases that occurred during this time was taken as the response. The velocity of the slow phases of latent nystagmus was measured when the patient looked at stationary stripes (response to zero velocity). The responses to temporally directed stimulus motion (filled circles) are much weaker than the responses to nasally directed stimulus motion (open circles), but the responses to nasally directed stimulus motion are also subnormal. Responses with a gain of 1.0 would have shown as two 45° lines, symmetrically above and below the zero line. Patient codes: AZ020874, UD110671, KH170470, MK201072, SP050469, AS291070. The patient represented in the uppermost panel is the same as in Fig. 20.5.

divergent strabismus from infancy (Roelofs, 1928; present writer's experience).

20.4 Dissociated vertical divergence

Dissociated vertical divergence occurs in subjects with otherwise normal binocularity, but is much more frequent in patients with early onset strabismus. There is one similarity between latent nystagmus and dissociated vertical divergence; both these ocular motor abnormalities depend on the balance of visual inputs coming through the right and left eyes. To illustrate the clinical findings in dissociated vertical divergence, a literal balance with two scales can be used (Fig. 20.6). If the right eye is fixing a bright picture and the left eye is occluded, the balance of visual inputs is shifted strongly to the right eye. This imbalance drives the left eye up. In the classical Bielschowsky test, the imbalance is decreased by placing a dark filter before the fixing right eye, thus reducing the dominance of the input through the right eye and allowing the left eye to come slightly

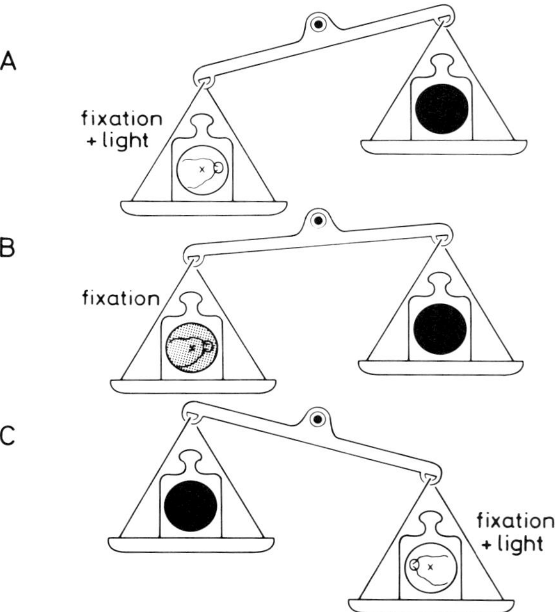

Fig. 20.6 Dependence of eye position on the balance of visual inputs in dissociated vertical deviation. (From Kommerell and Mattheus, 1984.) To describe the phenomena of DVD, the metaphor of a balance was used by Ohm (1928).

down (Bielschowsky, 1930). If the right eye is completely occluded and the left eye takes over fixation, the imbalance is reversed to a dominance of the input through the left eye which drives the right eye up.

The balance of the visual inputs can also be influenced by conscious effort. The more the patient tries to resolve a difficult acuity task, the more the squinting eye is driven up (Rüssmann and Albrecht, 1986).

Obviously, a balance is only a metaphor to demonstrate the phenomena of dissociated vertical divergence. It does not tell us very much about the neural mechanism which has remained obscure. The changes of vertical deviation on the alternate cover test are brought about by disjunctive movements, and they are not combined with vertical nystagmus (Helveston, 1980). Therefore, we cannot see any relationship to the vertical asymmetry of the smooth tracking systems present in patients with infantile strabismus. These patients indeed have a preference for upward tracking (Schor and Levi, 1980; Tychsen and Lisberger, 1986), but this asymmetry is most likely an associated abnormality, not related to dissociated vertical divergence.

Dissociated vertical divergence is not a variant of the so-called ocular tilt reaction (see Chapter 18), because the torsion that accompanies the vertical deviation is opposite in the two conditions. In dissociated vertical divergence, the upward-moving eye extorts, whereas in the ocular tilt reaction, the upward-moving eye intorts.

20.5 Congenital nystagmus

As opposed to latent nystagmus that regularly occurs together with infantile strabismus, the association of congenital nystagmus and strabismus is incidental, and the great majority of congenital nystagmus patients do not have strabismus (Dell'Osso, 1985). Nevertheless, because of the high prevalence of congenital nystagmus and strabismus, the association of the two conditions is frequently seen in specialist centres (Dell'Osso, 1985). Therefore, it may be appropriate to include congenital nystagmus in this article. The following comments will be focused on a recent hypothesis that might explain the pathogenesis of congenital nystagmus.

20.5.1 CHARACTERISTICS OF CONGENITAL NYSTAGMUS

1. The waveform is variable, and the slow phases often show the shape of increasing velocity exponentials (Dell'Osso and Daroff, 1975).
2. The nystagmus occurs mainly in the horizontal plane, even in up and down gaze.

3. The intensity of the nystagmus varies with the direction of gaze. In many cases, the minimum is not in the middle, but rather eccentric. To make use of the eccentric minimum, the patient has to turn his head to the opposite side.
4. Fixation effort intensifies the nystagmus, in contrast to vestibular nystagmus which is decreased by fixation.
5. An adequate optokinetic response is lacking.

20.5.2 PATHOPHYSIOLOGICAL CONSIDERATIONS

Patients with congenital nystagmus are unable to use slip of images across the retina to control their eye movements. The evidence for this assertion is their inability to respond normally to optokinetic stimuli (Jung and Kornhuber, 1964; Yamazaki, 1979; Halmagyi, Gresty and Leech, 1980; Yee, Baloh and Honrubia, 1980; Abadi, Dickinson and Lomas, 1982; Kommerell and Mehdorn, 1982; Abadi and Dickinson, 1985). Some patients do not respond at all. Others show slow phases directed opposite to the optokinetic stimulus. This so-called inverted optokinetic nystagmus does not serve to reduce the velocity of the image on the retina.

Recently, we advanced the hypothesis that the primary defect responsible for the development of congenital nystagmus might be the inability of the ocular motor system to make use of retinal slip as a control variable for the stabilization of the eyes (Kommerell and Mehdorn, 1982). This defect, present at an early sensitive period of ocular motor development, could permit the formation of abnormal synaptic connections that produce congenital nystagmus.

The clinical observation that congenital nystagmus is often not discovered until the third month of life fits well with the idea that it develops secondarily to a primary defect of retinal slip control. Only in the exceptional cases, where nystagmus has been observed since the first days of life, does a primary abnormality in the brain have to be postulated.

It may be argued that if patients with congenital nystagmus are capable of following moving targets with slow eye movements (Dell'Osso *et al.*, 1972; Dell'Osso, 1986), this does not support our assertion regarding the lack of retinal slip control but, in fact, this ability does not contradict our hypothesis. Experiments using paracentral after-images as targets for fixation suggest that the slow tracking movements may be executed by the control of target *position* on the retina rather than slip across the retina. Slow tracking movements, superimposed on an ongoing nystagmus, were elicited in seven patients when paracentral after-images were used as targets for fixation (Kommerell, 1986). An example is given in Fig. 20.7.

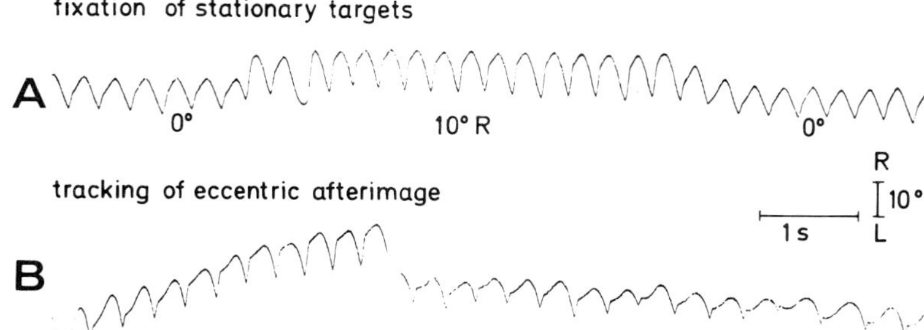

Fig. 20.7 Infrared-reflection-recording of an 18-year-old woman with congenital nystagmus. A. Refixations between two stationary targets at 0° and 10° on the right. B. When the patient's attention was focused on a paracentral after-image which appeared on the right, a slow tracking movement to the right of about 10°/s, superimposed on the patient's pseudocycloid congenital nystagmus waveform, was elicited. With an after-image on the left, a slow tracking movement of about 2°/s to the left was elicited. (From Kommerell, 1986.)

A further question arises. If the lack of a control system which prevents slip of the retinal image is the basic abnormality underlying the development of congenital nystagmus, it should be interesting to know where the defect is located. As patients with congenital nystagmus do not usually complain of difficulties in motion perception, we regard a sensory defect in the retinocortical pathway to be unlikely. As indicated in Fig. 20.8, we found patients with congenital nystagmus to be capable of distinguishing velocities in the range between 15°/s and 100°/s, although less precisely than normal controls (Kommerell, Horn and Bach, 1986). This result indicates that the lack of normal optokinetic responses typically encountered in patients with congenital nystagmus is not due to a sensory defect in the retinocortical pathway. Rather, a defect in the transmission of optokinetic signals to the brainstem has to be suspected.

20.6 Summary

The so-called infantile strabismus syndrome consists of strabismus, a defect of temporally directed pursuit and optokinetic tracking in monocular viewing, and latent nystagmus. The following causal relationship between these signs is suggested. Infantile strabismus impairs the development of binocularity in the visual cortex. The reduced binocularity prevents oculomotor maturation in that the nasal-temporal asymmetry of the smooth tracking systems which is a normal feature in the first few months of life remains as a permanent defect. Finally, the asymmetry

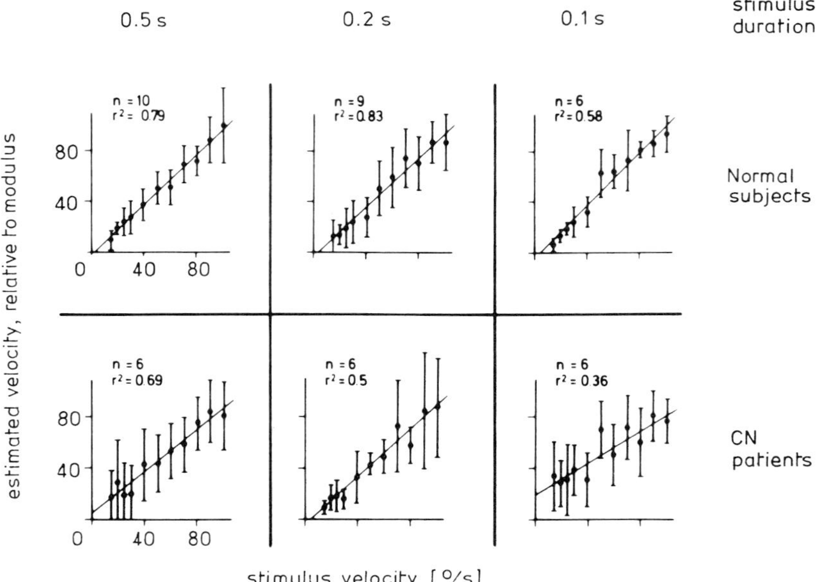

Fig. 20.8 Compound diagram of velocity estimates obtained from normal subjects (top) and congenital nystagmus patients (bottom). Stimulus durations decrease from the left to the right panel. The responses of all subjects belonging to the respective group were averaged. The vertical lines show the standard deviation, the oblique lines represent the regressions. The coefficient of determination (r^2) between estimated velocity (relative to the modulus) and stimulus velocity (before averaging) is indicated in each panel. (From Kommerell, Horn and Bach, 1986.)

of the smooth tracking systems produces latent nystagmus. The impairment of temporally directed tracking cannot be due to a defect in the retinocortical pathway because patients can perceive temporally directed object motion, and they have no difficulty in the distinction between various velocities. Rather, the visual cortex seems to lack the ability to transmit temporally directed object motion to the premotor structures of the brainstem if binocularity has failed to develop in the first months of life.

An unusual patient is described who was able volitionally to manifest his latent nystagmus. This case and other examples of cognitive influence on latent nystagmus reported in the literature are not at variance with the hypothesis that it is due to the asymmetry of the smooth tracking systems, because cognitive influence on the smooth tracking sytems has also been shown in normal subjects who can elicit optokinetic nystagmus in the dark by visual imagery.

Dissociated vertical divergence is another sign that frequently occurs together with early onset strabismus. As with latent nystagmus, dissociated vertical divergence depends on the balance of inputs coming through the right and left eyes but, other than this, its pathogenesis is unknown.

As opposed to latent nystagmus that regularly occurs together with infantile strabismus, the association of congenital nystagmus and strabismus is incidental. A hypothesis on the pathogenesis of congenital nystagmus is reported. The primary defect responsible for its development might be the inability of the ocular motor system to make use of retinal slip as a control variable for the stabilization of the eyes. This inability, present at an early sensitive period of ocular motor development, could permit the formation of abnormal synaptic connections that produce congenital nystagmus.

Acknowledgement

This investigation was supported by the Deutsche Forschungsgemeinschaft, SFB 70, B4.

References

Abadi, R.V. and Dickinson, C.M. (1985) The influence of preexisting oscillations on the binocular optokinetic response. *Ann. Neurol.*, **17**, 578–86.

Abadi, R.V., Dickinson, C.M. and Lomas, M.S. (1982) Inverted and asymmetrical optokinetic nystagmus, in *Functional Basis of Ocular Motility Disorders* (eds G. Lennerstrand, D.S. Zee and E.L. Keller). Pergamon, Oxford, pp. 143–6.

Abel, L.A., Grossman, G., Dell'Osso, L.F., Thurston, S.E. and Daroff, R.B. (1986) Abstract, in *Ocular Motor Minisymposium* (ed. S.E. Thurston). *Neuro-ophthalmology*, **6**, 137–8.

Atkinson, J. (1979) Development of optokinetic nystagmus in the human infant and monkey infant, in *Developmental Neurobiology of Vision* (ed. R.D. Freeman). Plenum, New York, pp. 277–87.

Atkinson, J. and Braddick, O. (1981) Development of optokinetic nystagmus in infants: an indicator of cortical binocularity?, in *Eye Movements: Cognition and Visual Perception* (eds D.F. Fisher, R.A. Monty and J.W. Senders). Erlbaum, Hillsdale, NJ, pp. 53–64.

Bielschowsky, A. (1930) Die einseitigen und gegensinnigen ('dissoziierten') Vertikalbewegungen der Augen. *Albrecht von Graefe's Arch. Ophthalmol.*, **125**, 493–553.

Cynader, M. and Harris, L. (1980) Eye movement in strabismic cat. *Nature*, **286**, 64–5.

Dell'Osso, L.F. (1985) Congenital, latent and manifest latent nystagmus – similarities, differences and relation to strabismus. *Jap. J. Ophthalmol.*, **29**, 351–68.

Dell'Osso, L.F. (1986) Evaluation of smooth pursuit in the presence of congenital nystagmus. *Neuro-ophthalmology*, **6**, 383–406.

Dell'Osso, L.F. and Daroff, R.B. (1975) Congenital nystagmus waveform and foveation strategy. *Doc. Ophthalmol.*, **39**, 155–7.

Dell'Osso, L.F., Gauthier, G., Liberman, G. and Stark, L. (1972) Eye movement recordings as a diagnostic tool in a case of congenital nystagmus. *Am. J. Opt. Am. Acad. Opt.*, **49**, 3–13.

Dell'Osso, L.F., Schmidt, D. and Daroff, R.B. (1979) Latent, manifest latent and congenital nystagmus. *Arch. Ophthalmol.*, **97**, 1877–85.

Doden, W. (1961) Latenter Nystagmus bei Strabismus concomitans alternans. *Ber. Dtsch. Ophthalmol. Ges.*, **63**, 486–90.

Flynn, J.T., Pritchard, C. and Lasley, D. (1984) Binocular vision and OKN asymmetry in strabismic patients, in *Strabismus* II (ed. R.D. Reinecke), Proceedings of the Fourth Meeting of the International Strabismological Association. Grune and Stratton, Orlando, pp. 35–43.

Hain, T.C., Kelman, S.E. and Zee, D.S. (1985) Pursuit and saccade asymmetries in latent nystagmus. *Soc. Neurosci., Abst.*, **11**, 231.

Hainline, L., Lemerise, E., Abramov, I. *et al.* (1984) Orientational asymmetries in small-field optokinetic nystagmus in human infants. *Behav. Brain Res.*, **13**, 217–30.

Halmagyi, G.M., Gresty, M.A. and Leech, J. (1980) Reversed optokinetic nystagmus (OKN), mechanism and clinical significance. *Ann. Neurol.*, **7**, 429–35.

Harris, L.R. and Cynader, M. (1981) The eye movements of the dark-reared cat. *Exp. Brain Res.*, **44**, 57–70.

Helveston, E.M. (1980) Dissociated vertical deviation. A clinical and laboratory study. *Trans. Am. Ophthalmol. Soc.*, **78**, 734–79.

Hoffmann, K.P. (1979) Optokinetic nystagmus and single cell responses in the nucleus tractus opticus after early monocular deprivation in the cat, in *Developmental Neurobiology of Vision* (ed. R.D. Freeman). Plenum, New York, pp. 63–73.

Hoffmann, K.P. (1982) Cortical versus subcortical contribution to the optokinetic reflex in the cat, in *Functional Basis of Ocular Motility Disorders* (eds G. Lennerstrand, D.S. Zee and E.L. Keller). Pergamon, Oxford, pp. 303–10.

Hoffmann, K.P. (1983) Neuronal responses related to optokinetic nystagmus in the cat's nucleus of the optic tract, in *Progress in Oculomotor Research* (eds A. Fuchs and W. Becker). Elsevier/North-Holland, New York, pp. 443–54.

Hoffmann, K.P. and Distler, C. (1986) The role of direction selective cells in the nucleus of the optic tract of cat and monkey during optokinetic nystagmus, in *Adaptive Processes in Visual and Oculomotor Systems* (eds E.L. Keller and D.S. Zee). Pergamon, Oxford, pp. 261–6.

Jung, R. and Kornhuber, H.H. (1964) Results of electronystagmography in man: the value of optokinetic, vestibular, and spontaneous nystagmus for neurologic diagnosis and research, in *The Ocular Motor System* (ed. M.B. Bender). Harper and Row, New York, pp. 428–88.

Keiner, G.B.J. and Roelofs, C.O. (1955) Optomotor reflexes and nystagmus, in *La Haye* (ed. M. Nijhoff), vol. 1, p. 224. Cited after Goddé-Jolly, D. and Larmande, A. (1973) *Les Nystagmus*, vol. 1. Masson and Cie, Paris, Chapter VIII, p. 632.
Kestenbaum, A. (1961) *Clinical Methods of Neuro-ophthalmologic Examination.* Grune and Stratton, New York, London, p. 366.
Kommerell, G. (1978) Beziehungen zwischen Strabismus und Nystagmus, in *Augenbewegungsstörungen, Neurophysiologie und Klinik* (ed. G. Kommerell). Bergmann, München, pp. 367–73.
Kommerell, G. (1986) Congenital nystagmus: control of slow tracking movements by target offset from the fovea. *Graefe's Arch. Clin. Exp. Ophthalmol.*, **224**, 295–8.
Kommerell, G. and Mattheus, S. (1984) Reversed fixation test (RFT); a new tool for the diagnosis of dissociated vertical deviation (DVD), in *Strabismus* II (ed. R.D. Reinecke). Grune and Stratton, Orlando, pp. 721–8.
Kommerell, G. and Mehdorn, E. (1982) Is an optokinetic defect the cause of congenital nystagmus?, in *Functional Basis of Ocular Motility Disorders* (eds G. Lennerstrand, D.S. Zee and E.L. Keller). Pergamon, Oxford, pp. 159–67.
Kommerell, G., Horn, R. and Bach, M. (1986) Motion perception in congenital nystagmus, in *Adaptive Processes in Visual and Oculomotor Systems* (eds E.L. Keller and D.S. Zee). Pergamon, Oxford, pp. 485–91.
Körner, F. and Dichgans, J. (1967) Bewegungswahrnehmung, optokinetischer Nystagmus und retinale Bildwanderung. *Albrecht v. Graefe's Arch. Klin. Exp. Ophthalmol.*, **174**, 34–48.
Kornhuber, H.H. (1960) Über Begleitschielen und latenten Nystagmus aus neurologischer Sicht, in *Sitzungsbericht* 102 (ed. K.A. Reiser). Versammlung Verein Rheinisch-Westfälischer Augenärzte, pp. 45–8.
Lang, J. (1968) *Squint Dating from Birth.* First International Congress of Orthoptists. Kimpton, London, pp. 231–7.
Loewer-Sieger, D.H. (1962) *Amblyopie. Een Studie over de Kenmarken en de Behandeling.* J. Ruysendaal, Amsterdam.
McKee, S.P. and Welch, L. (1985) Sequential recruitment in the discrimination of velocity. *J. Opt. Soc. Am. A*, **2**, 243–51.
Mehdorn, E. (1982) Nasal-temporal OKN-asymmetries after bilateral occipital infarction in man, in *Functional Basis of Ocular Motility Disorders* (eds G. Lennerstrand, D.S. Zee and E.L. Keller). Pergamon, Oxford, pp. 321–4.
Mehdorn, E. and Kommerell, G. (1983) Beziehungen zwischen latentem Nystagmus, asymmetrischem optokinetischem Nystagmus und defektem Binokularsehen. *Fortschr. Ophthalmol.*, **80**, 281–3.
Mein, J. (1983) The asymmetric optokinetic response. *Br. Orthoptic. J.*, **40**, 1–3.
Mohn, G., Sireteanu, R. and van Hof-van Duin, J. (1986) The relation of monocular optokinetic nystagmus to peripheral binocular interactions. *Invest. Ophthalmol. Vis. Sci.*, **27**, 565–73.
Naegele, J.R. and Held, R. (1982) The postnatal development of monocular optokinetic nystagmus in infants. *Vision Res.*, **22**, 341–6.
Nicolai, H. (1959) Differenzen zwischen optokinetischem Rechts- und Linksnystagmus bei einseitiger Schielamblyopie. *Klin. Monatsbl. Augenheilk.*, **134**, 245–50.

Ohm, J. (1928) Der latente Nystagmus im Stockdunkeln. *Arch. Augenheilkunde*, **99**, 417–37.

Ohmi, M., Howard, I.P. and Eveleigh, B. (1986) Directional preponderance in human optokinetic nystagmus. *Exp. Brain Res.*, **63**, 387–94.

Roelofs, C.O. (1928) Nystagmus latens. *Arch. Augenheilkunde*, **98**, 401–47.

Rüssmann, W. and Albrecht, J. (1986) Aufmerksamkeitsverlagerung und dissoziiertes Höhenschielen. *Klin. Monatsbl. Augenheilk.*, **188**, 245–7.

Schor, C.M. (1981) Directional anisotropies of pursuit tracking and optokinetic nystagmus in abnormal binocular vision, in *Ocular Motor Symposium* (eds D. Fender and B. Cooper). Cal-Tech Press, Pasadena, CA, pp. 83–104.

Schor, C.M. (1983) Subcortical binocular suppression affects the development of latent and optokinetic nystagmus. *Am. J. Optom. Physiol. Opt.*, **60**, 481–502.

Schor, C.M. and Levi, D.L. (1980) Disturbances of small field horizontal and vertical optokinetic nystagmus in amblyopia. *Invest. Ophthalmol. Vis. Sci.*, **19**, 668–83.

Sharpe, J.A., Lo, A.W. and Rabinovitch, H.E. (1979) Control of the saccadic and smooth pursuit systems after cerebral hemidecortication. *Brain*, **102**, 387–403.

Sorsby, A. (1931) Latent nystagmus. *Br. J. Ophthalmol.*, **15**, 1–18.

Sparks, D.L., Gurski, M.R., Mays, L.E. and Hickey, T.L. (1986) Effects of long-term and short-term monocular deprivation upon oculomotor function in the Rhesus monkey, in *Adaptive Processes in Visual and Oculomotor Systems* (eds E.L. Keller and D.S. Zee). Pergamon, Oxford, pp. 191–7.

Stevens, S. (1957) On the psychophysical law. *Psychol. Rev.*, **64**, 153–84.

Strong, N.P., Malach, R., Lee, P. and van Sluyters, R.C. (1984) Horizontal optokinetic nystagmus in the cat. Recovery from cortical lesions. *Dev. Brain Res.*, **13**, 179–92.

Tychsen, L. and Lisberger, St.G. (1986) Maldevelopment of visual motion processing in humans who had strabismus with onset in infancy. *J. Neurosci.*, **6**, 2495–508.

Tychsen, L., Hurtig, R.R. and Scott, W.E. (1985) Pursuit is impaired but the vestibulo-ocular reflex is normal in infantile strabismus. *Arch. Ophthalmol.*, **103**, 536–9.

van Hof-van Duin, J. (1976) Early and permanent effects of monocular deprivation on pattern discrimination and visuomotor behaviour in cats. *Brain Res.*, **111**, 261–76.

van Hof-van Duin, J. (1978) Asymmetry of optokinetic nystagmus observed in normal kittens and light deprived cats, in *Augenbewegungsstörungen, Neurophysiologie und Klinik* (ed. G. Kommerell). Bergmann, München, pp. 363–6.

van Hof-van Duin, J. and Mohn, G. (1986) Monocular and binocular optokinetic nystagmus in humans with defective stereopsis. *Invest. Ophthalmol. Vis. Sci.*, **27**, 574–83.

van Vliet, A.G.M. (1973) On the central mechanism of latent nystagmus. *Acta Ophthalmol. (Copenh.)*, **51**, 772–81.

Yamazaki, A. (1979) Abnormalities of smooth pursuit and vestibular eye movements in congenital jerk nystagmus, in *Ophthalmology* (ed. K. Shimizu), vol. 2. Excerpta Medica, Amsterdam, pp. 1162–5.

Yee, R.D., Baloh, R.W. and Honrubia, V. (1980) Study of congenital nystagmus: optokinetic nystagmus. *Br. J. Ophthalmol.*, **64**, 926–32.

Zee, D.S., Friendlich, A.R. and Robinson, D.A. (1974) The mechanism of downbeat nystagmus. *Arch. Neurol.*, **30**, 227–37.

Zee, D.S., Tusa, R.J., Herdmann, S.J., Butler, P.H. and Gucer, G. (1986) The acute and chronic effects of bilateral occipital lobectomy upon eye movements in monkey, in *Adaptive Processes in Visual and Oculomotor Systems* (eds E.L. Keller and D.S. Zee). Pergamon, Oxford, pp. 267–74.

Zikmund, V. (1966) Oculomotor activity during visual imagery of a moving stimulus pattern. *Stud. Psychol.*, **8**, 254–72.

CHAPTER 21

Electrophysiology of eye muscles

ALFRED HUBER

The peripheral oculomotor system, consisting of eyeballs, their external muscles and corresponding nerves, represents that neuromuscular system which probably until now has been one of the best examined. According to Robinson (Robinson, 1982), our knowledge of the mechanics and neurophysiology of this peripheral oculomotor apparatus is so far advanced that we are already able to predict the kind of oculomotor disorders resulting from lesions of muscles, orbital tissue and oculomotor nerves. Were it possible to implant an artificial eye muscle, one could indicate in a quantitative manner its exact physiological requirements. Among muscles of the human body, the extraocular muscles have a mechanical task which is unique both as regards speed and the accuracy required: their movements are not only very quick but also very precise. Correspondingly one can find a series of anatomical, pharmacological and electrophysiological properties by which this speed and precision of movements is attained, properties which differ from those of ordinary skeletal muscles more in a quantitative than in a qualitative manner.

The extraocular muscles are composed of several hundred muscle fibres, which are much smaller than those of most skeletal muscles. All six extraocular muscles manifest two different muscle portions: an orbital zone with small red fibres rich in mitochondria (slow fibres) and a global zone with large pale fibres (fast fibres) containing less mitochondria. In between exist intermediate zones. Contraction velocity is inversely related to mitochondrial quantity. Enzyme studies confirm slow, fast and intermediate fibre types. Both zones, the global and orbital, of the extraocular muscles are composed of singly or multiply innervated muscle fibres. Electrophysiology has developed the important notion that various histological muscle fibre types are functionally differentiated on the basis of the amount of work they do, rather than on the basis of the type of eye movement to which they contribute. It seems that the outer smaller red fibres of the orbital zone are recruited early in an eye movement, turned off in extreme gaze or large saccades, and maintain a steady, low-level force for the primary position of gaze. Later the deeper large pale fibres of the global zone, which have high output and short duration firing during saccadic movement, are recruited. Thus electrophysiological data indicate a continuous spectrum of fibre activity, suited to demand, rather than a sharp separation into fast and slow fibres, although there appears to be an orbital–global gradient. The organization of the orbital and global fibres of the extraocular muscles has some corollary in the central nervous system organization pattern: in the monkey brainstem, the third nerve dorso-medial nuclei are small motor neurones which innervate the orbital fibres (Büttner-Ennever and Akert, 1981).

Apart from the above-mentioned fibres the human extraocular muscles contain numerous muscle spindles, concentrated near the origin and insertion of the muscles, which receive motor innervation entirely from collaterals of motor fibres to extrafusal muscle fibres, rather than from a specific gamma efferent supply. The afferent fibres from the muscle spindles seem to enter the brainstem via the Vth nerve, though whether by the sensory or the motor root is uncertain. The role of the spindles as proprioceptors is not related to a conscious awareness of eye positions or eye movements. They may modify adversive movements initiated by retinal stimuli and play a part in maintaining fixation or in preventing unnecessary overshoot movements. Each extraocular muscle may be looked upon as an elastic spring, the tension of which can be varied with great rapidity and extremely fine graduation. There is no doubt that the localization of what we see does not ensue from the afferent stretch signals, but from the computing of the efferent muscle impulses.

Registration and analysis of electrical activity in the eye muscles goes back to the pioneer work of Björk and Kugelberg (1953), who first introduced electromyography of the extraocular muscles as a tool of investigation into neuro-ophthalmological diagnosis. Numerous authors have used this method since in clinical and research work (Kuboki, 1956, Kamouchi, 1957; Jampolsky, Tamler and Marg, 1959; Esslen and Papst, 1961; Breinin, 1962; Huber, 1973, 1977; Mitsui, 1986) and thus established an electrophysiology of the eye muscles.

21.1 Technique of electromyography

For registration of the muscular electrical activity one uses thin coaxial needle electrodes. After simple topical anaesthesia the sterilized electrode is inserted through the conjunctiva along the tendon into the belly of the eye muscle in a direction almost parallel to the muscle axis. The very low action potentials from the eye muscles picked up by the electrode are amplified and displayed on a cathode-ray oscilloscope.

21.2 Electrical activity of normal eye muscle

The electromyogram (EMG) is a record of the electrical discharge of the muscle, not of the nerve. It manifests itself in the form of action potentials which are the summation of the potentials of all the muscle fibres belonging to one motor unit. The discharge within the motor unit is nearly but not perfectly synchronous. On the oscilloscope each action potential is visible as an electric wave of bi- or tri-phasic character, in which the big upward deflection corresponds to the actual stimulation of the muscle fibres. Using the EMG, the activity of the alpha-motoneurones is recorded because their discharge is the ignition of the activity of the whole motor unit.

Eye muscles differ considerably from peripheral skeletal muscles: their motor units discharge with higher frequency (up to several hundred discharges per second), they have a much lower amplitude (averaging 20–200 μV) and exhibit a much shorter duration (1–2 ms). These electrophysiological qualities of extraocular muscles point to a motor unit of very small dimension, a fact which has its parallel in the anatomically proven low innervation ratio of the eye muscle (one axon distributed to only 5–10 muscle fibres in comparison with the skeletal muscles where one axon is distributed to 100–200 muscle fibres). Small size of motor units and low innervation ratio is characteristic of muscles involved in delicate, precise and finally graded, movements such as the eye muscles perform.

Whereas despite a certain tonus, skeletal muscles at rest manifest no recordable electrical acitivity, the extraocular muscles are rarely electrically silent: they show electrical activity even in versions out of the action field. In the primary position they have distinct electrical activity. There is practically no position of electrical rest: undoubtedly such a continuous 'tonic' activity is to a large extent responsible for the exact and precise position and excursions of the eyes.

In extraocular muscles the response to effort (identical with movement of the eye into the field of action of the recorded muscle) consists of two phenomena: (1) recruitment of new motor units and (2) increase in frequency of firing. The resulting electromyogram thus develops from the pattern of discharge of single units into a more complex pattern and finally into the so-called interference pattern (on maximum effort of the recorded muscles) in which, because of the overlapping of the activity, the individual motor units are no longer recognizable.

By recording two antagonistic extraocular muscles simultaneously, Sherrington's principle of reciprocal innervation can be beautifully demonstrated: the gradual increase of activity in the agonist runs parallel to progressive inhibition of activity in the antagonist (exemplified both in direct and contralateral antagonists). Synergists show a parallel increase of activity. Similar phenomena can be observed during symmetrical midline convergence: increasing firing rate and number of motor units in the medial recti is accompanied by corresponding reciprocal inhibition of the lateral recti. The exception to the reciprocity law, co-contraction occurs mainly under pathological circumstances.

During local and general anaesthesia a rapid loss of action potentials occurs up to complete electrical silence in the extraocular muscles. Sleep is therefore the only physiological process affording relaxation and rest of the eye muscles.

It is of considerable importance to mention that all electromyographic studies confirm the validity of Hering's law of distributed innervation throughout the physiological range of binocular movements; in other words the general principle that the outflow of innervation into the motor nerves of the extraocular muscles reveals the central adjustment of opposing innervations. According to Breinin another law of innervation exists: namely if the innervation does not alter, the eye does not move; and when the eye moves the innervation alters.

21.3 Abnormal electrical activity of eye muscle

The contribution of electromyography to pathophysiology of eye muscles and especially to the analysis of disturbances of eye motility is important. The EMG, carefully interpreted and sometimes repeated at different time intervals, can establish in most instances the topographic diagnosis of oculomotor disorders. The possibilities of topographic EMG differentiations are the following: (1) disease of the eye muscle itself (ocular myopathies); (2) disturbances of the neuromuscular transmission (myasthenias); (3) lesions of the peripheral neurone (neurogenic palsies); (4) disturbances of central innervation (supranuclear lesions). All these disturbances are reflected by alterations of the electric wave-form, the amplitude and frequency of the motor units and the pattern of electrical firing.

21.3.1 DISEASES OF EYE MUSCLES (MYOPATHIES)

Until recently a great number of affections of the eye muscles has been interpreted erroneously as being of neuropathic origin. Ocular myopathy is an affection of the eye muscle which can occur as a local manifestation of a generalized myopathy of skeletal muscles, but very often manifests as a condition confined only to the ocular muscles.

An ocular myopathy must be suspected if oculomotor palsies cannot be classified into a peripheral neurogenic or central (nuclear or supranuclear) scheme. The progressive affection of eye muscles supplied by more than one oculomotor nerve is also in favour of a myopathy. In many cases it will be practically impossible clinically to differentiate between the motility disturbances due to a lesion of oculomotor nerves and that due to an affection of muscle and only electromyography of the affected muscles will establish the differential diagnosis. The crucial criterion of myogenic palsy in the electromyogram is the striking disproportion between the high degree of electrical activity and the very poor effect on motility of the affected eye muscle even upon maximum effort. This phenomenon can be explained by the fact that the contractile mechanism of the muscle fibres is affected earlier and more intensively, whereas the electrical properties of the muscle cell membrane persist longer. This electromyographic pattern is in distinct contrast to that of the neuropathic palsy which is characterized by a diminution of the number of the motor units proportional to the degree of the paresis, reaching complete electrical silence with total interruption of impulse conduction. In skeletal muscles a further characteristic and constant sign of myopathy is the shortening of potentials with diminution in their amplitudes. Since the potentials of ocular muscles are already of short duration, it is very difficult if not impossible to register further shortening. On the other hand, in ocular myopathy the reduction of amplitude can usually be observed very distinctly. On the basis of clinical observations, electromyographic and histological findings, it has been possible to distinguish various forms of myopathic ophthalmoplegias: chronic progressive ocular muscle dystrophy (Graefe's disease), acute and chronic myositis, dysthyroid ophthalmoplegia, disturbance of eye motility in myotonia and myopathies due to general affections (metabolic diseases, congenital muscle diseases).

(a) Chronic progressive ocular muscle dystrophy (Graefe's disease). Graefe's disease (also called abiotrophic ophthalmoplegia) is an entity that was once called progressive nuclear ophthalmoplegia under the erroneous impression that the ocular motor nuclei were primarily involved. However, more recently it has been interpreted as a myopathy with

characteristic histopathological changes (mitochondrial abnormalities). It may or may not be associated with involvement of skeletal muscles elsewhere in the body (face, pharynx or neck). Ptosis is usually the first symptom noted, but restriction of eye movements also occurs early. The lids drop gradually and the eye movements are limited in such a way as not to fit into any one nerve pattern. There is no tendency for remission, and no diurnal variation; on the contrary, the disease generally progresses to complete immobility of both eyes. Because of the slow development of eye muscle palsies the patients practically never complain of diplopia. This ocular myopathy generally appears before the age of 30 and progresses gradually over the following decades. There are also congenital forms which simulate the end-stage of the disease. One particular form of chronic progressive external ophthalmoplegia is oculopharyngeal dystrophy, characterized by ptosis, dysphagia and autosomal dominant heredity. Sometimes external ophthalmoplegia can be observed in this oculopharyngeal syndrome, as well. In the classic form of this disease signs may develop after the fourth, but usually after the sixth, decade.

A combination of chronic progressive external ophthalmoplegia with retinal changes and/or cardiac disorders and/or neurological disorders is called Ophthalmoplegia-plus, or Kearns syndrome. Here the morphological and biochemical features demonstrate disturbed mitochondrial function, as well as visible changes in the mitochondrial structure (i.e. ragged-red fibres in the muscle biopsy specimen). Whereas Kearns syndrome consists of progressive external ophthalmoplegia, retinitis pigmentosa and heart block in young people, the neurogenic characteristics are most predominant in the severe, extensive infantile–juvenile form known as Kearns–Sayre syndrome, with spongy deterioration of the brain as a sign of involvement of intracerebral mitochondria.

(b) Ocular myositis. There are two clinical manifestations of the disease. An *acute* form with orbital pain, diplopia, exophthalmos, ptosis and often chemosis of the conjunctiva, oedema of the lids and distinct conjunctival irritation and multiple pareses of extraocular muscles, generally progressing to complete immobility of the affected eye; and a *chronic* form (oligosymptomatic ocular myositis) which affects only single eye muscles with signs of slight, or even no, conjunctival irritation. Ocular myositis shows alterations in the electromyogram similar to those of ocular muscle dystrophy, first of all an electrical activity out of proportion to the degree of paralysis but, in myositis, a reduction in amplitude of potentials is very seldom observed. In numerous cases, spontaneous myogenic activity (the result of a hypersensitivity of the muscle fibre membranes to depolarizing influences) can be registered; moreover, polyphasic action potentials in myositis are more frequent than in ocular muscle dystrophy.

The distinction between chronic myositis and myasthenia gravis, which clinically is sometimes impossible, can be made easily by the Tensilon test (positive only in myasthenia).

Both the acute and the chronic form of ocular myositis respond extremely well to general and local application of high doses of corticosteroids. Myositis is an allergic-hyperergic affection of the eye muscles and the orbital tissues.

(c) Dysthyroid ophthalmoplegia (endocrine ocular myopathy). There is now clinical and electromyographic evidence that eye muscle palsies occurring in thyroid disease are caused by contraction deficiency on the basis of a myopathy that is also observed in the skeletal muscles. The ophthalmoplegia preferentially manifests itself as unilateral or bilateral limitation of ocular motion in the upward direction, simulating upward gaze palsy, caused by restriction of the globe by the inferior recti muscles, rather than by weakness of the elevator muscles. This restriction can be confirmed by the forced duction test. Sometimes the medial or lateral recti are involved as well, thus producing the picture of horizontal gaze palsy. Even almost completely paralysed eye muscles show a myopathic pattern in the EMG, with a disproportion between the well-preserved electrical properties and the great deficiency of contractile strength. Only muscles paralysed for a long time show significant decreased amplitude and loss of whole motor units, signs of fibrosis.

Of great importance in the clinical diagnosis of dysthyroid ophthalmoplegia are the signs of hyperthyroidism, if present: more or less pronounced unilateral or bilateral exophthalmos, sometimes combined with congestive swelling of the lids and chemosis of the conjunctiva; Graefe's sign, lag of the upper lid when looking down; Dalrymple's sign, pathological retraction of the upper lid; Stellwag's sign, infrequent lid closure; and Moebius' sign, convergence weakness. There is no direct relationship between the degree of exophthalmos and the eye muscle palsies: they may even precede the appearance of the exophthalmos. Most frequently they occur within a few weeks after treatment of hyperthyroidism when the patient is hypothyroid, but they may occur concomitantly with hyperthyroidism or years later, when the patient is euthyroid. The dysthyroid ophthalmoplegia generally runs a self-limited course that has a duration varying from a few months to a year or more. Some myopathy may persist with consequent fixation of the eyes in an anomalous position.

(d) Ocular myotonias. The common denominator in the various myotonias is an inability of the muscles to relax easily from the contracted state. All myotonias are inherited in an autosomal dominant fashion with

complete or near complete penetrance. Disturbances of muscular activity and endocrine function are the cardinal lesions of myotonic disorders, which have a broad disease spectrum: at one end is myotonia congenita (Thomsen's disease) and at the other end periodic familial paralysis (also called familial hypokalaemic myotonia). In the middle of these extremes are the well-defined clinical entities of dystrophia myotonica (Steinert's disease) and paramyotonia congenita. Between these clinical groups, best maintained for clinical classification, there are certain transitional atypical cases which unite them into a composite whole. Dystrophia myotonica is characterized by distal muscle atrophy, myopathic facies, loss of hair, complicated cataract, atrophy of gonads and hearing loss; disorders of ocular motility are rather infrequent: ptosis, reduced frequency of lid movements, convergence spasms and sometimes also a pseudo-Graefe sign. In myotonia congenita (Thomsen's disease) the most characteristic symptom is the myotonic reaction of all striated muscles: after active contraction or electrical irritation, there is a distinctly delayed relaxation. The myotonic reaction can also be observed in the eye muscles, most frequently in the levator muscle. After prolonged upward gaze, there occurs a lid retraction on looking downward simulating Graefe's sign (so-called pseudo-Graefe sign). There may also be an inability to open the lid easily after forced lid closure. More infrequently one can observe a slowness of ocular movements or limitation of gaze. After a convergence movement a tonic after-contraction within the internal recti can make the patient unable to look straight for a short time and produce a temporary convergent strabismus with diplopia ('freezing of the gaze'), which relaxes only after a few seconds to the normal parallel position of the eyes. The electromyogram in ocular myotonias shows myotonic bursts of variable frequency, between 100 and 200 per second, discharges occurring as the so-called 'after-activity' at the end of voluntary innervation without relationship to will. These electrical phenomena are directly responsible for the inability of the muscles to relax from the contracted state. The myotonic reaction, consisting in involuntary after-discharges elicited by normal impulses, is due to an abnormal hypersensitivity of the muscle fibre itself.

In conclusion, one can say that ocular myopathies have an important place in neuro-ophthalmological diagnosis, representing about 12% of all eye muscle palsies. It is of utmost importance to differentiate ocular myopathies from neurogenic pareses, which may show a similar or identical clinical picture. Apart from clinical judgement, Tensilon testing and EMG of the affected muscles contribute much to correct diagnosis, hence to successful treatment. Sometimes the early findings of an ocular myopathy may be the presentation of a general myopathy that has been overlooked because of only minor symptomatology.

21.3.2 DISORDERS OF THE NEUROMUSCULAR TRANSMISSION

Myasthenia gravis is the prototype of a disorder of neuromuscular transmission within the area of the eye muscles. Nearly all patients with this disease will develop ocular signs sooner or later and may develop ptosis or diplopia as their first presenting symptoms. The most frequent ocular sign of myasthenia consists of a ptosis and a limitation of eye movements that does not fit into the pattern of a nerve lesion. Thus we may have a ptosis of one eye and an oculomotor palsy of the other eye or we may have a spotty involvement of muscles innervated by several oculomotor nerves. The involvement of the eye muscles may precede those of the general skeletal muscle system or remain the only myasthenic manifestation (ocular myasthenia). A predilection of myasthenia for the superior recti may sometimes simulate vertical gaze palsies. Myasthenia gravis may occur at any age from childhood to senescence. The characteristic sign of myasthenic pareses is the fact that they vary with the time of the day or with the state of the patient's fatigue: they are minimal when the person first awakes in the morning and become worse towards the end of the day. Spontaneous remissions alternate with unmotivated exacerbations. Pupillary and accommodation function always remain normal.

The most important diagnostic test for myasthenia gravis is the use of anti-cholinesterase agents. Prostigmine in appropriate doses is still the best test procedure for children. But for adults intravenous edrophonium chloride (Tensilon) gives a quicker and more certain response. It is customary to give 2 mg Tensilon within the first 15 s and the remaining 8 mg after the following 30 s. A positive Tensilon effect manifests itself within a minute but only lasts for a few minutes. The reaction may be recognized at the improved or even normalized function of the previously paretic eye muscles and the disappearance of the ptosis. In doubtful cases of ocular myasthenia electromyography is of greatest diagnostic value: here a positive Tensilon effect can be recognized at the distinct increase of the electrical activity even if the affected eye muscle manifests no or only slight improvement of its action. The electrical pattern of myasthenia in the extraocular muscles is that of a progressive decrease in activity of the muscle during sustained effort characterized by progressive fall out of motor units, such that the interference pattern disappears and only a few motor units remain in action with potentials of reduced amplitude and rate of discharge. This fatigue pattern does not occur in other forms of extraocular muscle diseases. Conclusive for myasthenia during electromyography is the pharmacological test with Tensilon: intravenous Tensilon produces after a few seconds a distinct increase in the electrical activity in the paretic muscle in such a way that upon maximum effort even the interference pattern may reappear, but only for a few minutes. The importance of this electrical response to Tensilon lies in the fact that the reaction appears pathognomonic of myasthenia and may occur in complete absence of visible ocular movement.

Recently, the method of single fibre electromyography has also been applied to myasthenic eye muscles. With the use of single fibre EMG, neuromuscular disturbances can be detected before impulse blocking occurs. The single fibre electrode is inserted into the slightly voluntarily activated paretic eye muscle, and a position is sought where action potentials from two fibres belonging to the same motor unit can be obtained. There is temporal variability, the so-called jitter, between the two action potentials at consecutive discharges. This is mainly due to a variation in the neuromuscular transmission time of the two motor end plates involved. In myasthenic eye muscles the jitter is increased to abnormal values, indicating a reduced safety factor: with progressing increase in jitter impulse blocking also occurs. Most important for diagnostic purposes is that in cases with purely ocular myasthenia in ocular, as well as in clinically not affected skeletal muscles (i.e. extensor digitorum communis), an increased jitter can be found; thus, single fibre electromyography may well become a most useful test for diagnosis of ocular or general myasthenia.

21.3.3 PERIPHERAL NEUROGENIC EYE MUSCLE PALSIES

Peripheral neurogenic eye muscle pareses or palsies are a consequence of a lesion of the neural part of the motor unit, i.e. a lesion which may have its site from the end-plate along the axon up to the ganglion cells in the ocular motor nuclei. Although the relationship of certain eye muscles to the oculomotor, the trochlear and the abducens nerve produces characteristic patterns of neurogenic palsies, and concomitant signs of other cranial nerves' involvement provide important information about the neurogenic nature of an eye muscle palsy, diagnostic difficulties are often present and not always easy to overcome. Electromyography here contributes to a distinct improvement of the diagnostic possibilities: a neurogenic paresis or paralysis manifests quite a different pattern of electrical activity of the affected muscle than a myogenic or myasthenic palsy. The most characteristic phenomenon in the EMG is the diminution in the number of motor units, a diminution which goes parallel to the degree of the paresis. This can proceed up to the stage where the totally interrupted and denervated eye muscle reveals no electrical activity at all. In cases of complete interruption of impulse conduction (irreversible block) there appear after two or three weeks fibrillation potentials which occur spontaneously and represent a sign of hypersensitivity of the denervated muscle fibres which discharge asynchronously. These fibrillations are of short duration (1 ms) and rather low discharge rate (1–5 per second); they are so similar to normal small single motor units that in cases of incomplete denervation they can be diagnosed only when the gaze is directed out of the field of action of the affected muscle, when they show no volitional increase in frequency. Whereas the totally denervated eye muscle reveals no electrical activity apart from the fibrillations (= total or complete palsy), the partially denervated muscle (= paresis) manifests diminution of the number of the motor units proportional to the degree of the paresis, which may fire at an increased frequency apparently attempting to compensate for the muscle weakness.

The reinnervation of paretic eye muscle manifests itself first by the disappearance of fibrillation potentials which are replaced by newly formed motor unit potentials of typically polyphasic character. Their amplitude is low, their discharge rate slow and their fatigability is great. Gradually the polyphasic waves disappear, and the amplitude and frequency of firing increase. Thus by means of electromyography it is possible to follow the different phases of reinnervation of a paralysed eye muscle. Moreover, it is important to know that electrical signs of reinnervation very often precede the clinically visible signs when motility of the paretic muscle reappears.

The EMG of the paretic eye muscle does not allow a topographic differentiation along the axon from the end plate to the nuclear region. Here we have to rely upon the neuro-ophthalmological symptomatology, in other words, the neurological signs which accompany the eye muscle palsies.

21.3.4 DISTURBANCES OF CENTRAL INNERVATION (SUPRANUCLEAR LESIONS)

Supranuclear lesions of the cerebral control mechanism of eye movements disturb the selection, distribution and spread of central innervational impulses to the motor units of the eye muscles. The EMG therefore is characterized by a disorder of the normal harmonic co-operation of agonist and antagonist, in other words by a disturbance of the law of reciprocal innervation (Sherrington, 1894).

In paralysis of lateral and vertical conjugate movements, the EMG manifests a pathological persistent increase of electrical activity independent of any intention to move the eyes. When placing electrodes simultaneously into agonist and antagonist, there is not only an exceptionally increased electrical activity of both muscles in the primary position, but this activity does not change either in agonist or antagonist during movements or efforts for movements in any direction. Such a disorder of reciprocal innervation represents a sort of spastic state in which the gaze palsies may be considered.

In Duane's retraction syndrome characterized by symptoms of a congenital abducens 'paralysis', retraction of the eye and narrowing of the palpebral fissure on adduction, the electromyographic investigation reveals as cause of this 'paralysis' a pathological synergistic innervation between muscles which work normally as antagonists. The EMG shows a fairly normal innervation of both internal and external rectus in the primary position, a strong co-innervation of the external rectus with the internal rectus during adduction and a very poor or complete lack of activity in the external rectus on intention to abduct the eye. The simultaneous contraction of both recti causes the phenomenon of retraction of the eyeball (Huber and Esslen, 1969). In this disorder the maximum innervation of the external rectus is during adduction, the minimum during abduction of the eye, which explains the abduction deficit. Such paradoxical innervation is due to an abnormal contact of oculomotor nerves with the external rectus.

Two post-mortem examinations of Duane's syndrome (Miller *et al.*, 1982) revealed absence of the abducens nuclei and the abducens nerves. The external recti muscles were innervated by aberrant branches from the inferior division of the oculomotor nerve.

Duane's syndrome is therefore a congenital anomaly (caused by a teratogenic event during the second month of gestation) consisting of absence or aplasia of the abducens nucleus and nerve and a substitute innervation of the external rectus muscle by extra branches of the oculomotor nerve.

Whether similar phenomena occur in cases of concomitant strabismus or not is not yet completely solved. In intermittent exotropia it has been demonstrated that on breaking into exotropia the lateral rectus activity was increased while the medial rectus activity was inhibited in the diverging eye. Whether these observations support an active divergence mechanism or not will not be discussed here, but the important fact is that divergence in intermittent exotropia is definitely associated with a corresponding alteration of innervation in the horizontal recti of the diverging eye. Similar observations have been obtained in cases of intermittent esotropia were an increased electrical activity takes place in the medial rectus whenever that eye breaks from fixation and deviates inwards. On the other hand, on the basis of electromyographic findings, there is no excessive innervation in the deviated eye in established constant esotropias or exotropias. One must therefore assume that the increased activity which brought about the deviation and which can be proved under conditions of intermittency, at some time disappears. In place of the excessive innervation which originally caused one eye to turn in or out, some structural changes must occur, in other words the primary innervational shortening of the squint agonist is replaced by a shortening on the basis of tissue factors (i.e. 'contracture'). Future research will certainly give more precise indications about the relation between the innervational (dynamic) and the structural (static) components which determine the position of the eyes in established concomitant strabismus.

21.4 Conclusion

Electromyography is an invaluable research tool in normal neurophysiology of extraocular muscle functions. Its most important contribution to daily clinical work is the diagnosis of ocular motility disorders on different levels. It makes possible the differential diagnosis between lesions of the peripheral neurone, disturbances of the neuromuscular junction, ocular myopathies and disorders of the central innervation, a differentiation so important for adequate treatment. In concomitant strabismus, electromyography will clarify the still obscure relationship between innervational and structural factors which bring about these deviations. Such a new approach to electrophysiology of the extraocular muscles under normal and pathological conditions provides much valuable and interesting insight into the activity of higher cerebral oculomotor centres and thus also facilitates the understanding of fundamental brain processes.

References

Björk, A. and Kugelberg, E. (1953) Motor unit activity in the human extraocular muscles. *Clin. Neurophysiol.*, **5**, 271–8.

Breinin, G.M. (1962) *The Electrophysiology of Extraocular Muscles.* University of Toronto Press, Toronto.

Büttner-Ennever, J.A. and Akert, K. (1981) Medial rectus subgroups of the oculomotor nucleus and their abducens internuclear input in the monkey. *J. Comp. Neurol.*, **197**, 17–27.

Esslen, E. and Papst, W. (1961) Bedeutung der Elektromyographie für die Analyse von Motilitätsstörungen der Augen. *Bibliotheca Ophthalmica*, Fasc. **57**.

Huber, A. (1973) L'intérêt clinique de l'électromyographie des muscles oculaires. *Oto.-Neuro-Ophthalmol.*, **45**, 303–14.

Huber, A. (1977) Elektromyographie der Augenmuskellähmungen, in *Bücherei des Augenarztes* (eds F.A. Hamburger and F. Hollwich). F. Enke, Stuttgart, pp. 74–112.

Huber, A. and Esslen, E. (1969) Die Duane-Syndrome. *Doc. Ophthalmol.*, **26**, 620–7.

Jampolsky, A., Tamler, E. and Marg, E. (1959) Artefacts and normal variations in human ocular electromyography. *Arch. Ophthalmol.* (*Chicago*), **61**, 402–13.

Kamouchi, T. (1957) Electromyogram of the palsied extraocular and levator muscles. *Jap. J. Ophthalmol.*, **1**, 30–4.

Kuboki, T. (1956) Electromyography of human extraocular muscles. *Acta Soc. Ophthalmol., Jap.*, **60**, 29–37.

Miller, N.R., Steven, M., Gree, R.G. and Clark, A.W. (1982) Unilateral Duane's retraction syndrome. *Arch. Ophthalmol.*, **100**, 1468–72.

Mitsui, Y. (1986) *Strabismus and the Sensorimotor Reflex.* Excerpta Medica, Amsterdam, Princeton, Geneva, Tokyo.

Robinson, D.A. (1981) Control of eye movements, in *American Physiological Society, The Nervous System, Handbook of Physiology*, Vol. II, Part 2 (ed. V.B. Brooks), Williams and Wilkins, Baltimore, pp. 1275–320.

Sherrington, C.S. (1894) Experimental note on two movements of the eyes. *J. Physiol.* (*Lond.*), **17**, 27–38.

Part III

The Pupil

CHAPTER 22

The afferent pupillary pathway

C.J.K. ELLIS

22.1 Introduction

An afferent pupillary defect (APD) is a valuable, objective sign of a lesion of the anterior visual pathway (Thompson, 1966) and has been described in disease of the retina (Bovino and Burton, 1980; Thompson, Watzke and Weinstein, 1980; Newsome, Milton and Gass, 1981; Thompson *et al.*, 1982), optic nerve (for a review, see Perkin and Rose, 1979), optic tract (Bell and Thompson, 1978) and superior brachium (Ellis, 1984).

Clinical testing for an APD depends upon asymmetrical involvement of the pupillary fibres from each eye and such asymmetry is demonstrated by alternately stimulating the eyes with light (the swinging light test (Thompson, 1966)). In the worse affected eye the amplitude of the initial pupillary constriction as the light falls on the eye is less and the subsequent pupillary dilatation (escape) whilst under the light is greater than in the less affected eye. Thus the pupillary abnormality is more accurately described as a relative afferent pupillary defect (RAPD) (Thompson, 1976).

The RAPD has been studied most extensively in optic neuritis in which serial observations of the pupillary reactions during the evolution and resolution of the acute phase have been correlated with loss of acuity and visual field. An afferent pupillary defect has been described on clinical assessment in between 6% (Lynn, 1959; Nikoskelainen, 1975) and 75% (Perkin and Rose, 1979) of patients with optic neuritis. Where infra-red pupillography is used in addition every patient with acute unilateral optic neuritis has been found to have an RAPD. This RAPD may remain as the only physical sign of a resolved episode of optic neuritis (Ellis, 1979; Cox, Thompson and Corbett, 1981).

22.2 Anatomy of the afferent pupillary light reflex pathway

The afferent pupillary light reflex pathway originates in the retinal photoreceptor layer and travels via axons of retinal ganglion cells. Both rods and cones contribute to the pupillary light reflex (Loewenfeld, 1966). The optic nerve fibres conveying the pupillary light reflex discharges in the cat are slow conducting (<10 m/s) (Hultborn, Mori and Tsukahara, 1978) and may correspond to the W-sustained group of retinal ganglion cells identified by Stone and Fukada (1974). These ganglion cells contain a subclass of cells that are luminance sensitive (firing tonically with sustained stimuli in response to varying luminance levels) and project to the pretectum (Cleland and Levick, 1974; Fukada and Stone, 1974). The ganglion cells of the W-sustained fibres constitute about 40% of the total cat ganglion cell population and are distributed throughout the retina but with a marked central predominance falling off sharply with eccentricity (Fukada and Stone, 1974). In the cat the neurophysiological properties of the X-transient group of retinal ganglion cells make them most likely to subserve visual acuity (Ikeda, 1979). There is indirect evidence therefore that in the cat the visual and pupillary afferent fibres may be separate throughout their course. The distribution of retinal receptors is not uniform across the retina being more dense in the nasal than temporal retina (Van Buren, 1963). There is a single post-mortem case report of quantitative histology of the optic chiasm in a patient with a previous complete unilateral optic nerve lesion, that indicates that there may also be asymmetrical decussation of fibres in the optic chiasm (ratio crossed : uncrossed 53 : 47) (Kupfer, Chumbley and Downer, 1967). Thus in the optic tract there may be more crossed than uncrossed fibres. This possible asymmetry may be of importance in understanding RAPD arising in post-chiasmal disease.

The pupillary afferent fibres leave the optic tract at its posterior third and travel around the superior colliculus via the superior brachium to reach the pretectal nucleus (Ransom and Magoun, 1930). Single cell recording of rat pretectal neurones has shown both luminance-sensitive and darkness-sensitive cells responding to changes in retinal illumination with tonic modulation in their discharge frequency (Clarke and Ikeda, 1985). Changes in single unit discharge frequency were associated with proportional changes in pupillary diameter. These findings further supported the suggestion that the pupillary light reflex is mediated via luminance-sensitive neurones.

22.3 The normal pupillary light reflex

Since the introduction of infra-red pupillometry (Lowenstein and Friedman, 1942) the physiological characteristics of the pupillary light reflex have been studied in detail (Lowenstein and Friedman, 1942; Alpern, McCready and Barr, 1963; Lowenstein and Loewenfeld, 1969; Ellis, 1981). All these workers agree that the direct pupillary light reflex amplitude increases from threshold to maximum amplitude with increasing stimulus intensity (Fig. 22.1). Latency from stimulus to onset of pupillary constriction decreases with increasing stimulus intensity (Fig. 22.2). Threshold pupillary responses may have latencies of up to 500 ms decreasing to a minimum of about 200 ms for maximum amplitude responses. This long latency is thought principally to be due to the delay in iris smooth muscle constriction. Stimulation of the cat ciliary ganglia

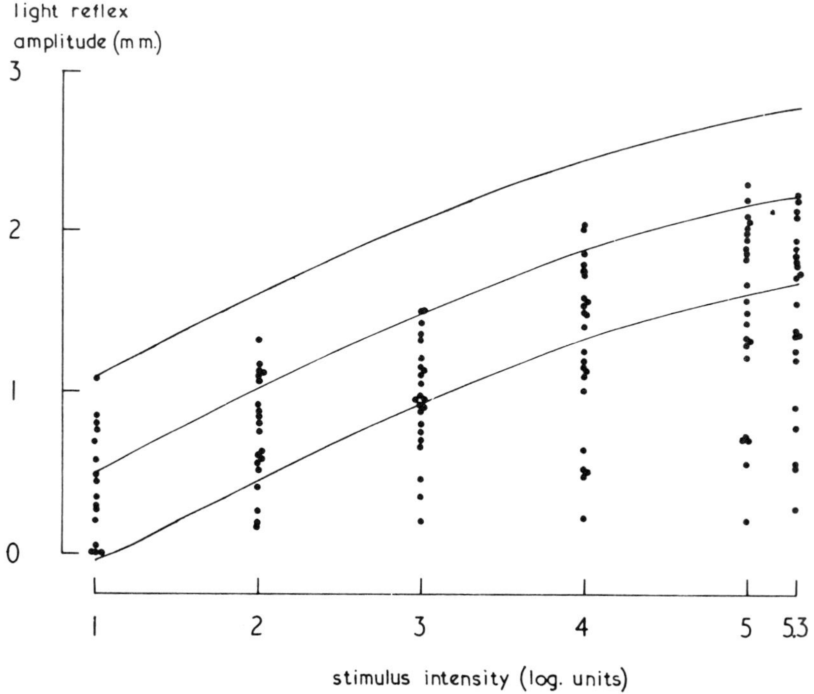

Fig. 22.1 The mean and 95% confidence limits of direct light reflex amplitude with increasing stimulus intensity (solid lines). This shows that in the normal condition direct light reflex amplitude increases with increasing stimulus intensity tending towards a maximum value. Dots indicate the reflex amplitude from the affected eye of 22 patients with acute unilateral optic neuritis. (All figures reproduced with permission from Ellis, 1979.)

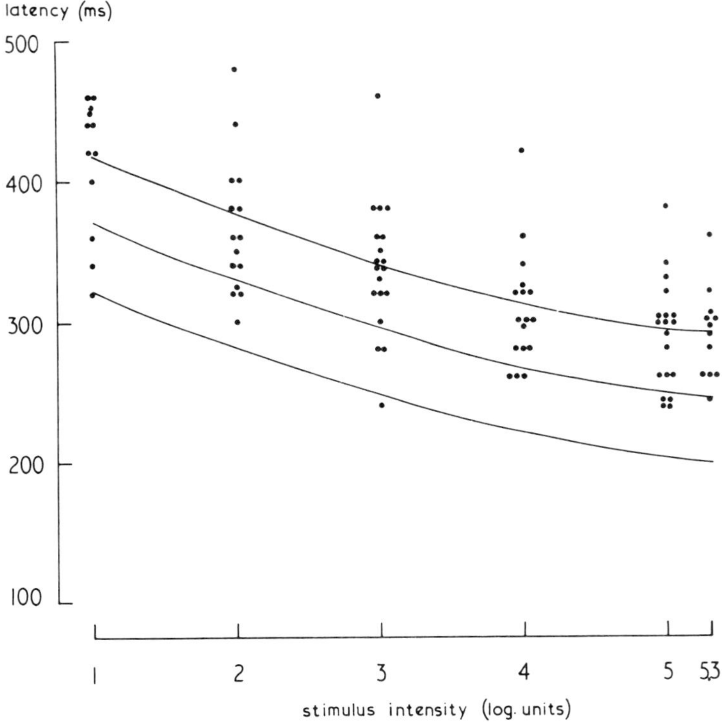

Fig. 22.2 The mean and 95% confidence limits of latency from stimulus to onset of response of the direct light reflex (solid lines). This shows that latency reduces with increasing stimulus intensity tending to a minimum value (solid lines). Dots indicate latencies from the affected eye of 22 patients with acute unilateral optic neuritis.

produces pupillary constriction with latencies of no less than 100 ms (Hultborn *et al.*, unpublished data) and in the pigeon with a striated muscle iris sphincter minimum latencies of around 60 ms have been recorded (Loewenfeld, 1966). A component of the pupillary response latency also arises in the retina, and electroretinography (ERG) in man shows that latency of discharge in some retinal ganglion cells may be up to 60 ms at low stimulus intensity in the cat (Ikeda and Wright, 1972).

Rates of pupillary constriction and dilatation also increase with increasing stimulus intensity (Fig. 22.3). Thus pupillary light reflexes elicited by high intensity light have larger amplitude, shorter latency and faster rates of constriction and dilatation than responses at lower stimulus intensity. However, it is evident from the 95% confidence limits shown (Figs 22.1–22.3) that the normal range for these parameters is wide due to uncontrol-

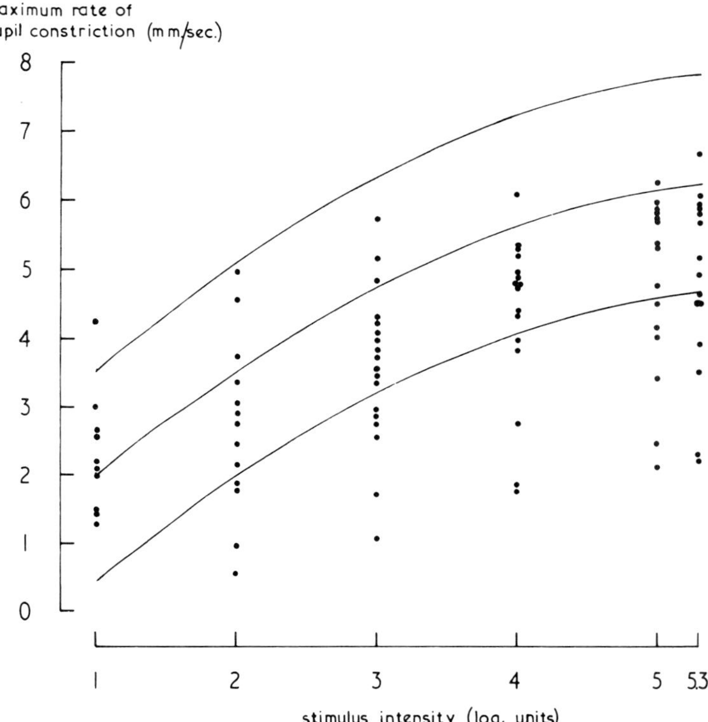

Fig. 22.3 The mean and 95% confidence limits of maximum rate of pupillary constriction of the direct light reflex amplitude (solid lines). This indicates that with increasing stimulus intensity the rate of pupillary constriction progressively increases tending toward a maximum. Dots indicate the rates of constriction from the affected eye of 22 patients with acute unilateral optic neuritis.

lable variables such as the level of supranuclear inhibition of the Edinger–Westphal nucleus (Lowenstein and Loewenfeld, 1969).

22.4 Afferent pupillary defects in acute optic neuritis

Infra-red pupillometry allows the pupillary light reflexes to be studied dynamically and in darkness. Where patients with unilateral acute optic neuritis have been studied with this technique and by careful clinical assessment an RAPD is found in every case (Ellis, 1979; Cox, Thompson and Corbett, 1981).

The RAPD in these patients was demonstrated clinically by the swinging light test (Levatin, 1959). Pupillography showed that the affected pupil had a smaller direct light reflex amplitude (Fig. 22.1), a longer latency (Fig. 22.2) and a slower rate of constriction (Fig. 22.3) than the unaffected pupil (Ellis, 1979). This asymmetry is the basis of the value of the swinging light test that facilitates comparison of the responses from the two eyes. However, when responses of equal amplitude from affected and unaffected eyes are compared there was no significant difference between the two except that a more intense light stimulus was required to elicit the reflex from the affected eye (Figs 22.4 and 22.5). Thus in an RAPD the latency, constriction and dilation velocities are appropriate to the amplitude of the light reflex and are the same as a response elicited from a normal eye at a lower stimulus intensity. This observation led Lowenstein and Friedman (1942) to describe the pupillary responses in optic nerve disease as low intensity reactions.

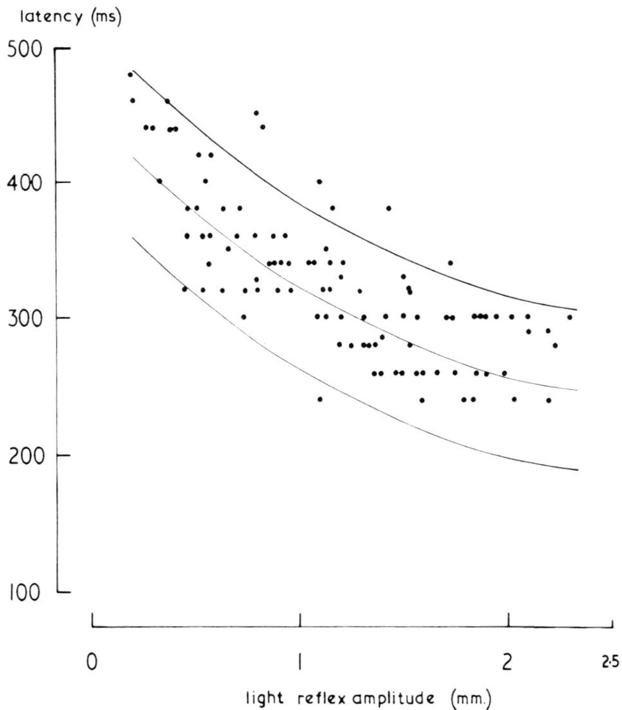

Fig. 22.4 The mean and 95% confidence limits of the relationship between latency and amplitude of the direct light reflex (solid lines). Dots are the latencies from 22 patients with acute unilateral optic neuritis.

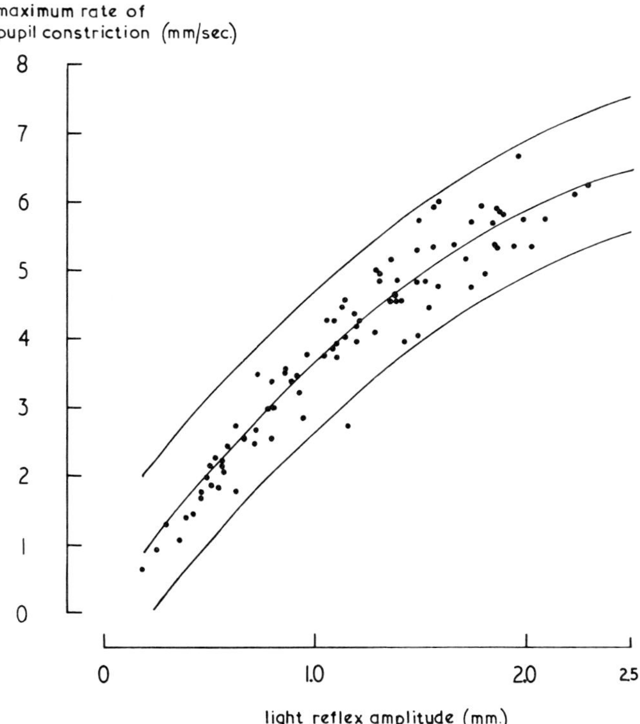

Fig. 22.5 The mean and 95% confidence limits of maximum rate of pupillary constriction against light reflex amplitude. The dots are the values from 22 patients with acute unilateral optic neuritis.

The magnitude of a patient's RAPD may thus be expressed as the difference in direct light reflex amplitude between the affected and unaffected eyes when stimulated with light of the same intensity. In one study this inter-ocular difference provided the basis of the definition of a relative afferent pupillary defect (Ellis, 1979) which was said to exist where inter-ocular difference in direct light reflex amplitude exceeded mean inter-ocular difference ±2 SD in a control group (Fig. 22.6). It is also possible to express magnitude of an RAPD as the value of neutral density filters that have to be placed over the normal eye to equate the amplitude of the pupillary reflexes (Thompson, Corbett and Cox, 1981).

In one study (Ellis, 1979) the magnitude of the RAPD in the acute phase of an episode of unilateral optic neuritis correlated with other evidence of

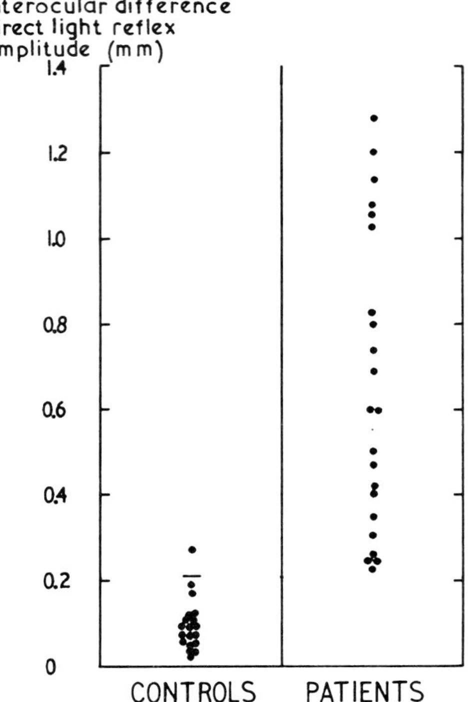

Fig. 22.6 The interocular difference in direct light reflex amplitude (magnitude of RAPD) in 22 patients with acute unilateral optic neuritis. This is compared with age-matched control values, the upper limit of normal, designated by the bar, being defined as mean plus two standard deviations. Every patient with an interocular difference in direct light reflex amplitude of more than 0.21 mm was designated as having a significant relative afferent pupillary defect.

optic nerve involvement such as impairment of visual acuity (Fig. 22.7), the size and density of field loss, and colour deficit. The greater the reduction of visual acuity, and the larger and more dense the central scotoma the greater the magnitude of the RAPD. This relationship also applied during recovery; as the visual acuity improved to normal the RAPD became smaller. However, in 13 of 22 patients with acute unilateral optic neuritis, a persistent RAPD, evident clinically as well as on pupillography, remained as the only residual clinical evidence of the previous optic neuritis. A persistent RAPD has also been reported by Cox, Thompson and Corbett (1981). In another study of optic neuritis the size

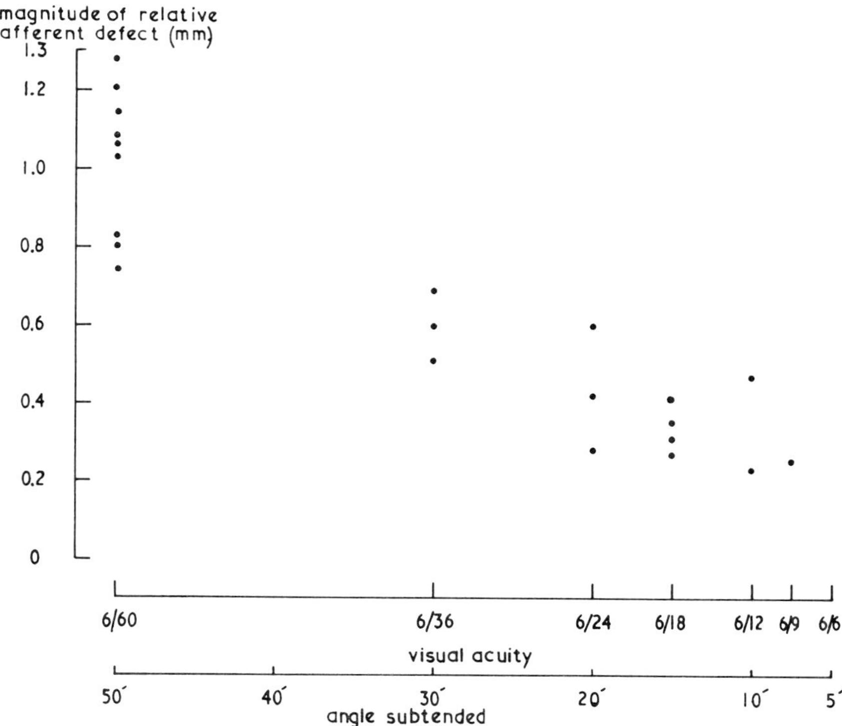

Fig. 22.7 Magnitude of the relative afferent pupillary defect related to visual acuity at presentation. The more impaired visual acuity the greater the RAPD associated with it.

and density of the field defect was found to be the most important factor relating to the presence of an RAPD (Thompson, Corbett and Cox, 1981). Small central field defects due to optic nerve disease correlate with large RAPD and marked impairment of visual acuity. Peripheral field loss has to be extensive to produce equivalent pupillary abnormality (Thompson *et al.*, 1982). It is evident from other studies that where visual acuity is assessed by contrast sensitivity (Galvin, Regan and Heron, 1976) persistent defects are seen in an apparently resolved case of optic neuritis. The pupillary abnormality may thus not be the only residual physical sign after an episode of optic neuritis but seems to be the most sensitive on clinical assessment. Indeed where a patient with a previous episode of unilateral optic neuritis has no relative afferent pupillary defect in that eye this should raise the possibility of subsequent involvement of the other eye thereby reducing the asymmetrical involvement of the optic nerves necessary for an RAPD to be evident (Cox, Thompson and Corbett, 1981).

Pupillary abnormality in optic neuritis has also been correlated with abnormalities of the visual evoked potential (VEP) to pattern reversal. There are three studies attempting to relate RAPD to the VEP in patients with optic neuritis. Bynke, Rosen and Sandberg-Wollheim (1980) studied pupillary reactions by the swinging light test but did not quantitate the RAPD. The principal VEP data related to the finding of a tendency of VEP latency to revert to normal during follow-up in a group of patients studied for a mean of five years after the clinical episode of visual loss. This group of cases had a less severe visual deficit at onset, but there was no correlation of latency with ultimate visual acuity. Patients whose VEP returned to normal generally had fewer remaining ocular signs. VEP amplitude was reduced in the acute phase and returned towards normal more quickly than VEP latency but 'there was a general tendency of the amplitude to return to a somewhat lower level than for the clinically healthy eye'.

In the study by Kirkham and Coupland (1981) of patients with optic neuritis, pupillary abnormality was assessed by pupil cycle time and the swinging light test. The pupil cycle time is a technique which measures the frequency of pupillary oscillations set up by a horizontal beam of light just grazing the lower margin of the pupil (Miller and Thompson, 1978). This study showed that in optic neuritis delay in VEP latency was likely to be associated with a relative afferent pupillary defect and delayed pupil cycle time. VEP amplitude was not included in this study.

Only in one study (Ellis, 1979) have VEP latency and amplitude been correlated with the magnitude of a relative afferent pupillary defect. In this study the magnitude of the RAPD correlated with reduction in VEP amplitude from the symptomatically affected eye in comparison with the unaffected eye (Fig. 22.8). The greater the magnitude of the RAPD the more reduced was the VEP amplitude in that eye relative to the amplitude from the other eye. This relationship also persisted during follow-up in 22 cases of acute optic neuritis. As the relative afferent pupillary defect lessened along with improvement in other aspects of visual deficit, the VEP amplitude in that eye progressively increased. Of the 22 cases 13 remained unilateral during the period of follow-up (mean length of follow-up five months) and in these 13 patients the magnitude of the relative afferent pupillary defect was associated with persistent reduction of VEP amplitude relative to the symptomatically unaffected eye. In some patients the relative afferent pupillary defect was the only clinically evident abnormality and the sensitivity and objectivity of pupillary assessment after optic neuritis was thereby demonstrated. However,

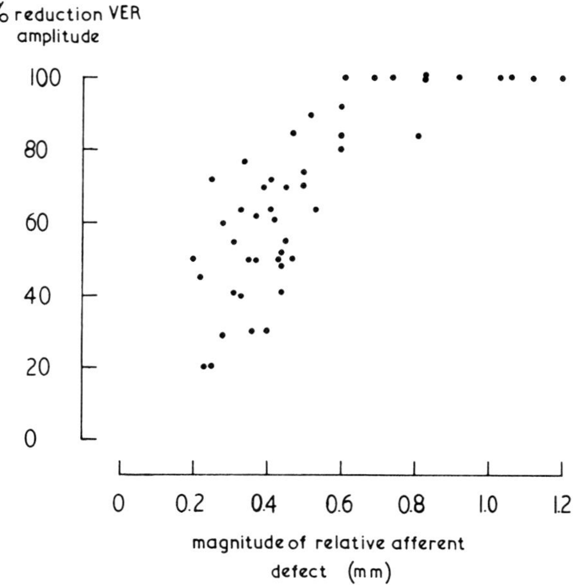

Fig. 22.8 The magnitude of the RAPD related to percentage reduction of VER amplitude. This is the proportional reduction of the VER amplitude in the affected eye when compared to VER amplitude from the unaffected eye. This shows that the larger the RAPD the greater the reduction in VER amplitude. 100% reduction implies abolition of the pattern evoked response.

nine of the 22 cases developed involvement of the other eye during follow-up and in these cases the relative afferent pupillary defect was either reduced, abolished or reversed to the other eye according to the severity of involvement of the initially unaffected eye. These findings stress the relative nature of the swinging light test in which the two eyes are compared and the more severely affected eye shown to be abnormal. There was no correlation in this study between VEP latency and the severity of the initial visual impairment or the presence or persistence of the relative afferent pupillary defect. In no case did the VEP latency show any significant reduction; indeed during the follow-up period an unchanging VEP latency from the symptomatically unaffected eye was taken as an indication of the reliability of this eye as a control for VEP amplitude and pupillary assessment during follow-up. Figure 22.9 provides an example of one patient from this study who developed a left optic neuritis with severe impairment of visual acuity and in whom a persistent relative afferent pupillary defect was associated with persistent reduction of the VEP amplitude from the affected eye.

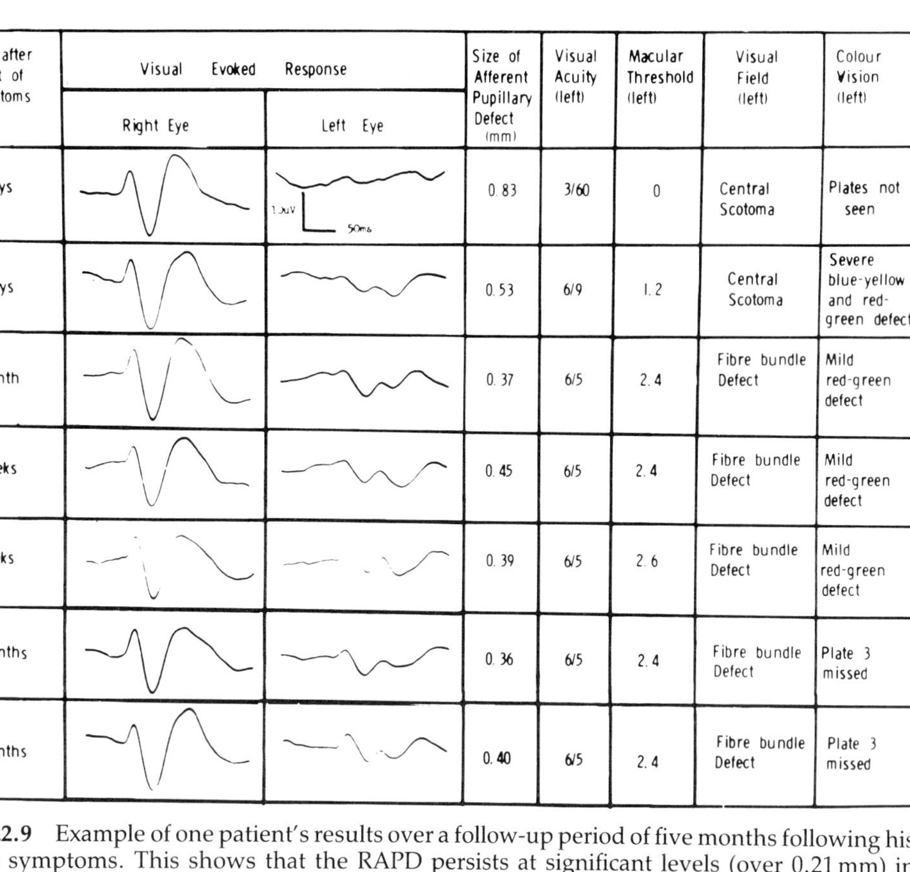

Time after onset of symptoms	Visual Evoked Response		Size of Afferent Pupillary Defect (mm)	Visual Acuity (left)	Macular Threshold (left)	Visual Field (left)	Colour Vision (left)
	Right Eye	Left Eye					
8 days		1.0µV 50ms	0.83	3/60	0	Central Scotoma	Plates not seen
16 days			0.53	6/9	1.2	Central Scotoma	Severe blue-yellow and red-green defect
1 month			0.37	6/5	2.4	Fibre bundle Defect	Mild red-green defect
6 weeks			0.45	6/5	2.4	Fibre bundle Defect	Mild red-green defect
9 weeks			0.39	6/5	2.6	Fibre bundle Defect	Mild red-green defect
3 months			0.36	6/5	2.4	Fibre bundle Defect	Plate 3 missed
5 months			0.40	6/5	2.4	Fibre bundle Defect	Plate 3 missed

Fig. 22.9 Example of one patient's results over a follow-up period of five months following his acute symptoms. This shows that the RAPD persists at significant levels (over 0.21 mm) in association with persistent reduction of VEP amplitude.

22.5 Pathophysiology of the relative afferent pupillary defect

Halliday and McDonald (1977) have speculated that the increase in VEP amplitude seen with clinical recovery following optic neuritis is due to progressive reduction in the number of optic nerve fibres reversibly blocked by nerve swelling and oedema. If the VEP amplitude does provide some indication of the number of fibres synchronously discharged in response to a pattern reversal, then the relationship with a relative reduction in pupillary light reflex amplitude suggests that the magnitude of an RAPD depends upon the disparity between the number of fibres synchronously discharged in the two optic nerves. The more fibres that are blocked on the affected side the greater is this disparity and the larger is the RAPD. How does this possible pathophysiological explanation relate to the observation made earlier that an RAPD appears to be related to apparent reduction in stimulus intensity in the affected eye? A direct experimental approach investigating the physiological changes in demyelinated nerves was first adopted in the peripheral nervous system but doubts about the relevance of these findings to conduction in nerve fibres of the central nervous system stimulated work on central fibres. McDonald and Sears (1970) produced demyelination in the spinal cord of the cat by injecting small amounts of diphtheria toxin in the dorsolateral sulcus. This resulted in a lesion with many of the histological characteristics of the optic nerve plaques seen in human optic neuritis, in particular focal demyelination with preservation of axonal continuity. Following stimulation of these demyelinated axons three principal abnormalities in conduction were discovered which form the basis of present knowledge of the pathophysiology of demyelination in central nerve fibres. Across large plaques of demyelination conduction block was observed. Smaller areas of demyelination allowed conduction to continue but this occurred at a slower rate and was sensitive to external influences such as temperature (Rasminsky, 1973) and extracellular fluid composition (Becker, Michael and Davis, 1974). The fibres in which conduction continued in this slow fashion showed an inability to conduct trains of impulses at physiological frequencies due to increased refractory period of the nerve. These findings, although an indication of pathophysiology of demyelination, were not easy to apply to the clinical situation in optic neuritis as there was no means of assessment of optic nerve conduction in that condition. However, with the introduction of the visual evoked potential to pattern reversal (Halliday, McDonald and Mushin, 1972), a reproducible and sensitive means of detecting such abnormalities was available.

It is interesting to speculate on whether the abnormalities described by

McDonald and Sears (1970) might be relevant in understanding the RAPD. Their observations that some fibres showed an inability to conduct trains of impulses may relate to the apparent reduction of stimulus intensity in an affected eye. One of the neurophysiological consequences of an increase in stimulus light intensity in cats is an increase in the frequency of spike discharge of the retinal ganglion cells (Ikeda and Wright, 1972). Could the apparent reduction in stimulus intensity in the affected eye be the consequence of a train of impulses initiated by a high intensity stimulus becoming slowed in frequency across a plaque of demyelination thus resulting in a spike frequency equivalent to a low intensity stimulus? McDonald (1974) has suggested that the desynchronizing effect of such a conduction disturbance may be the explanation of abnormalities in vibration sense seen in multiple sclerosis. Of the three principal abnormalities in conduction described by McDonald and Sears (1970) it is probable that conduction block is the most important factor in the production of an RAPD, but it is possible that impaired transmission of trains of impulses may also contribute, as discussed previously. Delay in latency does not seem to relate directly to the production of an afferent defect. This was also the conclusion of Halliday and McDonald (1977) in relation to symptoms in optic neuritis and it is clear from the latency studies in patients with RAPDs in optic neuritis that there is no correlation between prolongation of latency and the magnitude of an RAPD.

The observations by Clarke and Ikeda (1985) may also relate to this. They found that discharge spike frequency in luminance-sensitive pretectal neurones in the rat increased with increasing stimulus intensity, thus supporting the possibility that the basic abnormality resulting in an RAPD is an asymmetry between the two eyes of the discharge spike frequency in the pretectal nucleus. Such a conclusion has to be speculative as comparisons between results from various animal studies and even between VEP and pupillary information in man may be unjustified; the pupil response is elicited by changes in luminance, the VEP by changes in contrast. The fibres that conduct the VEP to pattern reversal and pupillary afferent fibres may not be the same. VEP amplitude has been found by many workers to be a relatively inconsistent variable, but there is, as described, some evidence, direct or indirect, to support the hypothesis proposed.

Future research may be directed towards a more accurate identification of the anatomy of the afferent pupillary pathway. If the pupillary afferent fibres are indeed smaller and slower conducting fibres than the visual fibres, there is the potential for differential involvement in a variety of neurological conditions and such differences might be of diagnostic importance.

References

Alpern, M., McCready, D.W. and Barr, L. (1963) The dependence of the photopupil response on flash duration and intensity. *J. Gen. Physiol.*, **47**, 265–78.

Becker, F.U., Michael, J.H. and Davis, F.A. (1974) Acute effects of oral phosphate on visual function in Multiple Sclerosis. *Neurology*, **24**, 601–7.

Bell, R.A. and Thompson, H.S. (1978) Relative afferent pupillary defects in optic tract hemianopia. *Am. J. Ophthalmol.*, **85**, 538–40.

Bovino, J.A. and Burton, T.C. (1980) Measurement of the relative afferent pupillary defect in retinal detachment. *Am. J. Ophthalmol.*, **90**, 19–21.

Bynke, H., Rosen, I. and Sandberg-Wollheim, P. (1980) Correlation of VEP, ophthalmological and neurological findings after unilateral optic neuritis. *Acta Ophthalmol.*, **58**, 673–87.

Clarke, R.J. and Ikeda, H. (1985) Luminance and darkness detectors in the olivary and posterior pretectal nuclei and their relationship to the pupillary light reflex in the rat. *Exp. Brain Res.*, **57**, 224–32.

Cleland, B.G. and Levick, W.R. (1974) Brick and sluggish concentrically organised ganglion cells in the cat's retina. *J. Physiol.*, **240**, 421–56.

Cox, T.A., Thompson, H.S. and Corbett, J.J. (1981) Relative afferent pupillary defects in optic neuritis. *Am. J. Ophthalmol.*, **92**, 685–90.

Ellis, C.J.K. (1979) The afferent pupillary defect in acute optic neuritis. *J. Neurol. Neurosurg. Psychiat.*, **42**, 1008–17.

Ellis, C.J.K. (1981) The pupillary light reflex in normal subjects. *Br. J. Ophthalmol.*, **65**, 754–9.

Ellis, C.J.K. (1984) Afferent pupillary defect in pineal region tumour. *J. Neurol. Neurosurg. Psychiat.*, **47**, 739–41.

Fukada, Y. and Stone, J. (1974) Retinal distribution and central projections of Y, X and W cells of the Cat's retina. *J. Neurophysiol.*, **37**, 749–72.

Galvin, R.J., Regan, D. and Heron, J.R. (1976) Impaired temporal resolution of vision after acute retrobulbar neuritis. *Brain*, **99**, 255–68.

Halliday, A.M. and McDonald, W.I. (1977) Pathophysiology of demyelinating disease. *Br. Med. Bull.*, **33**, 21–7.

Halliday, A.M., McDonald, W.I. and Mushin, J. (1972) Delayed visual evoked responses in optic neuritis. *Lancet*, **ii**, 982–5.

Hultborn, H., Mori, K. and Tsukahara, N. (1978) The neuronal pathway subserving the pupillary light reflex. *Brain Res.*, **159**, 255–67.

Ikeda, H. (1979) The physiological basis of amblyopia, in *Trends in Neurosciences*. Special Vision Issue, August, 209–12.

Ikeda, H. and Wright, M.J. (1972) Receptive field organisation of sustained and transient retinal ganglion cells which subserve different functional roles. *J. Physiol.*, **277**, 769–800.

Kirkham, T.H. and Coupland, S.G. (1981) Multiple regression analysis of diagnostic predictors in optic nerve disease. *Canad. J. Neurol. Sci.*, **8**, 67–72.

Kupfer, C., Chumbley, L. and Downer, J. (1967) Quantitative histology of optic nerve, optic tract and lateral geniculate nucleus of man. *J. Anat.*, **101**, 393.

Levatin, P. (1959) Pupillary escape in disease of the retina or optic nerve. *Arch. Ophthalmol.*, **62**, 768.

Loewenfeld, I.E. (1966) Pupillary movements associated with light and near vision. An experimental review of the literature. *Natl Acad. Sci.* N.R.C. Publication, **1272**, 17–105.

Lowenstein, O. and Friedman, E.D. (1942) Pupillographic studies. *Arch. Ophthalmol.*, **27**, 969–93.

Lowenstein, O. and Loewenfeld, I. (1958) Electronic pupillography. *Arch. Ophthalmol.*, **59**, 352–63.

Lowenstein, O. and Loewenfeld, I.E. (1969) The Pupil, in *The Eye, Muscular Mechanisms* (ed. H. Davson), Academic Press, London, pp. 255–337.

Lynn, B.H. (1959) Retrobulbar neuritis. *Trans. Ophthalmol. Soc. UK*, **79**, 701.

McDonald, W.I. (1974) Pathophysiology in multiple sclerosis. *Brain*, **97**, 179–96.

McDonald, W.I. and Sears, T.A. (1970) The effects of experimental demyelination on conduction in the central nervous system. *Brain*, **93**, 583–98.

Miller, S.D. and Thompson, H.S. (1978) Pupil cycle time in optic neuritis. *Am. J. Ophthalmol.*, **85**, 635–42.

Newsome, D.A., Milton, R.C. and Gass, J.D.M. (1981) Afferent pupillary deficit in macular degeneration. *Am. J. Ophthalmol.*, **92**, 396–402.

Nikoskelainen, E. (1975) Symptoms, signs and early course of optic neuritis. *Acta Ophthalmol.*, **53**, 254–72.

Perkin, G.D. and Rose, F.C. (1979) *Optic Neuritis*. Oxford University Press, Oxford.

Ransom, S.W. and Magoun, H.W. (1930) The central path of the pupilloconstrictor reflex in response to light. *Arch. Neurol. Psychiat.*, **30**, 1193–204.

Rasminsky, M. (1973) The effects of temperature on conduction in demyelinated single nerve fibres. *Arch. Neurol.*, **28**, 287–92.

Stone, J. and Fukada, Y. (1974) Properties of the cat retinal ganglion cells: a comparison of W-cells with X- and Y-cells. *J. Neurophysiol.*, **37**, 722–48.

Thompson, H.S. (1966) Afferent pupillary defects. *Am. J. Ophthalmol.*, **62**, 860–73.

Thompson, H.S. (1976) Pupillary signs in the diagnosis of optic nerve disease. *Trans. Ophthalmol. Soc. UK*, **96**, 377–81.

Thompson, H.S., Corbett, J.J. and Cox, T.A. (1981) How to measure the relative afferent pupillary defect. *Surv. Ophthalmol.*, **26**, 39–42.

Thompson, H.S., Watzke, R.C. and Weinstein, J.J. (1980) Pupillary dysfunction in macular disease. *Trans. Am. Ophthalmol. Soc.*, **78**, 311–17.

Thompson, H.S., Montague, P., Cox, T.A. and Corbett, J.J. (1982) The relationship between visual acuity, pupillary defect and visual field loss. *Am. J. Ophthalmol.*, **93**, 681–8.

Van Buren, J.M. (1963) *The Retinal Ganglion Cell Layer*. Charles C. Thomas, Springfield, p. 130.

Wyatt, H.J. and Musselman, J.F. (1981) Pupillary light reflex in humans. *Vision Res.*, **21**, 513–25.

CHAPTER 23

Pharmacology of the pupil

STEPHEN E. SMITH AND SHIRLEY A. SMITH

23.1 Introduction

This chapter will describe how drugs can aid in the diagnosis and localization of lesions to the iris innervation. For example, drug tests can be used in conjunction with clinical and physiological signs to identify the cause of a small pupil as sympathetic neuropathy and to determine whether the damage is pre- or postganglionic. One of the important principles utilized in such tests is that of denervation supersensitivity.

23.2 Iris pharmacology and the law of denervation supersensitivity

The human iris is composed of two smooth muscles, the sphincter and dilator pupillae. The sphincter is activated during the light and the near reflex to constrict the pupil by activation of its parasympathetic innervation. This releases acetylcholine which activates muscarinic cholinoceptors on the smooth muscle cells. Pharmacological evidence has shown these to be identical to the muscarinic receptors found elsewhere in the body of mammals, e.g. the gastrointestinal tract and the salivary glands (Smith, 1976; Kaumann and Hennekes, 1979). The dilator is activated during stress and in response to darkness to dilate the pupil by activation of its sympathetic innervation. This releases noradrenaline which stimulates alpha-adrenoceptors (Sneddon and Turner, 1969; Matheney, Carrier and Ahlquist, 1977) on the smooth muscle cells. There is evidence from experiments with irides isolated from mammalian species, including man, that each muscle of the iris receives a reciprocal innervation in addition. Thus the sphincter has beta-adrenoceptors which relax the muscle to aid sympathetically mediated pupillary dilatation (Kern, 1971) and the dilator has muscarinic receptors which relax the muscle during parasympathetically mediated pupillary constriction (Schaeppi, Rubin and Koella, 1966). The importance of these sphincter adrenoceptors and dilator cholinoceptors in human iris physiology remains to be established.

Canon and Rosenblueth (1949) formulated the law of denervation supersensitivity which describes how an organ, deprived of its normal innervation, becomes more sensitive to the chemical transmitter normally released from those nerves. This 'up-regulation', an attempt by the organ to overcome the effects of the denervation, is thought to be mediated by an increase in the number and activity of the special receptors on the end-organ which are activated by the transmitter during neurotransmission. This is a general principle applying to denervated voluntary muscle, smooth muscle and glands. It occurs not only with complete lesions to the directly connected nerve, but also to a lesser degree with partial lesions, lesions to more proximal nerves in the pathway and even with functional deficits. It is now understood to be one end of a regulatory spectrum, the other end of which is the decreased sensitivity or 'down-regulation' that occurs when an organ receives excessive excitation as, for example, during chronic drug treatment with high doses of receptor stimulant drugs such as pilocarpine. It has been shown that acute and chronic treatment with such cholinomimetic miotics in man causes a reduction in sensitivity to subsequent receptor stimulation (Smith and Smith, 1980). Thus the initial application of aceclidine, pilocarpine and eserine eye-drops in high doses has a bigger pupillary constricting effect than subsequent applications given within 48 hours.

23.3 Parasympathetic tests

These tests were originally developed to aid in the diagnosis of Adie's tonic pupils. A patient presenting with one large pupil of recent onset with accompanying accommodative paresis but in otherwise good health is likely to have an Adie's pupil. Clinical signs which aid the diagnosis are loss of deep tendon reflexes, slow small pupillary reflexes to light and near, and segmental sphincter palsy. Drug tests confirm it by establishing that the large pupil is due to neuropathic damage and not local iris damage. Application of a drug which mimics the transmitter acetylcholine will cause a supersensitive miosis in the affected eye in Adie's pupil due to the denervation caused by damage to the ciliary ganglion or short ciliary nerves. On the other hand, a large pupil associated with myopathic trauma will have no response to such a drug.

Originally methacholine 2.5%, a chemical derivative of acetylcholine, was used in these tests. This has been replaced by pilocarpine, an alkaloid which has much better corneal penetration than methacholine. Thompson (1977) recommends pilocarpine 0.125% which usually gives a small constriction to a healthy pupil and a larger constriction to an Adie's pupil. In unilateral cases, 80% of affected pupils constricted 0.2 mm more than the fellow eyes, measured 30 minutes after instillation of the drops.

Although less common, Adie's syndrome can present with both pupils affected in which case diagnostic drug tests are less sensitive without the patient's own healthy pupil to use for comparison. The response of the pupil to drugs is very variable between subjects, due to differences in corneal penetration, age, starting diameter and iris colour. These sources of variation are eliminated when comparing responses in both pupils of a subject. In bilateral cases, reference to a normal range is needed, which describes the average miosis obtained in a large number of healthy eyes with the sources of variation quantified as far as possible. Thompson's data from 25 unaffected eyes of unilateral cases can be used to construct a normal range. Analysis of his data shows that the average response of a normal pupil in the light to 0.125% pilocarpine is 0.84 mm, but the response is strongly dependent on how big the pupil is initially (Fig. 23.1). Thus the normal response for a 3 mm pupil is 0.33 mm but for a

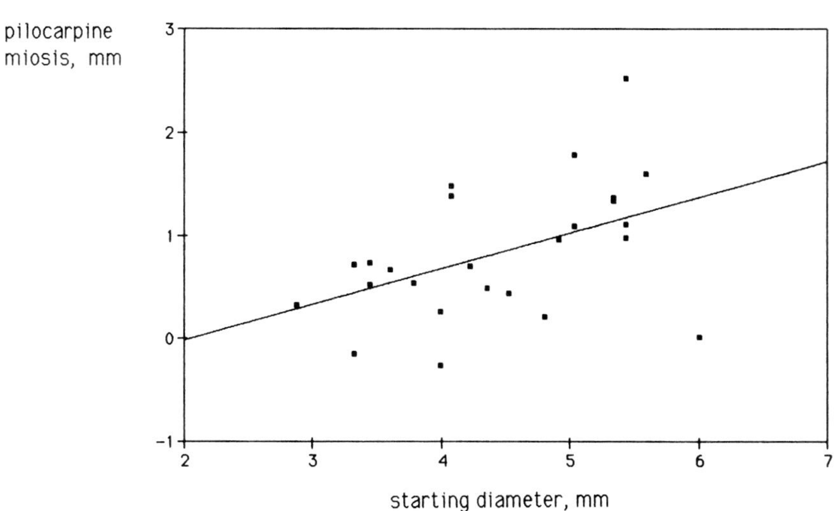

Fig. 23.1 Pilocarpine miosis increases with increasing starting pupil diameter. (Based on data in Thompson, 1977.)

6 mm pupil it is 1.37 mm. Since pupil size decreases with age, it follows that pilocarpine sensitivity declines with increasing age. More work is needed to define the normal range for this diagnostic drug test.

Many cases of Adie's pupils are investigated in the clinic some time after the initial onset of symptoms when the affected pupil is in fact smaller than the normal one. Adie's pupils only remain larger than the fellow one for about 2–6 months, after which aberrant regeneration of fibres subserving accommodation grow to innervate the affected sections of the sphincter pupillae (Thompson, 1977). The neuronal drive associated with ciliary muscle function then constricts the pupil via its aberrant nerves to give a small pupil. The Adie's pupil remains supersensitive compared with its fellow eye until the small starting diameter limits the pilocarpine miosis.

23.4 Sympathetic tests

Due to the re-uptake system for noradrenaline in the postganglionic sympathetic neurone, drug tests are more varied and useful in sympathetic dysfunction. Normally, when noradrenaline has been released from the nerve to act on the muscle its action is terminated by being taken up again into the nerve endings, unlike in parasympathetic neurotransmission when the action of acetylcholine is terminated by enzymatic destruction. Other amines can be taken into the nerve in this way or can block the uptake system, giving drugs which mimic sympathetic excitation. For example, hydroxyamphetamine dilates the pupil indirectly by getting into the nerve and displacing noradrenaline from its storage sites. Thus in postganglionic lesions it will have no effect, since there will be no noradrenaline for it to release and the agent itself has no direct agonist action on receptors. If the lesion is preganglionic or central in origin, hydroxyamphetamine will dilate the pupil, often by more than normal since decentralized nerves have increased stores of transmitter (Brown, Dearnaley and Geffen, 1967). This agent is therefore valuable in locating the site of the damage in the sympathetic pathway.

Cocaine is a drug which dilates the pupil by blocking the noradrenaline re-uptake process, so that the transmitter builds up in the neuromuscular junction and activates the adrenoceptors. Thus neuropathy anywhere in the sympathetic pathway will reduce or abolish the dilatory effect of cocaine. A supersensitive mydriasis to phenylephrine, a directly acting adrenoceptor stimulant, will also indicate that a lesion exists but does so by looking for an increased response, as opposed to a decreased response with cocaine. This combination allows one to exclude various non-specific causes for an increased phenylephrine effect such as increased corneal penetration due to corneal pathology.

The phenylephrine test, the sympathetic equivalent of the pilocarpine test in parasympathetic lesions, is positive in central, preganglionic and postganglionic damage in the sympathetic pathway. A patient with a central lesion may have had a medullary infarction or have cervical cord disease. Preganglionic lesions can arise when a lung or breast malignancy has spread to the thoracic outlet, or in connection with neck or chest surgery or trauma. Causes of postganglionic lesions include ipsilateral vascular headache syndromes, intraoral or retroparotid trauma, internal carotid artery pathology and tumours of the medial cranial fossa or the cavernous sinus.

As with the pilocarpine test, unilateral Horner's pupil is best investigated for supersensitivity by comparison with the fellow eye. In bilateral cases, reference can be made to the age-related normal range shown in Fig. 23.2. This range was constructed from measurements in 55 healthy individuals, one hour after instillation of 2 drops of 2% phenylephrine in a room with dim background light. Vertical pupil diameter was measured with television pupillometry, but a simple photographic method would suffice.

Regression analysis showed that mydriasis increases with advancing age and with decreasing starting pupil diameter in healthy subjects. However, the relationship with age is the important one, since the age-

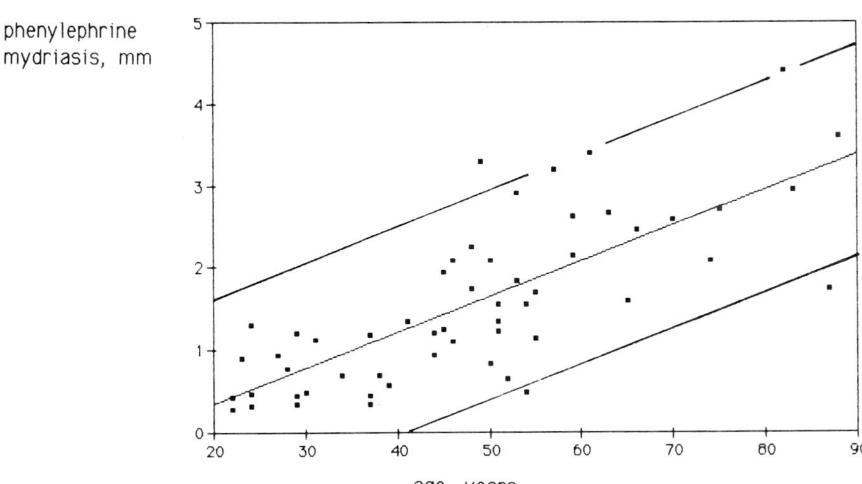

Fig. 23.2 Age-related normal range for 2% phenylephrine. The middle line shows the expected values for age and the outer ones show the upper and lower limits of normality.

dependent decrease in pupil size accounts for the effect of starting diameter. The effect of age is marked: the expected mydriasis for a 20-year-old is only 0.36 mm whereas for a 60-year-old it is 2.08 mm. The reason for the age effect is not known. One possibility is that age itself creates a supersensitive dilator due to an age-related decrease in sympathetic tone. In practical terms, it is pointless to use the phenylephrine diagnostic drug test without reference to an age-related normal range (Table 23.1).

Table 23.1 Age-related normal ranges for 2% phenylephrine and 0.5% hydroxy-amphetamine drug tests. Values are based on the 2.5 and 97.5 percentiles of the age regression (Smith and Smith, 1983)

Age range	*Mean*	*Phenylephrine mydriasis (mm)*			*Hydroxyamphetamine mydriasis (mm)*		
Years		*Lower*	*Expected*	*Upper*	*Lower*	*Expected*	*Upper*
16–25	20.5	–	0.36	1.6	0.45	1.64	2.8
26–35	30.5	–	0.79	2.0	0.6	1.77	2.9
36–45	40.5	–	1.22	2.4	0.7	1.9	3.0
46–55	50.5	0.4	1.65	2.85	0.8	2.03	3.1
56–65	60.5	0.8	2.08	3.3	0.9	2.16	3.2
66–75	70.5	1.25	2.51	3.7	1.05	2.29	3.3
76–85	80.5	1.65	2.94	4.1	1.15	2.42	3.45

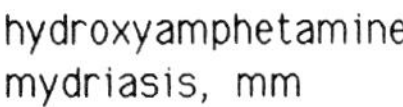

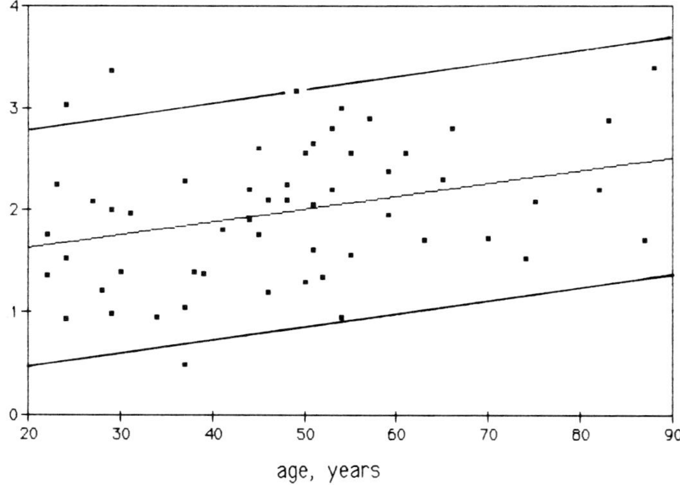

Fig. 23.3 Age-related normal range for 0.5% hydroxyamphetamine. The middle line shows the expected values for age and the outer ones show the upper and lower limits of normality.

Interestingly, the mydriasis to hydroxyamphetamine is far less dependent on age (Fig. 23.3 and Table 23.1). This appears to exclude a non-specific cause for the phenylephrine age dependency such as increased corneal penetration through an ageing cornea. If there is a decrease in sympathetic function with age it does not appear to be due to any gross peripheral dysfunction of the postganglionic nerves since they continue to release noradrenaline in response to hydroxyamphetamine. One can speculate that the postganglionic nerves are functionally decentralized with age, as this would explain the findings with the various sympathomimetic drugs.

A combination of the phenylephrine and hydroxyamphetamine tests, performed at least 2 days apart, can provide very useful information (Maloney, Younge and Moyer, 1980). For example, a patient presents with unilateral ptosis and miosis with few clues in the physical examination or history to indicate the cause except for a reference to occasional one-sided headaches. The phenylephrine test, and the cocaine test if desired, will confirm whether the ptosis and miosis are indeed due to sympathetic neuropathy. If the mydriasis to hydroxyamphetamine is reduced in the affected eye, compared to its fellow and the normal range shown in Table 23.1, it is good evidence that the site of the lesion is postganglionic and associated with the headache. If the response is normal or enhanced, the lesion is probably preganglionic and tests for malignancy should be considered.

23.5 Widespread neuropathies

Drug tests are used most in localized neuropathies affecting the ocular innervation but they can be useful in more generalized conditions such as diabetic neuropathy, familial dysautonomias, sarcoidosis, porphyria, alcoholic neuropathy and multiple system atrophy (Shy–Drager syndrome). In diabetic autonomic neuropathy the pupil fails to dilate adequately in darkness and the light reflexes may be slow and reduced in amplitude (Smith and Smith, 1983). While both branches of the autonomic nervous system are eventually affected, damage to the sympathetic pathway is more common and the dilator becomes supersensitive to phenylephrine. The response to hydroxyamphetamine is preserved, indicating that the postganglionic nerves are essentially operational.

The finding of sympathetic denervation supersensitivity in the diabetic patient with neuropathic and retinopathic complications has been utilized in an effective regimen for mydriasis for fundal inspection (Huber, Smith and Smith, 1985). Pupils of such patients are often difficult to dilate with conventional agents such as cyclopentolate or homatropine because there is inadequate sympathetic drive to activate the dilator despite the drug-induced sphincter paralysis. A combination of phenylephrine (10% or 2.5%) with 1% tropicamide is very effective because the supersensitive dilator reacts very well to phenylephrine allowing use of the weaker anticholinergic tropicamide. This has minimal post-clinic accommodative paralysis compared with the stronger cyclopentolate or homatropine.

23.6 Conclusions

Drug tests which utilize the law of denervation supersensitivity are useful aids in diagnosing neuropathies. There is a wider variety of drugs available for testing sympathetic compared with parasympathetic function due to the special uptake systems operating in the sympathetic nerve ending. These tests will be most effective when attention is paid to controlling the ambient lighting conditions, using the fellow eye as a control if possible, and using normal ranges which account for the variability in drug response due to such factors as age and starting pupil diameter. More work is needed to improve these normal ranges.

References

Brown, G.L. Dearnaley, D.P. and Geffen, L.B. (1967) Noradrenaline storage and release in the decentralised spleen. *Proc. R. Soc. Lond. B*, **168**, 48–56.

Canon, W.B. and Rosenblueth, A. (1949) *The Supersensitivity of Denervated Structures. A Law of Denervation*. Macmillan, New York.

Huber, M.J.E., Smith, S.A. and Smith S.E. (1985) Mydriatic drugs for diabetic patients. *Br. J. Ophthalmol.*, **69**, 425–7.

Kaumann, A.J. and Hennekes, R. (1979) The affinity of atropine for muscarine receptors in the human sphincter pupillae. *Naunyn Schmeidebergs. Arch. Pharmacol.*, **306**, 209–11.

Kern, R. (1971) The adrenergic receptors of the intraocular muscles in man. An in vitro study. *Exp. Eye Res.*, **11**, 145.

Maloney, W.F., Younge, B.R. and Moyer, N.J. (1980) Evaluation of the causes and accuracy of pharmacologic localization in Horner's syndrome. *Am. J. Ophthalmol.*, **90**, 394–402.

Matheney, J.L., Carrier, G.O. and Ahlquist, R.P. (1977) Roles of neuronal and extraneuronal uptake in responses of rabbit iris dilator muscle to levarterenol and phenylephrine. *J. Pharmaceut. Sci.*, **66**, 93–5.

Schaeppi, U., Rubin, R. and Koella, W.P. (1966) Electrical stimulation of the isolated cat iris. *Am. J. Physiol.*, **210**, 1165–9.

Smith, S.A. (1976) Factors determining the potency of mydriatic drugs in man. *Br. J. Clin. Pharmacol.*, **3**, 503–7.
Smith, S.A. and Smith, S.E. (1980) Subsensitivity to cholinoceptor stimulation of the human iris sphincter in situ following acute and chronic administration of cholinomimetic miotic drugs. *Br. J. Pharmacol.*, **69**, 513–18.
Smith, S.A. and Smith, S.E. (1983) Evidence for a neuropathic aetiology in the small pupil of diabetes mellitus. *Br. J. Ophthalmol.*, **67**, 89–93.
Sneddon, J.M. and Turner, P. (1969) The interaction of local guanethidine and sympathomimetic amines in the human eye. *Arch. Ophthalmol.*, **81**, 622–7.
Thompson, H.S. (1977) Adie's syndrome: some new observations. *Trans. Am. Ophthalmol. Soc.*, **75**, 587–626.

CHAPTER 24

Transsynaptic changes in the sympathetic and parasympathetic innervation of the pupil

JOEL M. WEINSTEIN, THOMAS J. ZWEIFEL
AND H. STANLEY THOMPSON

24.1 Transsynaptic changes in the oculosympathetic pathway

Over the past two decades pharmacological testing has become a valuable diagnostic adjunct in patients with abnormal pupils. In the sympathetic nervous system, cocaine has been useful in the confirmation of Horner's syndrome (Grimson and Thompson, 1975; Thompson, 1977; Thompson *et al.*, 1982) and hydroxyamphetamine has been useful in the localization of lesions within the oculosympathetic pathway (Thompson and Mensher, 1975; Maloney, Younge and Moyer, 1980). With a high degree of reliability, cocaine fails to dilate the pupil on the side of the oculosympathetic lesion in patients with Horner's syndrome (Grimson and Thompson, 1975; Thompson *et al.*, 1982). Hydroxyamphetamine, which releases endogenous norepinephrine from postganglionic sympathetic nerve endings, localizes the lesion by failing to dilate the pupil only when the oculosympathetic lesion affects the postganglionic neurone. In patients with central or preganglionic lesions, however, the pupil dilates normally to hydroxyamphetamine (Thompson and Mensher, 1975; Maloney, Younge and Moyer, 1980; Skarf and Czarnecki, 1982).

Recent observations, however, have suggested certain exceptions to this rule. Specifically, patients with congenital or early acquired Horner's syndrome often fail to dilate with hydroxyamphetamine, despite lesions that seem to originate in the preganglionic neurone (Weinstein, Zweifel and Thompson, 1980; Weinstein and Cutler, 1983). In addition, these patients often display marked supersensitivity to phenylephrine hydrochloride. This paradox can be explained by postulating an orthograde transsynaptic dysgenesis of the postganglionic neurone following preganglionic injury in early life. This hypothesis is consistent with observations of animals with preganglionic sympathectomy who undergo dramatic biochemical and anatomical changes in the postganglionic neurone after preganglionic injury (Black, Hendry and Iversen, 1972a,b; Black and Geen, 1973; Black, Joh and Reis, 1974; Black and Mytilineau, 1976; Black, Bloom and Hamill, 1976; Hamill, Bloom and Black, 1977). This response probably reflects normal mechanisms for neuronal plasticity, which is important in the development of the immature nervous system. In order to clarify these mechanisms in humans, we examined 13 patients with unilateral Horner's syndrome that was congenital or acquired within the first three years of life. In each case, an effort was made to clarify the pathogenesis and anatomic site of the lesion based on: (1) clinical history and examination, (2) pupillary pharmacology, and (3) pattern of facial anhidrosis.

24.1.1 METHODS

Obstetric and neonatal histories were obtained for all patients. Each patient had an ophthalmological examination as well as a neurological examination. Pupillary size was recorded using flash Polaroid photography. The presence of Horner's syndrome was confirmed with 5 or 10% cocaine or by pupillography. Pharmacological localization was performed with 1% hydroxyamphetamine hydrobromide and by 1% phenylephrine hydrochloride. Patients were classified as postganglionic if dilation of the normal eye was 1 mm or more greater than that of the affected eye. Patients were classified as postganglionic by the phenylephrine test if constriction of the affected eye was 2 mm or more greater than the normal eye. In all cases results of the two tests were in agreement.

Sweating was induced by exercise or heat lamp; if a response was not clinically detectable, quinizarin or starch-iodide powder was applied for more careful testing.

24.1.2 RESULTS

Results of the study are given in Table 24.1. It was possible to categorize patients into three groups based on clinical history, pupillary pharma-

Table 24.1 Clinical data of 13 patients with Horner's syndrome

Patient No.	*Obstetric and neonatal history*	*Age at initial exam*	*Results of neurological exam*	*Hypochromia*	*Hydroxy-amphetamine hydrobromide test*	*Phenylephrine hydrochloride supersensitivity*
Group I						
1	Prolonged ineffective labour, difficult forceps delivery	46 yr	Normal	Yes	Postganglionic	Yes
2	Rotation performed for fetal malposition; difficult delivery; head trauma; opisthotonus	22 mo	Normal	Yes	Postganglionic	Yes
3	Difficult delivery; high forceps	12 yr	Normal	Yes	Postganglionic*	Yes
4	32 wk gestation; weight, 2170 g; 4.5 min to deliver head; resuscitation required	16 mo	Normal	Yes	Postganglionic*	Yes
Group II						
5	Normal	13 mo	Normal	Yes	Postganglionic*	Yes
6	Normal (hyperbilirubinaemia)	18 mo	Normal	Yes	Postganglionic*	Yes
7	Normal	3 yr	Normal	Yes	Postganglionic	Yes
8	Normal	6 mo	Normal	Yes	Postganglionic	Yes
Group III						
9	Repair of tracheo-oesophageal fistula	13 mo	Normal	No	Preganglionic*	No
10	Surgery at age 12 mo on thoracic sympathetic chain for neuroblastoma	6 yr	Normal	Yes	Postganglionic*	Yes
11	C-8-T-1 ventral root injury (Klumpke's palsy)	3 yr	Weakness of muscles innervated, by C-8-T-1	No	Postganglionic*	Yes
12	Surgery age 3 for thoracic neuroblastoma	26 yr	Normal	Yes	Postganglionic	Yes
13	Thoracic surgery Blalock–Taussig shunt	5 wk	Normal	Yes	Postganglionic	Yes

* Partial postganglionic lesion.

cology, and sweating pattern. Patients 1 to 4 (Group I) had postganglionic pharmacology and normal sweating (or only a small patch of sweating deficit on the ipsilateral forehead), implicating a lesion of the postganglionic neurone distal to the superior cervival ganglion (a lesion of the superior cervical ganglion would have included complete hemifacial anhidrosis). All four patients had evidence of obstetric trauma to the neck (difficult forceps extraction, etc.), suggesting that the pathogenesis of the lesion may have been trauma to the internal carotid plexus. Four patients (Group II) had postganglionic pharmacology with complete hemifacial anhidrosis, placing the lesion at the superior cervical ganglion. None of these patients had notable birth trauma. Five patients (Group III) had well-documented surgical or obstetric injury to the preganglionic sympathetic pathway. Four of the five patients, however, had postganglionic pharmacology.

24.1.3 DISCUSSION

Comments on patient Groups I and II are presented elsewhere with further discussion of the pathogenesis of congenital Horner's syndrome in these patients (Weinstein, Zweifel and Thompson, 1980). We will turn our attention to Group III. As shown in Table 24.1, patients 9 to 13 had postganglionic pharmacology. They had both failure to dilate with hydroxyamphetamine and supersensitivity to phenylephrine, despite an initial injury of the preganglionic neurone. Patients 9 and 12 did not have complete hemifacial anhidrosis as might have been predicted from the preganglionic site of their lesions. This may reflect a limitation in our testing procedure related to inability to detect the small differences in sweating. Patients in Group III illustrate the variable response to injury of the immature sympathetic nervous system. An isolated preganglionic defect may persist, as in patient 13, or transsynaptic changes may take place, as in patients 9 to 12. These patients illustrate the phenomenon of transsynaptic impairment of the postganglionic neurone following neonatal preganglionic injury.

Two alternative explanations exist, which do not invoke transsynaptic phenomena, for the postganglionic pharmacology in our patients with preganglionic injury. First, it is possible that responses of these patients to hydroxyamphetamine and phenylephrine are consistent with preganglionic injury. This is clearly not the case, as demonstrated by the study of Thompson and Mensher (1975). Although Maloney, Younge and Moyer (1980) reported mydriatic failure to hydroxyamphetamine in a small minority of patients with preganglionic lesions, the authors failed to elaborate the clinical criteria by which the lesion was localized to a preganglionic site. Did some of these patients have congenital Horner's syndrome? Without further data, it is difficult to accept these patients as true exceptions to the rule. A second possibility is that some or all of the preganglionic neurones in these children synapsed at a site other than the superior cervival ganglion but we are unaware of evidence that this can occur, and indeed abundant evidence exists demonstrating absence of synapse of oculosympathetic neurones at other sites along the sympathetic chain.

In neonatal animals the presence of intact preganglionic sympathetic fibres is necessary for the normal structural and biochemical maturation of postganglionic neurones in the superior cervical ganglion and their axon terminals in the iris (Black, Hendry and Iversen, 1972a,b; Black and Mytilineau, 1976). This phenomenon of orthograde transsynaptic regulation of sympathetic nerve development has been extensively studied in an experimental model by Black and his associates (Black, Hendry and Iversen, 1972a,b; Black and Geen, 1973; Black, Joh and Reis, 1974; Black and Mytilineau, 1976; Black, Bloom and Hamill, 1976) and by Hamill, Bloom and Black (1977). Surgical transection of the preganglionic fibres in the neonatal rat or mouse results in: (1) impaired maturation of enzyme systems, e.g. tyrosine hydroxylase in postganglionic (superior cervical ganglion) cells and diminished supplies of catecholamines in their axon terminals in the iris (Black, Hendry and Iversen, 1972a; Black, Joh and Reis, 1974; Black and Mytilineau, 1976); (2) decreased density of innervation in the iris with decreased branching and ramification of surviving adrenergic neurones (Black and Mytilineau, 1976); and (3) a slightly decreased number of cells in the superior cervical ganglion primarily due to failure of pre-existing cells to replicate (Black, Hendry and Iversen, 1972a).

Some of our patients with congenital Horner's syndrome showed a partial response to hydroxyamphetamine, characterized by incomplete mydriasis (less than the normal pupil) and very slight improvement in ptosis. This partial response is not ordinarily seen in adults with postganglionic lesions but is predicted by the experimental model of transsynaptic dysgenesis. Even in neonatal animals with complete preganglionic lesions, some postganglionic axon terminals are present to respond to hydroxyamphetamine, though deafferented postganglionic fibres are diminished in number and relatively depleted of catecholamines. This results in a characteristic partial postganglionic response. In addition, these patients showed a definite supersensitivity to direct-acting adrenergic substances, which may be attributed to defective postganglionic innervation as well as to deafferentation.

The pattern of heterochromia in this series is noteworthy. Hypochromia of the iris developed in all but two patients. Patient 11 had very light blue irides, so iris hypochromia would not have been clinically evident. In patient 9, who had preganglionic injury and did not develop postganglionic changes, iris hypochromia on the affected side did not develop. Although we can ascribe only limited importance to this observation in a single patient, it is interesting to speculate that the absence of hypochromia is in some way related to the preganglionic site of the patient's lesion, as opposed to the postganglionic (transsynaptic) involvement in all the other patients.

Since cells in the sympathetic ganglia and iris melanocytes are both neural crest derivatives and share many biochemical similarities (Lerner, 1971), it is appropriate to ask whether melanocytes are innervated. In fact, both biochemical and electron microscopic studies support the concept of neural regulation of ocular melanocytes (Laties, 1978; Laties and Lerner, 1978). Given the biochemical and embryological similarities between melanocytes and ganglion cells, both of which are neural crest derivatives, it is conceivable that both are subject to transsynaptic influence during development. Failure of iris melanocyte development in congenital Horner's syndrome may be analogous to the transsynaptic changes that take place in the superior cervical ganglion following lesions of the preganglionic neurone. Lesions of the postganglionic pathway (either primary or secondary to transsynaptic changes) lead to neurotropic dysgenesis of iris melanocytes. Lesions limited to the preganglionic pathway, as in patient 9, spare the innervation of the melanocyte, leaving the melanocyte third neurone relationship intact, so that hypochromia does not develop.

24.2 Transsynaptic changes and denervation supersensitivity in the parasympathetic pathway to the pupillary sphincter

Although denervation supersensitivity apparently occurs after preganglionic lesions, it is unclear whether this phenomenon reflects transsynaptic changes in the postganglionic neurone or whether it merely represents a regulatory phenomenon at the motor end plate related to a lower frequency of stimulation. Since topical agents that release acetylcholine from postganglionic neurones (analogues to hydroxyamphetamine) are not available in the parasympathetic system to resolve this issue, the question of transsynaptic changes must be discussed in the context of studies of denervation supersensitivity after preganglionic lesions.

The evidence for transsynaptic influences on the parasympathetic innervation of the pupil has accumulated over the last decade. The earliest experimental studies related to denervation supersensitivity of the pupil were those of Anderson (1905a,b), who found denervation supersensitivity to dilute cholinergics after preganglionic denervation in the cat. These conclusions were apparently ignored after the studies of Adler and Scheie (1940), who concluded from experimental studies in the cat that cholinergic supersensitivity occurred with postganglionic, but not with preganglionic, lesions. These authors do not describe their experimental procedure in detail, however, and the site of their 'preganglionic' and 'postganglionic' lesions is unclear (Adler and Scheie, 1940). Subsequent studies have firmly established the existence of denervation supersensitivity after decentralization in the parasympathetic innervation of other organs. It would be surprising if the pupil was an exception to this rule. The work of de Haas (1960), for example, demonstrated that denervation supersensitivity occurs with either pre- or postganglionic parasympathetic lesions, for the lacrimal gland. The confusing history of the experimental literature (prior to 1982) related to the pupil is discussed at length by Ponsford, Bannister and Paul (1982).

Prior experimental studies must now be viewed in light of recent evidence suggesting a direct parasympathetic pathway to the eye, at least in the rabbit (Parelman, Fay and Burde, 1984). If such a pathway exists and provides partial innervation to the pupillary sphincter, supersensitivity resulting from third nerve palsy may not represent a transsynaptic phenomenon related to decentralization but rather the more common type of denervation supersensitivity. The concept of direct innervation of the intrinsic ocular muscles had been supported by earlier studies by Westheimer and Blair (1973), who nicotinized the ciliary ganglion and found intact accommodation but not pupillary constriction after stimulation of the third nerve. This concept has been vigorously contested by Loewenfeld (1973).

Long-standing ideas about cholinergic supersensitivity of pre- and postganglionic pupillary lesions were questioned by Mindel (1981), who applied topical echothiophate to both eyes of seven patients who had unilateral third nerve paralysis or paresis. Miosis was greater in the affected eye in three subjects, greater in the normal eye in two subjects, and equal in two subjects. The author interprets his results conservatively and suggests three possible interpretations for the increased miosis in some patients: (1) denervation supersensitivity of the sphincter pupillae muscle; (2) concomitant paresis of the dilator pupillae muscle on the side of the third nerve palsy; and (3) increased drug penetration through the cornea of the paretic eye, due to corneal changes related to ptosis. There is good reason to suspect that cholinergic denervation was not the only factor involved in the three patients who showed increased miosis in the paretic eye. One of the three patients had a traumatic carotid-cavernous fistula, making involvement of the oculosympathetic pathway a reasonable possibility. Another patient who demonstrated greater miosis of the paretic eye had no corneal sensation making an increased drug penetration quite likely. The third patient who demonstrated increased miosis to echothiophate had a congenitally small anterior segment with a smaller cornea on the affected side. Once again it is not possible to be certain about penetration of drug through this abnormal cornea.

Ponsford, Bannister and Paul (1982) also found evidence of 'denervation supersensitivity' to methacholine in 14 patients with third nerve palsies associated with aneurysmal compression of the third nerve. Eleven patients had associated subarachnoid haemorrhage. Their criterion for denervation supersensitivity was constriction of ≥1.0 mm after methacholine. All 14 patients demonstrated supersensitivity in the affected eye, as did 13 out of 14 patients with Adie's tonic pupil but, for reasons that are not satisfactorily explained, the contralateral control eye also showed supersensitivity in seven out of 12 patients, despite the absence of clinical evidence of third nerve palsy. It seems likely that the authors' criterion of ≥1.0 mm of constriction after methacholine was far too sensitive and included false positive results in many normal eyes. In fact, 10 out of 58 (17%) of Ponsford's neurological patients with no evidence of third nerve palsy or pupillary abnormality demonstrated denervation supersensitivity by this criterion. Four out of 17 (24%) patients with subarachnoid haemorrhage alone and no evidence of third nerve involvement also showed supersensitivity. The authors attributed the apparent supersensitivity of the normal contralateral pupil in patients with third nerve palsy to transsynaptic changes in neuronal pathways connecting the two third nerves. Despite these confusing results, pupillary constriction in the eyes with third nerve palsy was significantly greater than in neurological controls or in patients with subarachnoid haemorrhage without third nerve palsy.

Further clinical pharmacological evidence for denervation supersensitivity after third nerve palsy has been found by J.N. Currie (Neuro-Ophthalmology Section, National Eye Institute, Bethesda, MD) and S. Lessell (Department of Ophthalmology, Harvard University) (unpublished data). They evaluated pupillary responses in 62 normals, 10 patients with third nerve palsy, and 17 patients with postganglionic lesions (7 Adie's, 10 others). The investigators employed solutions of 1/20% pilocarpine (except one patient who had 1/128%) and developed norms for pupillary response to topical drug administration, including (1) millimetres of constriction, (2) percentage change of diameter, and (3) intereye difference in constriction (expressed either as a percentage or in millimetres). Employing these criteria, the investigators found that *all* 10 eyes with third nerve palsy had changes in diameter (absolute denervation supersensitivity) as well as intereye difference (relative denervation supersensitivity) that were more than 2 SD greater than the mean. Moreover, the responses of the eyes with third nerve palsy were statistically indistinguishable from those of eyes with postganglionic lesions, suggesting a comparable degree of supersensitivity.

It appears from these clinical and experimental studies that denervation supersensitivity does occur after decentralization of the parasympathetic innervation of the iris sphincter. The magnitude of these changes, the pharmacological mechanisms involved, and the relative importance of changes at pre- and postsynaptic sites remain to be elucidated.

References

Adler, F.H. and Scheie, H.G. (1940) The site of disturbance in tonic pupils. *Trans. Am. Ophthalmol Soc.*, **38**, 183–92.

Anderson, H.K. (1905a) The paralysis of involuntary muscle: II. On paralysis of the sphincter of the pupil with special reference to paradoxical constriction and the functions of the ciliary ganglion. *Acta Neurol. Scand.*, **48**, 510–19.

Anderson, H.K. (1905b) The paralysis of involuntary muscle: III. On the action of pilocarpine, physostigmine and atropine upon the paralysed iris. *J. Physiol. (Lond.)*, **33**, 414–38.

Black, I.B. and Geen, S.C. (1973) Transsynaptic regulation of adrenergic neuron development: inhibition by ganglionic blockade. *Brain Res.*, **63**, 291–302.

Black, I.B. and Mytilineau, C. (1976) Transsynaptic regulation of development of end-organ innervation by sympathetic neurons. *Brain Res.*, **101**, 503–21.

Black, I.B., Bloom, E.M. and Hamill, R.W. (1976) Central regulation of sympathetic neuron development. *Proc. Natl Acad. Sci. USA*, **73**, 3575–8.

Black, I.B., Hendry, I.A. and Iversen, L.L. (1972a) Transsynaptic regulation of growth and development of adrenergic neurons in a mouse sympathetic ganglion. *Brain Res.*, **34**, 228–40.

Black, I.B., Hendry, I.A. and Iversen, L.L. (1972b) Effects of surgical decentralization and nerve growth factor on the maturation of adrenergic neurons in a mouse sympathetic ganglion. *J. Neurochem.*, **19**, 1367–77.

Black, I.B., Joh, T.H. and Reis, D.J. (1974) Accumulation of tyrosine hydroxylase molecules during growth and development of the SCG. *Brain Res.*, **75**, 133–44.

de Haas, E.B.H. (1960) Lacrimal gland response to parasympathicomimetics after parasympathetic denervation. *Arch. Ophthalmol.*, **64**, 34–43.

Grimson, B.S. and Thompson, H.S. (1975) Drug testing in Horner's syndrome, in *Neuro-Ophthalmology Symposium* (eds J.S. Glaser and J.L. Smith), vol. 8. C.V. Mosby, St Louis, pp. 265–70.

Hamill, R.W., Bloom, E.M. and Black, I.B. (1977) The effect of spinal cord transection on the development of cholinergic and adrenergic sympathetic neurons. *Brain Res.*, **134**, 269–78.

Laties, A.M. (1978) Ocular melanin and the adrenergic innervation to the eye. *Trans. Am. Ophthalmol. Soc.*, **72**, 560–604.

Laties, A.M. and Lerner, A.B. (1978) Iris color and relationship of tyrosinase activity to adrenergic innervation. *Nature*, **255**, 152–3.

Lerner, A.B. (1971) Neural control of pigment cells, in *Biology of Normal and Abnormal Melanocytes* (eds T. Kawamura, T.B. Fitzpatrick and M. Seyi). University Park Press, Baltimore, pp. 3–16.

Loewenfeld, I.E. (1973) Discussion of Westheimer, G. and Blair, S.M.: The parasympathetic pathways to the internal eye muscles, from *Invest. Ophthalmol.*, 1973, **12**, 193–7. *Surv. Ophthalmol.*, **18**, 242–8.

Maloney, W.F., Younge, B.R. and Moyer, N.J. (1980) Evaluation of the causes and accuracy of pharmacologic localization in Horner's syndrome. *Am. J. Ophthalmol.*, **90**, 394–402.

Mindel, J.S. (1981) Miosis from echothiophate in patients with total oculomotor nerve paralysis from intracranial abnormalities. *Am. J. Ophthalmol.*, **91**, 373–80.

Parelman, A.J., Fay, M.T. and Burde, R.M. (1984) Confirmatory evidence for a direct parasympathetic pathway to internal eye structures. *Trans. Am. Ophthalmol. Soc.*, **LXXXII**, 371–80.

Ponsford, J.R., Bannister, R. and Paul, E.A. (1982) Methacholine pupillary responses in third nerve palsy and Adie's syndrome. *Brain*, **105**, 583–97.

Skarf, B. and Czarnecki, J.S.C. (1982) Distinguishing postganglionic from preganglionic lesions: studies in rabbits with surgically produced Horner's syndrome. *Arch. Ophthalmol.*, **100**, 1319–22.

Thompson, B.M., Corbett, J.J., Kline, L.B. and Thompson, H.S. (1982) Pseudo-Horner's syndrome. *Arch. Neurol.*, **39**, 108–11.

Thompson, H.S. (1977) Diagnosing Horner's syndrome. *Trans. Am. Acad. Ophthalmol. Otolaryngol.*, **83**, 840–2.

Thompson, H.S. and Mensher, J.H. (1975) Hydroxyamphetamine test in Horner's syndrome. *Am. J. Ophthalmol.*, **79**, 523–6.

Weinstein, J.M. and Cutler, J.I. (1983) Observations on transsynaptic changes in acquired Horner's syndrome. *Am. J. Ophthalmol.*, **95**, 837–8.

Weinstein, J.M., Zweifel, T.J. and Thompson, H.S. (1980) Congenital Horner's syndrome. *Arch. Ophthalmol.*, **98**, 1074–8.

Westheimer, G. and Blair, S.M. (1973) The parasympathetic pathways to internal eye muscles. *Invest. Ophthalmol.*, **12**, 193–7.

Part IV

The Fundus and Optic Nerve

CHAPTER 25

Pathogenesis of optic disc oedema

SOHAN SINGH HAYREH

25.1 Introduction

Optic disc oedema is a common ophthalmoscopic finding and is seen in a variety of conditions, which include the following:

1. Raised intracranial pressure of any aetiology.
2. Lesions of the anterior part of the optic nerve, such as anterior ischaemic optic neuropathy, optic neuritis, drusen, optic disc vasculitis, granulomatous and other inflammatory lesions, and compression by a variety of retrobulbar orbital or optic nerve lesions.
3. Ocular lesions, which include central retinal vein occlusion, ocular hypotony, retinal vasculitis, uveitis and a number of other ocular inflammatory disorders.
4. Systemic diseases, including malignant arterial hypertension, and methanol or triethyl tin intoxication.

While optic disc oedema is seen in all these conditions, the question arises whether its pathogenesis is the same in them all. We have investigated the subject, experimentally (in rhesus monkeys) and clinically, in a number of conditions during the past 25 years (Hayreh, 1964, 1965, 1968, 1977a; Hayreh and Baines, 1972; Baumbach *et al.*, 1977, 1978; Hayreh and Hayreh, 1977a,b; Hayreh *et al.*, 1977, 1981; Tso and Hayreh, 1977a,b; Martin-Amat *et al.*, 1978; Hayreh and Chopdar, 1982; Kishi, Tso and Hayreh, 1985; Hayreh, Servais and Virdi, 1986). Table 25.1 lists the various conditions studied by us experimentally, and summarizes the materials and methods used in these studies.

Table 25.1 Materials and methods of the various experimental studies on pathogenesis of optic disc oedema, conducted by the author

Cause of optic disc oedema	*No. of monkeys (m)/eyes*	*Method used to produce optic disc oedema*	*Investigations performed*	*Reference*
Raised intracranial pressure (Fig. 25.1)	66 m	Intracranial balloon	SCFF, SFFA, LM, EM, axoplasmic flow, HRP	Hayreh, 1964, 1965, 1968, 1977a; Hayreh and Hayreh, 1977a,b; Tso and Hayreh, 1977a,b
Anterior ischaemic optic neuropathy (Fig. 25.2)	117 eyes	Post. ciliary artery occlusion	SCFF, SFFA, LM	Hayreh and Baines, 1972; Hayreh and Chopdar, 1982
Demyelinating optic neuritis (Fig. 25.3)	6 m	Allergic encephalomyelitis	SCFF, SFFA, LM, VEP, neurologic and ophthalmic examination	Hayreh *et al.* 1981
Malignant arterial hypertension (Fig. 25.4)	57 m	Goldblatt's procedure	SCFF, SFFA, LM, EM, HRP, blood pressure recording	Kishi, Tso and Hayreh, 1985; Hayreh, Servais and Virdi, 1986
Toxic optic neuropathy (Fig. 25.5)	10 m	Oral methyl alcohol/i.v. formate	SCFF, SFFA, LM, EM, HRP, biochemical evaluation	Baumbach *et al.*, 1977; Hayreh *et al.*, 1977; Martin-Amat *et al.*, 1978
Traumatic optic neuropathy (Fig. 25.6)	4 m	Burn on retrobulbar ONH	SCFF, SFFA, LM, EM, HRP	Baumbach *et al.*, 1978

Abbreviations: EM, electron microscopy; HRP, horseradish peroxidase; i.v. intravenous; LM, light microscopy; ONH, optic nerve head, Post., posterior; SCFF, stereoscopic colour fundus photography; SFFA, stereoscopic fluorescein fundus angiography; VEP, visual evoked potential.

Our experimental studies and other recently available evidence in the literature strongly suggest that, in most of these conditions, optic disc oedema is due to stasis of axoplasmic transport in the axons of the optic nerve head, although certainly there are conditions where this mechanism probably has no role to play, e.g. in central retinal vein occlusion and many of the inflammatory conditions. Axoplasmic flow stasis produces axonal swelling at the level of the optic disc and consequently swelling of the disc itself. The mechanism of axoplasmic flow stasis, however, varies, depending on the condition.

25.2 Role of axoplasmic flow in the pathogenesis of optic disc oedema

Weiss in 1944 described a continuous flow of axoplasm in axons. There are two types of axoplasmic transport: *anterograde* (from the cell body, along the axon, to its terminals) and *retrograde* (from the terminals of an axon, along the axon, to its cell body). In anterograde axoplasmic transport, the material is transported down the axon at different rates – at least two (fast and slow), probably more, each comprising different materials. Axoplasmic flow can be blocked by a variety of causes, including anoxia, ischaemia, cyanide poisoning, colchicine, methyl alcohol, local anaesthetics, compression, section of axon and temperature ≤11°C. I reviewed this subject some time ago (Hayreh, 1978a).

Based on our experimental studies, the following are the causes of axoplasmic flow stasis in the various conditions.

25.2.1 RAISED INTRACRANIAL PRESSURE

Our experimental studies (Hayreh, 1964, 1965, 1968, 1977a; Hayreh and Hayreh, 1977a,b; Tso and Hayreh, 1977a,b) on raised intracranial pressure associated with optic disc oedema (Fig. 25.1) provided definite proof that (a) there is axoplasmic flow stasis in the optic nerve head, involving both the fast and slow axoplasmic flows (Tso and Hayreh, 1977b); and (b) a rise in cerebrospinal fluid pressure in the sheath of the optic nerve is essential for the production of optic disc oedema. The proof of this fact is that when the sheath was decompressed (by cutting a window in the dura and arachnoid of the bulbous part of the sheath of the optic nerve), the optic disc oedema on that side resolved, in spite of the persistence of raised cerebrospinal fluid pressure intracranially in the majority of cases. This has since been confirmed amply in patients with optic disc oedema due to raised intracranial pressure (Davidson, 1969; Smith, Hoyt and Newton, 1969; Galbraith and Sullivan, 1973; Burde, Karp and Miller,

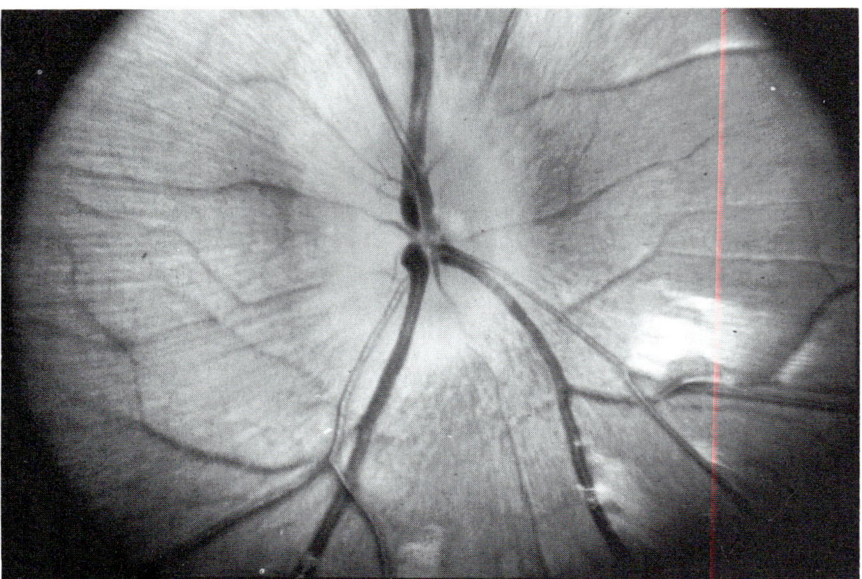

Fig. 25.1 Fundus photograph of a rhesus monkey, showing optic disc oedema with a progressively inflated intracranial balloon (situated in the right temporal lobe), 3 months after the introduction of the balloon. (Reproduced from Hayreh, 1968.)

1974; Billson and Hudson, 1975; Keltner *et al.*, 1977; Kaye, Galbraith and King, 1981; Kilpatrick *et al.*, 1981; Gutgold-Glen, Kattah and Chavis, 1984). The rise in the cerebrospinal fluid pressure in the sheath of the optic nerve is due to transmission of the raised intracranial cerebrospinal fluid pressure through the trabecular meshwork in the optic canal (Hayreh, 1984). This in turn produces axoplasmic flow stasis. How the raised cerebrospinal fluid pressure in the sheath of the optic nerve produces axoplasmic flow stasis is still not definitely known. Some studies have shown that a rise in the cerebrospinal fluid pressure in the sheath of the optic nerve causes a rise in the tissue pressure in the retrobulbar optic nerve (Ernest and Potts, 1968; Hedges and Zaren, 1973). I feel it is logical to attribute axoplasmic flow stasis in the optic nerve axons to the rise in the tissue pressure in the optic nerve (Hayreh, 1977a).

Thus, in optic disc oedema with raised intracranial pressure there is a stasis of the slow and fast components of the axoplasmic flow at the lamina cribrosa (Tso and Hayreh, 1977a,b). There is only mild interstitial oedema, and occasionally a small amount of extracellular fibrin in the vicinity of swollen axons. There is always a latency of 1–7 days between the raised intracranial pressure and development of optic disc oedema

(Hayreh and Hayreh, 1977a). This may be due to the fact that the bulk of the axoplasm moves as a part of the slow component and in optic disc oedema the block is mainly in the slow flow, so that it would take some time for the axoplasmic stasis to produce swelling of the axons.

25.2.2 ANTERIOR ISCHAEMIC OPTIC NEUROPATHY

This was produced experimentally in rhesus monkeys by occlusion of the posterior ciliary arteries, and the optic disc during the acute phase showed oedema (Fig. 25.2) and later on optic atrophy. We have also studied prospectively over 500 patients with anterior ischaemic optic neuropathy in our clinic.

As mentioned above, anoxia and ischaemia block axoplasmic flow. The optic nerve head is supplied essentially by the posterior ciliary arteries, mainly via the peripapillary choroid and to a much less extent by recurrent branches from the short posterior ciliary arteries (Hayreh, 1978b) (Fig. 25.7). Our experimental (Hayreh and Baines, 1972; Hayreh and Chopdar, 1982) and clinical (Hayreh, 1974a,b, 1975, 1980, 1981a,b; Hayreh and Zahoruk, 1981) studies have shown that anterior ischaemic

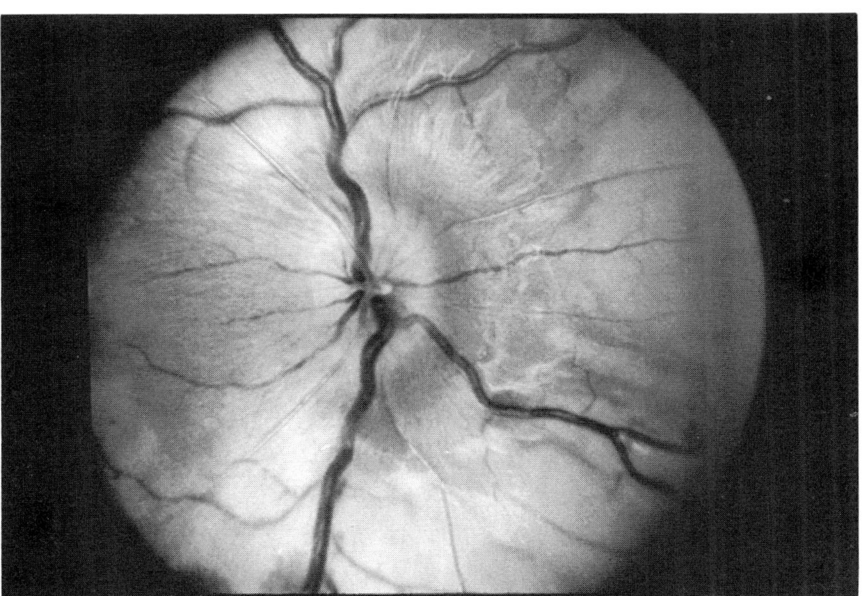

Fig. 25.2 Fundus photograph of a rhesus monkey, showing optic disc oedema one day after occlusion of the posterior ciliary arteries. Note also the presence of white outer retinal infarcts, which do not involve the peripapillary retina. (Reproduced from Hayreh and Chopdar, 1982.)

optic neuropathy is due to interference with the blood supply to the optic nerve head. Block of rapid and slow orthograde axoplasmic flow in the optic nerve head in this condition has been demonstrated (McLeod, Marshall and Kohner, 1980).

25.2.3 DEMYELINATING OPTIC NEURITIS

The demyelinating type of optic neuritis was produced by production of experimental allergic encephalomyelitis (Hayreh *et al.*, 1981). All eyes developed optic disc oedema (Fig. 25.3). Pathological studies in this type of optic neuritis show evidence of axoplasmic flow block (Rao, Tso and Zimmerman, 1977; Rao, 1981). On histopathology the optic nerve in this condition showed perivascular inflammatory cellular infiltration, and demyelination, and even loss of axons. Thus it would seem the

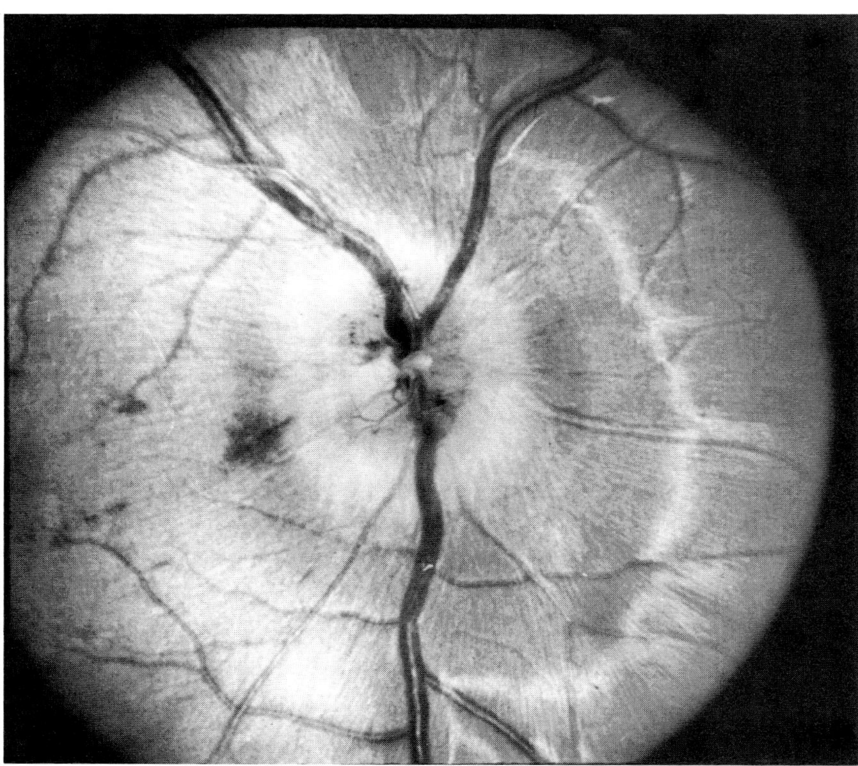

Fig. 25.3 Fundus photograph of a rhesus monkey, showing optic disc oedema with experimental allergic encephalomyelitis. (Reproduced from Hayreh *et al*, 1981.)

axoplasmic flow block in this condition is due to compression of the axons or their disruption, resulting in optic disc oedema.

25.2.4 MALIGNANT ARTERIAL HYPERTENSION

Clinical and pathological studies (Kishi, Tso and Hayreh, 1985; Hayreh, Servais and Virdi, 1986) on experimental renovascular malignant arterial hypertension have revealed that optic disc oedema (Fig. 25.4) in this condition is not due to raised intracranial pressure, nor a part of hypertensive encephalopathy or retinopathy, but to optic nerve head ischaemia. In our experimental studies, the clinical pattern of evolution of optic disc changes, i.e. optic disc oedema first and optic disc pallor about 2–3 months later (Hayreh, Servais and Virdi, 1986), is typical of that seen by us in over 500 patients with anterior ischaemic optic neuropathy followed prospectively in our clinic. Light and electron microscopic findings clearly demonstrated the ischaemic nature of the hypertensive optic neuropathy (Kishi, Tso and Hayreh, 1985). This was also suggested by electron microscopic studies by Garner *et al.* (1975). We postulated the following

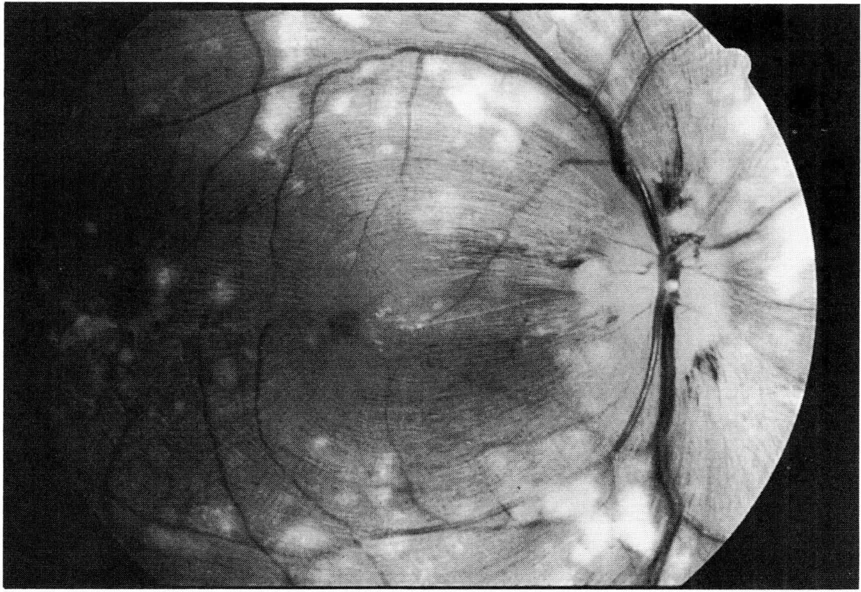

Fig. 25.4 Fundus photograph of a rhesus monkey, showing optic disc oedema and other hypertensive fundus changes with renovascular malignant arterial hypertension and systolic blood pressure of 190 mm Hg. (Reproduced from Hayreh, Servais and Virdi, 1986.)

mechanism as the cause of the optic nerve head ischaemia in these eyes (Hayreh, Servais and Virdi, 1986).

Renin–angiotensin–aldosterone plays an important role in the development and maintenance of renovascular malignant hypertension (Hayreh *et al.*, 1986). Angiotensin II (liberated by the action of renin on angiotensinogen) is the most powerful vasopressor substance known. Angiotensin leaks into the choroidal interstitial fluid from the leaky choriocapillaris and causes vasoconstriction of the choroidal vascular bed. Since peripapillary choroid is the main source of blood supply to the optic nerve head (Hayreh, 1978b), its vasoconstriction and occlusion would secondarily produce ischaemia of the optic nerve head. Also angiotensin from the choroidal interstitial fluid would diffuse into the optic nerve head through the Border Tissue of Elschnig and produce vasoconstriction by direct action on the capillaries and other vessels in the optic nerve head.

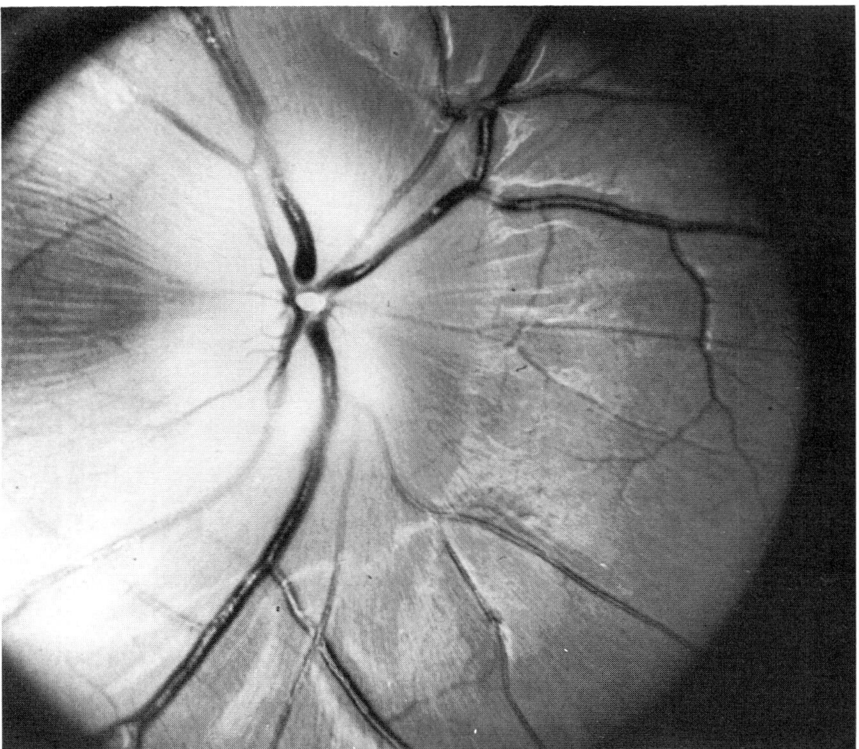

Fig. 25.5 Fundus photograph of a rhesus monkey, showing optic disc oedema but no other fundus lesion after methyl alcohol poisoning.

25.2.5 TOXIC OPTIC NEUROPATHY

In our studies of methyl alcohol toxic optic neuropathy, optic disc oedema (Fig. 25.5) was the only ophthalmoscopic finding during the acute poisoning (Hayreh *et al.*, 1977; Martin-Amat *et al.*, 1978), and electron microscopic studies revealed evidence of axoplasmic transport obstruction in the optic nerve head (Baumbach *et al.*, 1977). The axoplasmic flow block was due to inhibition of ATP formation by formates in the optic nerve head and also to axonal compression in the retrolaminar optic nerve by the swollen oligodendroglia and astrocytes.

25.2.6 TRAUMATIC OPTIC NEUROPATHY

By cautery we produced thermal burns on the retrolaminar region of the optic nerve (Baumbach *et al.*, 1978). The disc developed oedema (Fig. 25.6) in the involved region. Electron microscopy revealed axonal swell-

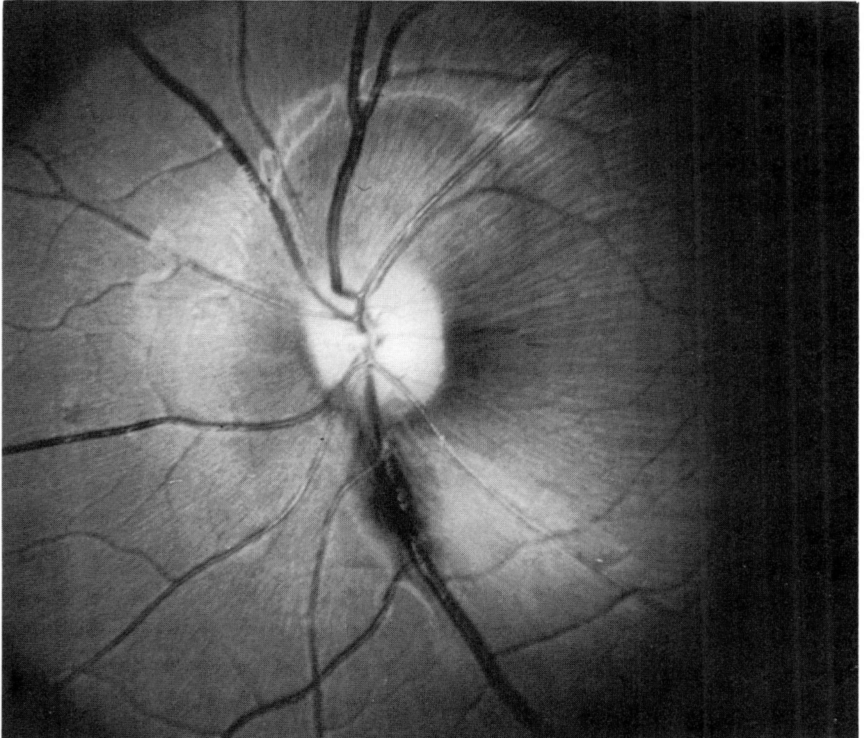

Fig. 25.6 Fundus photograph of a rhesus monkey, showing optic disc oedema of the superior part of the optic disc 29 hours after a cautery burn on the superior temporal part of the optic nerve immediately behind the eyeball.

ing and marked increase in mitochondria anterior to the site of injury – findings suggesting axoplasmic flow blockage in that region, and axonal destruction.

In addition to our studies (described above), which showed axoplasmic flow stasis in optic disc oedema, there are other studies in the literature showing axoplasmic flow stasis in optic disc oedema due to the following causes.

25.2.7 OCULAR HYPOTONY

In this there is blockage of the fast and slow components of anterograde (Minckler and Tso, 1976; Minckler, Tso and Zimmerman, 1976; Minckler and Bunt, 1977) and retrograde (Minckler and Bunt, 1977) axoplasmic flow at the level of lamina cribrosa.

25.2.8 COMPRESSION OF THE RETROBULBAR OPTIC NERVE

This may be due to tumours or other causes. In such cases electron microscopic studies have revealed evidence of axoplasmic transport blockage anterior to the site of compression (Wirtschafter, Rizzo and Smiley, 1975; Tso and Fine, 1976).

25.2.9 TRIETHYL TIN POISONING

In this, intramyelinic swelling in the optic nerve has been shown (Hedges, 1975). Myelin swelling would compress the axons in the retrolaminar region, produce axoplasmic flow obstruction and consequent optic disc oedema.

In conclusion, this brief account shows that axoplasmic flow blockage in the optic nerve head is the common pathway for production of optic disc oedema in many diseases; however, the actual mechanism of axoplasmic flow obstruction in different conditions varies markedly. Since axoplasmic flow stasis is the primary factor responsible for axonal swelling and development of optic disc oedema in these conditions, the part of the optic disc showing optic atrophy does not develop optic disc oedema because there are no axons to swell in that area.

25.3 Secondary vascular changes

The account given above indicates that the primary change in optic disc oedema is the swelling of the axons in the optic nerve head, mainly in front of the lamina cribrosa. In the unyielding optic nerve head, particularly in the prelaminar region, the swollen axons, by compression of the fine vessels lying among the axons, produce secondary vascular changes (Fig. 25.8), if the disc swelling lasts for some time (Hayreh, 1977a). Since the venous channels are thin-walled, fine vessels and a low pressure system, they are most easily compressed, resulting in venous statis in the optic disc and in the distribution of the long radial peripapillary capillaries, which drain into the retinal veins on the optic disc (Fig. 25.7). The venous stasis could produce three types of vascular changes:

1. Capillary dilatation, microaneurysms and haemorrhages on the disc as well as in the neighbouring retina, mainly in the distribution of the long radial peripapillary capillaries (Hayreh, 1969, 1977b) (Fig. 25.8).
2. In the prelaminar region, dilatation of fine vessels, venous stasis and slow filling of the capillaries.
3. Since the central retinal vein, a thin-walled vessel, also travels through the optic nerve head (Fig. 25.7), it is also compressed by the surrounding swollen axons; this produces retinal venous engorgement.

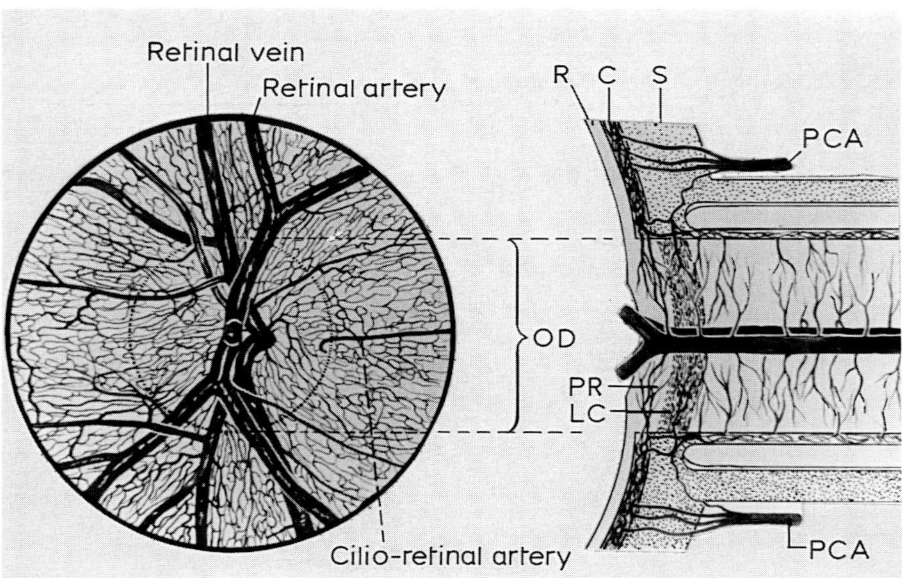

Fig. 25.7 Diagrammatic representation (on right side) of blood supply of anterior part of the optic nerve in man; figure on left represents ophthalmoscopic view of the blood vessels on the optic disc and adjacent retina. C, choroid; LC, lamina cribrosa; OD, optic disc; PCA, posterior ciliary artery; PR, prelaminar region; R, retina; and S, sclera. (Reproduced from Hayreh, 1977a.)

(a)

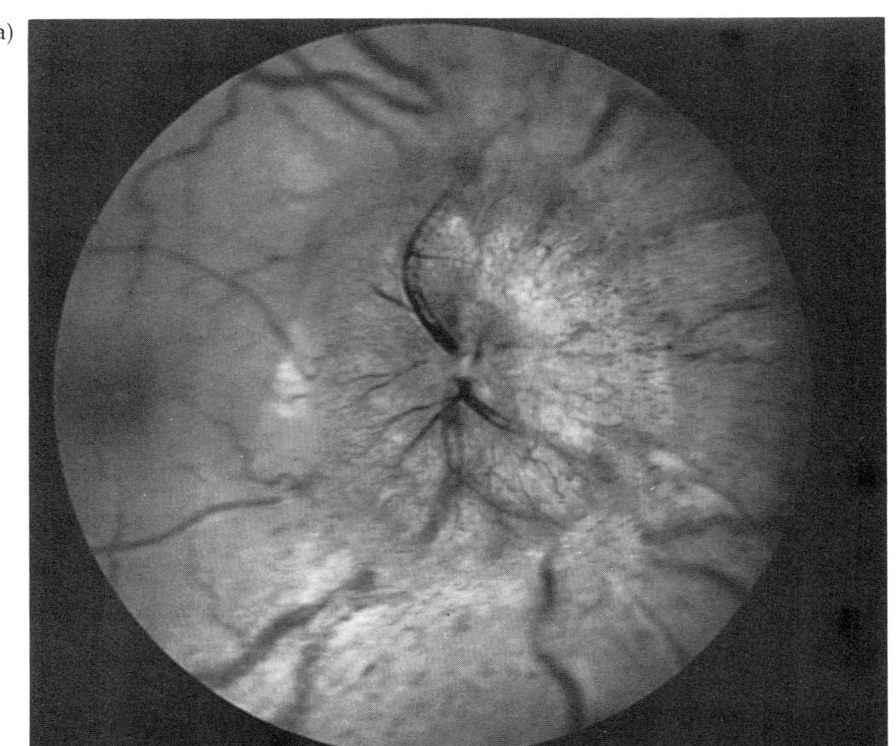

(b)

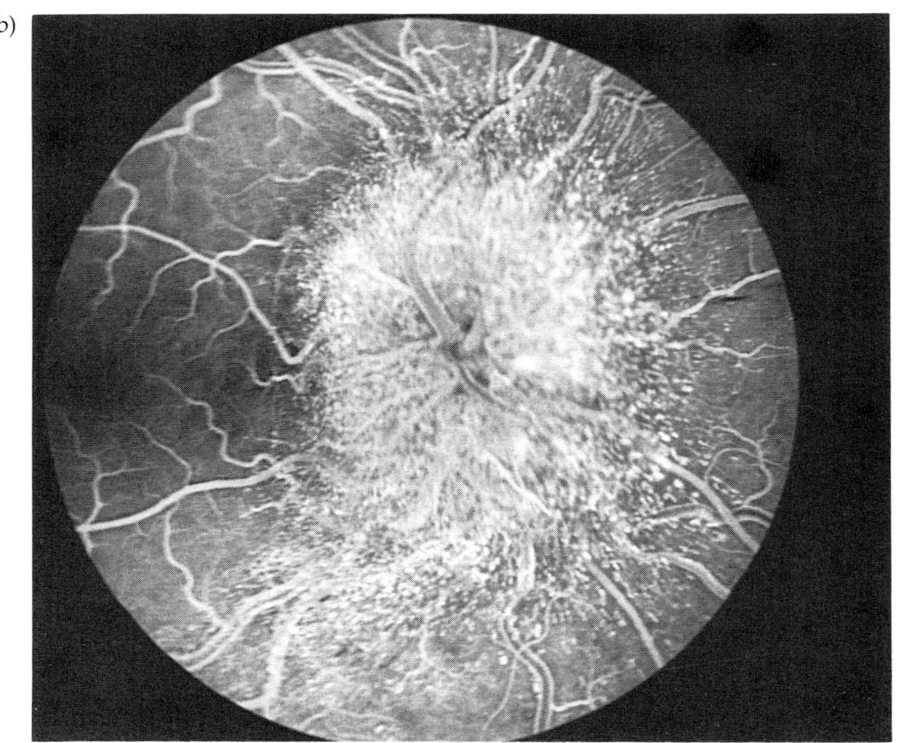

(c)

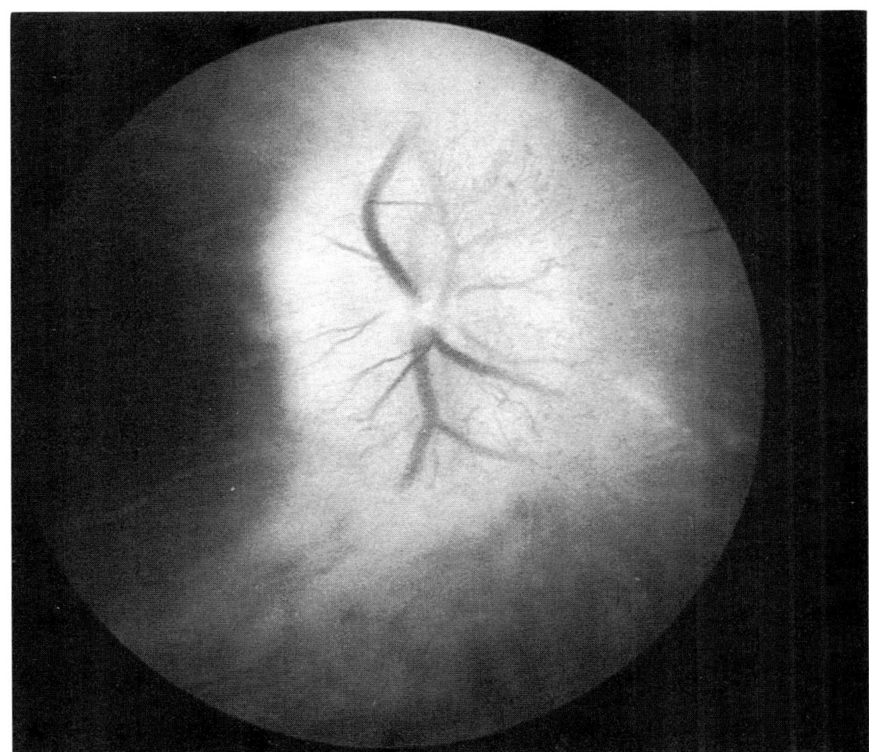

Fig. 25.8 Fundus photograph (a) and fluorescein angiograms (b,c) of an obese 20-year-old woman with benign intracranial hypertension, cerebrospinal fluid pressure of 410 mm water, and bilateral optic disc oedema. Fluorescein angiograms show (b) during the retinal arteriovenous phase, dilated capillaries and microaneurysms on optic disc surface and adjacent retina in the distribution of radial peripapillary capillaries, and (c) late fluorescein staining 15 minutes after the dye injection. (Reproduced from Hayreh, 1977b.)

The severity of the secondary vascular changes in these eyes depends upon the extent and duration of swelling of the optic disc – the longer the duration and greater the disc swelling, the more marked are the vascular changes. Thus in very mild and very early disc oedema, there may be no apparent vascular changes. These vascular changes in the optic nerve head may produce a breakdown of the normal blood vascular barrier in the optic nerve head and lead to accumulation of extracellular fluid, reported on electron microscopy in well-developed optic disc oedema (Tso and Hayreh, 1977a). Similarly, fluorescein leakage seen on angiography (Fig. 25.8c) is a manifestation of breakdown of the blood–optic nerve and blood–retinal barriers, most probably due to separation of endothelial cells in the capillaries, caused by distension of the capillaries. In the past, the vascular changes were erroneously thought to be the primary cause of the optic disc oedema.

25.4 Conclusions

Thus, in the various conditions described above, the primary mechanism in the production of optic disc oedema is the axoplasmic flow stasis, while the vascular changes are secondary phenomena. In view of this, it would seem that while the very early optic disc oedema is due to swelling of the nerve fibres, the marked optic disc oedema seen later on may represent swollen nerve fibres, extracellular fluid accumulation and vascular engorgement in the optic nerve head. These findings also clearly show that to advocate the use of the term 'papilloedema' for optic disc swelling in raised intracranial pressure and 'optic disc oedema' for disc swelling due to other causes (Walsh and Hoyt, 1969), is totally illogical.

Acknowledgements

This research project was supported by research grants from the Beit Memorial Research Foundation, London, the US National Institutes of Health (EY-01576, EY-01151, NS-03354, GM-12675, GM-19420), American National Multiple Sclerosis Society (RG 1087-A, RG 1220-A), and unrestricted grant from Research to Prevent Blindness, Inc., New York. I am grateful to my wife Shelagh for her help in the preparation of this manuscript, to Mrs Ellen Ballas and Mrs Georgiane Parkes-Perret for secretarial help, and to the Ophthalmic Photography Department for illustrations.

References

Baumbach, G.L., Cancilla, P.A., Hayreh, M.S. and Hayreh, S.S. (1978) Experimental injury of the optic nerve with optic disc swelling. *Lab. Invest.*, **39**, 50–60.

Baumbach, G.L., Cancilla, P.A., Martin-Amat, G. *et al.* (1977) Methyl alcohol poisoning – IV. Alterations of the morphological findings of the retina and optic nerve. *Arch. Ophthalmol.*, **95**, 1859–65.

Billson, F.A. and Hudson, R.L. (1975) Surgical treatment of chronic papilloedema in children. *Br. J. Ophthalmol.*, **59**, 92–5.

Burde, R.M., Karp, J.S. and Miller, R.N. (1974) Reversal of visual deficit with optic nerve decompression in long-standing pseudotumor cerebri. *Am. J. Ophthalmol.*, **77**, 770–2.

Davidson, S.I. (1969) A surgical approach to plerocephalic disc oedema. *Trans. Ophthalmol. Soc. UK*, **89**, 669–90.

Ernest, J.T. and Potts, A.M. (1968) Pathophysiology of the distal portion of the optic nerve: I. Tissue pressure relationships. *Am. J. Ophthalmol.*, **66**, 373–80.

Galbraith, J.E.K. and Sullivan, J.H. (1973) Decompression of the perioptic meninges for relief of papilledema. *Am. J. Ophthalmol.*, **76**, 687–92.

Garner, A., Ashton, N., Tripathi, R., Kohner, E.M., Bulpitt, C.J. and Dollery, C.T. (1975) Pathogenesis of hypertensive retinopathy: an experimental study in the monkey. *Br. J. Ophthalmol.*, **59**, 3–44.

Gutgold-Glen, H., Kattah, J.C. and Chavis, R.M. (1984) Reversible visual loss in pseudotumor cerebri. *Arch. Ophthalmol.*, **102**, 403–6.

Hayreh, M.S. and Hayreh, S.S. (1977a) Optic disc edema in raised intracranial pressure – I. Evolution and resolution. *Arch. Ophthalmol.*, **95**, 1237–44.

Hayreh, M.S., Hayreh, S.S., Baumbach, G.L. *et al.* (1977) Methyl alcohol poisoning – III. Ocular toxicity. *Arch. Ophthalmol.*, **95**, 1851–8.

Hayreh, S.S. (1964) Pathogenesis of oedema of the optic disc (Papilloedema): a preliminary report. *Br. J. Ophthalmol.*, **48**, 522–43.

Hayreh, S.S. (1965) Pathogenesis of oedema of the optic disc (Pappilloedema). Thesis, London University.

Hayreh, S.S. (1968) Pathogenesis of oedema of the optic disc. *Doc. Ophthalmol.*, **24**, 289–411.

Hayreh, S.S. (1969) Blood supply of the optic nerve head and its role in optic atrophy, glaucoma and oedema of the optic disc. *Br. J. Ophthalmol.*, **53**, 721–48.

Hayreh, S.S. (1974a) Anterior ischaemic optic neuropathy – I. Terminology and pathogenesis. *Br. J. Ophthalmol.*, **58**, 955–63.

Hayreh, S.S. (1974b) Anterior ischaemic optic neuropathy – II. Fundus on ophthalmoscopy and fluorescein angiography. *Br. J. Ophthalmol.*, **58**, 964–79.

Hayreh, S.S. (1975) *Anterior Ischemic Optic Neuropathy*. Springer-Verlag, New York.

Hayreh, S.S. (1977a) Optic disc edema in raised intracranial pressure – V. Pathogenesis. *Arch. Ophthalmol.*, **95**, 1553–65.

Hayreh, S.S. (1977b) Optic disc edema in raised intracranial pressure – VI. Associated visual disturbances and their pathogenesis. *Arch. Ophthalmol.*, **95**, 1566–79.

Hayreh, S.S. (1978a) Fluids in the anterior part of the optic nerve in health and disease. *Surv. Ophthalmol.*, **23**, 1–25.

Hayreh, S.S. (1978b) Structure and blood supply of the optic nerve, in *Glaucoma* (eds K. Heilmann and K. Richardson). Thieme, Stuttgart, pp. 78–96.

Hayreh. S.S. (1980) Anterior ischemic optic neuropathy – IV. Occurrence after cataract extraction. *Arch. Ophthalmol.*, **98**, 1410–16.

Hayreh. S.S. (1981a) Anterior ischemic optic neuropathy – V. Optic disc edema: an early sign. *Arch. Ophthalmol.*, **99**, 1030–40.

Hayreh, S.S. (1981b) Anterior ischemic optic neuropathy. *Arch. Neurol.*, **38**, 675–8.

Hayreh, S.S. (1984) The sheath of the optic nerve. *Ophthalmologica*, **189**, 54–63.

Hayreh, S.S. and Baines, J.A.B. (1972) Occlusion of the posterior ciliary artery – III. Effects on the optic nervehead. *Br. J. Ophthalmol.*, **56**, 754–64.

Hayreh, S.S. and Chopdar, A. (1982) Occlusion of the posterior ciliary artery – V. Protective influence of simultaneous vortex vein occlusion. *Arch. Ophthalmol.*, **100**, 1481–91.

Hayreh, S.S. and Hayreh, M.S. (1977b) Optic disc edema in raised intracranial pressure – II. Early detection with fluorescein fundus angiography and stereoscopic color photography. *Arch. Ophthalmol.*, **95**, 1245–54.

Hayreh, S.S. and Zahoruk, R.M. (1981) Anterior ischemic optic neuropathy – VI. In juvenile diabetics. *Ophthalmologica*, **182**, 13–28.

Hayreh, S.S., Massanari, R.M., Yamada, T. and Hayreh, S.M.S. (1981) Experimental allergic encephalomyelitis – I. Optic nerve and central nervous system manifestations. *Invest. Ophthalmol. Vis. Sci.*, **21**, 256–69.

Hayreh, S.S., Servais, G.E. and Virdi, P.S. (1986) Fundus lesions in malignant hypertension – V. Hypertensive optic neuropathy. *Ophthalmology*, **93**, 74–87.

Hayreh, S.S., Servais, G.E., Virdi, P.S., Marcus, M.L., Rojas, P. and Woolson, R.F. (1986) Fundus lesions in malignant hypertension III. Arterial blood pressure, biochemical, and fundus changes. *Ophthalmology*, **93**, 45–59.

Hedges, T.R. (1975) Papilledema: its recognition and relation to increased intracranial pressure. *Surv. Ophthalmol.*, **19**, 201–23.

Hedges, T.R. and Zaren, H.A. (1973) The relationship of optic nerve tissue pressure to intracranial and systemic arterial pressure. *Am. J. Ophthalmol.*, **75**, 90–8.

Kaye, A.H., Galbraith, J.E.K. and King, J. (1981) Intracranial pressure following optic nerve decompression for benign intracranial hypertension: case report. *J. Neurosurg.*, **55**, 453–6.

Keltner, J.L., Albert, D.M., Lubow, M., Fritsch, E. and Davey, L.M. (1977) Optic nerve decompression: a clinical pathologic study. *Arch. Ophthalmol.*, **95**, 97–104.

Kilpatrick, C.J., Kaufman, D.V., Galbraith, J.E.K. and King, J.O. (1981) Optic nerve decompression in benign intracranial hypertension. *Clin. Exp. Neurol.*, **18**, 161–8.

Kishi, S., Tso, M.O.M. and Hayreh, S.S. (1985) Fundus lesions in malignant hypertension – II. A pathologic study of experimental hypertensive optic neuropathy. *Arch. Ophthalmol.*, **103**, 1198–206.

Martin-Amat, G., McMartin, K.E., Hayreh, S.S. and Tephly, T.R. (1978) Methanol poisoning: ocular toxicity produced by formate. *Toxicol. Appl. Pharmacol.*, **45**, 201–8.

McLeod, D., Marshall, J. and Kohner, E.M. (1980) Role of axoplasmic transport in pathophysiology of ischaemic disc swelling. *Br. J. Ophthalmol.*, **64**, 247–61.

Minckler, D.S. and Bunt, A.H. (1977) Axoplasmic transport in ocular hypotony and papilledema in the monkey. *Arch. Ophthalmol.*, **95**, 1430–6.

Minckler, D.S. and Tso, M.O.M. (1976) Experimental papilledema produced by cyclocryotherapy. *Am. J. Ophthalmol.*, **82**, 577–89.

Minckler, D.S., Tso, M.O.M. and Zimmerman, L.E. (1976) A light microscopic, autoradiographic study of axoplasmic transport in the optic nerve head during ocular hypotony, increased intraocular pressure and papilledema. *Am. J. Ophthalmol.*, **82**, 741–57.

Rao, N.A. (1981) Chronic experimental allergic optic neuritis. *Invest. Ophthalmol. Vis. Sci.*, **20**, 159–72.

Rao, N.A., Tso, M.O.M. and Zimmerman, L.E. (1977) Experimental allergic optic neuritis in guinea pigs: preliminary report. *Invest. Ophthalmol.*, **16**, 338–42.

Smith, J.L., Hoyt, W.F. and Newton, T.H. (1969) Optic nerve sheath decompression for relief of chronic monocular choked disc. *Am. J. Ophthalmol.*, **68**, 633–9.

Tso, M.O.M. and Fine, B.S. (1976) Electron microscopic study of human papilledema. *Am. J. Ophthalmol.*, **82**, 424–34.

Tso, M.O.M. and Hayreh, S.S. (1977a) Optic disc edema in raised intracranial pressure – III. A pathologic study of experimental papilledema. *Arch. Ophthalmol.*, **95**, 1448–57.

Tso, M.O.M. and Hayreh, S.S. (1977b) Optic disc edema in raised intracranial pressure – IV. Axoplasmic transport in experimental papilledema. *Arch. Ophthalmol.*, **95**, 1458–62.

Walsh, F.B. and Hoyt, W.F. (1969) *Clinical Neuro-ophthalmology.* Williams and Wilkins, Baltimore, p. 567.

Weiss, P. (1944) Damming of axoplasm in constricted nerve: a sign of perceptual growth in nerve fibers. *Anat. Rec.*, **88**, 464.

Wirtschafter, J.D., Rizzo, F.J. and Smiley, B.C. (1975) Optic nerve axoplasm and papilledema. *Surv. Ophthalmol.*, **20**, 157–89.

CHAPTER 26

The differential diagnosis of the swollen optic disc

M.D. SANDERS

Swelling of the optic disc is a physical sign of importance and may signify serious underlying neurological or systemic disease. The classification is of importance, for the terminology varies in different countries and amongst different subspecialities. Initially in the last century optic disc swelling with raised intracranial pressure was called optic neuritis by both neurologists and ophthalmologists. Sir Herbert Parsons in 1908 introduced the term papilloedema, which he ascribed to optic disc oedema with raised intracranial pressure. Subsequent publications have used the term papilloedema to represent optic disc swelling from any cause, irrespective of whether the underlying cause lay in the eye, the brain or reflected some systemic disorder. Refinements in diagnosis became possible in the 1960s and 1970s with the advent of fluorescein angiography which enabled precise documentation of the microcirculation of the disc and assessed the permeability of the vessels. Fundus photography also established the swelling of retinal axons. Thus a more precise and clinically relevant classification emerged which has been upheld by distinguished neuro-ophthalmologists (Walsh and Hoyt, 1969).

The essentials of the revised classification are to limit the term papilloedema to indicate raised intracranial pressure, and to separate two further subgroups into those where the optic discs appear swollen as a congenital anomaly (pseudopapilloedema) and finally a group with visual loss and other ocular signs (local causes of disc oedema). These three subgroups will now be discussed: (1) papilloedema; (2) pseudo-papilloedema; (3) local causes of disc swelling.

26.1 Papilloedema

The clinical poignancy of the diagnosis of papilloedema has been partially ameliorated by the evolution of CT and MRI scanning, which enable the rapid diagnosis of intracranial masses. However, visual loss can occur in benign intracranial hypertension which has a visual morbidity of almost 50%. Prevention of visual loss depends on careful monitoring of the degree of papilloedema and assessment of the visual fields.

26.1.1 CLASSIFICATION OF PAPILLOEDEMA

The observed changes at the optic disc when the intracranial pressure is elevated depends on the predetermined shape and size of the optic disc, the degree and duration of elevation of CSF pressure, intraocular pressure, systemic blood pressure, the state of the optic nerve and disc vessels, and the patency of the optic nerve sheath. The inter-relationship of these varied factors provides a scale of changes at the optic disc which can be subdivided into five groups (Sanders, 1969).

(a) Early papilloedema. No haemorrhages or infarcts but capillary dilatation with leakage of fluorescein and early swelling of neurones. Venous pulsation may be absent and the blind spot is often enlarged (Fig. 26.1).

(b) Acute onset papilloedema. The disc is swollen with haemorrhages and infarcts indicating both vascular and neuronal decompensation (Fig. 26.1).

(c) Chronic papilloedema. Long-standing but mild elevation of the CSF pressure produces compensating vascular changes at the disc. There may be no haemorrhages or exudates but a dilated capillary plexus is seen on the surface of the disc, and the peripapillary neurones may have a waxy appearance (Fig. 26.1).

(d) Vintage papilloedema. The importance of this term is that it may signify potential visual loss, and has to be distinguished from Drusen of the disc. The disc shows pallor, dilated capillaries and small punctate refractile bodies on the surface of the disc which may represent neuronal degradation (corpora amylacea) (Fig. 26.1).

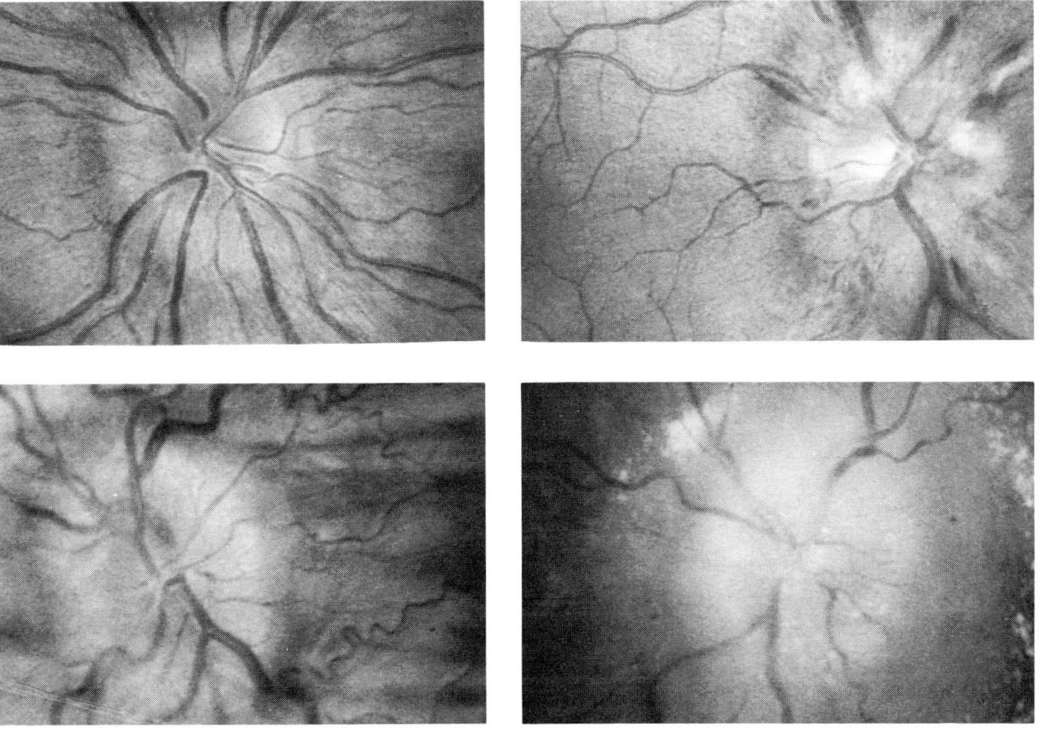

Fig. 26.1 Papilloedema. Early papilloedema (top left); acute papilloedema (top right); chronic papilloedema with choroidal folds (bottom left); vintage papilloedema with punctate opacities at lower pole of disc (bottom right).

(e) Atrophic papilloedema. The end stage of untreated papilloedema is the result of ischaemia of all tissues of the disc, so the disc is flat and pale: there is marked loss of neuronal pattern, and the vessels are attenuated with perivascular sheathing.

26.1.2 PERIPAPILLARY CHANGES

In addition to the changes seen at the optic disc, the increased pressure in the optic nerve sheath produces indentation and distortion of the posterior pole of the eye. The changes include: choroidal folds (Bird and Sanders, 1973), peripapillary disciform degeneration, vascular changes with retinociliary shunt vessels.

26.1.3 PATHOGENESIS AND TREATMENT

Papilloedema is due to raised pressure in the optic nerve sheath which, when sufficiently high, impairs perfusion of the deeper disc tissues, resulting in axoplasmic distension. The reduced perfusion of the deeper disc tissues induces compensatory dilatation of the retinal capillary plexus situated on the surface of the disc. One effect of this hypoxia of the deeper disc tissues is dilatation of the retinal axons with the retardation of normal axoplasmic flow. Treatment of papilloedema consists of reducing the pressure in the optic nerve sheath either medically (Diamox) or surgically, by (1) optic nerve sheath decompression, (2) lumboperitoneal shunt, or decompression of the temporal or occipital regions of the brain.

26.2 Pseudopapilloedema (Fig. 26.2)

Any congenital condition that mimics disc elevation, neuronal thickening or dilatation of superficial disc capillaries may be considered to simulate papilloedema and thus fall into the broad group termed 'Pseudopapilloedema'. The degree of similarity between 'true' and 'pseudo' papilloedema obviously depends on the skill of the observer but, in a clinical context of a young person with headaches, the differentiation may be difficult and fluorescein angiography and CT scanning may be mandatory.

There are two important aspects of pseudopapilloedema.

1. The commonest group of patients referred to a neuro-ophthalmologist have small optic discs. These may be associated with tortuous/dilated peripapillary vessels, and a prominent neuronal sheen. Fluorescein angiography does not show dilated peripapillary

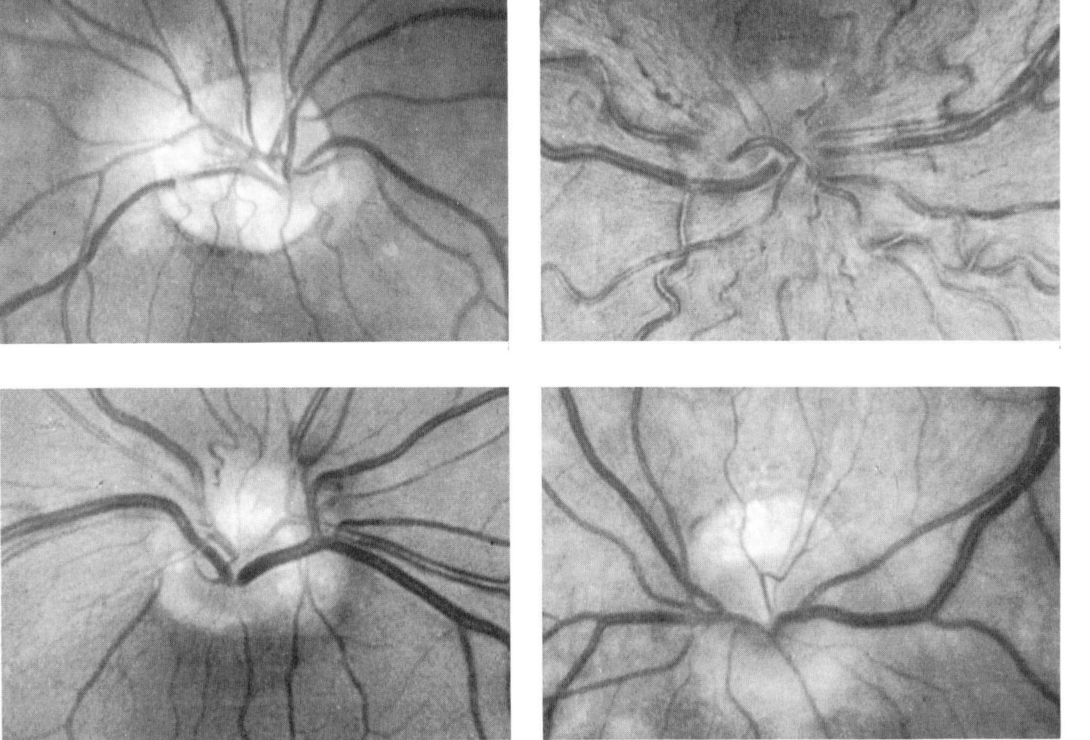

Fig. 26.2 Pseudopapilloedema. Small full disc with tortuous vessels (top left); small full disc with myopia (top right); tilted disc with inferior hypoplasia (bottom left); small disc with exposed drusen and anomalous vessels (bottom right).

(a)

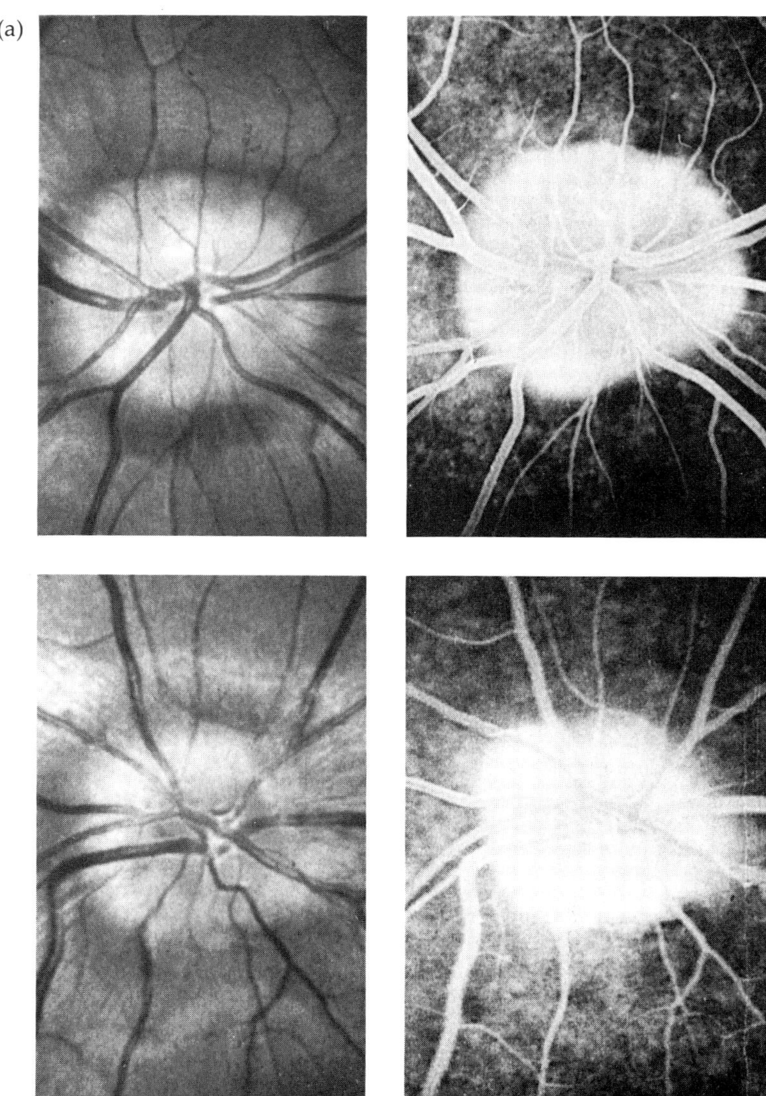

capillaries in the early stages and residual leakage of fluorescein does not occur in late pictures. These two features are the most important signs in differentiating pseudopapilloedema from papilloedema. In papilloedema both dilated and 'leaking' capillaries are an important feature.

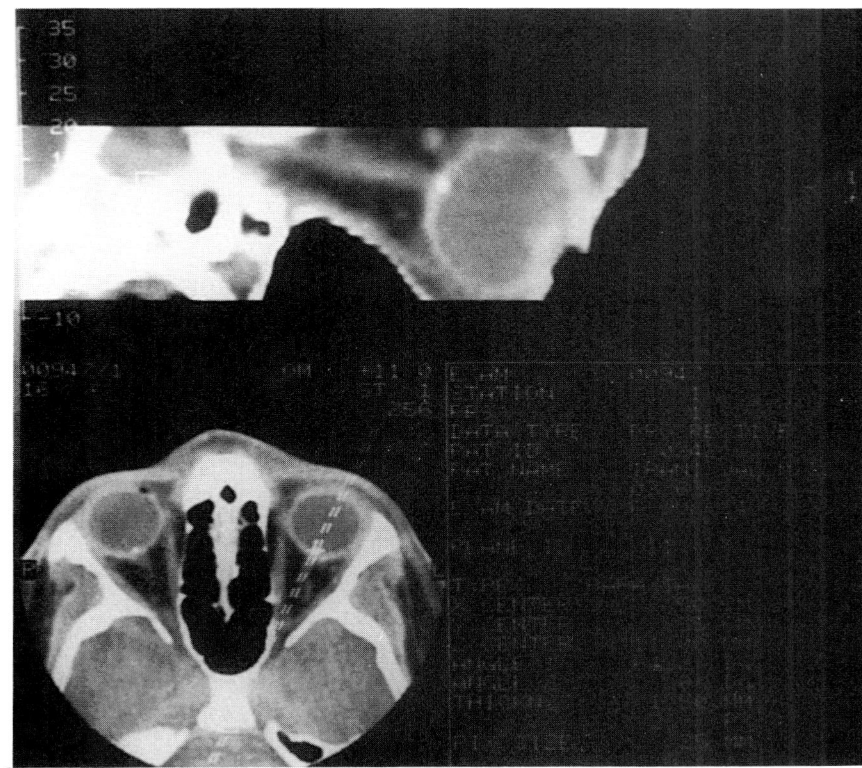

Fig. 26.3 Buried drusen. (a) Copy of colour photographs of right and left eyes to demonstrate fullness of the discs and absence of physiological cups (top). Residual photographs of fluorescein angiograms 10 minutes after injection to show leakage of dye (bottom). (b) CT scan shows calcification at both optic disc on both axial and parasagittal cuts.

2. Optic disc drusen: the group of pseudopapilloedema that most closely mimics papilloedema is due to drusen of the disc – particularly when buried. Patients with buried drusen even have leakage of fluorescein in late pictures. (Fig. 26.3a). The optic discs are invariably small, have associated vascular anomalies and may show peripapillary pigmented epithelial changes. The CT scan shows characteristic calcified bodies at the optic discs (Fig. 26.3b) and the affinity of extruded axonal material for calcium has been emphasized (Tso, 1981).

The diagnosis of a congenital anomaly at the optic disc should not close the mind to the concept that these patients may in addition have a co-existing intracranial mass.

26.3 Local causes of disc oedema (Fig. 26.4)

The local conditions that may affect the optic disc are extremely varied and only the major subgroups will be considered. One of the features that serves to distinguish this group from papilloedema is the presence of visual loss in the early stages, and usually at presentation.

1. Inflammatory	papillitis uveitis
2. Vascular	arterial (ischaemic papillopathy) venous (CRV occlusion)
3. Tumours	primary (of optic nerve or nerve sheath) secondary
4. Infiltrations	e.g. sarcoid, lymphoma
5. Local ocular lesions	i.e. angiomas of the disc, low intraocular pressure

26.3.1 INFLAMMATORY

Inflammatory disease of the optic nerve and optic disc are both associated with central visual loss.

(a) Optic nerve. Optic neuritis presents a clinical picture of rapid visual loss, pain on ocular movements, tenderness of the globe and ultimate recovery. Demyelination situated in the retrobulbar portion of the optic nerve is usually the cause and produces papillitis with mild disc swelling and fluorescein leakage. In some cases marked optic disc swelling occurs with haemorrhages and the term neuro-retinitis has been applied. Papillitis may also be seen in sarcoidosis.

(b) Optic disc, choroid and retina. Disc swelling is seen in most cases of retinal vasculitis and choroiditis. The common systemic diseases producing disc swelling are sarcoidosis, Behçet's disease and autoimmune retinal vasculitis. Characteristic fluorescein angiographic changes include:

1. paucity of capillary dilatation of the disc;
2. extensive fluorescein leakage from all capillaries of the posterior pole, and particularly extending to the macula (in marked contrast to papilloedema).

Recently an acute optic neuropathy has been recognized with marked disc oedema, visual loss and vitreous inflammation due to syphilis, HIV disease and hepatitis B.

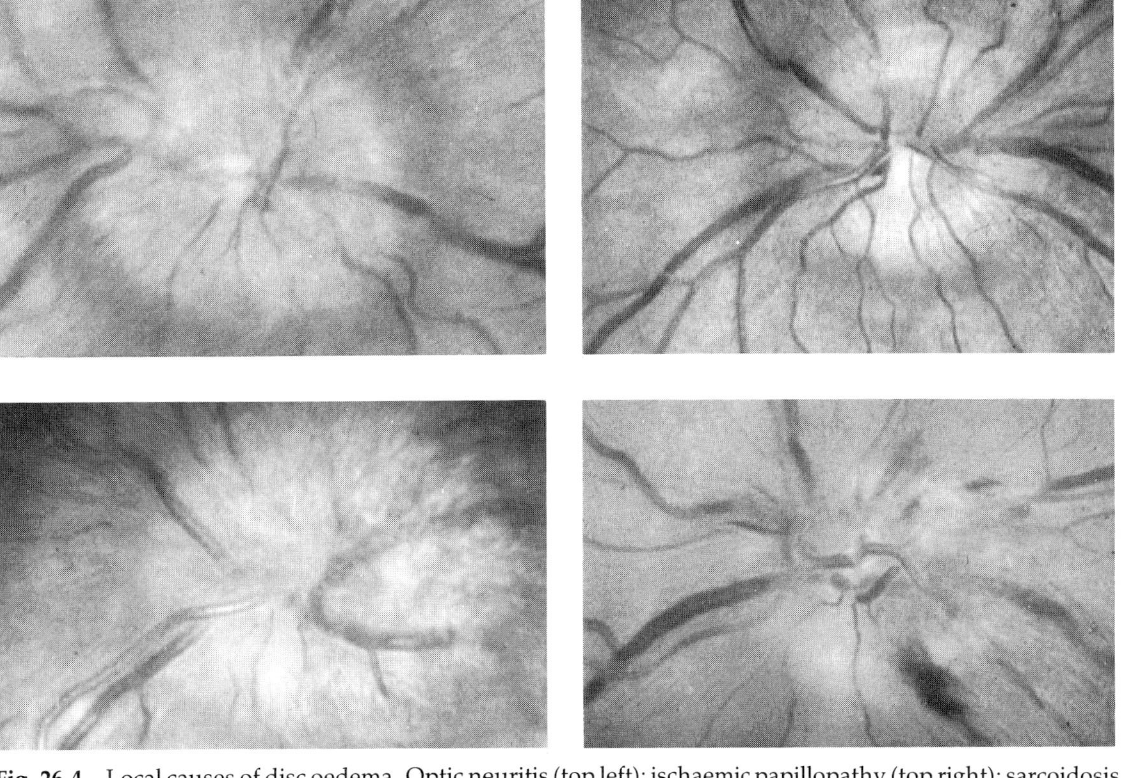

Fig. 26.4 Local causes of disc oedema. Optic neuritis (top left); ischaemic papillopathy (top right); sarcoidosis (bottom left); optic nerve glioma (bottom right).

26.3.2 VASCULAR

Optic disc swelling occurs in occlusion of either the arterial or venous supplies to the disc. Thus in central retinal vein (CRV) occlusion there is almost invariably low grade disc oedema. Arterial involvement produces disc oedema particularly when the ciliary branches to the optic disc are involved. This produces a classical clinical syndrome with the following features:

1. rapid visual loss;
2. arcuate, altitudinal pattern of loss;
3. absence of pain;
4. pallid swelling of the optic disc;
5. asymmetric capillary dilatation and fluorescein leakage on fluorescein angiography. The condition is termed ischaemic optic neuropathy or ischaemic papillopathy.

Two subgroups have been defined, one occurring in elderly patients with giant cell arteritis, and the second in middle-aged males with a less severe form. Multifactorial causes have been considered which may involve the vessel wall (i.e. arteriosclerosis, migraine), or the blood constituents (i.e. hyperviscosity) or the perfusion pressure (i.e. sudden blood loss, carotid disease, Takayasu's disease, etc.).

26.3.3 TUMOURS

Tumours of the optic nerve produce disc swelling as one aspect of a general picture which includes proptosis, ophthalmoplegia and visual loss. Optic nerve gliomas and meningiomas are the commonest group, and the nerve sheath meningioma produces characteristic diagnostic signs. The optic disc signs may be subdivided into three groups which reflect the duration of the meningioma.

1. Mild disc oedema, or pallor with visual loss.
2. Chronic/vintage disc oedema, with optico-ciliary shunt vessels and peripapillary changes.
3. Optic atrophy, sometimes with optico-ciliary shunt vessels.

26.3.4 INFILTRATIONS

Mild or chronic disc swelling may be seen in any condition that involves the superficial or deeper disc tissues. These conditions include sarcoidosis, leukaemia (particularly lymphoblastic) and lymphomas.

26.4 Conclusion

This brief review has served to categorize the various causes of disc oedema. A full ophthalmic assessment is essential with careful evaluation of the vitreous and peripheral retina for signs of inflammatory disease. The ophthalmologist continues to have a major diagnostic role, and fluorescein angiography and CT and MRI scanning have expanded clinically available tests.

References

Bird, A.C. and Sanders, M.D. (1973) Choroidal folds in association with papill-oedema. *Br. J. Ophthalmol.*, **57**, 89–97.

Hoyt, W.F. and Beeston, D. (1966) *The Ocular Fundus in Neurological Diseases.* C.V. Mosby, St Louis.

Sanders, M.D. (1969) A classification of papilloedema based on a fluorescein angiographic study of 69 cases. *Trans. Ophthalmol. Soc. UK*, **89**, 177.

Tso, M.O.M. (1981) Pathology and pathogenesis of drusen of the optic nerve head. *Ophthalmology*, **88**, 1066.

Walsh, F.B. and Hoyt, W.F. (1969) *Clinical Neuro-ophthalmology*, vol. 1. Williams and Wilkins Co. (1984) Baltimore, 3rd edn.

CHAPTER 27

Failure of retinal vascular homeostasis and its clinical consequences

R. ROSS RUSSELL

The retina maintains a continuously high metabolism and requires a large and constant blood supply. There are two main sources, the posterior ciliary system and the central retinal artery; both of these derive originally from the ophthalmic artery.

The ciliary system which comprises 80% of the total ophthalmic blood flow supplies the choroid, optic nerve head and outer retina including the photoreceptors. There is a rich vascular innervation and the capillaries have normal fenestrated junctions. The central retinal artery is unusual in having no vascular nerves and in having tight non-fenestrated junctions between the endothelial cells. The area of supply includes the nerve fibre layer and the inner retina including the ganglion cells.

In common with brain and other tissues retinal blood vessels have autoregulatory properties capable of functioning without nervous control. An increased pressure gradient across the vessel wall produced, for example, by a rise in intraluminal pressure or a fall in intraocular pressure results in vasoconstriction both in arteries and veins (Dollery, Hill and Hodge, 1963; Ross Russell, 1973). Conversely, a decreased pressure gradient results in vasodilatation. The effect is to match any change in perfusion pressure to a similar change in retinal vascular resistance and to minimize any alteration in retinal blood flow. There are limits to this homeostatic mechanism and, at both the lower limit and the upper limit of the autoregulatory range, blood flow becomes pressure dependent.

Metabolic stimuli produced by alterations in blood gas tensions can also be shown to affect the calibre of the retinal arteries (Hickham, Frayser and Ross, 1963). Hypoxia and hypercarbia, for example, produce vasodilatation. The function of vascular nerves in the choroidal circulation by analogy with the brain is probably to modify the range of pressure autoregulation and in addition to modulate the response to metabolic stimuli (Alm and Bill, 1973).

These homeostatic mechanisms may be modified by the effects of disease. It is known, for instance, that retinal arteries in patients with chronic hypertension show a decreased response to metabolic stimuli such as CO_2 and also have a reduced ability to dilate when intraluminal pressure is lowered (Hickham, Frayser and Ross, 1963). In the brain it has been shown that the capacity for autoregulation may also be affected or lost in ischaemia or in some states of increased blood viscosity (Rees *et al.*, 1970).

An important cause of disturbed retinal vascular regulation is occlusive disease of the extracranial arteries. In such patients the perfusion pressure in the retinal arteries is chronically reduced and, although the homeostatic mechanisms may suffice to maintain adequate blood flow for much of the time, any fall in systemic blood pressure may be followed by a temporary reduction in retinal flow. In the brain it has been shown that the ability of cerebral vessels to dilate in response to hypercapnic stimuli is reduced or lost, probably because the vessels are already in a state of maximal vasodilatation. The cerebral blood volume shows a marked increase and in some cases the levels of cerebral venous oxygen are reduced showing that the metabolic requirements of the brain can only be met by increased extraction of oxygen from the blood. These features indicate a critical perfusion state or reduced cerebrovascular reserve (Gibbs *et al.*, 1984).

Patients with this condition usually have extensive and multiple extracranial artery occlusion which may be atherosclerotic or arteritic in type. In the severest cases three or even four main arteries may be occluded and the brain and eyes may be supplied entirely by tortuous collateral pathways. The perfusion pressure in the eye is low and the patients are liable to suffer attacks of visual loss on one or both sides, should the perfusion pressure fall or the intraocular pressure rise. Actions such as rapidly standing up, beginning to exercise, sustained upward gaze or sometimes exposure to bright light or heat may provoke an attack (Russell and Page, 1983). These attacks have a less abrupt onset and a longer duration than amaurosis fugax caused by retinal embolism. The loss of vision is less complete and the patients describe a dazzling or 'contrasty' sensation rather than complete blackness or shutter effect (Table 27.1).

Table 27.1

Name	*Sex*	*Age*	*Arterial lesion*	*Transient visual symptoms*	*Provocation*	*Other features*
FA	M	70	Atheroma: LIC occlusion, RIC stenosis	daily, uniocular L eye fragmentation, excessive contrast	light, heat, standing, exertion	no cerebral symptoms, cerebral border-zone infarct on CT
MM	F	59	Atheroma: LCC occlusion	1–2/day, uniocular L eye blurring	light, standing, walking	tonic L pupil, L hemisphere, TIA and completed stroke
AD	M	72	Atheroma: bilateral ICA occlusion	both eyes dazzle	light	TIA unilateral, L tonic pupils
LS	M	62	Atheroma: LCC occlusion, RIC stenosis	×2 weekly, uniocular L eye flashing, lights, frosted glass	light, looking upwards	TIA L hemisphere
AE	F	53	Atheroma: RIC occlusion	daily, uniocular R eye, central coloured, flashing, fragmentation	light	TIAs and completed stroke, CT border-zone infarct
RS	M	59	Atheroma: RIC occlusion, REC stenosis	recurrent, uniocular R eye blurring	nil	localized infarct R hemisphere
LR	M	54	Atheroma: LCC occlusion, RIC stenosis	daily, dazzling, L eye contrasting kaleidoscope, contraction of field	heat, sunshine, looking upwards, neck extension, hot meal	TIA L hemisphere

The characteristic type of retinopathy may develop consisting of peripheral haemorrhages, microaneurysms and retinal oedema. Fluorescein angiography shows leakage from small veins, many microaneurysms and retarded blood flow (Russell and Page, 1983). In its early stages, it is compatible with normal visual acuity and visual fields but, if prolonged, there may develop retinal neovascularization, recurrent vitreous haemorrhages, vascular closure and eventually retinal detachment. Chronic ischaemia may also affect the anterior segment of the eye causing hypotony, rubeosis of the iris, neovascular glaucoma and ischaemia of the lens and cornea.

An abnormally low retinal artery pressure is the most reliable clinical sign, the central retinal artery of the disc collapsing with the lightest digital pressure on the globe. Delayed recovery of visual acuity after photostress is also a frequent finding especially in patients whose attacks are provoked by bright light. A most sensitive test, however, is an abnormal delay in the recovery of the b-wave of the ERG after photostress (Ross Russell and Ikeda, 1986).

The evolution and progression of hypotensive retinopathy have not been systematically studied. In its early stages it is symptomless and minor abnormalities consisting of a few peripheral haemorrhages and leakage from the veins may be seen in about 25% of patients on the side of complete carotid occlusion. It is possible that in some the condition may regress spontaneously while others progress to the state of intermittent cerebral and visual symptoms. At this stage there are a number of reports of regression of symptoms and of retinopathy following carotid endarterectomy or transcranial bypass (Neupert *et al.*, 1976; Kearns, Young and Piepgras, 1980). Untreated cases may progress to permanent loss of sight usually from retinal haemorrhage, neovascularization and detachment or from neovascular glaucoma. In the brain cerebral infarction may occur affecting the hemisphere border zones between the territories of the main cerebral arteries. These are the regions where perfusion pressure is normally at its lowest level and where autoregulation tends to break down under the conditions of systemic hypotension (Russell and Page, 1983). Infarction is often haemorrhagic in its early stages.

It is interesting to speculate on the mechanism of visual failure in response to bright light which is a characteristic symptom in many patients with retinal insufficiency. It has been suggested that the retinal blood supply may be unable to meet the increased demands of the retina under conditions of increased metabolism (Furlan, Whisnant and Kearns, 1979). This is unlikely, however, since the retinal oxygen consumption is actually higher in the dark than in the light. A second explanation postulates a run off or steal effect, the retinal blood flow being diverted to a dilated vascular bed in the face to the extent that the perfusion pressure to the retina is reduced. Some support for this was provided by a single patient with carotid occlusion (Russell and Page, 1983) who developed attacks of unilateral visual loss when his face was heated and in whom retinal perfusion pressure measured by ophthalmodynomometry was lowered still further by this manœuvre. Perhaps the most likely explanation is that the symptom is a non-specific indicator of mild choroidoretinal damage. A further study of the photostress ERG effect in other retinal disorders and in patients whose retinal insufficiency has been relieved surgically may throw further light on this question.

The recognition of low pressure retinopathy is a reliable indication of impaired carotid blood flow and of a haemodynamically significant extracranial artery occlusion. Because it may be present at a stage when symptoms are minimal the retinopathy may prove to be a valuable way of selecting patients for arterial surgery.

References

Alm, A. and Bill, A. (1973) The effect of stimulation of the cervical sympathetic chain on retinal oxygen tension and on uveal, retinal and cerebral blood flow in cats. *Acta Physiol. Scand.*, **88**, 84–94.

Dollery, C.T., Hill, D.W. and Hodge, J.V. (1963) The response of normal retinal blood vessels to angiotensin and noradrenaline. *J. Physiol.*, **165**, 500–7.

Furlan, A.J., Whisnant, J.P. and Kearns, T.P. (1979) Unilateral visual loss in bright light: an unusual symptom of carotid artery occlusive disease. *Arch. Neurol.*, **36**, 375–6.

Gibbs, J.M., Wise, R.J.S., Leenders, K.L. and Jones. T. (1984) Evaluation of cerebral perfusion reserve in patients with carotid artery occlusion. *Lancet*, **i**, 310–14.

Hickham, J.B., Frayser, R. and Ross, J.C. (1963) A study of retinal venous blood oxygen saturation in human subjects by photographic means. *Circulation*, **27**, 375–85.

Kearns, T.P., Young, B.R. and Piepgras, D.G. (1980) Resolution of venous stasis retinopathy after carotid bypass surgery. *Mayo Clin. Proc.*, **55**, 342–6.

Neupert, J.P., Brubaker, R.F., Kearns, T.P. and Sundt, T.M. (1976) Rapid resolution of venous stasis retinopathy after carotid endarterectomy. *Am. J. Ophthalmol.*, **81**, 600–2.

Rees, J.E., du Boulay, G.H., Bull, J.W.D., Marshall, J., Ross Russell, R.W. and Symon, L. (1970) Regional cerebral blood flow in transient ischaemic attacks. *Lancet*, **ii**, 1210–13.

Ross Russell, R.W. (1973) Evidence for autoregulation in human retinal circulation. *Lancet*, **ii**, 1048–50.

Ross Russell, R.W. and Ikeda, H. (1986) Clinical and electrophysiological features of low pressure retinopathy. *Br. J. Ophthalmol.*, **70**, 651–6.

Russell, R.W. and Page, N.G.R. (1983) Critical perfusion of brain and retina. *Brain*, **106**, 419–34.

CHAPTER 28

Vascular pathophysiology in optic neuritis

W.I. McDONALD

The usual approach to the pathophysiology of demyelinating disease in general, and optic neuritis in particular, has been through the study of conduction defects and psychophysical disturbances with a view to understanding the origin of symptoms. From this perspective, the correlations are fairly crude, and we can say little more than we could ten years ago. The conjectures made then are as valid as they were, but little has been added to our fundamental understanding of the neural pathophysiology: there are no new data which permit firm conclusions to be drawn about the origin of the long delays in visual evoked potentials seen at presentation with optic neuritis, the mechanism of recovery of function or the necessary relationships between disordered structure and disordered function (McDonald, 1983). Rather than rehearse these well-known propositions, I shall in this chapter consider another aspect of disordered physiology in optic neuritis: that of the blood–brain and blood–retinal barriers, and I shall do so not in relation to the origin of symptoms, but to the nature of the disease process and the mechanism of tissue damage.

Two critical questions in assessing the patient with optic neuritis are whether the disease process is localized to the optic nerve or is more widespread, and whether it is the clinical expression of a self-limited condition or the first manifestation of a continuing disease process. In other words: Is the pathological process unifocal or multifocal? Is the process monophasic or multiphasic? At present it is virtually impossible to answer these questions at presentation. Our recent exploration of the properties of the blood–brain barrier and the blood–retinal barrier offer the promise that it may soon be possible to do so.

28.1 Retinal vascular abnormalities

It has been known since the work of Rucker (1944) that retinal perivenous sheathing may be seen in multiple sclerosis. Because there had been no study of the retinal blood vessels in optic neuritis, we undertook a systematic investigation in 50 consecutive cases of isolated acute optic neuritis presenting to the Moorfields Eye Hospital (Lightman *et al.*, 1987). None of the patients had a history of previous neurological symptoms and none had evidence of abnormal neurological signs. All patients were examined with the indirect ophthalmoscope, with the slit lamp, and by fluorescein angiography.

Perivenous sheathing was present in six patients, and focal fluorescein leakage from peripheral venules was present in four of them; in six further patients there was leakage in the absence of sheathing. Fluorescein leakage sometimes occurred from the sheathed sites and sometimes from ophthalmoscopically apparently normal venules. Cells were detected in the media with the slit lamp in six patients, in four of whom there was also sheathing or fluorescein leakage. The perivenous sheathing was confined to the periphery of the retina (explaining the rarity with which it is observed by neurologists) in all but one patient in whom it was visible at the posterior pole.

These results indicate involvement of the retinal blood vessels and/or cellular exudation into the media in one-quarter of the patients in the present series with optic neuritis. When the retinal vascular abnormalities or cellular infiltration of the media were present in the symptomatic eye it might be argued that the changes simply reflected an extension of the pathological process from the optic nerve, although it was noteworthy that there were always substantial lengths of normal-appearing vessels between the optic nerve head and the sites of sheathing. In four patients the retinal abnormalities were in the clinically unaffected eye, and in one they were present in both eyes. These observations provide stronger evidence that in these patients at least the pathological process was multifocal at presentation.

The dissociation between the ophthalmoscopic sign of sheathing and the functional changes in the blood–retinal barrier, and/or the presence of cells in the media, raises the possibility that the events in the optic nerve and in the retina occurred at different times in some patients. Fluorescein leakage provides evidence for recent damage to the endothelium, and sheathing in the absence of leakage is usually interpreted as evidence of an older lesion. We did not carry out serial angiography in the patients with optic neuritis, but serial ophthalmoscopic examination of the fundus after 6–24 months showed that sheathing persisted in all throughout this time. These observations suggest that, in the patients with sheathing but without cells or leakage of fluorescein, the retinal abnormalities are old, and consequently that in the patients with a recent acute onset of symptoms of optic neuritis, the pathological changes occurred at different times: i.e. that the disease process was multiphasic. Support for this interpretation comes from the follow-up of our patients. Forty-six of the 50 (including all 14 patients with additional ocular abnormalities) were reassessed after a mean of 3.5 years. One of the latter patients and two of the patients without additional ocular abnormalities had had previous episodes of optic neuritis and were therefore excluded in assessing the risk of developing multiple sclerosis after the first clinical episode. Eight of the 13 remaining patients with additional ocular abnormalities have already developed clinically definite multiple sclerosis compared with three of the remaining 30. The difference between the two groups is highly significant ($P < 0.005$; relative risk 14.4).

28.2 Nuclear magnetic resonance (NMR) imaging in optic neuritis

Stronger supporting evidence for the existence of a multiphasic disease process at presentation in some patients with optic neuritis comes from the application of NMR technology to the study of the pathophysiology of the cerebral vessels in optic neuritis. Young *et al.* (1981) established that NMR imaging (MRI) is very sensitive in detecting abnormalities in the brain in multiple sclerosis. The abnormal images in the brain in multiple sclerosis correspond with plaques and there is good evidence that the abnormal signals in chronic lesions are at least in part a consequence of the astrocytic gliosis (Ormerod *et al.*, 1987). We have used MRI to determine the frequency with which the disease process is multifocal at presentation in acute optic neuritis. Seventeen of another series of 28 patients with acute isolated optic neuritis had multiple lesions at presentation, distributed in the same way as in multiple sclerosis (Ormerod *et al.*, 1986a). This frequency is similar to that of multiple sclerosis after optic neuritis in the United Kingdom (reviewed by McDonald, 1983) and it is tempting to suggest that the patients with multiple lesions at presentation already have multiple sclerosis. While it is likely that many of them do, that interpretation is not permissible on the MRI evidence alone because it is not known how often optic neuritis is the sole symptomatic expression of a multifocal but nevertheless monophasic disease process – i.e. a monosymptomatic form of acute disseminated encephalomyelitis. Such cases occur in childhood (Meadows, 1969).

It is known from studies of the brain in multiple sclerosis using X-ray CT scanning with enhancement by iodine-containing compounds that there is an increase in permeability of the blood–brain barrier in 'new' lesions (i.e. lesions appropriate anatomically to the neurological deficit occurring in a recent relapse) and that this increase in permeability subsides as clinical resolution occurs. MRI is much more sensitive than CT scanning in detecting lesions in multiple sclerosis (Young *et al.*, 1981) and we have begun to use gadolinium-DTPA as a marker for the blood–brain barrier in optic neuritis and multiple sclerosis.

Figure 28.1 shows MRIs of the brain in a patient with acute isolated optic neuritis. The scan is taken in the inversion-recovery mode in which lesions appear black. It is obvious that this patient has multiple periventricular and discrete white matter lesions. Comparison of Fig. 28.1(a), which was taken before the injection of gadolinium, and Fig. 28.1(b), which was taken after, shows little change in the appearance of the lesions. Comparison of another lesion indicated by the arrow in Fig. 28.1(c) in this same patient (before) and after gadolinium (Fig. 28.1d) shows that its magnetization characteristics are changed profoundly, indicating that gadolinium had leaked into the tissue; the lesion now appears white. If, as seems probable, the conclusions about permeability of the blood–brain barrier in relation to the age of lesions in multiple sclerosis derived from the CT scanning data are applicable to the NMR data, the patient of Fig. 28.1 has one recent and multiple older lesions present at the time of development of optic neuritis. Follow-up studies are required to establish that the presence of lesions both with and without blood–brain barrier breakdown at the time of presentation indicates that the patient has multiple sclerosis. We do not yet have adequate follow-up data on patients who have been studied with gadolinium, but it is worth noting that in another group of 25 patients who have been scanned serially after 5–20 months, additional cerebral lesions have been found in five, providing strong supporting evidence for the diagnosis of multiple sclerosis (D. Miller, unpublished observations).

Another way of distinguishing between acute and more chronic lesions in the brain is provided by determining the ratio of the relaxation times T1 and T2 in the lesions, the values of which are influenced by the amount of water in the tissue and the relative protein concentration in different compartments (Barnes *et al.*, 1987). Ormerod *et al.* (1986b) have shown that it is possible to distinguish between acute and chronic brainstem lesions in multiple sclerosis in this way; it seems likely that the differences are due to differing amounts of extracellular oedema and gliosis in the two

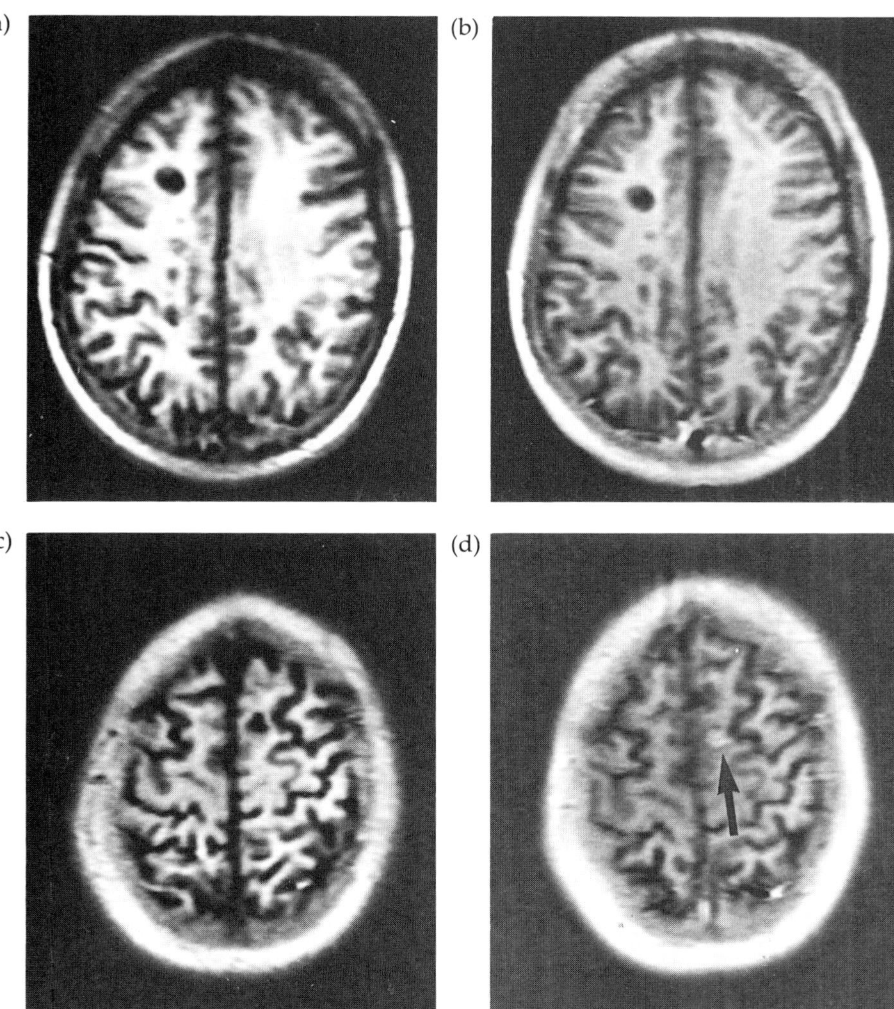

Fig. 28.1 MRI from a patient with 'isolated' acute optic neuritis (inversion-recovery mode), before (a,c) and after (b,d) injection of gadolinium–DTPA.

types of lesion.

Thus NMR techniques can provide evidence not only for a multifocal disease process in patients with acute isolated optic neuritis, but by studying the blood–brain barrier and the magnetization characteristics of lesions, of a multiphasic disease process as well.

28.3 Pathogenetic implications of retinal venous sheathing

There is now good evidence for the existence of immune deviations in patients with optic neuritis and multiple sclerosis (reviewed by McDonald, 1986). An unresolved question, however, is whether the immunological abnormalities are primary or whether they are secondary to myelin breakdown produced by some other mechanism. Specifically, it has been argued that the perivascular cuffing, which is characteristic of the active lesion in multiple sclerosis, is a reaction to myelin breakdown products. The observations on the retina in optic neuritis and multiple sclerosis help to resolve this issue. An immune reaction is preceded by a vascular event – immunologically competent cells leave the circulation to reach the target tissue and are accompanied by exudation of fluid. Histologically, the sheathed retinal vessels and the venules in the plaque of multiple sclerosis both show perivascular cuffing with mononuclear cells. In multiple sclerosis, the vascular events resulting in an increase in permeability of the blood–brain and blood–retinal barriers and perivascular cuffing occur where there are certain anatomical peculiarities: continuous tight junctions between the endothelial cells, and investment of the endothelium by glial processes are derived from cells which express the same protein (glial fibrillary acidic protein – GFAP), i.e. the astrocyte in the brain and the Mueller cell in the retina. In some locations where these events occur (the retinae) there is neither myelin nor oligodendrocytes; in others (in the normal-appearing white matter of the brain) the myelin is intact; and in yet others, there is demyelination. That the vascular events occur in the absence of myelin breakdown products provides strong evidence that they are not a reaction to them. A more likely alternative is that they precede demyelination and lead to it as they do in experimental allergic encephalomyelitis.

References

Barnes, D., McDonald, W.I., Johnson, G., Tofts, P.S. and Landon, D.N. (1987) Quantitative nuclear magnetic resonance imaging: characterization of experimental cerebral oedema. *J. Neurol. Neurosurg. Psychiat.* **50**, 125–33.

Lightman, S., McDonald, W.I., Bird, A.C., Francis, D.A., Hoskin, A., Batchelor, J.R. and Halliday, A.M. (1987) Retinal venous sheathing in optic neuritis: its significance for the pathogenesis of multiple sclerosis. *Brain*, **110**, 405–14.

McDonald, W.I. (1983) The significance of optic neuritis. Doyne Lecture. *Trans. Ophthalmol. Soc. UK*, **103**, 230–46.

McDonald, W.I. (1986) The mystery of the origin of multiple sclerosis. Gowers Lecture. *J. Neurol. Neurosurg. Psychiat.*, **49**, 113–23.

Meadows, S.P. (1969) Retrobulbar and optic neuritis in childhood and adolescence. *Trans. Ophthalmol. Soc. UK*, **89**, 603–38.

Ormerod, I.E.C., McDonald, W.I., du Boulay, G.H., Kendall, B.E., Moseley, I.F., Halliday, A.M., Kriss, A., Kakigi, R. and Peringer, E. (1986a) Disseminated lesions at presentation in patients with optic neuritis. *J. Neurol. Neurosurg. Psychiat.*, **49**, 124–7.

Ormerod, I.E.C., Bronstein, A. Rudge, P., Johnson, G., MacManus, D., Halliday, A.M., du Boulay, E.P.G.H., Kendall, B.E., Moseley, I.F., Jones, S.J., Kriss, A. and Perringer, E. (1986b) Nuclear magnetic resonance imaging in clinically isolated lesions of the brain stem. *J. Neurol. Neurosurg. Psychiat.*, **49**, 737–43.

Ormerod, I.E.C., Miller, D.H., McDonald, W.I., du Boulay, E.P.G.H., Rudge, P., Kendall, B.E., Moseley, I.F., Johnson, G., Tofts, P.S., Halliday, A.M., Bronstein, A., Scaravilli, F., Harding, A.E., Barnes, D. and Zilkha, K.J. (1987) The role of NMR imaging in the assessment of multiple sclerosis and isolated neurological lesions: a quantitative study. *Brain* (in press).

Rucker, C.W. (1944) Sheathing of the retinal veins in multiple sclerosis. *Proc. Staff Meet. Mayo Clin.*, **19**, 176–8.

Young, I.R., Hall, A.S., Pallis, C.A., Legg, N.J., Bydder, G.M. and Steiner, R.E. (1981) Nuclear magnetic resonance imaging of the brain in multiple sclerosis. *Lancet*, **ii**, 1063–6.

Index

Page numbers in italic refer to illustrations